CANCER GENETICS

CANCER
GENETICS

Edited by

HENRY T. LYNCH, M.D.

Professor and Chairman

Department of Preventive Medicine and Public Health

The Creighton University School of Medicine

Omaha, Nebraska

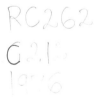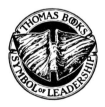

CHARLES C THOMAS • PUBLISHER

Springfield • Illinois • U. S. A.

Published and Distributed Throughout the World by
CHARLES C THOMAS · PUBLISHER
Bannerstone House
301–327 East Lawrence Avenue, Springfield, Illinois, U.S.A.

© *1976 by* CHARLES C THOMAS · PUBLISHER
ISBN 0–398–03222–X
Library of Congress Catalog Card Number: 74-8275

Library of Congress Cataloging in Publication Data
Lynch, Henry T.
Cancer Genetics.
1. Cancer—Genetic Aspects. I. Title.
RC262.L9   616.9′94′042   74-8275
ISBN 0–398–03222–X

Printed in the United States of America
BB-14

To my wife Jane, and my children, Patrick, Kathleen, and Ann

CONTRIBUTORS

EDWARD CHAPERON, Ph.D.

Associate Professor
Department of Medical Microbiology
Creighton University School of Medicine
Omaha, Nebraska

JAMES E. CLEAVER, Ph.D.

Associate Professor of Radiology
University of California
San Francisco, California

HARVEY DOSIK, M.D.

Chief Division of Hematology
Jewish Hospital and Medical Center
of Brooklyn
Assistant Professor of Medicine
State University of New York
Downstate Medical Center
Brooklyn, New York

HAROLD F. FALLS, M.D.

Professor of Ophthalmology
Research Associate
Department of Human Genetics
University of Michigan
Ann Arbor, Michigan

RICHARD A. GATTI, M.D.

Research Fellow in Immunology
Department of Pediatrics
University of Minnesota Medical School
Minneapolis, Minnesota

ROBERT A. GOOD, M.D., Ph.D.

President
Sloan Kettering Cancer Institute
New York City, New York

HODA A. GUIRGIS, Ph.D.

Associate Professor
Department of Preventive Medicine and
Public Health
Creighton University School of Medicine
Omaha, Nebraska

WILLIAM L. HARLAN, M.D.

Neurologist
Evansville, Indiana

CLARK W. HEATH, JR., M.D.

Chief
Leukemia Section
Epidemiology Program
Center for Disease Control
Public Health Center
Atlanta, Georgia

CHARLES E. JACKSON, M.D.

Chief, Genetic Section
Department of Medicine
Henry Ford Hospital
Detroit, Michigan

Research Associate,
Department of Human Genetics
Clinical Associate Professor
of Medicine
University of Michigan
School of Medicine
Ann Arbor, Michigan

ARNOLD R. KAPLAN, Ph.D.

Visiting Professor
Department of Preventive Medicine and
Public Health
Creighton University School of Medicine
Omaha, Nebraska

CAROL KRAFT, B.S., R.N.

Department of Preventive Medicine and
Public Health
Creighton University School of Medicine
Omaha, Nebraska

LAWRENCE KRAIN, M.D.

Resident
Department of Internal Medicine
University of California School of Medicine
Los Angeles, California

ANNE J. KRUSH, M.S.

Assistant Professor
Moore Clinic
John's Hopkins University
Baltimore, Maryland

SYLVIA D. LAWLER, M.D.
M.R.C.P., FRC.

Pathologist
Department of Clinical Research
The Royal Marsden Hospital and the
Institute of Cancer Research
London, England

JANE LYNCH, B.S., R.N.

Instructor
Department of Preventive Medicine and
Public Health
Creighton University School of Medicine
Omaha, Nebraska

BARUCH MODAN, M.D.

Head
Department of Clinical Epidemiology
Tel Aviv University Medical School
Chaim Medical Center
Chairman
Department of Epidemiology
Tel Aviv University
Faculty of Continuing Medical Education
Tel Hashomer, Israel

GABRIEL M. MULCAHY, M.D.

Director
Department of Pathology
Jersey City Medical Center
Jersey City, New Jersey

NORMAN C. NEVIN, B.Sc., M.D.,
M.R.C.P.Ed.

Senior Lecturer
Human Genetics
The Queens University of Belfast
Consultant in Human Genetics
The Northern Ireland Hospitals Authority

MASAHARU SAKURAI, M.D.

Roswell Park Memorial Institute
Buffalo, New York

AVERY A. SANDBERG, M.D.

Chief of Medicine C
Roswell Park Memorial Institute
Buffalo, New York

MITSUO TAKASUGI, Ph.D.

Adjunct Assistant Professor of Surgery
University of California School of Medicine
Los Angeles, California

PAUL I. TERASAKI, Ph.D.

Professor of Surgery
University of California School of Medicine
Los Angeles, California

JERZY TETER, M.D.

Professor
Department of Clinical Endocrinology
Medical Academy
Warsaw, Poland

ROBERT J. THOMAS, Ph.D.

Assistant Professor
Department of Anatomy
Assistant Professor and Director
Section of Computer Sciences
Operations and Management
Department of Preventive Medicine and
Public Health
Creighton University School of Medicine
Omaha, Nebraska

GEORGE J. TODARO, M.D.

Chief
Viral, Leukemia and Lymphoma Branch
National Cancer Institute
National Institutes of Health
Bethesda, Maryland

GEORGE K. TOKUHATA, Dr. P.H., Ph.D.

Director
Division of Reaearch and Biostatistics
Commonwealth of Pennsylvania
Department of Health
Harrisburg, Pennsylvania
Professor of Biostatistics
University of Pittsburg Graduate School of
Public Health
Associate Professor of Community
Medicine—Epidemiology
Temple University College of Medicine

LESTER WEISS, M.D.

Chief, Cytogenetic Laboratory
Director, Genetics Counselling Clinic
Henry Ford Hospital
Detroit, Michigan 48202
Clinical Associate Professor
of Pediatrics
University of Michigan
School of Medicine
Ann Arbor, Michigan

PREFACE

THE ETIOLOGIC ROLE OF GENETICS in human cancer is enigmatic. However, significant strides toward its resolution are being made in laboratories and cancer centers in several areas of the world. Genetics is only one of many disciplines concerned with solving some of the riddles of cancer etiology and carcinogenesis. However, cancer genetics has been a controversial science, undoubtedly reflecting in part the complexity of performing genetic studies on a subject as complicated as man. For example, man's matings cannot be controlled; he has relatively few progeny; and his generation span is longer than that found in most other animal species. It is often difficult to obtain histological confirmation of cancer, especially 20 or more years after a patient's death, and yet, pathologic confirmation is mandatory for accurately assigning disease status in pedigree recording. Finally, contacting patients and informing them about the goals and objectives of the studies, particularly with respect to such an emotionally charged subject as cancer, may prove to be a formidable task; indeed psychological factors may cause an individual to cease cooperation in the very midst of an investigation. Obstacles to procuring this vital information, as well as the performing of longitudinal studies in order to learn about the natural history of the particular familial cancer problem, often plague cancer geneticists. Therefore, it is no small wonder that the greatest number of cancer genetic investigations have been performed at the infrahuman level.

This book was written primarily as an attempt to contribute order, breadth, and scope to the overall problem of cancer genetics in humans, with due consideration to the above-mentioned limitations. Thus, chapters range from basic science problems in cancer immunology, histocompatibility with particular reference to the HL-A system, oncogenic viruses, DNA problems as found in xeroderma pigmentosum, and cytogenetic problems, to more clinical-genetic-epidemiologic issues. The latter include such subjects as ethnic considerations concerned with cancer occurrence and distribution in Israel, problems in genetics, tobacco and lung cancer, genetics and specific cancers including those involving the breast, endometrium, ovary, colon, stomach, prostate, and skin, a variety of cancer syndromes, and finally a discussion of genetic counseling with implications for all of the above problems. Emphasis was given to the highlights of each of these subjects in the respective chapters. However, in the chapter by Drs. Mulcahy and Harlan, dealing with genetics, cancer, and the nervous system, an attempt was made to present this subject in a comprehensive manner emphasizing an indepth view of this entire field. This particular chapter is therefore designed to serve as the prototype for detailed coverage in a specific defined area of cancer genetics.

Emphasis has been placed upon clinical correlation of existing knowledge in the hope that the predictability of familial cancer risk might be more frequently utilized in clinical practice, i.e. for identifying patients at genetically high or low cancer risk for specific anatomic target organs in the hope of earlier diagnosis. Hopefully, genetic methodologies in due time may lead to the discovery of genetic markers which might facilitate more accurate prediction of specific cancer risks and identify patients prone to cancer sufficiently early for improved cancer control. This information should also be useful in the construction of clinical models to be utilized in the experimental design of studies of carcinogenesis.

Cancer genetics is an exceedingly broad subject, and its complete elucidation would require many volumes prepared by countless contributors. Therefore, by necessity, this book is limited in scope to selected subjects which the editor hopes will provide at least a small measure of insight into ongoing research on genetics and carcinogenesis. Concurrently, an attempt has been made to provide a frame of reference about genetic etiology in cancer for the basic scientist, the human geneticist, the clinical investigator, the practicing clinician, and the clinical oncologist.

Henry T. Lynch

ACKNOWLEDGMENTS

C OUNTLESS INDIVIDUALS HAVE WORKED tirelessly in the preparation of this book during the past five years of its evolution. If I began mentioning these individuals by name, I would undoubtedly miss some, and this would be very painful to me. I would, therefore, prefer to express my deepest appreciation to all of you for your kindness and your generosity of time, effort, and energy.

This book could not possibly have been written without the help of many dedicated members of cancer-prone families. These patients were truly our cancer genetics and epidemiology *laboratory* from which we have gained knowledge to allow us to incorporate facts and theories into this book. The dedication of these individuals has been profound, and only those of you who have worked with families will really be able to appreciate the generosity of these dedicated subjects and the gratitude which I experience.

I am especially indebted to the several contributing authors to this book. All are individuals who have been extremely productive in their respective clinical and research disciplines and in spite of their hectic schedules, they took time out to prepare material for this book. Words cannot possibly express my personal gratitude.

Finally, I wish to acknowledge the Creighton University School of Medicine for the fine facilities, support, and whole hearted backing of this project.

H.T.L.

CONTENTS

CANCER GENETICS

CHAPTER 1

INTRODUCTION TO

CANCER GENETICS

HENRY T. LYNCH

Historical Background

IN SPITE OF countless investigations in laboratories throughout the world, the etiology of cancer remains an enigma. Throughout the ages many different issues, events, and circumstances in the lives of men have been considered to be of etiologic significance in carcinogenesis. These conceptions have ranged from witchcraft and folklore to an indictment of physical events such as thunder and lightning, proximity to volcanoes and other major natural events and calamities. Consideration has also been given to psychological factors including fear and anxiety, man's personal habits and characteristics such as his food and dietary patterns including smoking, alcohol consumption, and other idiosyncrasies, and his familial or hereditary background including his particular race or ethnic group. Thus, when reviewing the history of cancer epidemiology in man, one finds the literature replete with "observations," many of which may or may not have been subjected to sophisticated scientific inquiry, supporting or rejecting these various hypotheses for cancer etiology [1]

For many years, physicians and scientists have considered that hereditary factors may be etiological in human cancer. However, early observations in this field were hampered significantly by two major problems: 1) lack of controlled investigations; and 2) severe limitations in the overall problem of cancer diagnosis. Nevertheless, as early as 100 A.D., a Roman physician entertained considerable curiosity about the increased occurrence of breast cancer in the family of one of his patients; however, practically no progress was made in the area of disciplined inquiry during the next 17 centuries. In 1866, Broca,[2] the renowned French surgeon, reported an increased occurrence of carcinoma of the breast in his wife's family (Fig. 1-1) which he believed must be explained on the basis of hereditary factors. In addition, he was interested in the possibility of a general cancer diathesis, since he was also struck by his observation of an increased frequency of cancer of *other* anatomic sites in this family.

Genetic and Environmental Interaction

The role of the host in the etiology of disease depends upon genetic-environment interactions. No characteristic or trait, normal or abnormal, is inherited. It is only the genetic material that is inherited; and it is this that sets the individual's range of potential reactions, i.e. the character and extent of reactions to environmental influences. At any given time, the host's constitution is the summation of his life experiences and exposures as realized within the limits of responses set by his genetic endowment. At one extreme, there are single gene alterations (mutations) that apparently impart their effects in all known genetic backgrounds and in all known environments. These are the situations to which terms such as *genetic disease* and *genetic trait* are commonly applied as a shorthand convenience. At the other

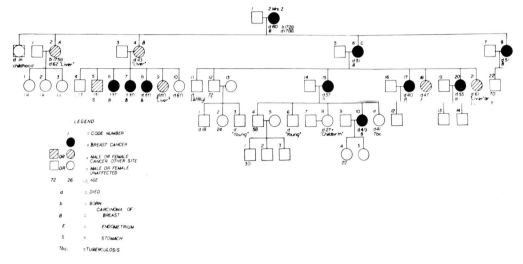

Figure 1–1. A pedigree of the family which Broca ascertained.

extreme, the effects of genotypic differences may be detectable only by statistical methods, and then, only within a limited environmental constellation. Despite the shorthand designations that geneticists may use in referring to genes and in equating gene action with specific genetic traits, many (and probably most) traits are affected by more than one gene,[3] particularly at the level of biological organization in which the majority of common disease states (such as cancer) are defined. At this level of biological organization, it is particularly important to evaluate the action of hereditary factors as strictly as possible within the context of the environments in which they are expressed.[4]

Family studies provide one of the best means for investigating genetic-environmental interactions in cancer etiology. Environmental differences may be compared between the members of high-risk families, i.e. those with remarkably high familial cancer frequencies, who have developed the disease and those who have not. The establishment of constitutional markers to identify those individuals who are particularly at risk for familial cancer may profoundly enhance the significance of such studies.[5]

Different types of cancers are sometimes aggregated in the same kindred.[1] The existence of familial aggregations of these disease entities suggests the involvement of an underlying etiological unity to them.[6]

Animal Studies

As might be expected, the greatest impetus and stimulus to cancer genetic studies in man were based upon genetic investigations in laboratory animals.[7] Some of these earliest observations were based simply upon the recognition of a clustering of neoplasms in certain groups of animals as opposed to the lack of clustering in other members of the same species. Later studies revealed that cancer was not contagious in the usual usage of this term, and that certain cancers were under the influence of heredity.[1] Thus, armored with these facts, vigorous attempts were made to delineate specific hereditary tumor patterns in these animals. One of the crucial studies in this area was that of Lathrop and Loeb[7] who demonstrated that certain familial aggregations in animals manifested characteristic types of tumors and, moreover, when certain strains were inbred, it was demonstrated that specific types of tumors were inherited as separate characters. One of the stumbling blocks which confronted these early investigators in animal cancer genetics was the heterogeneity of their animal stocks. Subsequently, homozygous strains of animals were developed for use in cancer genetic research. It was then possible to segregate particular types of tumors within these specific strains so that meaningful genetic data could be compiled and critically analyzed.

Of all laboratory animals used in these genetic studies, the common laboratory mouse has contributed most to research in cancer genetics. Its many biological and genetical advantages have been discussed at great length by Green and his staff at the Jackson Laboratory at Bar Harbor, Maine.[8] Indeed, mice have been used extensively for cancer research ever since C. C. Little established the DBA strain in 1909. Many genetic hypotheses have been tested through the years such as the relationship of disease incidence among different mouse strains and the evaluation of host factors and exogenous factors. Selective inbreeding studies with careful evaluation of new mutations in these animals have subsequently contributed to the comprehension of the etiology of a variety of diseases including cancer in man.

More than 70 strains of homozygous mice are now available for study by cancer geneticists, some of which include: 1) strain BALB/C which developed a high incidence of pulmonary tumors and lymphatic leukemia; 2) strain C57 Black, a tumor resistant strain in which few mammary or pulmonary tumors develop; and 3) strain C3H in which a high incidence of mammary tumors and hepatomas occurs.[8]

Studies of cancer genetics at the infra-human level have had the advantage of controlled experimentation, the lack of which is obvious and of course poses a serious deterrent in human studies. Thus, the development of highly inbred strains of animals has made it possible to evaluate the genotype of the host with a high degree of precision. In turn, the role of environment and its interactions with the genotype has made it possible to evaluate the exigencies of this interplay with a high degree of accuracy. Thus, in certain well designed animal experiments, it is possible to draw conclusions for a genetic hypothesis for cancer etiology; namely, we can evaluate the relative roles of genetics and environment in carcinogenesis. The general conclusion stemming from numerous studies of this nature, i.e. wherein genetic and extra-genetic factors can be controlled, has been that the individual's genotype plays a major role in response to carcinogens; thus, it is obviously mandatory that carcinogenic factors be evaluated critically in their relationship and/or interaction with host factors. However, one must realize at the outset that an all-or-none law as a frame of reference in terms of quantifying genetic and environmental carcinogenic factors is not possible when interpreting animal data, and in the case of humans, the problem is considerably more complex. For example, leukemia can be produced invariably in certain animals and in man through massive doses of radiation. Similarly, an excess of chemical carcinogens such as methylcholanthrene, urethane, and nitrogen mustard will invariably induce cancer in animals and probably in man. However, when such a massive exposure to carcinogens is administered, the investigator is hampered in his understanding of the role of host factors since these are literally overwhelmed by the massive carcinogenic dose. Contrariwise, certain animal strains can be highly inbred so that they manifest an exquisite genetic susceptibility to cancer; in this case it becomes difficult if not impossible to evaluate the relative importance of nongenetic factors. Thus, in some of the simple Mendelian inherited precancerous syndromes in man such as the multiple nevoid basal cell carcinoma syndrome and familial polyposis coli, the genetic "carcinogenic" component may be so strong that it is difficult to study the possible interacting role of environmental factors in cancer etiology.[1]

The above considerations notwithstanding, Heston[9] generalized that every variety of neoplasm, regardless of the species in which it is manifested, is probably to some degree under the influence of genes. Thus, he viewed genetic factors as crucially important even when nongenetic factors such as an oncogenic virus is known to be involved. He stated, for example,

> When an oncogenic virus is involved, the genotype of the host may control the propagation and transmission of the virus or the malignant response of the cell to the virus. When a chemical or physical carcinogen is introduced, the genotype of the organism may control the malignant response of the cell to the carcinogen and determine in which tissue or tissues this response will occur. But the importance of the genotype may be most clearly shown in the occurrence of the so-called spontaneous tumors—those with which no external biologic, physical, or chemical carcinogen has been identified.

Successful genetic investigations have been made using specific strains of these laboratory mice in which susceptibility to certain malignant neoplasms has been developed, characterized and now catalogued. These include strains which have been bred for susceptibility to practically every histologic variety of cancer including leukemias, mammary tumors, lung tumors, osteogenic sarcomas, and a variety of carcinomas. Other laboratory animals of different species, including the rat and chicken, have also been bred for susceptibility to specific malignant

neoplasms. However, in spite of the relative ease in producing and maintaining inbred strains of laboratory animals for susceptibility to specific malignant neoplasms, the genetic mechanism in many cases appears to be complex. For example, in mice, Heston[9] stated that of all the types of tumors for which evidence of genetic influence has been found, not one example has been observed to be due to a *single* gene. Rather, these tumors appear to be inherited in terms of threshold characters[10] or so-called quasi-continuous characters as suggested by Grüneberg[11] and used interchangeably with the threshold concept by Heston.[9] This term signifies that these tumors can be influenced by a multitude of genetic and extra-genetic factors. However, alternative expression may occur because of differences in thresholds for development of cancer. In addition, this term does not imply that the characters are necessarily found in all or none of the individuals of a particular inbred strain, but rather that they occur in certain incidences characteristic of the particular strain. Finally, Heston[9] stated that when the strain is inbred to fix the genotype, the genotype will then establish the incidence of the specific malignant neoplasm. In turn, a variety of extra-genetic factors will interact with this specific genotype and this specific interaction will then determine the expression of the development of the tumor. This line of reasoning is supported by abundant laboratory experiments at the infra-human level and it certainly has many implications for the study of cancer genetics in man.

The concept of threshold character in cancer epidemiology is perhaps best seen in the case of mammary tumors in the mouse. In this particular tumor, the role of genetic factors has been firmly established; it is known that specific genes on specific chromosomes can materially alter the incidence as well as the average age for the occurrence of this tumor. However, in addition to the role of specific genes in the etiology of this tumor, it is just as firmly established that a mammary tumor virus as well as other factors including chemical carcinogens, radiation, endogenous hormonal stimulation, and administered estrogens play a critical role in its production. When the majority of these influences are present, we can expect a high tumor response by altering these factors.

In context with threshold factors and the inherited susceptibility of cancer, single genes may have an exceedingly potent effect on the incidence of certain tumors. This is seen clearly in the case of ovarian tumors which may be increased from virutally 0 percent to 100 percent by the dominant spotting gene.[12] However, we must realize that spontaneous ovarian tumors may still occur in the absence of this particular gene and that incidence may be influenced by the presence of other genes. Furthermore, such factors as radiation may also influence the expression of this tumor.

While several cancer and precancerous diseases in man appear to be under the control of a single gene, simple inheritance of cancer in laboratory animals has been encountered infrequently. One example involves renal adenoma in the rat as described by Eker and Mossige.[13] However, as in experimental animals, the majority of tumors in man that appear to be under hereditary control do not show simple inheritance; rather they appear to be due to complex genetic mechanisms, involving multiple genes in interaction with a variety of environmental factors. In these cases, the risk for cancer to close blood relatives of the cancer proband may be given in statistical terms by so-called empirical risk figures; these risk estimates by themselves do not provide firm knowledge of the true significance of genetic and/or extragenetic factors. In short, they do not necessarily shed light on cause-effect relationships in carcinogenesis. While the complex nature of inheritance of cancer in man poses a challenge to the ingenuity of cancer epidemiologists, obviously it leaves the door wide open for scrutiny of how genotypic factors in association with extra genetic factors, i.e. biological and chemical carcinogens, operate dynamically in the production of cancer.

An example of the importance of threshold concepts of inheritance of cancer in animals, with implications for man, is seen in pulmonary tumors. The relationship between genes and chemical carcinogens in pulmonary tumors in the mouse, has been studied in depth. The rate of spontaneous pulmonary tumors in specific inbred strains of mice increases through chemical induction by methylcholanthrene, dibenzanthracene, urethane, and nitrogen mustard, but the strains nevertheless retain their relative rate of incidence of spontaneous pulmonary tumors.[14,15] Interesting parallels are found in humans as evidenced by the work of Tokuhata and Lilienfeld.[16] Specifically, cigarette smoking has caused an increase in pulmonary cancer in almost epidemic proportions, and has permitted studies of the genetics of this disease in concert with the role of inhaled carcinogens. A genetic component has been determined which appears to be more potent among nonsmokers than among smokers; however, there appears to be a synergistic interaction between host factors and inhaled carcinogens much in keeping with the models established in experimental animals.[16] Thus, from this particular example, we see clearly that in studying the epidemiology of tumors in man, we must weigh carefully the relative importance of both genetic and nongenetic factors.

The role of viral factors in the etiology of cancer in man is of utmost interest. Nevertheless we must not lose sight of the fact that genetic factors may also be of critical importance in these problems. Thus, there are many examples of host specificity in tumor viruses. For example, mammary tumor virus is readily propagated and transmitted by genetically susceptible strains, but when introduced into a resistant strain, such as C57BL mice, it dies out within one or two generations.[17] Genetic factors are also important in Rous sarcoma virus which is controlled by a single gene with its susceptibility being dominant.[18] The significance of host-viral factors could be of profound importance in humans wherein oncogenic viruses might conceivably be under genetic control comparable to the situation in mice [19] or the Rous sarcoma virus in chickens; thus, according to Heston,[9] "The genotype of the individual may be as important a factor (or possibly a more important one) as exposure to the viruses in determining whether cancer will occur."

Animal experimentation has provided a wealth of information concerning the specific site of action of the gene(s) which leads to tumor production. These have involved the transplantation of organs. One of the earliest experiments showing clear results involved pulmonary tumors.[20][21] Specifically, lung transplants were placed in genetically susceptible and genetically resistant strains of mice. Results indicated that the action of genes in the production of lung neoplasms, in which the parent strains differed, was localized in the end organ, namely, the lung.

Other approaches determining malignant transformation at the gene or molecular level have involved tissue culture experiments.[22] Thus, it has been observed that

> cells from cultures may readily under-
> go immediate transformation and
> through transplanting them at succes-
> sive times back into mice of the inbred
> strain of origin, the time of this
> transformation can be identified with-
> in limits of a few days. This is the
> critical time and through intensive
> observation of the cells from changes
> in nutritional requirements, now
> identifiable with the chemically de-
> fined media, for antigenic changes as

shown through transplantations, and for directly observed chromosomal changes, it may be possible to associate some of these changes . . . with a malignant change.[9]

Problems in Human Studies

The combination of epidemiology and human genetics involves studies of phenomena that occur naturally in human populations, in addition to those based upon experimental methods. Characteristically, data are collected concerning various types of statistical associations between different diseases, or between a disease and individual characteristics, or between diseases and characteristics within particular kinships. One can never be completely certain that all of the relevant variables have been taken into account.[23] The cogency of data on familial incidence as evidence for the significant etiological implication of genetic factors rests ultimately upon the thoroughness with which it has been possible to exclude environmental factors as responsible for the associations found.[24]

Numerous problems are encountered in human cancer genetics which collectively contribute to considerable confusion and controversy. Foremost is the fact that *Homo sapiens* is a heterogeneous species and not amenable to the type of experimentation leading to inbred strains so readily accomplished in laboratory animals. In addition, some of the emotional problems, many of which are related to cultural and societal differences, and at the personal level, where fear of cancer is rampant, increase the difficulty of studying human cancer. Compounding the issue even further is the complexity of the cancer problem from a medical standpoint; diagnosis with pathologic verification is mandatory in order to appraise specific anatomic sites of cancer predilection in patients and their relatives. Cancer may metastasize widely thereby confounding the original site and causing problems in diagnosis unless meticulous pathological evaluations have been made; indeed, even when pathological studies are made, the answer may still remain unclear so far as the primary site is concerned.

In addition, the usual late age of onset of cancer may also obscure an understanding of its expression within kindreds since some individuals at genetic risk for the disease may die at an *earlier* age from causes other than cancer and thus, cancer would not be recorded in the pedigree. In addition, it is often difficult to obtain medical records of patients who received treatment many years prior to the initiation of a genetic study. Indeed, in many cases, when records have been secured, the investigator may find that they are too incomplete to arrive at a sufficiently accurate diagnosis to be used for genetic analysis. For example, many hospital records are destroyed after a certain number of years, thus erasing forever the very type of information which the human cancer geneticist requires for his studies. On the other hand, death certificates have been utilized by many investigators who unfortunately may *not* have appreciated the number of errors that these documents may contain. Indeed, it is the opinion of this writer that many studies in human cancer genetics have been hampered significantly by some of the above problems, particularly those in which cancer diagnoses have been reported inaccurately. Such errors have led to some very harsh and obviously legitimate criticisms about the role of genetics in human cancer.[1]

Broad Epidemiologic Approach: Population Studies

Genetics studies of human diseases go back at least to the early Mendelian days,

but most of them dealt with clear monofactorial modes of transmission. Human geneticists have made relatively little progress in etiological elucidations of multifactorial traits. One area of significant progress in this category involves empirical studies of relative risks, i.e. ratios of two conditional probabilities.

In considering the problem of carcinogenesis, the cancer epidemiologist must take into account every conceivable epidemiologic clue which might be contributing in even a small way to the problem at hand. He must view his patient in context with myriad genetic and nongenetic factors as well as their interactions, and he must relate these complex issues to each specific histologic variety of cancer. When he studies cancer incidence and prevalence in a specific population, he must appraise not only the genetic background, including racial factors, family history, and degree of consanguinity, but he must also scrutinize critically the patients' environmental exposures. The latter include x-rays, actinic radiation, abnormalities in soil content, animal and floral characteristics indigenous to the particular area, as well as the social, economic, and psychological peculiarities of the area's inhabitants including their cultural and dietary idiosyncracies, i.e. such problems as smoking habits and drinking patterns including specific types of alcoholic and nonalcoholic beverages consumed, and occupational pursuits with special attention to specific carcinogenic exposures in these particular industries. Finally, the cancer epidemiologist must even study the personal and physical practices of these individuals, even including sexual customs such as the time of first sexual intercourse, whether or not promiscuity is prevalent, and circumcision rites. These have been related etiologically to uterine cervical carcinoma and penile cancer.

The necessity for an eclectic approach to the study of carcinogenesis in man has become realized fully during the past century, stemming in part from the results of the compilation of statistics on cancer incidence and prevalence from different parts of the world. These statistics have established clearly that cancer is *not* uniformly distributed in any population; indeed wide variations in the frequency of specific anatomic varieties of cancer from one population to the next is the rule rather than the exception! For example, studies of the incidence of cancer among workers employed in the gold mining industry of South Africa have revealed wide variations in the frequency of specific malignant neoplasms. The most frequently occurring cancers among these individuals were cancer of the liver, esophagus, respiratory system, and urinary bladder. However, when specific geographical and tribal factors were analyzed critically, it was found that in the Mozambique population, cancer of the liver and urinary bladder were most frequent while esophageal cancer was the most commonly occurring malignant neoplasm among the Xhosas from the Transkei. Respiratory tract cancer showed the highest rate among the Natal population, predominantly among the Zulu.[25-27] These observations suggest strongly that variations in cancer incidence must in some way be a function of the complex interaction of host and environmental factors, i.e. geographical area including the general physical environment, the customs and habit patterns of each specific tribe, as well as the very basic genetic makeup of the members of these tribes.

Cancer genetics, then, is just one aspect of the science of cancer epidemiology in which major attention is focused upon host factors and family history and their interaction with the patient's total environmental milieu. Thus, in keeping with this reasoning, the cancer geneticist must evaluate his patient carefully, paying attention to all possible incriminating factors which could play an etiologic role in the problem at hand. These problems, as one can readily appreciate, may in fact be exceedingly complex. For example, in the study of testicular cancers in children, Li and Fraumeni[28] found little in the way of positive family history in the evaluation of 70 medical records of children with testicular cancer from fourteen institutions. However, they found one child with testicular cancer and Down's syndrome which represented the fourth reported instance of the association between these two relatively rare disorders. While theirs was only a single case, nevertheless, the frequency for this association may exceed chance.[29] It was also of interest not only that cryptorchidism was present in their patient with Down's syndrome but that it was also present in excess in other patients with Down's syndrome.[30] Thus, these observations suggest that "the link with testicular cancer may result from a shared association with testicular maldevelopment."[28] Cryptorchidism occurs in about 10 percent of adults with testicular cancer, which represents nearly a 50-fold excess frequency for its association with testicular cancer.[31] In addition, orchiopexy may not protect against testicular cancer since the scrotal testis contralateral to a cryptorchid gonad has an increased risk for the development of cancer.[28] In addition, atrophic or hypoplastic testes in the scrotum are also at an increased risk for the development of cancer.[32] Thus, Li and Fraumeni conclude that the evidence including that of morphologic defects in cryptorchid testis from early life "suggest that gonadal dysgenesis rather than ectopy per se increases the risk of cancer in a cryptorchid testis."[28] Further evidence to support the possibility that gonadal dysgenesis is involved in the pathogenesis of testicular tumors is the fact that a positive sex chromatin pattern has been observed in testicular teratoma and embryonal carcinoma.[33] Testicular tumors also occur in testicular feminization syndrome,[34] inherited as a sex limited autosomal dominant (sex linked recessive transmission cannot be excluded).

The study of cancer genetics may provide clinical investigators with insight into human clinical models which might be studied profitably. For instance, Klinefelter's syndrome should be of interest not only to geneticists and cytogeneticists, but because of its frequent association with cancer, particularly breast cancer, it should be of interest to clinical oncologists as well. Thus, a patient with Klinefelter's syndrome who developed breast cancer and an interstitial cell tumor of the testis, also was found to have a high urinary estriol.[35] Interestingly, interstitial cell tumors have also developed in animals treated with estrogen compounds.[36] Although the role of hormones in the pathogenesis of testicular tumors and other cancers in childhood is unknown, recently the administration of estrogen to a woman during pregnancy was linked to the later occurrence of adenocarcinoma of the vagina in her daughter.[37]

Thus, from these brief comments we recognize immediately the importance of an in-depth inquiry in cancer genetic studies which could in many circumstances involve the interplay of genetic and extra genetic factors.

In order to obtain maximum information about the etiology of cancer and in turn achieve a better understanding of carcinogenesis, we must exploit every conceivable clue. One area could be the study of a variety of diseases which may be associated either with cancer susceptibility or cancer resistance. Possibly, one of the reasons why so little attention has been given to this problem is because it requires an inordinate effort to establish a cancer relationship in a specific disease, particularly those in which the cancer relationship may be subtle. Questions raised immediately are the obvious ones, foremost of which is "Why does cancer occur in association with disease 'X' with greater or lesser frequency than that expected in the general population?" Extending this point further, one wonders about the role of biochemical, physiologic, and histologic characteristics of the cancer, and of course, genetic characteristics of the host with a particular disease which render him more susceptible to cancer. Thus, determining the nature of these specific factors could provide us with useful and meaningful information about cancer etiology.

In some diseases, the cancer association may be unusually strong; and certain features of the particular disease may provide a tissue site which harbors a proclivity for cancer, i.e. familial polyposis coli (autosomal dominant), polyposis coli in Gardner's syndrome (autosomal dominant), polyposis of the colon in Turcot's syndrome (autosomal recessive), each condition showing an increased risk for colonic carcinoma; exostoses of bone in multiple hereditary exostoses, (autosomal dominant) with an increased risk for development of chondrosarcoma in any of these bony exostoses; skin cancer risk in xeroderma pigmentosum (autosomal recessive); or the cancer susceptibility may be less specific such as occurs in the risk for sarcoma and meningioma in Werner's syndrome (autosomal recessive).[1] Recognition of site specific cancer risks in such disorders may provide useful models for the study of carcinogenesis. Indeed, the study of skin in xeroderma pigmentosum patients through the use of highly sophisticated organ culture techniques and biochemical studies has led to the possible implication of an endonuclease deficiency[38] which in due time may provide new insight about carcinogenesis in this disease (Chapt. 8).

Several of the commonly occurring cancers, including carcinoma of the breast, prostate, colon-rectum, (polyposis coli syndromes and cancer family syndrome excepted), stomach and endometrium show an increased empiric risk (about 3-fold increase) on a site-specific basis to first degree relatives of cancer probands.[1]

A listing of cancerous and precancerous diseases with either a clearcut or suggested hereditary etiology is presented in Tables 1-I through 1-V. These tables provide a cursory view of cancerous and precancerous disorders, aggregations of which have led to various hereditary etiological hypotheses in families. These tables should be used cautiously, with full knowledge of the fact that multiple etiologic factors may be involved in any one particular condition. Thus, in

TABLE 1-I

CANCEROUS AND PRECANCEROUS DISEASES SHOWING AUTOSOMAL DOMINANT
INHERITANCE PATTERNS

Disorder	Predominant Cancers
Neurofibromatosis	Sarcoma, acoustic neuroma, pheochromocytoma
Gardner's Syndrome	Adenocarcinoma of the colon, thyroid carcinoma, sarcoma
Multiple Nevoid Basal Cell Carcinoma Syndrome	Multiple basal cell carcinomas; medulloblastoma
Cutaneous Malignant Melanoma*	Cutaneous malignant melanoma
Tylosis and Esophageal Carcinoma (Keratosis Palmaris et Plantaris)	Esophageal Cancer
"Sclerotylosis"*	Skin cancer; several visceral carcinomas (tongue, tonsil, breast, uterus) reported, but no esophageal carcinoma
Tuberous Sclerosis (Bourneville's Disease)	Intracranial neoplasms (astrocytomas, glioblastomas)
Von Hippel-Lindau's Syndrome	Hemangioblastoma of cerebellum, hypernephroma, and pheochromocytoma
Peutz-Jegher's Syndrome	Adenocarcinoma of duodenum, colon, and ovary
Epidermolysis Bullosa Dystrophia (Congenital Traumatic Pemphigus)	Carcinoma of mucous membranes, multiple basal and squamous cell carcinoma of the skin
Kaposi's Sarcoma (Multiple Idiopathic Hemorrhagic Sarcoma of Kaposi)*	Sarcoma; high incidence of coexistent lymphoma
Porphyria Cutanea Tarda	Basal cell carcinoma of skin, hepatoma
Generalized Keratoacanthoma	Rare occurrences of squamous cell carcinoma
Pachynychia Congenita	Carcinoma of mucous membranes
Hereditary Multiple Endocrine Adenomatosis Syndrome (Multiple Endocrine Neoplasia Type I)	Tumors of the pituitary gland, parathyroid gland and pancreatic islet cells
Multiple Mucosal Neuromata Syndrome	Medullary carcinoma of the thyroid, pheochromocytoma, and parathyroid tumors
Sipple's Syndrome (Multiple Endocrine Neoplasia Type II)	Medullary carcinoma of the thyroid, pheochromocytoma, and parathyroid disease
Testicular Feminization Syndrome†	Seminoma
Blue Rubber-Bleb Nevus Syndrome	Cerebellar medulloblastoma (a single case)
Cowden's Disease (Multiple Hamartoma Syndrome)*	Carcinoma of breast and thyroid
Celiac Disease (Nontropical Sprue; Gluten-Induced Enteropathy)	Lymphoma; esophageal carcinoma
Familial Fibrocystic Pulmonary Dysplasia	Bronchogenic carcinoma
Stein-Leventhal Syndrome*	Endometrial Carcinoma
Hereditary Multiple Benign Cystic Epithelioma (Epithelioma Adenoides Cysticum of Brooke)	Baso-squamous cell carcinoma in at least one confirmed case
Carcinoma of breast* in association with other Malignant Neoplasms‡	Breast cancer, associated malignant neoplasms including soft tissue sarcomas, leukemia, brain tumors, and a variety of adenocarcinomas.
Retinoblastoma	Retinoblastoma

*Possible autosomal dominant, based upon a limited number of observations.

†Sex-limited autosomal dominant though sex-linked recessive mode of inheritance cannot be excluded.

‡This is recorded here tentatively in the dominant catalogue based upon limited family investigations by Li and Fraumeni, "Soft Tissue Sarcoma, Breast Cancer, and Other Neoplasms: A Familial Syndrome?," *Annals of Internal Medicine,* 71:747–752, (1969) and Lynch *et al.,* "Tumor Variations in Families with Breast Cancer," *Journal of the American Medical Association,* 222:1631–1635, 1972.

TABLE 1-II
CANCER AND PRECANCEROUS DISEASES SHOWING AUTOSOMAL RECESSIVE INHERITANCE
PATTERNS AND THOSE SHOWING SEX-LINKED INHERITANCE

Autosomal Recessive Inheritance	
Disorder	*Predominant Cancers*
Xeroderma Pigmentosum	Basal and squamous cell carcinoma of skin and malignant melanoma (3%)
Xeroderma and Mental Retardation (DeSanctis-Cacchione Syndrome)	Basal and squamous cell carcinoma of skin
Werner's Syndrome (Progeria of the Adult)	Sarcomas, meningiomas
Ataxia-Telangiectasia (Louis-Bar Syndrome)	Acute leukemia and lymphoma, possible gastric carcinoma
Bloom's Syndrome (Congenital Telangiectatic Erythema and Stunted Growth)	Acute leukemia
Chediak-Higashi Syndrome	Lymphoma
Albinism	Basal and squamous cell carcinoma of skin
Fanconi's Aplastic Anemia	Leukemia and lymphoma
Glioma-Polyposis Syndrome (Turcot's Syndrome)	Brain tumors, (glioblastoma multiforme, medulloblastoma) and adenocarcinoma of colon secondary to polyposis coli
Beckwith-Wiedemann Syndrome*	Adrenal cortical carcinoma, nephroblastoma, embryonal tumors of liver, gonadoblastoma
Alpha-1-Antitrypsin Deficiency	Hepatoma†

Sex-Linked Recessive Inheritance	
Disorder	*Predominant Cancers*
Aldrich Syndrome (Wiskott-Aldrich Syndrome)	Leukemia, lymphoma
Bruton's Agammaglobulinemia	Acute leukemia
Dyskeratosis Congenita	Squamous cell carcinoma of skin and mucous membranes
Reticuloendothelial Syndrome with Hyperglobulinemia	Reticuloendothelial cancer

* Autosomal dominant inheritance with reduced penetrance and variable expressivity cannot be excluded. M.M., Cohen, *et al., American Journal of Diseases of Children*, 122:515–519, 1971.
† Rare examples of this association have been recorded. N.O. Berg, "Liver Disease in Adults with Alpha$_1$-antitrypsin Deficiency," *New England Journal of Medicine*, 287:1264–1267, 1972.

TABLE 1-III
SITE-SPECIFIC MALIGNANT NEOPLASMS
WITH POSSIBLE FAMILIAL OCCURRENCE

Breast
Colon
Stomach
Prostate
Endometrium
Hodgkin's disease
Waldenstrom's macroglobulinemia
Multiple myeloma
Leukemia
Lymphoma
Hepatocellular carcinoma
Carcinoid tumor
Carcinoma of the duodenum
Testicular tumors
Neuroblastoma
Wilms' tumor
Burkitt's lymphoma
Bronchogenic carcinoma
Ovarian carcinoma
Nasopharyngeal carcinoma

the case of carotid body tumors one should realize that while autosomal dominant inheritance has been shown in families with this tumor, the overwhelming majority of occurrences are due to apparent nongenetic factors; specifically about 97 percent of occurrences are on a sporadic basis with unknown etiology. Similarly, retinoblastoma has a classical genetic etiology in between 20 and 40 percent of the cases; however, certain undefined nongenetic factors (fresh genetic mutations cannot be excluded) may also be of etiologic importance. On the other hand, though heredity appears to play a significant role in lupus erythematosis, the exact genetic mechanism has not yet been determined. In addition, the significance

TABLE 1-IV
PRECANCEROUS DISEASES WHEREIN GENETIC FACTORS HAVE BEEN UNDER
CONSIDERATION BUT HAVE NOT YET BEEN CLEARLY ELUCIDATED

Disorders	*Predominant Cancers*
Scleroderma (Progressive Systemic Sclerosis)	Bronchiolar carcinoma, malignant carcinoid
Dermatomyositis (adult form)	Adenocarcinoma of viscera
Sjogren's Syndrome (Keratoconjunctivitis Sicca)	Lymphoma
Systemic Lupus Erythematosus	Thymic tumors, leukemia, and lymphoma
Giant Pigmented Nevi* (Bathing Trunk Nevi)	Melanomas in children
Klinefelter's Syndrome (XXY)	Breast cancer
Turner's Syndrome Exhibiting 45X/46XY Mosaicism or other Chromosomal Complements with the Presence of a Y chromosome	Gonadoblastoma
Down's Syndrome	Leukemia
Paget's Disease (Osteitis deformans)	Osteogenic sarcoma
Ulcerative Colitis	Colon cancer
Nevus Sebaceous of Jadassohn	Basal cell carcinoma of skin; salivary adenocarcinoma

*Hereditary etiology has not yet been established, but the congenital basis and known hereditary factors of certain melanomas raise suspicion about genetic etiology.

of malignant transformation in this disease must be critically scrutinized so that its full relationship to this immune reactive disorder may be comprehended. In all events, these tables reflect the fact that considerable knowledge about cancer genetics has been accrued during the past several decades as evidenced by the number of listings in the several categories presented. By the same token the incompleteness of this listing attests to the need for continued diligent genetic investigations concerning carcinogenesis. Reviews of the subject have been compiled by Lynch, *et al.*[1,39,40,41] Cytogenetics and cancer[42-45] (Table 1-V) is discussed by Sandberg and Sakurai in Chapter 9.

Genetic Markers in Human Cancer Studies

When an individual has two or more distinct types of cells as in cellular mosaicism, it is possible to study the origin and development of cancers which may occur. In the case of mammalian females two different cells result as a consequence of the inactivation of one of the two X chromosomes; this event occurs early in embryo-genesis in every somatic cell and it is believed that the event is random but once it occurs all of the descendants of that particular cell will have the same inactivated X chromosome. Several X-linked disorders of man including glucose-6-phosphate dehydrogenase (G-6-PD) have been clearly linked with the activated X chromosome. Thus, individuals heterozygous at this locus will have the following two possibilities: An "A" gene and a "B" gene each of which controls enzyme types determined through electrophoretic studies. When skin fibroblasts from a patient who is heterozygous at this locus are grown in tissue culture it is possible to identify both varieties of enzymes. However, it is also possible to remove single cells from the cell mixtures and develop clones based on the descendants of a single cell and thereby identify a single enzyme in each clone. In 1964 DeMars and Nance[46] identified this phenomenon clearly. Other investigators have also investigated tumors having this specific genetic marker. For example, in 1965 Linder and Gartler[47] applied this system to the study of uterine leiomyomas in patients who were heterozygous at the G-6-PD locus. Their experiments disclosed that normal uterine muscle adjacent to the

TABLE 1-V
CYTOGENETIC ABERRATIONS IN CANCERS AND PRECANCEROUS DISEASES

Disorders	Chromosome Defect	Associated Neoplastic Disease and/or Comment
Carcinoma	Aneuploidy, tetraploidy, marker chromosomes	—
Acute leukemia	Karyotypes normal in as many as 50% of reported cases	—
Acute lymphocytic leukemia	When karyotype abnormal, find hyperdiploidy	—
Acute myeloblastic leukemia	When karyotype abnormal, find hypo- or hyperdiploidy	—
Chronic lymphocytic leukemia (CLL)	Christchurch (Ch) chromosome-deletion of small arms of small acrocentric chromosome believed to be No. 21; pseudodiploidy also reported	CLL found in several relatives with this chromosome defect in two families
Chronic granulocytic leukemia (CGL)	Philadelphia (Ph) chromosome-deletion of approximately half of long arms of small acrocentric chromosome believed to be No. 21	CGL shows Ph¹ chromosome in majority of patients; may be "acquired," as opposed to "genetic"
Mongolism (Down's syndrome)	Trisomy 21, or translocation 15/21	Acute leukemia
Turner's syndrome	XO/XY	Gonadoblastoma
Klinefelter's syndrome	XXY or mosaicism	Breast carcinoma, leukemia and reticulum cell sarcoma
Trisomy D	13–15 trisomy	Myelogenous leukemia
Fanconi's aplastic anemia	Inherited as autosomal recessive, but shows chromosome breakage and rearrangement in cultured leukocytes	Leukemia and lymphoma
Bloom's syndrome	Inherited as autosomal recessive and shows chromosome breakage and rearrangement in cultured leukocytes	Leukemia and carcinoma
Waldenstrom's macroglobulinemia	Supernumerary chromosome which is metacentric or slightly submetacentric, as large or larger than the No. 1 chromosome	This supernumerary chromosome has been found to be present in several cases of Waldenstrom's macroglobulinemia
Ataxia-telangiectasia	Inherited as an autosomal recessive but shows chromosome breakage and rearrangement in cultured cells	Lymphoreticular malignancies believed to result from failure of the immune mechanism
Congenital abnormalities, cancer, increased incidence of fetal wastage, and chromosomal aberrations; suggestive relationship, but more studies will be required	Chromosomal breakage, structural variation changes in modal number	Solid and hematopoietic cancer
Di Guglielmo's syndrome (erythroleukemia, erythremic myelosis)	Aneuploidy and structural alterations	Acute leukemia
Myelofibrosis and myeloid metaplasia (myeloproliferative syndrome)	Early have normal karyotype; prior to development of acute leukemia may see abnormality in chromosome number and morphology	Predisposes to polycythema vera and acute leukemias

leiomyomas had both "A" and "B" enzyme varieties. The tumor, itself, showed only one specific type, i.e. either "A" or "B" but not *both*, thereby suggesting a single-cell origin for each neoplasm. On the other hand, Gartler and his associates[48] identified both types of enzymes in tissue culture in their study of patients with hereditary multiple

trichoepithelioma. This suggests a multicellular origin for these tumors.

Chronic myelogenous leukemia (CML) was similarly studied[49] in a group of heterozygous patients, extracts of whose peripheral blood (granulocytes) contained only a single enzyme type. It was, therefore, concluded that this event which "occurred in preparations derived from millions of granulocytes strongly favors a clonal origin of the leukemia cells in CML and supports the likelihood that the clone arises as a result of a rare event occurring in a single cell." A similar event may also occur in the Philadelphia (Ph[1]) chromosome, a marker in CML which has also suggested a clonal origin for CML. This specific chromosome is a G-group marker which is found consistently in dividing bone marrow cells from practically all patients with typical findings of CML but the chromosome is not found in other cells in these patients such as in lymphocytes and fibroblasts.

There is a paucity of studies involving the G-6-PD system in patients with carcinoma. Fialkow[49] reported squamous cell carcinoma of the maxillary antrum in a patient showing Gd[A]/Gd[B] (heterozygous) in whose blood cells he observed two enzyme types, but in whose tumor cells only one enzyme type which suggested a clonal origin for this particular neoplasm. However, in reviewing other types of carcinomas which included two originating in the colon, one in the liver, and one in the breast, he found both "A" and "B" enzyme types. He concluded that it was possible that these particular carcinomas had a multicellular origin and he was concerned with the possibility that distant metastases might originate from several primary tumor cells. For example, 28 metastatic nodules were studied in a patient with carcinoma of the colon and it was found that the majority contained only one or the other type of G-6-PD, thus suggesting ". . . that they originated from single malignant cells." However, in a patient with metastatic tumor nodules from primary liver cancer it was found that both enzyme types existed. Additional study will, therefore, be necessary in order to better comprehend the significance of the marker systems in carcinoma, particularly with respect to the G-6-PD system.

Finally, G-6-PD deficiency is discussed in Chapter 22 in context with cancer resistance and in diabetics with reduced cancer risk.

Childhood Cancer: Population Studies, Family Studies

The quest for etiology of cancer in childhood poses a challenge to the epidemiologist, geneticist, pediatrician, and clinical oncologist.[1,50] The traditional approach to the problem has been primarily retrospective[51,52] based upon statistical surveys of the incidence of childhood cancer in one or more large populations. A specific example of this approach is found in the Oxford Survey of Childhood Cancers reported by Stewart and Barber[51] wherein epidemiologic studies were made of patients with childhood cancers in comparison with a control population. Differences between patients and controls were not striking though initial results revealed that the sibship position, maternal age, findings of mongolism, and recent attacks of pneumonia were likely to be associated with leukemia in children. It was also suspected that children who had been X-rayed in utero, children whose mothers had had several abortions, and children who had brothers and sisters with cancer, were more likely to develop cancer than were children in whose families none of these events had occurred.[51]

A population survey was made of pineal tumors in childhood in Japan,[53] which revealed an eleven-fold increase over those which would be expected in the United States. However, when evaluating these data one should always consider the relative significance of racial, genetic, cultural, geographic, as well as other unexplained variables and/or their interaction.

While population surveys are of unquestionable value to the cancer epidemiologist, studies of individual cancer prone families may also provide a rich source of information about cancer etiology.[1,39,40,54] The family study approach may provide the cancer researcher with an opportunity to search extensively for genealogic relationships, cytogenetic aberrations, medical peculiarities, histologic documentation of cancer, as well as for unusual cultural and habit idiosyncracies. Carcinogenic exposures can be studied within the context of the family and its environmental milieu. Admittedly, this is time consuming when considering the limited number of experimental subjects available when compared with the vast numbers involved in population surveys; in addition, the success of the investigation is dependent in large part upon the cooperative attitude of the family. We believe, nevertheless, that this particular approach to cancer epidemiology is worthwhile; and in certain circumstances, it may provide clues which could eventually aid significantly in the comprehension of carcinogenesis. Many recent studies document the merit of this approach to cancer epidemiology.[1,39,40,50,54–58] The example described by Li and Fraumeni,[50] an apparently new syndrome involving a variety of cancers in children including brain tumors, leukemia, and soft tissue sarcomas, as well as an excess of cancer occurring in adults, including breast cancer and multiple primary malignant neoplasms illustrates our point well. In another family study Lynch and Green[57] described a child who manifested bilateral Wilms' tumor in association with congenital heart disease (Ebstein's anomaly). His mother had a polyendocrine cancer syndrome with four primary carcinomas (medullary thyroid carcinoma, bilateral pheochromocytoma, and carcinoma of the breast). An excess of similar cancers in other relatives from this same family has been confirmed recently.[59]

Evidence now exists in several autosomal recessive diseases associated with cancer in childhood showing that heterozygotes in these families manifest an increased frequency of cancer.[60] For example, in Fanconi's anemia which is inherited as an autosomal recessive, cytogenetic abnormalities occur including a high incidence of chromatid breaks, exchanges, and endoreduplications. Heterozygous carriers of the gene for Fanconi's anemia also show an increased frequency of cancer and interestingly, fibroblasts from these patients show increased transformation induced by SV40 virus in tissue culture preparations (to be discussed in greater detail shortly). Thus, Swift[60] has suggested that on the basis of an estimated frequency of Fanconi's heterozygotes that cancer occurrence among them is about three times that expected for the general population; and it is estimated that approximately 1 in 20 will develop acute leukemia.

Results from these epidemiologic surveys of childhood cancer,[1,51–53] as well as from family studies,[39,40,55–58] indicate a need for the development of theories about carcinogenesis which implicate as well as characterize host factors in childhood cancer. Specifically, existing theories are primarily oriented to adult cancer but their hypotheses and conclusions cannot always be transferred meaningfully to the problems of cancer in infants and children. For example, the fact that children are more susceptible to certain specific histological varieties of cancer is in marked variance with the statement that cancer susceptibility invariably increases with age from birth. In addition, present theories of carcinogenesis consider extrinsic factors more important than intrinsic or host factors, probably because an overwhelming majority of epidemiologic surveys have been concerned with the appraisal of known carcinogenic factors such as smoking, radiation, and certain occupational exposures, all of which are more characteristic of adult populations.

They have been far less concerned with intrinsic factors in the host which could harbor significant associated etiologic importance in determining cancer development in infants and children.

A Family with Childhood Cancer

A major responsibility of the cancer geneticist is to evaluate occurrences of cancer within families. As discussed, he must discern the specific histologic varieties of cancer and relate their mode of distribution in the kindred to known or presumptive etiologic mechanisms. Occasionally a particular condition might be recognized immediately as following a classical Mendelian inheritance pattern such as occurs in familial polyposis coli (autosomal dominant). However, in the overwhelming majority of cases, the type of inheritance may not be simple or clear-cut; rather, due to a paucity of knowledge about associations of one specific histologic variety of cancer with others, problems of ascertainment due to unavailability of relatives, or incomplete pathologic confirmation of medical disorders, the study will necessarily be less well-defined.

An example of the type of clinical cancer problem occasionally encountered by clinicians and cancer geneticists will be discussed briefly. This concerned a family wherein the proband (Fig. 1–2) received a diagnosis of pleiomorphic sarcoma of the right thigh (AFIP 1367196) at age 20 months and died from metastases at age two years and six months. The child's sister received a diagnosis of medulloblastoma of the right cerebellum at age six and died two months postoperatively with metastases confirmed at autopsy (A-64-247). Two other siblings, a boy age five and a girl age one year five months were alive without evidence of cancer. The father had sarcoma (histologic confirmation) at age 36. The mother, also

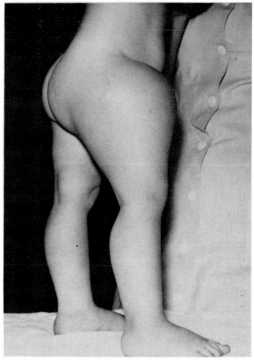

Figure 1–2. A child with sarcoma of the leg. (This family was made available through the courtesy of D. Hoefnagel, M.D., Dept. of Pathology, Dartmouth Medical School, Hanover, New Hampshire.)

age 36, had not had past or present evidence of cancer. There was no consanguinity. However, the proband's father's sister (the proband's paternal aunt) died of cancer of the liver at age two years and four months though unfortunately the biopsy specimen was unavailable. The father's brother was age 33 and was free of cancer. The proband's paternal grandfather had a mixed tumor of the left parotid gland (salivary type) at age 22 and underwent a radical resection because of a recurrence six years later, at which time he received radiation therapy. He died at age 40 from chondrosarcoma of the skull which may well have been related to the radiation therapy. The paternal grandmother died of choriocarcinoma at age 40. The proband's paternal great grandmother died at age 43 of cancer of the uterus (histology was not available). Except for the radiation exposure in the proband's paternal grandfather, there was no other relative who had experienced carcinogenic exposures.

In summary, the findings in this family showed histologically verified cancer in two siblings (sarcoma of the thigh in the proband and medulloblastoma of the right cerebellum in his six year old sister), sarcoma in their father, and cancer of the liver by history in the two year old paternal aunt of the proband. Both paternal grandparents had histologically verified cancer.

It is not possible to categorize the findings in this kindred in terms of any currently recognizable hereditary cancer syndrome. However, in due time, with careful follow-up of the family, a more meaningful comprehension of the problem might emerge. In short, the familial aggregation of cancer in this family appears to be significant though at this moment it does not fit any recognizable hereditary cancer syndrome. Laboratory studies, including cytogenetics and viral investigations might help elucidate etiology. The family does pose a challenge and is the type of problem encountered by those interested in cancer genetics.

New Methodologies

Newly developing research methodologies are making it possible to determine the existence of identifiable biological determinants in patients with certain genetic and/or cytogenetic disorders associated with cancer susceptibility. For example, through the use of such oncogenetic viruses as SV40,[61-69] human cells in tissue culture can be transformed into neoplastic cells.[62,63] Quantitative assay methods are now available for estimating the frequency of transformation for a particular cell strain; thus, cells from individuals with certain genetic anomalies who show a high risk for cancer have in turn shown increased frequencies of transformation of cells following infection with SV40. These have been confirmed in fibroblasts from patients with Down's syndrome,[63,64] Fanconi's anemia,[65,66] Klinefelter's syndrome,[67] and from a patient with XY-gonadal dysgenesis.[68] These methodologies have also been applied to members of certain cancer-prone families,[69] to patients with cancer of the colon,[70] and to patients with acute myelogenous leukemia[71] among whom a variable range of transformation was observed. These findings suggest that transformation frequency determination might harbor a powerful potential for the detection of individuals who are genetically predisposed to cancer, and thereby enable the physician to use this information profitably for closer surveillance of his patients in order to achieve earlier cancer diagnosis (Chapt. 7).

The oncogene theory[19,72] hypothesizes that quiescent genes present at conceptus are subsequently triggered by certain outside "signals," i.e. hormones, environmental chemicals, X-ray, solar radiation and countless other potentially incriminating carcinogenic events, to produce uncontrollable cellular reproduction and tumor formation. Thus, these environmental factors, appearing during critical periods of growth and development, activate genes which turn cells in a specific target organ into a cancer cell. This theory could also explain the differing tumor aggregations in specific hereditary cancer problems. Thus, when "genetic" factors are discussed in differing contexts in this book we wish to admonish the reader to consider the fact that genes may be influenced to a variable degree by other factors, including oncogenic viruses. Thus, the issue of genetic etiology is an exceedingly complex one, and demands a broad and eclectic approach if we are to make significant progress in this discipline.

Experiments in Allophenic Mice: Cancer Genetic Implications

We have already emphasized the fact that practically every inbred strain of mice shows a characteristic profile of malignant neoplasms wherein breeding experiments have strongly suggested that the susceptibility to most of these tumors is probably polygenic. Nevertheless, the basic mechanisms involving genetic factors in cancer research remain unclear.

While considerable information has been obtained relevant to genetic factors in cancer through *in vitro* studies, it is reasonable to assume that additional answers in the area of cancer genetics might ultimately be found through *in vivo* studies involving the growth of tissues within the context of the dynamically integrated and functioning organism so that interactions between tissue systems can be critically analyzed. Thus, questions pertaining to cancer susceptibility relevant to whether the carcinogenic events are initiated on a local level in a particular tissue or whether it is from some generalized aberration within the organism can be more profitably pursued. It is in this area that the utilization of allophenic mice have proven to be most useful, especially in testing hypotheses pertaining to whether specific genetic loci influence vulnerability to tumors through selectively expressing this susceptibility in specific tissues. Thus, manipulation of cellular genotypes in terms of high and low susceptible cellular genomes through their differential distribution among tissues has been developed to provide answers to these questions.

Mintz[73] has pioneered in the development of a novel form of mammalian genetic manipulation which has opened new horizons for *in vivo* studies of the genetic basis of neoplasia through the development of a laboratory artifact, namely, the allophenic mouse. An allophenic mouse is a genetic mosaic produced by aggregating the blastomeres of two embryos with differing genotypes into a single cluster during cleavage stages. This complex is then implanted into the uterus of a surrogate mother. Surviving embryos result in a living adult mouse with cells which harbor immunogenetically distinct constitutions and which coexist in the living animal. Thus, the allophenic mouse

. . . contains different phenotypic subpopulations of cells, because of dissimilarities in cellular genotypes. One such animal has four (or even more) parents instead of two, since it is derived by joining together two (or more) cleavage-stage embryos *in vitro,* each with its own set of parents and thus its own genetic constitution. About a third of all the artificial composites, after transfer to an incubator mother, continue their development to birth and become healthy, long-lived adults. Since the birth . . . of the first mosaic mouse, over 1,000 quadriparental individuals had been produced and have survived (in Mintz's laboratory). The two different cellular genotypes can be found in any or all tissues, because of the early stage at which the cells are aggregated. In addition, the total level of retained mosaicism, and the tissue distributions and proportions of the respective genotypes, vary greatly from one animal to another, even within the same paired combination . . . . Allophenic animals are permanently immunologically tolerant of any immunogenetic differences in their component cells and have never developed runt disease. They nevertheless possess full immunological competence to respond to and reject *foreign antigens* such as skin grafts of another histocompatibility type.

Thus, utilizing allophenic animals it is possible to experiment with this system so that cells from a high-tumor strain can now be made to coexist with cells of an unrelated low-tumor strain, starting prior to cell differentiation. The permutations and combinations in tissue distributions of cellular genotypes constitute the experiment. The animals bring to light those biological relationships that are relevant to genetic control of tumor susceptibility and to the progress of malignancy and metastasis.

Thus, Mintz has been able to conduct numerous experiments on a variety of tumors for which there is evidence of genetic predisposition. Her aims in these experiments were to identify whether the heredity of the potentially malignant cells, of other organs, or of the host as a whole, is responsible for susceptibility; and, ultimately, to define in molecular terms the means by which the susceptible cell phenotype is produced.

Studies showed that loci controlling susceptibility to mammary tumors appear to express themselves chiefly in the mammary glands cells themselves, and those controlling susceptibility to hepatomas become active mainly in liver cells. Intracellular rather than intercellular events seem paramount in the origin of these specific histologic varieties of cancer.

The allophenic mouse model also has implications for virological experiments. For example, according to Mintz,[73] "Gene control of susceptibility to viral tumors may also involve a significant measure of control of viral infectivity via the target cell itself, depending upon the cellular phenotype. Allophenic mice afford new avenues for genetic analysis of this possibility *in vivo* under conditions in which genetically different cells are exposed to the virus within a shared set of systemic influences."

This novel method merits continuing attention as we search for clues to the role of genetics in carcinogenesis.

Biological Correlates with Cancer

Inquiry into the identification of potentially important biological correlates with cancer have been popular for several decades, though unfortunately, to date, their significance and utilization has been limited. We shall limit our discussion to only three of these methodologies, namely blood group antigens, Australia antigen, and HL-A histocompatibility antigens.

The ABO Blood Groups and Cancer Associations

The search for a possible etiologic relationship between ABO blood groups and cancer was initiated through the studies of Buchanan and Higley[74] in 1921, in the same year, by Alexander[75] and by Johansen in 1925.[76] In 1953, Aird and associates[77] were probably the first investigators to demonstrate a significant association between gastric carcinoma and blood group A. This observation was verified by other investigators who also confirmed a statistical association between blood group A and pernicious anemia.[78-80] Interestingly, blood group A has also been found to be statistically associated with carcinoma of the genital tract,[81] tumors of salivary gland tissue in general,[82] and with mucinous secreting tumors in particular.[83] Blood group A has also been shown to be associated with multiple primary malignant neoplasms.[84] While blood group A is seemingly the most frequent blood group antigen associated with cancer, there is evidence showing that a classically inherited (autosomal recessive) precancerous disease, namely xeroderma pigmentosum, has a statistical correlation with blood group O.[85]

Recently, Marcus[86] has updated this entire subject and expanded it to include other diseases in addition to cancer and has discussed existing knowledge of the biochemistry, genetics, and physiologic factors relevant to the ABO and Lewis blood group systems and their associations with human disease.

When considering noncancerous diseases, we find that diseases such as duodenal ulceration show a high statistical association with blood group O;[80] in turn, duodenal ulceration is also more likely to occur in nonsecretors of blood group substances than in secretors.[87] Other investigators[88,89] have demonstrated that blood group O patients have an excessive rate of bleeding, perforations, and stomach ulcers. These complications were not found to be correlated with secretor status.

Other cancers showing increased associations with blood group A include cancer of the ovary,[81,90] cancer of the pancreas,[91] prostate,[92] gallbladder,[93] and lip.[94] Astrocytoma of the brain, particularly when the patient is less than 20 years of age, was found to show a statistical association with blood group O.[95] Interestingly, in face of the preponderance of blood group A and its association with a variety of cancers, Clifford[96] found that in Kenya, patients with blood group A were seemingly at low risk for nasopharyngeal carcinoma.

Buckwalter and associates[97] found a correlation of blood group O with lung cancer though other investigators[75,98,99] were not able to find any blood group association with lung cancer. Other tumors lacking significant correlation with blood group antigens have included cancer of the colon and rectum,[92,97] esophagus,[91,94,100] larynx,[101] liver,[102] tongue,[94] uterus,[103] and chromophobe adenoma.[91]

Lee[104] reviewed the literature on blood group associations in cancer of the uterine cervix, endometrium, and breast, and concluded that the results in these particular tumors were too conflicting to arrive at any conclusive impressions so far as blood group antigens and their association with these diseases were concerned.

The study of blood group antigens and their associations with cancer nevertheless harbors a research potential for cancer epidemiologists and for geneticists. Some of the problems encountered in these studies perhaps have been compounded by the profound racial admixtures in many populations with concomitant variable assortments of blood group antigens, problems in statistical sampling of the populations, and of course, the occasional problem of laboratory error in assessment of blood group antigens as well as inadequate histologic evaluation of malignant neoplasms. These problems notwithstanding, the full etiologic meaning of the mentioned associations of blood groups with malignancies is unclear. Thus, Buckwalter comments as follows:

> The full implications of the observed association remain to be realized. Interested clinical and basic scientists alike have regarded this association as perhaps the frontier of a new field of investigation, development of which may lead to an understanding of fundamental considerations having to do with the cause of gastric cancers, cancers in general, and the broader aspects of heredity and disease.[78]

Australia Antigen (Au [1] or HAA)

In 1965, Blumberg and associates[105] described a *new* antigen in the serum of patients with leukemia, now referred to as Australia antigen. Since this report numerous investigations have been conducted upon this antigen from the standpoint of its epidemiology, genetics, and its physical and chemical characteristics. The first significant epidemiologic clue about the antigen was that it was either closely associated with or possibly could be a causal agent in viral hepatitis.[106,107] Indeed it is estimated that millions of asymptomatic patients harbor this antigen, as *carriers*.[106]

The Australia antigen was first found in the serum of an Australian Aborigine and hence it has been referred to as Australia antigen (phenotype Au [1] and also as hepatitis associated antigen (HAA).

The Australia antigen is relatively rare in normal individuals in the United States occurring only in about 1 in 1,000 normal people; however, it occurs in about 27 percent of persons with acute viral hepatitis (post-transfusion hepatitis, 41 percent; infectious hepatitis, 22 percent).[106,107] On rare occasions the antigen disappears with clinical improvement. Other terminology for this antigen has included, "SH antigen."[108]

Under electron microscopy it has been observed that the antigen is a particle of about 200 Angstroms in diameter which contains knoblike subunits on its surface. This approximates the suspected size of the hepatitis virus.[108]

The antigen has been observed in patients with Down's syndrome in which interesting variations of its prevalence are found based upon the type of ascertainment. For example, the antigen is found in about 30 percent of institutionalized (large institutions) patients with Down's syndrome; contrariwise, the antigen is extremely rare in other mentally retarded patients in the same institution and is almost uniformly absent in the employees.

In contrast with the institutionalized Down's syndrome patients, the antigen is infrequently found in outpatients with Down's syndrome and it is also rare in patients with Down's syndrome found in small institutions. This has led to the impression that a host factor in patients with Down's syndrome results in a high susceptibility to chronic infection with the Australia antigen.[108]

Data from several areas of the world show varying frequencies of Australia antigen. Thus, it is present in about 3 percent of Indians from south India, 6 percent in Vietnamese, and 6 percent in Filipinos.[108]

In addition, a family study in Cebu, in the Phillipines and another in Bougainville Territory in New Guinea revealed familial clustering of the antigen consistent with inheritance of the trait as an autosomal recessive.[106]

Patients with Down's syndrome and Australia antigen have been found to have moderate increases in serum glutamic pyruvic transaminase (SGPT) and liver biopsy has shown evidence of chronic hepatitis.[108]

Of additional interest, Australia antigen has been shown to occur in excess in affected individuals in families with familial cryptogenic cirrhosis, and in two families with multiple occurrences of chronic liver disease and hepatoma.[109] Denison and associates[110] have also presented an example of familial hepatoma with Australia antigen and Bancroft and associates[111] described a family with hepatitis and Australia antigen. Finally, Ohbayashi has presented the combined results of a study of three families[112] which has included a new family in addition to the two families they previously studied.[109]

The study by Ohbayashi and associates[112] is based on sera from 54 persons from three families noteworthy for increased occurrences of chronic liver disease and hepatoma. Australia antigen and the antibodies against Australia antigen were tested through the use of the immune adherence hemagluttination method. Results showed that Australia antigen was positive in 14 (93 percent) out of 15 of the affected members and their siblings and this antigen was also positive in 20 (83 percent) out of the 24 children of the female siblings. These findings were contrasted with the fact that Australia antigen was negative in seven out of the eight children of the male siblings and it was also negative in six spouses of the siblings that were tested. Anti-Australia antigen was detected in only one of the wives of the Australia antigen positive males.

Conclusions drawn from these families as well as from a review of familial cirrhosis from the Japanese literature suggested that in certain kindreds, Australia antigen or an Australia antigen-infective agent is transmitted from mother to child and is also responsible for the development of the carrier state, chronic hepatitis, cirrhosis of the liver, and eventual development of hepatoma.

HL-A System in Human Cancer

Antigens of the HL-A system are widely distributed throughout the body and are under genetic control by two linked loci which are believed to be located adjacent to a separate locus that controls the mixed lymphocyte reaction.[113] The HL-A system is of crucial importance in influencing histocompatibility reactions in man.

This system harbors a potential for the study of genetic linkage of histocompatibility antigens to cancer. This could prove to be of clinical value should certain HL-A antigens be found to correlate with findings of histologically confirmed cancer or with patients who are genetically susceptible to cancer by pedigree evaluations; and contrariwise, it would be of equal interest should large numbers of patients who are free of cancer, or who come from families noteworthy for a paucity of cancer, have specific HL-A antigens in common. Thus, the method would have merit in identifying cancer prone or cancer resistant histocompatibility antigens in these respective clinical categories. However, too few population and family studies have been performed to glean meaningful results.[114]

As in so many other investigations in cancer genetics, animal studies have provided an initial stimulus for developing methods for later application to humans. Hence, initial interest in the distribution of HL-A antigens in patients with cancer stems primarily from the demonstration of an association between the major histocompatibility system of mice (H-2) and susceptibility and resistance to certain forms of leukemia.[115]

Several differing types of human cancer have been studied including choriocarcinoma,[113,116] Hodgkin's disease,[117] and other lymphoid tumors in general.[118] Several suggestive associations have been made with these various cancer problems, but it is too early to establish a precise cause effect type of correlation between HL-A types and specific varieties of cancer. For example, in the case of Hodgkin's disease an increased incidence of HL-A5 has been shown by some investigators;[117] and in acute lymphatic leukemia of childhood an increased incidence of HL-A2-12 has been identified.[119] Our own studies of the cancer family syndrome are too preliminary for definitive analysis, though we have identified a trend in the direction of HL-A2-12 in patients who have either had cancer or who are at genetic risk for the development of cancer in Family "N".

The primary importance of the utilization of the HL-A system in human cancer genetic studies appears to rest in the potential it harbors for linkage studies for defining risk factors for cancer susceptibility. Since a reliable marker indicating cancer proneness is virtually lacking at the moment it will behoove us to continue to add to the body of accumulating knowledge about the HL-A system in the hope that it might prove of value as an adjunct to cancer genetic investigations. This subject is discussed in greater detail in Chapters 5 and 6.

Somatic Mutation Hypothesis —

The somatic mutation hypothesis suggests that tumors are derived from single mutant cells. Recent genetic, cytogenetic, and virologic evidence has lent credence to this hypothesis. Early studies by Tyzzer[120] in experimental animals provided impetus for the concept of somatic mutation as being a critical event in carcinogenesis. Specifically, Tyzzer showed that marked differences occurred in the behavior of tumors when transplanted in certain mice. This even occurred when tumors arose in homogeneous strains, providing evidence that such differences might be explained by the acquisition of new characteristics by the soma during tumorigenesis. During the course of artificial propagation, these characteristics would persist, and were regarded by Tyzzer as a modification of somatic tissue which he referred to as somatic mutation.

Acceptance of the somatic mutation hypothesis does not conflict with the growing body of knowledge which favors the role of primary genetic factors for certain cancers and precancerous disorders affecting humans. Knudson[121,122] has described a two mutation model for cancer etiology. His first clinical example pertained to retinoblastoma. According to his hypothesis, a certain fraction of occurrences of retinoblastoma are non-hereditary and are the result of two somatic mutational events in one cell which is thereby transformed into a tumor cell which eventually produces a solitary tumor (i.e., retinoblastoma). The other fraction of individuals affected with this disease involves hereditary occurrences, in individuals who have inherited one of the mutational events and are relatively predisposed to the malignant neoplasm, which may then occur from a single somatic mutation in any of such an individual's cells. The first mutational event in the hereditary variety is a germinal one arising as a fresh dominant mutation in a parental germinal cell.[123] The hereditary variety of retinoblastoma has an earlier age of onset and is much more likely to be bilateral than the non-hereditary occurrence.

Association between the germinal mutation and bilateral (and some unilateral occurrences of retinoblastoma does not imply that every retinal cell will undergo malignant transformation. The germinal mutation does contribute to heightened susceptibility of retinal cells to the malignant transformation,

because the retinal cells and all other cells are already affected with one of the two mutations necessary for the malignant transformation. Knudson's simple model hypothesized that a second mutational event must occur in an appropriate somatic cell before the cancer occurs. Non-hereditary cases also involve two separate mutations, both of which are postulated to occur in the same somatic cell. According to Knudson's theory, retinoblastoma results from two mutations, both in the hereditary and in the non-hereditary forms of the disease. In the hereditary form, the first mutation is germinal and the second one is somatic. The hypothesis is consistent with the excess of bilateral retinoblastomas observed in the hereditary category, since every retinal cell is affected with the first of the two hypothetically required mutations and is thereby more prone to being affected by the two mutations than a somatic cell lacking the germinally-transmitted mutation.

According to this hypothesis, non-hereditary (primary somatic) occurrences, showing predominance of unilateral disease, have acquired only the single tumor, due to the fact that the probability that two rare events would both occur by chance in two different cells in the same individuals is extremely small.

Knudson[121] has shown that certain individuals who inherit the first mutation (one to ten percent) do not develop any tumor, presumably due to non-occurrence of the somatic mutation and/or non-penetrance of the gene. Therefore, three possibilities exist in the hereditary form of this disease: 1) no tumor may occur; 2) unilateral disease may occur; 3) more than one tumor may occur.

Knudson subsequently extended his model to include Wilms' tumor,[122] neuroblastoma and pheochromocytoma,[123] conditions wherein the familial forms also are often bilateral and are diagnosed at an earlier age than non-familial occurrences.

Knudson's theory for somatic mutation and hereditary cancer gains additional support from certain characteristics which appear almost repeatedly in the natural history of genetic varieties of human cancer. These include the fact that the hereditary varieties more often occur at an earlier age, and are more likely to show bilateral involvement and/or an excess of multiple primary malignant neoplasms.[1,39-41]

Summary

These introductory statements cannot possibly reflect the full scope and breadth of this book. Rather, they are designed primarily to provide the reader with a frame of reference, background, and philosophy of cancer genetics. Coupled with a selective literature review, the reader may peruse more profitably any of these several aspects of cancer genetics.

Obviously, a complete coverage of the subject of cancer genetics could not possibly be accomplished in a single volume. Thus, an attempt has been made to select carefully a variety of subjects which reflect major activity in this rapidly moving discipline; hopefully, these issues will stimulate further inquiry into this perplexing and often baffling field.

REFERENCES

1. Lynch, H.T.: *Hereditary Factors in Carcinoma* in *Recent Results in Cancer Research*, New York, Springer-Verlag, 1967, pp. 186.
2. Broca, P.P.: *Traité des Tumeurs*, Paris, P. Asselin, 1866, Vol. 1, pp. 80.
3. Dobzhansky, T.: *Evolution, Genetics, and Man*. New York, 1955.
4. Osborne, R.H.: The "host factor" in disease: genetic and environmental interaction, *Ann NY Acad Sci 91*:602–607, 1961.
5. Naik, S.N., and Anderson, D.E.: The association between glucose-6-phosphate dehydrogenase deficiency and cancer in American Negroes, *Oncology, 25*:356–364, 1971.
6. Burnet, M.: *The Clonal Selection Theory of Acquired Immunity*. Nashville, Vanderbilt U P, 1959.
7. Lathrop, A.E.C., and Loeb, L.: The incidence of cancer in various strains of mice, *Proc Soc Exp Biol Med, 11*:34–38, 1913.
8. Green, E.L. (Ed): *Biology of the Laboratory Mouse*. 2nd ed. New York, Blakiston Division, McGraw, 1966.
9. Heston, W.E.: Genetic factors in the etiology of cancer. *Cancer Res, 25*:1320–1326, 1965.
10. Falconer, D.S.: *Introduction to Quantitative Genetics*. New York, Ronald, 1960.
11. Grüneberg, H.: Genetical studies of the skeleton of the mouse. IV. quasicontinuous variations. *J Genet, 51*:95–114, 1952.
12. Russell, E.S., and Fekete, E.: Analysis of w-series pleiotropism in the mouse: effect of W^vW^v substitution on definitive germ cells and on ovarian tumorigenesis. *J Nat Cancer Inst, 21*:365–381, 1958.
13. Eker, R., and Mossige, J.: A dominant gene for renal adenomas in the rat. *Nature* (Lond), *189*: 858–859, 1961.
14. Heston, W.E.: Effects of genes located on chromosomes III, V, VII, IX, and XIV on the occurrence of pulmonary tumors in the mouse, *Proc Int Genet Symp* Tokyo, Kyoto, 1956.
15. Lynch, C.J.: Lung tumors following intraperitoneal injection of 1:2:5:6-dibenzanthracene into young mice of three strains. *Proc Soc Exp Biol Med, 52*:368–371, 1943.
16. Tokuhata, G.K., and Lilienfeld, A.M.: Familial aggregation of lung cancer in humans. *J Natl Cancer Inst, 30*:289–312, 1963.
17. Andervont, H.B.: Fate of the C3H milk influence in mice of strains C and C57 black. *J Natl Cancer Inst, 5*:383–390, 1945.
18. Waters, N.F., and Burmester, B.R.: Mode of inheritance of resistance to rous sarcoma

virus in chickens. *J Natl Cancer Inst, 27:* 655–661, 1961.

19. Meier, H., and Huebner, R. J.: Host-gene control of C-Type tumor virus expression and tumorigenesis: relevance of studies in inbred mice to cancer in man and other species. *Proc Natl Acad Sci* U.S.A., *68:* 2664–2668, 1971.

20. Heston, W.E., and Dunn, T.B.: Tumor development in susceptible strain A and resistant strain L lung transplants in LA F$_1$ hosts. *J Natl Cancer Inst, 11:*1057–1071, 1951.

21. Shapiro, J.R., and Kirschbaum, A.: Intrinsic tissue response to induction of pulmonary tumors. *Cancer Res, 11:*644–647, 1951.

22. Evans, V.J., Parker, G.A., and Dunn, T.B.: Neoplastic transformations in C$_3$H mouse embryonic tissue *in vitro* determined by intraocular growth. I. Cells from chemically defined medium with and without serum supplement. *J Natl Cancer Inst., 32:* 89–121, 1964.

23. Lilienfeld, A.M.: Problems and areas in genetic-epidemiological field studies. *Ann NY Acad Sci, 91:*797–805, 1961.

24. David, P.R., and Snyder, L.H.: Genetics and Disease. *Proc Second Natl Cancer Conf, 2:*1128, 1952.

25. Robertson, M.A., Harington, J.S., and Bradshaw, E.: The cancer pattern in African gold miners. *Br J Cancer, 25:*395–402, 1971.

26. Robertson, M.A., Harrington, J.S., and Bradshaw, E.: The cancer pattern in Africans of the Transvaal Lowveld. *Br J Cancer, 25:*385–394, 1971.

27. Robertson, M.A., Harington, J.S., and Bradshaw, E.: The cancer pattern in Africans at Baragwanath Hospital, Johannesburg. *Br J Cancer, 25:*377–384, 1971.

28. Li, F.P., and Fraumeni, J.F.: Testicular cancers in children: epidemiologic characteristics. *J Natl Cancer Inst, 48:*1575–1581, 1972.

29. Miller, R.W.: Neoplasia and Down's Syndrome. *Ann NY Acad Sci, 171:*637–644, 1970.

30. Penrose, L.S., and Smith, G.F.: *Down's Anomaly*. Boston, Little, 1966, p. 31.

31. Campbell, H.E.: Incidence of malignant growth of the undescended testicle: a critical and statistical study. *Arch Surg, 44:*353–369, 1942.

32. Hausfeld, K.F., and Schrandt, D.: Malignancy of testis following atrophy: report of three cases. *J Urol, 94:*69–72, 1965.

33. Koch, F.: The occurrence of sex chromatin in testicular tumours. *Acta Pathol Microbiol Scand (A) [Suppl], 212:*45–49, 1970.

34. Volpe, R., Knowlton, T.G., Foster, A.D., and Conen, P.E.: Testicular feminization: a study of two cases, one with a seminoma. *Can Med Assoc J, 98:*438–445, 1968.

35. Dodge, O.G., Jackson, A.W., and Muldal, S.: Breast cancer and interstitial-cell tumor in a patient with Klinefelter's Syndrome, *Cancer, 24:*1027–1032, 1969.

36. Andervont, H.B., Shimkin, M.B., and Canter, H.Y.: Susceptibility of seven inbred strains and the F$_1$ hybrids to estrogen-induced testicular tumors and occurrence of spontaneous testicular tumors in strain BALB/c mice. *J Natl Cancer Inst, 25:*1069–1081, 1960.

37. Herbst, A.L., Ulfelder, H., and Poskanzer, D.C.: Adenocarcinoma of the vagina. *New Engl J Med, 284:*878–881, 1971.

38. Cleaver, J.E.: Defective repair replication of DNA in xeroderma pigmentosum. *Nature, 218:*652–656, 1968.

39. Lynch, H.T.: *Skin, Heredity, and Malignant Neoplasms*, New York, Med Exam, 1972, pp. 299.

40. Lynch, H.T., and Krush, A.J.: Cancer genetics. *South Med J, 64:*26–40, 1971.

41. Lynch, H.T., Anderson, D.E., Krush, A.J., and Larsen, A.L.: Heredity and carcinoma. *Ann NY Acad Sci, 155:*793–800, 1968.

42. Sandberg, A.A., and Sakurai, M.: The role of chromosomal studies in cancer epidemiology. In Lynch, Henry T. (Ed.): *Cancer Genetics*. Springfield, Thomas. To be published.

43. Sandberg, A.A., and Hossfeld, D.K.: Chromosomal abnormalities in human neoplasia. *Annu Rev Med, 21:*279–408, 1970.

44. Sandberg, A.A.: The chromosomes and causation of human cancer and leukemia. *Cancer Res, 26:*2064–2081, 1966.

45. Koller, P.C.: *The Role of Chromosomes in Cancer Biology,* New York, Springer-Verlag, 1972.

46. DeMars, R., and Nance, W.E.: Electrophoretic Variants of Glucose-6-Phosphate Dehydrogenase and the Single-Active-X in Cultivated Human Cells, *Retention of Functional Differentiation in Cultured Cells.* The Wistar Institute Monograph No. 1, Philadelphia, The Wistar Institute Press, 1964, pp. 35–48.

47. Linder, D., and Gartler, S.M.: Glucose-6-Phosphate dehydrogenase mosaicism: utilization as a cell marker in the study of leiomyomas. *Science, 150:*67–69, 1965.

48. Gartler, A.M., Ziprkowski, L., Krakowski, A., Ezra, R., Szeinberg, A., and Adam, A.: Glucose-6-Phosphate dehydrogenase mosaicism as a tracer in the study of hereditary multiple trichoepithelioma. *Am J Hum Genet, 18:*282–287, 1966.

49. Fialkow, P.J.: Genetic marker studies in neoplasia. In *Genetic Concepts and Neoplasia: A Collection of Papers Presented at the 23rd Annual Symposium on Fundamental Cancer Research.* Baltimore, Williams and Wilkins, 1970, pp. 112–137.

50. Li, F.P., and Fraumeni, J.F.: Soft-tissue sarcomas, breast cancer, and other neoplasms: a familial syndrome? *Ann Intern Med, 71:*747–752, 1969.

51. Stewart, A., and Barber, R.: The epidemiological importance of childhood cancers. *Br Med Bull, 27:*64–70, 1971.

52. Stewart, A., Webb, J., and Hewitt, D.: A survey of childhood malignancies. *Br Med J 1:*1495–1508, 1958.

53. Araki, C., and Matsumoto, S.: Statistical re-evaluation of pinealoma and related tumors in Japan. *J Neurosurg, 30:*146–149, 1969.

54. Davies, J.M.P., and Miller, R.W.: Childhood cancer, U.I.C.C., *Cancer Bull, 8:*1–3, 1970.

55. Chatten, J., and Voorhess, M.L.: Familial neuroblastoma: report of a kindred with multiple disorders, including neuroblastomas in four siblings. *New Engl J Med, 277:*1230–1236, 1967.

56. Miller, R.W., Fraumeni, J.F., and Manning, M.D.: Association of Wilms' tumor with aniridia, hemihypertrophy, and other congenital malformations. *New Engl J Med, 270:*922–927, 1964.

57. Lynch, H.T., and Green, G.S.: Wilms' Tumor and congenital heart disease: report of a case and family. *Am J Dis Child, 115:*723–727, 1968.

58. Reisman, M., Goldenberg, E.D., and Gordon, J.: Congenital heart disease and neuroblastoma: case report and brief comment, *Am J Dis Child, 111:*308–310, 1966.

59. Hill, S.: Personal Communication, 1970.

60. Swift, M.: Fanconi's anaemia in the genetics of neoplasia. *Nature, 230:*370–373, 1971.

61. Aaronson, S.A., and Lytle, C.D.: Decreased host cell reactivation of irradiated SV_{40} virus in xeroderma pigmentosum. *Nature, 228:*359–361, 1970.

62. Koprowski, H., Ponten, J.A., Jensen, F., Ravdin, R.G., Moorhead, P., and Saksela, E.: Transformation of cultures of human tissue infected with Simian Virus SV_{40}. *J Cell Comp Physiol, 59:*281–292, 1962.

63. Todaro, G.J., and Martin, G.M.: Increased susceptibility of Down's syndrome fibroblasts to transformation by SV_{40}. *Proc Soc Exp Biol Med, 124:*1232–1236, 1967.

64. Young, D.: The susceptibility to SV_{40} virus transformation of fibroblasts obtained from patients with Down's Syndrome. *Eur J Cancer, 7:*337–339, 1971.

65. Todaro, G.J., Green, H., and Swift, M.R.: Susceptibility of human diploid fibroblast strains to transformation by SV_{40} Virus. *Science, 153:*1252–1254, 1966.

66. Young, D.: SV_{40} transformation of cells from patients with Fanconi's Anaemia, *Lancet, 1:*294–295, 1971.

67. Mukerjee, D., Bowen, J., and Anderson, D.E.: Simian Papovavirus 40 transformation of cells from cancer patient with XY/XXY Mosaic Klinefelter's Syndrome. *Cancer Res, 30:*1769–1772, 1970.

68. Mukerjee, D., Bowen, J.M., Trujillo, J.M., and Cork, A.: Increased susceptibility of cells from cancer patients with XY-Gonadal Dysgenesis to Simian Papovavirus 40 Transformation. *Cancer Res, 32:*1518–

69. Todaro, G.J.: Variable susceptibility of human cell strains to SV_{40} Transforma-

tion. *Natl Cancer Inst Monogr, 29*:271–275, 1968.

70. Mukerjee, D., and Burdette, W.J.: Transformation of fibroblasts from patients with colonic cancer by oncogenic virus *in vitro*. In *Carcinoa of the Colon and Antecedent Epithelium*. Springfield, Thomas, 1970, pp. 314–318.

71. Snyder, A.L., Henderson, E.S., Li, F.P., and Todaro, G.J.: Possible inherited leukaemogenic factors in familial acute myelogenous leukaemia. *Lancet, 1*:586–589, 1970.

72. Huebner, R.J., and Todaro, G.J.: Oncogenes of RNA tumor viruses as determinants of cancer. *Proc Natl Acad Sci U.S.A., 64*: 1087–1094, 1969.

73. Mintz, B.: Neoplasia and gene activity in allophenic mice. In *Genetic Concepts and Neoplasia: A Collection of Papers Presented at the 23rd Annual Symposium on Fundamental Cancer Research*. Baltimore, Williams and Wilkins, 1970, pp. 477–517.

74. Buchanan, J.A., and Higley, E.T.: The relationship of blood-groups to disease. *Br J Exp Pathol, 1-2*:247–255, 1921–1922.

75. Alexander, W.: An inquiry into the distribution of the blood groups in patients suffering from malignant disease. *Br J Exp Pathol, 2*:66–69, 1921–1922.

76. Johannsen, E.W.: Blood grouping of cancer subjects. *Soc Biol* (Paris), *92*:112–115, 1925.

77. Aird, I., Bentall, H.H., and Roberts, F.J.A.: A relationship between cancer of stomach and the ABO blood groups. *Br Med J, 1*:799–801, 1953.

78. Buckwalter, J.A., Wohlwend, C.B., Colter, D.C., Tidrick, R.T., and Knowler, L.A.: The association of the ABO blood groups to gastric carcinoma. *Surg Gynecol Obstet, 104*:176–179, 1957.

79. Clarke, C.A.: Correlations of ABO groups with peptic ulcer, cancer, and other diseases. *J Med Educ, 34*:400–404, 1959.

80. Roberts, J.A.F.: Some associations between blood groups and disease. *Br Med Bull, 15*:129–133, 1959.

81. Osborne, R.H., and DeGeorge, F.V.: The ABO blood groups in neoplastic disease of the ovary. *Am J Hum Genet, 15*:380–388, 1963.

82. Cameron, J.M.: Blood groups in tumours of salivary tissue. *Lancet, 1*:239–240, 1958.

83. Osborne, R.H., and DeGeorge, F.V.: The ABO blood groups in parotid and submaxillary gland tumors. *Am J Hum Genet, 14*:199–209, 1962.

84. Fadhli, H.A., and Dominquiz, R.: ABO blood groups and multiple cancers. *JAMA, 185*:757–759, 1963.

85. el-Hefnawi, H., Smith, S.M., and Penrose, L.S.: Xeroderma Pigmentosum—its inheritance and relationship to the ABO blood group system. *Ann Hum Genet, 28*: 273–290, London, 1965.

86. Marcus, D.M.: The ABO and lewis blood-group system. *New Engl J Med, 280*:994–1006, 1969.

87. Clarke, C.A., Edwards, J.W., Haddock, D.R.W., Howel-Evans, A.W., McConnell, R.B., and Sheppard, P.M.: ABO blood groups and secretor character in duodenal ulcer; population and sibship studies. *Br Med J 2*:725–731, 1956.

88. Horwich, L., Evans, D.A.P., McConnell, R.B., and Donohoe, W.T.A.: ABO blood groups in gastric bleeding. *Gut, 7*:680–685, 1966.

89. Langman, M.J.S., Doll, R., and Saracci, R.: ABO blood group and secretor status in stomal ulcer. *Gut, 8*:128–132, 1967.

90. Milunicovà, A., Jandovà, A., Laurovà, L., and Skoda, V.: Hereditary blood and serum types, PTC test and level of the fifth fraction of serum lactatedehydrogenase in females with gynecological cancer (II Communication). *Neoplasma*, (Bratisl.) *16*:311–316, 1969.

91. Aird, I., Lee, D.R., and Roberts, J.A.F.: ABO blood groups and cancer of oesophagus, cancer of pancreas, and pituitary adenoma. *Br Med J 1*:1163–1166, 1960.

92. Bourke, J.B., and Griffin, J.P.: Blood-groups in benign and malignant prostatic hypertrophy. *Lancet, 2*:1279–1280, 1962.

93. Schmauss, A.K., Perlin, L., and Küpferling, E.: Distribution of ABO blood groups among patients who have gall stones and

carcinoma of the gall bladder. *Dtsch Z Verdau Stoffwechselkr, 28:*317–321, 1968.

94. Hartmann, O., and Stavem, P.: ABO bloodgroups and cancer. *Lancet, 1:*1305–1306, 1964.

95. Pearce, K.M., and Yates, P.O.: Blood groups and brain tumours. *J Neurol Sci, 2:*434–441, 1965.

96. Clifford, P.: Blood groups and nasopharyngeal carcinoma. *Lancet, 2:*48–49, 1970.

97. Buckwalter, J.A., Wohlwend, E.B., Colter, D.C., Tidrick, R.T., and Knowler, L.A.: ABO blood groups and disease. *JAMA, 162:*1210–1215, 1956.

98. Aird, I., Bentall, H.H., Mehigan, J.A., and Roberts, J.A.F.: The blood groups in relation to peptic ulcertaion and carcinoma of colon, rectum, breast, and bronchus. *Br Med J, 2:*315–321, 1954.

99. McConnell, R.B., Clarke, C.A., and Downton, F.: Blood groups in carcinoma of the lung. *Br Med J, 2:*323–325, 1954.

100. Beasley, W.H.: The ABO blood groups of carcinoma of the oesophagus and of benigh prostatic hyperplasia. *J Clin Pathol, 17:*42–44, 1964.

101. Bruchmuller, W., and Eggemann, G.: Kehlkopfkrebs und Blutgruppen. *Z Laryngol Otol, 47:*958–962, 1968.

102. Sankalé, M., Divetain, C., Vessereau, M., and Diop, B.: Distribution of blood groups in 120 African patients with primary cancer of the liver. *Pathol Biol* (Paris), *16:*1071–1073, 1968.

103. Janus, Z.L., Bailar, J.C., III, and Eisenberg, H.: Blood group and uterine cancer. *Am J Epidemiol, 86:*569–578, 1967.

104. Lee, Y.N.: The ABO blood groups and cancer. *Surg Gynecol Obsete, 132:*1093–1097, 1971.

105. Blumberg, B.S., Alter, H.J., and Visnich, S.: A "new" antigen in leukemia sera. *JAMA, 191:*541–546, 1965.

106. Blumberg, B.S., Sutnick, A.I., and London, W.T.: Hepatitis and leukemia: their relation to Australia antigen. *Bull NY Acad Med, 44:*1566–1586, 1968.

107. Blumberg, B.S., *et al.:* A serum antigen (Australian Antigen) in Down's Syndrome, leukemia, and hepatitis. *Ann Intern Med, 66:*924–931, 1967.

108. Blumberg, B.S., Sutnick, A.I., and London, W.T.: Australia antigen and hepatitis. *JAMA, 207:*1895–1896, 1969.

109. Ohbayashi, A., Matumi, M., and Okochi, K.: Australia antigen in familial cirrhosis. *Lancet, 1:*244, 1971.

110. Denison, E.K., Peters, R.L., and Reynolds, T.B.: Familial hepatoma with hepatitisassociated antigen. *Ann Intern Med, 74:*391–394, 1971.

111. Bancroft, W.H., Warkel, R.L., and Talbert, A.A., *et al.:* Family with hepatitis-associated antigen. *JAMA, 217:*1817–1820, 1971.

112. Ohbayashi, A., Okochi, K., and Mayumi, M.: Familial clustering of asymptomatic carriers of Australia antigen and patients with chronic liver disease or primary liver Cancer. *Gastroenterology, 62:*618–625, 1972.

113. Lawler, S.D., Klouda, P.T., and Begshawe, K.D.: The HL-A system in trophoblastic neoplasia. *Lancet, 2:*834–837, 1971.

114. McDevitt, H.O., and Bodmer, W.F.: Histocompatibility antigens, immune responsiveness and susceptibility to disease. *Am J Med, 52:*1–8, 1972.

115. Lilly, F.: The Histocompatibility-2 Locus and susceptibility to tumor induction. *Natl Cancer Inst Monogr, 22:*631–641, 1966.

116. Rudolph, R.H., and Thomas, E.D.: HL-A antigens and choriocarcinoma. *Lancet, 2:*408–409, 1971.

117. Falk, J., and Osoba, D.: HL-A antigens and survival in Hodgkins Disease, *Lancet, 2:*1118–1120, 1971.

118. Dick, F.R., Fortuny, I., Theologides, A., Greally, J., Wood, N., and Yunis, E.J.: HL-A and lymphoid tumors. *Cancer Res, 32:*2608–2611, 1972.

119. Walford, R.L., Finkelstein, S., Neerhout, R., Konrad, P., and Shanbrom, E.: Acute childhood leukaemia in relation to the HL-A human transplantation genes. *Nature, 225:*461–462, 1970.

120. Tyzzer, E.E.: Tumor Immunity. *J Cancer Res, 1:*125–156, 1916.

121. Knudson, A.G.: Mutation and Cancer: Statistical study of retinoblastoma, *Proc Nat Acad Sci USA, 68:*820–823, 1971.

122. Knudson, A.G., and Strong, L.C.: Mutation and Cancer: A model for Wilms' tumor of the kidney. *J Natl Cancer Inst, 48*:313–324, 1972.

123. Knudson, A.G. Jr., and Strong, L.C.: Mutation and Cancer: Neuroblastoma and pheochromocytoma, *Am J Hum Genet, 24*:514–532, 1972.

CHAPTER 2

FUNDAMENTALS OF

HUMAN GENETICS

Arnold R. Kaplan

Introduction

INDIVIDUAL DIFFERENCES in predisposition to acquire a particular disorder in any specific environment are the consequences of individual constitutional differences effected by interacting genetic and nongenetic factors. The etiology of a pathological condition may be evaluated in terms of the interactions of genetically-transmitted diatheses and exposures to precipitating factors. A particular property in an organism derives from series of complex biochemical reactions and biochemically-determined developmental processes. Interference with these at any of many different levels may affect the final end product. The complexity of metabolic activities within each cell is such that vast numbers of genes influence almost any activity. A particular gene or group of genes determines an indefinite but limited assortment of effects, the different effects being associated with differences in environment and/or with differences in other aspects of the total genetic make-up or genotype. Thus, one's genetic material, derived from one's parents, is a set of potentialities and not a set of already-formed or predetermined characteristics.

Controversy over the relevance of genetic differences to disease etiology may be instigated by concern for the patients' prognoses and therapies. The involvement of gene-transmitted constitutional differences in different diatheses does not necessarily imply a poor prognosis or negate therapy. The occurrence of even a primary relevance of genetic differences regarding different pre-dispositions to a disease category does not mean that the disease is any less amenable to therapy than it would be if all the principle etiological variables for the same disease were environmental.

A disorder or disease is an effect of, and may be affected by, genetic and/or environmental alterations. Theoretically, no disorder or disease is necessarily unpreventable or incurable; but the environmental/therapeutic changes which must be introduced in order to affect prevention, control, or cure, may be unknown. Identification of the gene-transmitted differences which are relevant to a disease's etiology may facilitate that disease's prevention or amelioration by purely environmental methods. The more it becomes possible to precisely characterize an individual's genotype, and the potential range of phenotypic, i.e. trait, variation resulting from interactions of that genotype with different environmental variables, the more likely are we to learn how to select and modify environments according to the different individuals' needs. Identification of genotypes which manifest particular diatheses in particular environmental milieux provides a basic step in the direction of effective prevention and control. Determination of the environmental differences between the genetically-predisposed individuals who develop the disease and those who do not will characterize the environmental modifications necessary to prevent and control the disease. Determination of the constitutional differences associated with the specific genes related to different diatheses for a disease will contribute to knowledge of the disease's etiology and the therapeutic modifications necessary to prevent and control that disease.

Phenotypes, Genotypes, Phenocopies, and Genocopies

The term phenotype refers to an individual's observable properties, physiological and pathological, structural and functional, which are effects of the interactions between his genotype and his environment. The sum total of an individual's genetic material, the total genetic constitution, is his genotype. The characteristics of an individual's development and growth, from conception to birth to maturity to death, are effects of the interactions of his genotype with his environment.

A trait or disorder which is usually associated with a particular gene or group of genes may, in response to particular environmental variables, be manifested without that gene or group of genes. Nonhereditary phenotypic modifications, which are caused by special environmental conditions, and which mimic similar phenotypes characteristically associated with particular genes, have been termed phenocopies. Specific effects of genic action can be imitated by certain environmental influences, interacting with genotypes which norms of reaction or phenotypic flexibilities include the potentials for such manifestations, even though the genotypes do not include the particular gene(s) which is/are characteristically associated with these effects. Series of grades of phenocopies may occur, to resemble effects characteristically associated with various combinations of multiple genes. A trait or disorder which is characteristically associated with a particular gene or group of genes may also occur in the absence of such gene(s), effected by other, i.e. different, genes. The effects of such *mimetic genes* have been termed genocopies.

Certain phenocopies are only inducible when a particular environmental influence is applied during a specific, or within a limited, period of development. That is, for some effects, there is a limited sensitive or critical period during which the effects may be determined. This suggests that, during such critical stages in development, there exist alternative paths which lead to different effects, and the path which is to be followed may be determined by genetic and/or environmental factors. The existence of a particularly sensitive period in development, during which a specific disorder is most easily initiated, means that induction of a phenocopy may depend upon the stage of development during which the environmental influence occurs, as well as upon the interacting genotype, i.e. the potential responsiveness or norm of reaction of that genotype, and the nature and intensity and duration of the environmental influence. Only a part of the population segment consisting of individuals who are genetically predisposed to a particular pathology actually do develop that pathology.

Many criteria have been studied for indications of the significance of genetic factors in etiologies of various pathologies, including elevated morbidity risks in relatives of index cases compared with the general population, increasing morbidity risks associated with increasing degrees of genetic kinship to index cases, greater concordance in monozygotic than in dizygotic pairs of twins, and variation in frequencies of the disorders in different populations. These observations, alone, are not rigorous and conclusive evidence of genetic etiology. Environmental factors common to relatives can simulate genetic determinants. It is not possible to conclusively prove that a trait is genetic except by showing that it could be due to one of several modes of inheritance. The genetic method consists in attempting to extract, from a possibly heterogeneous trait. One or more genetic entities due, in increasing order of refinement, to a single inheritance pattern, locus, or allele. Sometimes genetic traits depend on the presence of several genes, i.e. complementary epistasis. If the effect of each gene is recognizable, each component may be studied separately. Otherwise, the analysis may be beyond the limits of available methods in human genetics. The only unequivocally reliable approach to a nonexperimental system is to defer final determination of mode of inheritance until the relevant genes are individually recognizable. Traits determined by many genes, not individually recognizable, are unfavorable for genetic analysis.

The occurrence of multiple etiologies and associated multiple morbidity risks may be masked by a diagnostic system which is based upon the clinical symptoms or effects of a disease rather than its etiology. Thus, multiple morbidity risks involving clinically heterogeneous populations may be combined to indicate a composite morbidity risk figure which is invalid and misleading.[1]

Relatives of index cases can grossly be divided into categories according to their memberships in high-risk versus low-risk families, if such a division of particular data can be statistically supported by segregation analysis.[2] Such a dichotomy could be based, for example, upon familial versus nonfamilial or sporadic index cases, or upon concordant versus discordant pairs of monozygotic twins. Even if the disorders in most or many of the affected individuals were associated with simple modes of genetic transmission, some cases could be sporadic due to occurrence of phenocopies, genocopies, diagnostic errors, *etc*. The assumption of the occurrence of sporadic cases may lead to recognition of heterogeneity in data previously regarded as homogeneous, and may even show that the risk in some high-risk families is great enough to suggest a simple genetic hypothesis.[3] Genetic ratios within sibships may

be utilized to test for Mendelian modes of genetic transmission, based upon observations of individuals in only a single generation. Pedigree analysis, however, which utilizes available data regarding individuals in various generations of the family tree, is far more informative and is the principal method of genetic study in man.

Pedigree Analysis

Essentially, pedigree analysis involves utilization of basic Mendelian principles for extrapolation of genotypes from information on phenotypes and genetic relationships.

The term, family, is usually applied to a pair of parents and their children. The term may also be used to refer to a more extensive association of relatives, although a larger group of individuals who are related to each other genetically and through marriage is usually called a kindred. Females are usually symbolized by circles, and males by squares; but sometimes other symbols are used, e.g. the symbol for Mars to indicate a male, the one for Venus to indicate a female (See Fig. 1).

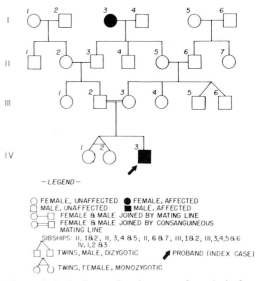

Figure 2–1. Pedigree showing use of symbols for communication of relationships within a kindred.

The symbols of a pair of parents are joined by a horizontal mating line, and their off-springs' symbols are located in a horizontal row below that line. Double horizontal mating lines indicate a consanguinous combination. The offsprings' symbols are connected by vertical lines to a horizontal line above them, which is connected further above by a single vertical line to the horizontal mating line. The children of a parental pair form a *sibship;* and the children in a sibship, regardless of sex, are *siblings* or *sibs* of each other. Possession of the trait being examined in the pedigree is designated by shading the symbol, e.g. circle or square, of the individual involved, and an unshaded symbol denotes absence of the character or disease. Twins are designated by lines extending from the two symbols involved to a common point on the horizontal sibship line. The affected individual with whom a particular pedigree study was initiated may be identified as the index case or proband or propositus. Generations are customarily identified with Roman numerals, ranging from the earliest at the top of a pedigree schematic to the most recent at the bottom. Within each generation, the individuals are numbered from left to right with Arabic numerals. Thus, each individual in a particular pedigree may be identified by the combination of a Roman number and an Arabic number.

Pedigree patterns characteristically provide information on the Mendelian principles of segregation and independent assortment, and they may also provide information on allelism and linkage.[10] A specific pedigree pattern depends upon whether effects of the gene involved are manifested in single dosage or only in double dosage, and upon whether the gene is located on one of the autosomes or on a sex chromosome. An individual who possesses an identical pair of genes on a particular locus of a pair of homologous chromosomes is homozygous for the locus; and an individual whose pair of genes on a particular locus are different from each other is heterozygous for the locus. In a heterozygous individual, if one of the pair of genes is recognizably manifested while the other one is suppressed, the former gene is termed dominant and the latter one is recessive. Genetic dominance is a manifestation of a gene's ability to be expressed in the phenotype of a genetically heterozygous individual. The failure of a gene to be expressed in the phenotype, when it occurs in a genetically heterozygous genotype, is genetic recessivity. A recessive gene may be carried and transmitted through innumerable generations without being manifested. A dominant gene, however, is characteristically manifested in the phenotypes of the individuals who possess either one (i.e. in the heterozygous individual) or a pair (i.e. in the homozygous individual) of them.

The manifestation of a trait transmitted by a single autosomal dominant gene with complete penetrance is indicated in a pedigree in which the trait does not skip generations. An individual with the trait has a parent with the trait, and approximately one-half the offspring of couples in which one of the parents is affected are similarly affected. A trait which is transmitted by a pair of autosomal recessive alleles, by contrast, may occur without any previous family history of the trait in either the maternal or the paternal side. Children born subsequent to an index case, establishing both parents as heterozygous carriers of the recessive gene for the trait, will include approximately one-fourth affected; and approximately two thirds of the unaffected siblings will be heterozygous *carriers* of the recessive gene. In the case of a very rare trait (in the population) transmitted by a pair of autosomal recessive alleles, consanguinity may be expected to occur more frequently in affected families than in the general population.

Genes which are located on the X chromosome, like those on autosomes, may be dominant or recessive. A female, with two X chromosomes, may be either homozygous or heterozygous for a particular locus on the X chromosome. A male, with only one X chromosome, is *hemizygous* for any X-linked gene. Such a gene may be dominant or recessive in the female. In the hemizygous male, with no other gene at the locus, an X-linked gene is always expressed. X-linked genetic transmission is characterized by the absence of male-to-male transmission, because a son necessarily inherits a Y chromosome from his (XY) father and an X chromosome from his (XX) mother. The X chromosome of a male is characteristically transmitted to none of his sons but to all of his daughters.

One's sex may affect the expression of a gene, and a trait transmitted by a gene which is manifested differently in the two sexes is sex-influenced. That is, a sex-influenced trait is one in which phenotypic manifestations are different in the two sexes. If the gene is completely suppressed in one of the two sexes, then it is sex-limited. A sex-influenced or sex-limited gene (i.e. regarding its manifestation in the phenotype) may occur on an autosome or on an X chromosome.

Genetic *linkage* involves the occurrence of different genetic loci on the same chromosome. If two loci occur on separate non-homologous, i.e. not pairing at meiosis, chromosomes, then independent assortment occurs. If two loci occur on the same chromosome, and particularly if they occur relatively close to each other, then the genes occurring on the two loci would usually tend to be transmitted in the same combination, i.e without independent assortment, from generation to generation. Close genetic linkage of different loci may be difficult to distinguish from allelism, *i.e.* occurrence of alternate gene forms at a single locus on a particular chromosome. The term, X-linked, refers to the location of a gene on the X chromosome. A gene whose locus occurs on the Y chromosome is termed Y-linked or holandric. Such a gene would characteristically affect only males, and would be transmitted only from father to sons.

Penetrance, Expressivity, and Heritability

A trait or disorder may be regarded as the dependent variable which has resulted from interactions of independent variables, i.e. environmental factors and the organism with its intervening variables (e.g. morphological and biochemical characteristics). The intervening variables do not remain constant, but are themselves modified by the independent variables which affect the organism. The penetrance of a gene or group of genes and the nature of its/their expressivity, observed as phenotypic manifestations, differ in different milieux, environmental and/or genetic. Thus, there are differences in penetrance of the gene(s) associated with predisposition to a disease, which are associated with different environmental milieux and different genetic milieux (i.e. the complete genotypes). When the gene(s) is/are penetrant, these differences affect variability in expressivity. Complete penetrance is shown by a genotype which is always associated with a particular phenotype. Even when a genotype associated with predisposition to a particular pathology is penetrant, there may be clinical differences between different affected individuals. Thus, even when penetrant, a genotype may show variable expressivity. Environmental as well as ancillary genetic variables interpose numerous influences between primary gene products and the final mechanisms by which genetic manifestations are actuated. Environmental variables may affect reductions in correlations between genotypes and observable phenotypic effects, causing variable expressivity and/or incomplete penetrance.

Heritability determinations are estimates of the proportion of the total phenotypic variance, i.e. individual differences, shown by a trait, that can be attributed to genetic variation in some particular population at a single generation under one set of conditions. The heritability of a particular pathology may be defined as the extent to which the variation in individual risk of acquiring the pathology is due to genetic differences. A trait will show a greater-than-zero heritability if two or more segregating alleles, which manifest different effects upon the trait, occur on at least one genetic locus. A relevant genetic locus, which is associated with phenotypic variation in one population because it is represented there by two or more different segregating alleles, might show no variation in another population because the same locus involves only a single allele, i.e. identical genes on homologous loci in that other population. One environment may activate a particular gene, while another may not. Thus, a trait may show a particular greater-than-zero heritability in one allele-segregating population, but other heritabilities in other populations which involve population-genetic differences and/or environmental differences. The different heritabilities shown for a particular trait in different populations do not indicate that any particular gene manifests different degrees of heredity in the different populations involved. The ontogeny of an individual's phenotype, i.e. observable outcome of development, has a norm or range of reaction which is not predictable in advance. Even in the most favorable investigations, only an approximate estimate can be obtained for the norm of reaction, when, as in plants and some animals, an individual genotype can be replicated many times and its development studied over a range of environmental conditions. The more varied the conditions, the more diverse might be the phenotypes developed from any one genotype. Different genotypes do not have the same norm of reaction. Therefore, the limits set by a particular gene or group of genes cannot be entirely specified. These limits are plastic within each individual but differ between individuals.

Extreme environmentalists have been wrong to hope that one law or set of laws might describe universal features of modifiability, and extreme hereditarians have been wrong to ignore the norm of reaction.[4] In its strictest sense, a heritability measure provides an estimate of the proportion of the variance in a trait, i.e. phenotype, expression and which is correlated with segregation of independently-acting alleles of a relevant genetic locus or of relevant genetic loci. Heritability is a property of a specific population and not of a trait (i.e. in all populations or in all milieux). In any particular population, heritability coefficients are based on observed correlations among individuals with different degrees of genetic kinship. Many published twin, family, twin-family, and extended-pedigree studies of disease incidence have essentially been studies of heritability, because they have not indicated a clearly-defined mode of heredity, i.e. a specific mode of genetic transmission. Heritabilities may vary between different groups because of different environmental contexts, as well as because of numerous secondary genetic (in addition to the genetic factors predominantly associated with the liability to the pathology) differences.

Thus, the findings from different studies of heritability, for any category of disorder which does not involve a clear and simple mode of genetic transmission with complete penetrance, may be expected to vary from each other. The demonstration of significant heritability for a pathology, in one particular group, indicates the major relevance of genetic differences for different predispositions to the pathology. The demonstration of lower heritability for the same pathology, in another group, may indicate that the effects of these genetic factors, i.e. within the genetically-defined norm or range of reaction, may be profoundly modulated by other genetic factors and/or by nongenetic influences.[5] Different combinations of different genetic and nongenetic factors may manifest similar phenotypes. The same genetic or nongenetic factor affecting different individuals, who differ with regard to other genetic factors and/or environmental influences, may show different manifestations. Thus, different genes may be associated with the same phenotype, and different phenotypes may be associated with the same gene(s), depending upon the total interacting genetic and environmental contexts. If the incidence of a particular pathology varies from one population to another, and the difference is not due solely to diagnostic inconsistencies, the variance can be ascribed to differences of mean liability, or to differences of variance of liability, or to combinations of both.[6] If there is a difference between two populations in the pathology's heritability, then two or more (rather than only one) predisposing genotypes are involved, and/or the lower heritability is associated with environmental circumstances which increase the nongenetic differences of the liability.

The relative contributions of heredity and environment for a trait may differ with different overall heredities, i.e. total genotypes, and with different environments. The reaction-norm concept is of fundamental importance to an understanding of gene action. Modification of a gene's environment, either by nongenetic environmental influences or through the effects of other genes, may affect the expression of any specific gene within the limits characteristic of that gene's phenotypic potential.

Statistics in Genetics

Inference or reasoning is a mode of thinking by which one starts from something known and proceeds to form a belief that there exists a fact hitherto unknown. The basic assumption is that one's methods of reasoning are reliable and lead to conclusions which correspond with facts. Many of the reasoned conclusions can then be checked and verified by perceptions of objective investigations. Every perception is received by a mind already made up of memories, interests, expectations, and bias. Therefore, the resultant new state of consciousness is derived in part from the observations and in part from what is in the mind already. Even at the times of observations, there are natural tendencies to confuse one's preconceptions with what is actually perceived. The most useful hypotheses are those which are testable, and testability is associated with simplicity and directness. As hypotheses increase in their complexity, and as they involve secondary hypotheses, their testabilities diminish.

The contributions of additional hypotheses which cannot be subjected to conclusive tests, which cannot be proved or disproved, provide little more than exercises for their contributors. The many relevant variables cannot always be entirely controlled, and some of them may not even be recognized. One may measure the overall variation, which is due to all the uncontrolled variables, as well as the differences relatable to the factors one is evaluating. Then, by comparing the two, one may judge whether the latter are statistically significant to provide confidence that they are not just the misleading expression of some uncontrolled or even unrecognized source of variation.[7] Scientific conclusions necessarily emerge as statements of probability. There is always the risk that particular results do not facilitate a sound or unbiased basis for a general statement, as reflected in the statement of probability which the analysis yields. The conclusions drawn from any study or combination of studies are not immutable or certain but, as the body of observational experience grows, the level of uncertainty is decreased.

Statistical Significance

A deviation from the expected ratio, in the observed ratio of unaffected and affected individuals, may be due to chance or to some relevant variable. The meaning of the statistical significance of a deviation can be calculated in terms of statistical probability that it may occur due only to chance. Statistical probability, the mathematical evaluation of chance, may be defined as the ratio of the number of occurrences of a specified combination of events to the total number of all possible combinations of the events. The term, statistical significance, relates to whether or not some specific reason or reasons, and not only chance, underlies the observed deviation. The probability level which is regarded as significant is somewhat arbitrary and depends upon the judgment of the investigator involved. If the probability that a deviation may occur between two populations, or between the observed and expected findings, is lower than one percent, then the findings would generally be regarded as statistically significant. A probability level above 1 percent but below 5 percent is sometimes considered significant, but more conservative investigators tend to consider such a figure as only of doubtful or questionable significance. The choice of which statistical test might most appropriately be utilized for any particular evaluation depends upon many factors, including the sizes of the samples involved, the parametric or nonparametric character of the data distributions, etc.[8,9]

One of the simplest and most commonly used tests in genetics is the *chi-square test*: the value of chi-square equals the sum of the squares of the absolute differences between the observed and expected categories divided by the respective expected values being compared; and the probability value may be determined from a corresponding chi-square value listed in standard tables.[10] The happenings of nature involve probability laws rather than predetermined causality. A scientific investigator only determines his best posits from the available information.[11] The addition of more specifically relevant information facilitates more accurate judgments. A genetic factor may be manifested only by appropriate genotype-environment combinations. The determination of whether a gene is harmful or useful or indifferent is related to the bearer's environment. The genetic epidemiologist functions as a kind of ecologist seeking significant correlations between a disorder and one or another variable from the great array of environmental influences. His success in these efforts will be related to the uniqueness of the variable involved and the directness of its effect, to the frequency of the basic defect, and to the ease of detection of the disorder under consideration.

The Hardy-Weinberg Principle

Hardy[12] and Weinberg[13] independently developed the principle that genotypic frequencies within a population in any generation depend solely upon the frequencies in the previous generation, if none of the genotypes was affected by selective factors and if the population was random-mating. The fundamental idea of gene distribution in populations, based on the assumption of random mating and no differential selection and no significant contribution from new mutations, is a deduction from the Mendelian principles of segregation and recombination. In a large population, if A_1 and A_2 are alleles for one particular locus, and the frequency of the gene A_1 in the population is p_1, and the frequency of the gene A_2 is p_2, then the genotypic frequencies after one or more random matings will be: for genotype (A_1A_1), $(p_1)^2$;

for genotype (A_1A_2), $(2p_1p_2)$; and for genotype (A_2A_2), $(p_2)^2$. The proportions may be determined by expansion of the binomial, $(p_1 + p_2)^2$. The genotypic frequencies may be determined for any number of alleles on a single locus, by expansion of the appropriate binomial. Thus, for three alleles—with the genes A_1, A_2 and A_3 occurring in the population, respectfully, at frequencies p_1, p_2, and p_3—$(p_1 + p_2 + p_3)^2$ equals $p_1^2 + p_2^2 + p_3^2 + 2p_1p_2 + 2p_1p_3 + 2p_2p_3$. The frequencies, then, would be: for (A_1A_1), $(p_1)^2$; for (A_2A_2), $(p_2)^2$; for (A_3A_3), p_3^2; for (A_1A_2), $(2p_1p_2)$; for (A_1A_3), $(2p_1p_3)$; and for (A_2A_3), $(2p_2p_3)$.

Selection, Drift, and Mutation

If individuals of differing genotypes should differ in their viabilities, then there would be differences in the relative contributions of different genotypes to the succeeding generation. That is, selection would occur in different degrees for the different phenotypes. The alleles in individuals whose genotypes are characterized by higher reproductive fitness will be represented in higher proportions than the alleles associated with the individuals of lower reproductive fitness. Selection can cause alterations in gene frequencies from one generation to the next.

The process of genetic drift[14] may lead to the establishment of a trait which is neutral and nonadaptive or even unfavorable. It involves the random fluctuation of gene frequencies due to chance, and is particularly important for small isolated populations. The probability of genetic drift affecting the gene frequencies of a population depends largely upon the size of the population: with a greater number of parents, the likelihood of loss and fixation are lower, because of the decreased probability that the same chance loss will occur consistently for the different parents. When an isolated population is small, the speed of drift may be high from one generation to the next, but, when a population is large, the process of drift would tend to be a slow one.

Mutations are changes in the genetic material, which are irreversible except for subsequent mutations. Chromosomal mutations involve genetic changes which are visible with present cytogenetic techniques and which involve duplication, deletion, or translocation of a complete chromosome or discernible chromosomal fragment. Gene mutations or point mutations involve changes which are not cytologically visible and which are identifiable only by their phenotypic manifestations. The estimated frequency of a gene mutation may be calculated. One method for such a calculation, primarily applicable to dominant mutations, is based simply on a census of the frequency of children with the particular dominant trait under study who are born to parents without the trait.[15] The underlying assumptions for such a direct calculation involve complete penetrance of the gene, and the occurrence of no other genetic locus or mode of genetic transmission associated with the trait.

An indirect method for calculating a particular mutation rate may be based upon the hypothesis that recurrent mutations from normal to abnormal balance the loss in fitness associated with the mutation. Thus, the number of new mutants would depend on the total number of normal alleles and the frequency with which they can mutate.[15] For a dominant mutant, the mutation rate equals $1/2(1 - f)x$ when f equals the fraction of mutant genes which are lost because of reduced reproductive fitness, and x is the frequency of the abnormality in the parent generation. The mutation rate for a recessive mutant may be approximated, using the same concept of equilibrium between new mutations and *loss* from the following formula: mutation rate equals $(1 - f)x$. An adaptation of the latter formula may be used for estimating the mutation rate for an X-linked recessive mutant. Since hemizygous males have one third of the X-linked abnormal alleles in the population, one third of the X-linked abnormal alleles are exposed to reduced reproductive fitness and some *loss*. Thus, in an equilibrium between mutation and elimination, the mutation rate equals $(1/3) (1 - f)x_m$ when x_m is the frequency of the abnormality among the males of the parent generation.[15]

Linkage

Genetic linkage is indicated by the occurrence of a greater association in inheritance of two or more nonallelic genes than would be expected with independent assortment. Genes are linked to each other when they occur on the same chromosome. In studying possible genetic linkage, it is first necessary to exclude the various other causes of positive or negative nonrandom associations of different traits, include multiple effects of a gene, allelism, population heterogeneity, and inbreeding.

A high frequency of association between different traits is often simply due to multiple effects of the same gene. This is clearly so when the association is absolute, that is, when the two traits are always found together as, for example, the excretion of phenylpyruvic acid and the absence of phenylalanine oxidase. The influence of allelism on associations of different traits is the converse of that of a gene with multiple effects. In a heterogeneous population, in which mating occurs at random with regard to the loci involved, and which is at equilibrium, associations of traits due to separate unlinked genes occur at random. On the other hand, nonrandom association of two genetic traits and the presence of a random association of either of these with a third genetic trait, within a heterozygous population, may

under certain conditions be indicative of linkage.[15] Inbreeding, i.e occurrence of more marriages between relatives than in panmixis, is another cause for occurrence of a frequency of association of traits that exceeds random expectations in a population.

Direct analysis for linkage is possible if the genotypic phase of a double heterozygotic parent is known. The genotypes of the parents of sibships that provide information on linkage can sometimes be deduced with certainty from genetic information on the sibs' grandparents, investigations of the kinds of children occurring in large sibships, and inspections of the parental phenotypes.

Indirect approaches to analyze for linkage make use of statistical phenomena that are consequences of linkage. The data for such analyses may even be found in collections of pedigrees where the genotypes of parents are incompletely known. One may construct a table of mean values for the whole range of recombination values, from complete linkage to independence, adjusted for any number of sibs in each sibship. Such a table can then be consulted for the detection and estimation of linkage. The sib-pair method provides another independent technique for analysis of linkage, which utilizes data from only a single generation. This method provides a means for distinguishing between independent recombination and linkage of different genes without knowledge of the parental genotypes. Accordingly, entries of paired sibs in a fourfold table will show a random distribution when there is no linkage; but, when linkage exists, an excess of sib pairs will occur in those tabulation cells where the two sibs are alike in both traits or unlike in both. A third method for the detection and estimation of the strength of linkage, conceptually the simplest, consists of determining the amount of information available in a collection of data on two loci, and comparing the probability of obtaining such data if the two loci are linked, with the probability if they are not. The ratio of these two probabilities to each other indicates the odds for or against linkage. For example, when the probability of obtaining the observed distribution of two traits in a pedigree is much higher if the genes are linked than if they are not, then the odds are obviously in favor of linkage. Conversely, when the probability of obtaining the information given by a pedigree is much higher if the genes are not linked than if they are, then the odds are against linkage. The probability of obtaining the particular distribution of traits shown by a given pedigree or collection of pedigrees may be expressed as a function of the recombination value, and different degrees of probability correspond to different degrees of linkage. The recombination value that gives the highest probability that the observed distribution would be obtained also provides the best estimate of the degree of linkage between the two loci.

Multifactorial Inheritance

Multifactorial or *polygenic* inheritance refers to the mode of genetic transmission involving traits which are associated with more than a single genetic locus, i.e. with more than a single pair of alleles. There is, as yet, no conclusive proof for multifactorial determination of alternative-trait development in man. Multifactorial inheritance could account for many abnormal traits that seem to have a genetic basis but have no regular sequence of generations or clear-cut Mendelian ratios. A multifactorial theory may be involved in an attempt to account for inheritance of graded characters within a basic Mendelian framework, or in association with the concept of a genetic-threshold effect. Characteristically, such theories have been applied to problems which were obviously insoluble in terms of major genes. The principal fault associated with multifactorial

theories is the fact that they are not specifically testable or refutable. A multifactorial device can be adapted to explain anything, with components which cannot be independently checked by observation.[16]

The Nature of the Genetic Material

The genotype interacts continuously throughout development, maturity, and senescence, with the nongenetic materials from within and without the cell. Pathology may develop in response to genotype, to environmental factors, or to a combination of both. The effects of the genetic material depend upon the structure and composition of the deoxyribonucleic acid (DNA) molecules which, together with proteins and histones, comprise the bulk of the chromosomal material within a cell's nucleus. Protein syntheses occur at the ribosomes in the cytoplasm, controlled by soluble ribose nucleic acid (RNA) particles formed by the nuclear DNA apparently acting at templates. Three classes of RNA molecules have been defined according to their activities in the transfer and translation of genetic information: messenger RNA, transfer RNA, and ribosomal RNA. A messenger RNA particle, formed on a segment of a DNA molecule in the nucleus, moves out into the cytoplasm, carrying in its molecular structure the information that determines the correct sequence of the assembly of amino acids in the synthesis of a specific protein. Ribosomal RNA molecules from the nucleus also move into the cytoplasm, and they combine with protein to form the ribosomes of the cytoplasm. Several ribosomes become attached to each molecule of messenger RNA to form the polysomes that are attached to the membranes of the cell's endoplasmic reticulum. There is a special transfer RNA for each of the 20 amino acids. Each one attaches to its own specific type of amino acid, selected from among those entering the cell from the blood, and transports this amino acid to a ribosome. There, the transfer RNA meets and attaches itself to the appropriate complementary site on the messenger RNA molecule and inserts its amino acid into the protein molecule developing on the ribosome. Each protein or polypeptide synthesis occurs at a ribosome site, after which the messenger RNA is broken down. Presumably, constant renewal of the messenger RNA is required for continued protein synthesis. Variations in the activity code of RNA, like those of DNA, are associated with variations in the sequence of purine-pyrimidine bases in the molecular chains.

Mutations, which are irreversible changes, i.e. except for subsequent mutations, in the genetic material, may occur in any living cell. Chromosomal mutations are those genetic changes in a cell line which are cytologically visible and involve acquisition or loss or transposition of a complete chromosome or a discernible chromosomal fragment. Gene mutations or point mutations, however, involve genetic changes which are not cytologically visible in the chromosomes. Gene mutations are identified only by their phenotypic manifestations, and they presumably include chemical and/or structural changes on the molecular level. The identifiability of a gene mutation depends upon identifiability of the phenotypic effect which results from various interactions within the total genetic and nongenetic context. Thus, a particular mutation may show a characteristic trait or defect in one particular context or with a particular test, but not in other contexts or with other tests.

Cytogenetics

The normal human chromosome number, 46, was first demonstrated by Tjio and Levan in 1956.[17] Since then, numerous chromosomal anomalies have been recognized. At least 0.5 percent of all newborns have been described as being affected with morphological abnormalities associated with currently detectable chromosomal anomalies.[18,19] Significant chromosomal peculiarities may occur in as much as 1.0 percent of the newborn population.[20]

A chromosomal disorder involving mosaicism, which is characterized by an individual possessing both normal and abnormal cell lines (i.e. a cell line with normal and one or more cell lines with abnormal chromosome complements) may result from mitotic misdivision during embryogenesis.[21,22] Such events appear to generally be isolated and without enhanced predisposition for repetition in future offspring produced by the same parents or by genetic relatives of the affected individuals. The probability of a chromosomal mosaic transmitting his/her chromosomal anomaly to his/her offspring does not depend upon occurrence or extent of the phenotypic syndrome, but upon whether or not the gonadal tissue has the chromosomal anomaly. If the gonadal tissue is affected, then the probability of transmitting the chromosomal anomaly and associated syndrome to his/her offspring depends upon the tendency to produce gametes (i.e. ova, spermatozoa) with the chromosomal anomaly. This would be essentially the same for the fertile mosaic whose gonadal tissue is affected as it would be for the individual whose tissues in general are affected with the chromosomal anomaly. The probability of transmitting an anomalous chromosome complement to a zygote directly, through an anomalous gamete, generally depends upon the probability of producing such a gamete. There are specific variations, however, regarding gamete viability and fertilizability, and zygote viability. Thus, the probability of transmitting an anomalous chromosomal complement to a zygote via the gamete, *in some cases*, varies markedly from the probability of producing such a gamete, and sometimes varies between the two sexes. Such variations regarding particular anomalies of specific chromosomes may be determined by examination of epidemiological and incidence data from relevant studies of the specific chromosome anomaly involved.

Numerical abnormalities of chromosome number (i.e. aneuploidies) most commonly result from nondisjunction (i.e. nonseparation) of a pair of chromatids during cell division. Meiotic nondisjunction produces gametes with abnormal chromosome complements (e.g. haploid number plus or minus the nondisjoined chromosome), and fertilization with such a gamete produces an abnormal zygote in which all of the cells have the same anomalous chromosomal complement. A mitotic error during embryogenesis, on the other hand, produces mosaicism, i.e. at least two distinct cell populations or lines in the affected individual. Mosaicism may also result from double fertilization. This may occur through fertilization with two independent spermatozoa, each one combining with one of two (i.e. already divided) nuclei within an undivided oocyte.

The viabilities of zygotes, fetuses, and children affected with particular chromosomal anomalies vary according to the severities of the anomalies. Chromosomal complements involving aneuploidies for the larger autosomes are generally inviable. At least 20 to 30 percent of spontaneous abortions or miscarriages have been shown to involve gross chromosomal anomalies,[23] and the incidence may be considerably higher.[24] Normal individuals with histories of repeated spontaneous abortions have been observed to contain significantly higher proportions of cells with chromosomal duplications and deletions than are generally observed.[25]

Aneuploidies in general, and *trisomies* in particular, do not occur as strictly random events. Their incidences have been associated with various pathological, physiological, and environmental variables.[26] The recurrence of chromosomal anomalies in some families may be related to the persistence of specific peculiarities affecting maternal or paternal gametogenesis. One possibility, which may be rejected in each individual case only after karyotyping cells from cultured gonadal tissues of both parents, is that one of the two parents may be a mosaic in whom the gonadel tissue is affected with the anomalous condition involved. Most karyotype analyses are based solely on leukocytes of peripheral blood, obtaining samples of which involves the least risk and the greatest ease compared to obtaining samples of other living tissues. The rare occurrence of a mosaic with generally normal phenotype and normal karyotypes based on cultured leukocytes, but with anomalous gonadal tissue, would not be diagnosed with standard karyotype analyses based only on leukocytes of peripheral blood. This rare possibility, and the relevant recurrence risk, is often overlooked or ignored.

Evidently, specific genes may sometimes affect mechanisms which regulate duplication of specific chromosomes. Chromosomal aberrations have been observed to occur at a high frequency in peripheral leukocytes in some individuals in the absence of exposure to known mutagenic agents.[27] Diverse chromosomal anomalies within the same family have been observed.[28] Parents of trisomic children have been observed to show a relatively high incidence of chromatid breaks, suggesting an impairment in their chromatid-breakage repair mechanisms.[29] Several studies have shown familial, and evidently genetic, differences in susceptibility or resistance to chromosomal changes or the disease processes associated with such changes.[26]

Sex Chromatin and the Sex Chromosomes

Sex-chromatin bodies occur in interphase nuclei of some female mammalian cells.[30] The maximum number in any particular nucleus is one less than the number of X chromosomes in that nucleus. After the single-X nature of the sex-chromatin body was demonstrated,[31] Lyon[32] postulated that only one X chromosome continues to be active in each mammalian cell, and that each sex-chromatin body is derived from one of the cell's inactivated X chromosomes. Differences in morphology and in quantitative distributions of sex-chromatin bodies have been associated with antibiotic medication[33] and other variables,[24] as well as with the different investigators' particular criteria for positive and negative designations.[35] Thus, interpolation of simple X-chromosome aneuploidies based solely upon qualitative sex-chromatin designations in buccal smears is not entirely reliable.[35]

Figure 2-2 is a photograph of the stained nucleus of a buccal cell, showing two distinct sex-chromatin masses adjacent to the nuclear periphery. The occurrence of two intranuclear sex-chromatin masses in some of an individual's cells indicates the presence of three X chromosomes in those cells. The presence of only one sex-chromatin mass is

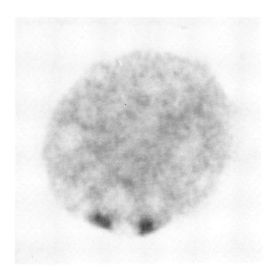

Figure 2–2. Photograph of stained nucleus of a buccal cell, showing two sex-chromatin masses adjacent to the nuclear periphery.

consistent with a chromosome complement that includes two X chromosomes, the normal female complement. The occurrence of only a single X chromosome (e.g. in a chromosomally-normal male, or in a female with the one-X or Turner syndrome), is indicated by the lack of any intranuclear sex-chromatin mass.

The X chromosome exists normally in the monosomic or hemizygous condition in the male (i.e. XY), whereas effects of deletion of one member of any autosomal pair are generally lethal or semilethal. The one-X condition is present in patients having Turner's syndrome with a count of 45 chromosomes. A variant of this chromosomal syndrome occurs in which the female has one normal X chromosome and another one partially deleted. Many of the symptoms which characterize Turner's syndrome have been observed in affected individuals with X isochromosomes, i.e. anomalous structures involving deletion of the short arm and duplication of the long arm in some, deletion of the long arm and duplication of the short arm in others. Thus, factors on both the short and the long arm are needed in duplicate for normal female development. Mosaics have been observed, whose tissues include cells with more than one genotype, e.g. both one-X and XX cells.

The XXX female has a total of 47 chromosomes. Mosaics have been observed, whose cell lines include more than a single genotype, e.g. XX and XXX cells. Phenotypic females with three instead of two X chromosomes, and two (instead of only one) sex-chromatin bodies in some nuclei, differentiate psychosexually as females and are not characterized by manifestations of gross morphological abnormalities. The reported clinical observations are variable, and most of the observed affected individuals are phenotypically normal females, with pubescence, ovulation, and fertility. Incidence of the XXX syndrome is greater than that of the one-X syndrome, being approximately

1.2/1,000 among live-born females.[18] The XXX genotype is evidently the most common sex-chromosome abnormality observed in newborn females.

The occurrence of more than a single X chromosome in association with a Y chromosome is most commonly known as Klinefelter's syndrome, testicular dysgenesis, and chromatin-positive microorchidism. The XXY karyotype is the most usual variety associated with this syndrome. Combinations involving other multiples of X chromosomes with one or more than one Y chromosome have also, but relatively rarely, been observed. Mosaics involving cells with characteristic Klinefelter karyotypes, as well as mosaics involving more than one kind of Klinefelter karyotype, have been described. Generally, no clinical abnormalities are observed in affected boys prior to puberty. Relatively long limbs have been described in many affected individuals, and enlarged breast development has been described in at least 25 to 30 percent of those diagnosed as affected with Klinefelter's syndrome; but there is no consistent pattern of stigmata and many affected individuals are known to be normal in appearance. The outstanding clinical feature is the presence of small testes, which is generally detected only after puberty when the testes have failed to enlarge. MacLean, *et al.*[18] found that the incidence of sex-chromatin positive individuals among unselected newborn males was about 2.0/1,000. Nearly three fourths of the observed group had simple XXY karyotypes, and all

but one of the remaining one-fourth in the Scottish survey were XY/XXY mosaics.

The incidence of XYY individuals is not definitely known, but it is much lower than that of XXY individuals and is quite rare in the general population. Males who are characterized by possession of a supernumerary Y chromosome, e.g. XYY and XXYY males, *etc.*, and mosaics who possess one or more cell lines with a supernumerary Y chromosome or a duplication of part of a Y chromosome (i.e. in the 'big Y' syndrome), tend to show increased frequencies of antisocial and aggressive behavior, very tall stature, and mild mental retardation.[22]

Autosomal Abnormalities

Figure 2–3 is a schematic representation of the various human chromosomes, arranged according to their relative sizes. When cells are cultured for chromosome analysis, they are stimulated to start dividing; and they are arrested at metaphase, when they can be stained and observed microscopically. Figure 2–4 is a schematic representation of the various human metaphase chromosomes, arranged sequentially in standard[36] groups. Each metaphase chromosome depicted in Figure 2–4 is actually a pair of chromatids, i.e. duplicated daughter chromosomes still connected to each other at the centromere. The chromosomes, as schematized in Figure 2–3, are inferred from the visible metaphase structures of pairs of chromatids i.e. as schematized in Figure 2–4. Figure 2–5 in-

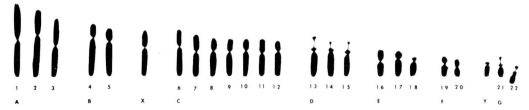

Figure 2–3. Schematic representation of the various human chromosomes arranged according to their relative sizes.

cludes, in the upper half, an example of metaphase chromosomes as photographed from a stained cultured peripheral-blood leukocyte. The lower half of Figure 2–5 shows a karyotype derived from the metaphase plate in the upper half: the chromosomes shown in an enlarged photographic print were cut out and sorted according to

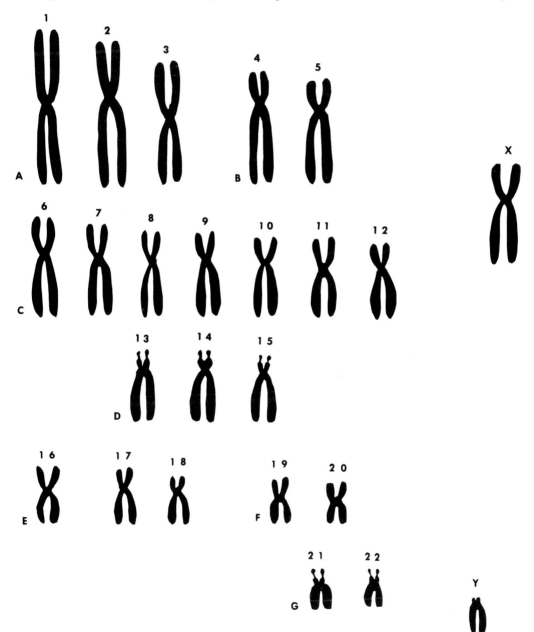

Figure 2–4. Schematic representation of the various human metaphase chromosomes, arranged according to Denver System[36] organization of groups.

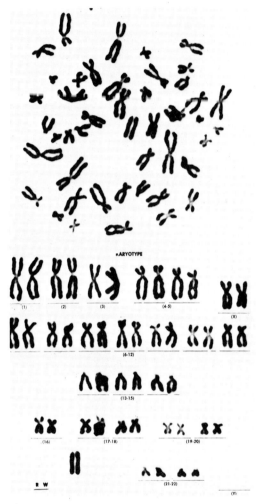

Figure 2–5. Photograph of metaphase chromosomes of a stained cultured peripheral-blood leukocyte (upper half) and a karyotype of that plate (lower half).

relative size and shape. The metaphase plate shown in Figure 2–5 includes a normal complement of autosomes (i.e. 22 pairs), a normal female complement of sex chromosomes (i.e. two X chromosomes), and an abnormal pair of acentric chromosomal fragments.[35]

The first proven[37] human autosomal anomaly associated with a well-known syndrome is the one associated with the G_1-trisomy syndrome (i.e. erroneously and anachronistically referred to as *mongolism* in English-speaking countries). Numerous autosomal abnormalities have since been described, including various duplications, deletions, and translocations.[21,26]

Chromosomal Abnormalities, Associations, and Clusterings

Inductions of chromosome anomalies have been associated with various factors: genetically-transmitted pathological conditions, infectious agents, radiation, and numerous chemical agents. There have been reports of family clusters and of community clusters with leukemia, with other malignancies, and with malformations associated with cytogenetic abnormalities. The high correlation between increasing maternal age and increasing incidence of the autosomal aneuploidy involved in the G_1-trisomy syndrome has been well established. The association between increasing maternal age and increasing incidence of an anomaly is not confined to the G_1-trisomy syndrome, but has also been observed for pregnancies terminating in miscarriage, for stillbirths, placenta previa, anencephaly, hydrocephaly, spina bifida, and for pregnancies producing normal infants who develop leukemia later in childhood.[21,26]

Epidemiological studies of the G_1-trisomy syndrome, which have shown annual fluctuations in incidence, multiannual periodicity, and regional clustering, may be interpreted as indicating the possible relevance of a virus or other infectious agent. Periodic fluctuations in incidence, which are characteristic of recurrent epidemics, have also been reported for other congenital anomalies, such as anencephaly, spina bifida, and hydrocephaly.[21,26] There have been well-documented reports of familial clusterings of leukemia and of other malignancies, and reports of seasonal variation in leukemia incidence.[26] Observations of associations between the G_1-

trisomy syndrome and leukemia incidence suggest an etiological relationship between the two conditions. Similarly, associations have been observed between the congenital aneuploidies involved in Klinefelter's syndrome and leukemia and other malignancies.[47,48] Increased incidence of cancer in general has been observed in families in which chronic lymphocytic leukemia and lymphosarcoma had occurred.[49] Patients affected with Bloom's syndrome and those with Fanconi's syndrome have shown abnormally high frequencies of chromosomal abnormalities in their somatic cells. They have also shown strikingly increased incidences of malignancies.

These observations suggest that the two diseases, each of which may involve simple Mendelian genetic transmission, induce abnormal frequencies of chromosomal rearrangements in the somatic cells of affected individuals. Abnormally high frequencies of chromosome breaks have been observed to occur in patients with serum hepatitis[50] and in patients with aseptic meningitis.[51,52] The induction of chromosome breaks by viruses has been well documented.[26] A specific virus, adenovirus 12, may be incorporated into the genetic material of a specific host cell and transform the normal cell into a malignant-type cell.[53] Chromosome anomalies in circulating leukocytes have been found in patients following their subjection to X-irradiation, to gamma ray and proton exposure, and to therapeutic doses of radioactive iodine.[26] Chromosome breakages have been induced by numerous chemical compounds.[54-56]

Various chromosomal abnormalities—chromosome and chromatid breaks and gaps, aneuploidies, translocations, duplications, deletions—represent effects of exogenous and/or endogenous mutagenic factors. Their associations with particular pathological entities need not necessarily involve cause-and-effect relationships: etiological factor(s) relevant to increasing the incidence of a pathological category may also affect occurrence of discernible mutations. The demonstrated association of two abnormal effects, a particular clinical pathology with significantly-increased discernible chromosomal changes, provides a clue toward solving the problems involving etiology of the pathology. Laboratory methods are available for relatively simple tests of suspected mutagenic agents,[54-56] to screen factors for possible etiological involvement with the pathology and the associated mutations.

Concluding Remarks

As the genotype operates within its intracellular and extracellular environment, many different environmental factors may affect expression of the genotype as well as induction of changes in the genotype (i.e. mutations). Numerous environmental factors have been identified as mutagens, and some as carcinogens. The continued elucidation of mechanisms by which these agents interact with the genotype will continue to expand our understanding of the dynamics of normal cellular differentiation as well as our understanding of neoplastic processes.[57]

REFERENCES

1. Kaplan, A.R.: Genetic counseling in mental retardation and mental disorder. In Lynch, H.T. (Ed.): *Dynamic Genetic Counseling For Clinicians.* Springfield, Thomas, 1969.

2. Morton, N.E.: Genetic tests under incomplete ascertainment. *Am J Hum Genet, 11:*1, 1959.

3. Morton, N.E.: Segregation and linkage. In

Burdette, W.J. (Ed.): *Methodology in Human Genetics*. San Francisco, Holden-Day, 1962.

4. Hirsch, J.: Behavior-genetic analysis and its biosocial consequences. *Seminars in Psychiatry, 2:*89, 1970.

5. Kaplan, A.R.. Concluding remarks: genetics and schizophrenia. In Kaplan, A.R. (Ed.): *Genetic Factors in "Schizophrenia."* Springfield, Thomas, 1972.

6. Falconer, D.S.: The inheritance of liability to diseases with variable age of onset, with particular reference to diabetes mellitus. *Ann Hum Genet, 31:*1, 1967.

7. Mather, K.: *Human Diversity*. Edinburgh, Oliver and Boyd, 1964.

8. Mather, K.: *Statistical Analysis in Biology*, 4th ed. London, Methuen, 1965.

9. Burdette, W.J. (Ed.): *Methodology in Human Genetics*. San Francisco, Holden-Day, 1962.

10. Fisher, R.A., and Yates, F.: *Statistical Tables for Biological, Agricultural, and Medical Research*, 6th ed. New York, Hafner, 1963.

11. Reichenbach, H.: Predictive knowledge. In Jarrett, J.L., and McMurrin, S.M. (Eds.): *Contemporary Philosophy*. New York, 1954.

12. Hardy, G.H.: Mendelian proportions in a mixed population. *Science, 28:* 49, 1908.

13. Weinberg, W.: Uber den Nachweis der Vererbung beim Menschen. *Jahreshefte Verein f. veterl. Naturk. in Würtemberg, 64:*368, 1908.

14. Wright, S.: Classification of the factors of evolution. *Cold Spring Harbor Symposium on Quantitative Biology, 20:*16, 1965.

15. Stern, C.: *Principles of Human Genetics*, 2nd ed. San Francisco, Freeman, 1960.

16. 'Espinasse, P.G.: The polygene concept. *Nature, 149:*732, 1942.

17. Tjio, J.H., and Levan, A.: The chromosome number of man. *Hereditas, 42:*1, 1956.

18. MacLean, N., Harnden, D.G., Court-Brown, M.W., Bond, J., and Mantle, D.J.: Sex-chromosome abnormalities in newborn babies. *Lancet, 1:*286, 1964.

19. Robinson, A., and Puck, T.T.: Studies in chromosomal nondisjunction in man. II. *Am J Hum Genet, 19:*112, 1967.

20. Lejune, J.: Chromosome studies in psychiatry. In: Wortis, J. (Ed.): *Recent Advances in Biological Psychiatry*. New York, Plenum Pr, 1967.

21. Kaplan, A.R.: The use of cytogenetical data in heredity counseling. *Am J Ment Defic, 73:* 636, 1969.

22. Kaplan, A.R.: Chromosomal aneuploidy, genetic mosaicism, occasional acentric fragments, and schizophrenia: association of schizophrenia with rare cytogenetic anomalies. In Kaplan, A.R. (Ed.): *Genetic Factors in "Schizophrenia."* Springfield, Thomas, 1972.

23. Thompson, H.: Abnormalities of the autosomal chromosomes associated with human disease: selected topics and catalogue. *Am J Med Sci, 250:*140, 1965.

24. Waxman, S.H., Arakaki, D.T., and Smith, J.B.: Cytogenetics of fetal abortions. *Pediatrics, 39:*425, 1967.

25. McKay, R.J., Witte, E.H., and Hodgkin, W.E.: Partially trisomic cells in chromosomal analyses. Paper read at Sixth Conference on Mammalian Cytology and Somatic Cell Genetics, Asilomar, California, 1967.

26. Kaplan, A.R., and Kelsall, M.A. (Eds.): Leukocyte chemistry and morphology correlated with chromosome anomalies. *Ann NY Acad Sci, Vol. 155, Art. 3*, 1968.

27. Gooch, P.C., and Fischer, C.L.: High frequency of a specific chromosome abnormality in leukocytes of a normal female. *Cytogenetics, 8:*1, 1969.

28. Atkins, L., Bartsocas, C.S., and Porter, P.J.: Diverse chromosomal anomalies in a family. *J Med Genet, 5:*314, 1968.

29. Kahn, J., and Abe, K.: Consistent and variable chromosome anomalies in parents of children with Down's syndrome. *J Med Genet, 6:*137, 1969.

30. Barr, M.L., and Bertram, E.G.: A morphological distinction between neurones of the male and female, and the behavior of the nuclear satellite during accelerated nucleoprotein synthesis. *Nature, 163:*676, 1949.

31. Ohno, S., Kaplan, W.D., and Kinosita, R.: Formation of the sex chromatin by a single

X-chromosome in liver cells of *Rattus norvegicus. Exp Cell Res, 18:*415, 1959.

32. Lyon, M.F.: Gene action in the X-chromosome of the mouse (*Mus musculus L.*). *Nature, 190:*372, 1961.

33. Sohval, A.R., and Casselman, W.G.B.: Alteration in size of nuclear sex-chromatin mass (Barr body) induced by antibiotics. *Lancet, 2:*1386, 1961.

34. Kaplan, A.R.: Association of a quantitative variable, Barr body score, with length of confinement in state mental hospitals. *J Nerv Ment Dis, 143:*449, 1966.

35. Kaplan, A.R., and Cotton, J.E.: Chromosomal abnormalities in female schizophrenics. *J Nerv Ment Dis, 147:*402, 1968.

36. Denver Report: A proposed standard system of nomenclature of human mitotic chromosomes. *Am J Hum Genet, 12:*384, 1960.

37. Lejeune, J., Gautier, M., and Turpin, R.: Les chromosomes humains en culture de tissus. *Compt R Acad Sci, 248:*602, 1959.

38. Shapiro, S.: A life table of pregnancy terminations and correlates of fetal loss. *Milbank Mem Fund Quart, 40:*7, 1962.

39. Parson, P.A.: Maternal age and development variability. *J Exp Biol, 39:*251, 1962.

40. Steward, A., Webb, J., and Hewitt, D.: Survey of childhood malignancies. *Br Med J, 1:* 1495, 1958.

41. Collmann, R.D., and Stoller, A.: A survey of mongoloid births in Victoria, Australia, 1942–1957. *Am J Pubic Health, 52:*813, 1962.

42. Collmann, R.D., and Stoller, A.: A survey of mongolism and congenital anomalies of the central nervous system in Australia. *NZ Med J, 61:*24, 1962.

43. Gordon, J.E.: Chickenpox: an epidemiological review. *Am J Med Sci, 244:*362, 1962.

44. Alter, M.: Anencephalus, hydrocephalus, and spina bifida epidemiology, with special reference to a survey in Charleston, S.C. *Arch Neurol, 7:*411, 1962.

45. Guthkelch, A.N.: Studies in spina bifida cystica. III. Seasonal variations in the frequency of spina bifida births. *Br J Pre Soc Med, 16:*159, 1962.

46. Slater, B.C.S., Watson, G.I., and McDonald, J.C.: Seasonal variation in congenital abnormalities. *Br J Prev Soc Med, 18:*1, 1964.

47. Robinson, L.R.: Neoplastic liability in Klinefelter's syndrome. *Br J Psychiatry, 112:*713, 1966.

48. Miller, R.W.: Relation between cancer and congenital defects in man. *New Engl J Med, 275:*87, 1966.

49. Morganti, C., and Cresseri, A.: Neuvelles recherches génétiques sur les lancé mies. *Sang, 25:*421, 1954.

50. Aya, T., and Makino, S.: Notes on chromosome abnormalities in cultured leukocytes from serum hepatitis patients. *Proc Japan Acad, 42:*648, 1966.

51. Makino, S., Yamada, K., and Kajii, T.: Chromosome aberrations in leukocytes of patients with aseptic meningitis. *Chromosoma, 16:*372, 1965.

52. Makino, S., Aya, T., Ikeuchi, T., and Kasahara, S.: A further study of chromosomes in cultured leukocytes from aseptic meningitis patients. *Proc Japan Acad, 42:* 270, 1966.

53. Fujinaga, K., and Green, M.: The mechanism of viral carcinogenesis by DNA mammalian viruses: viral-specific RNA in polyribosomes of adenovirus tumor and transformed cells. *Proc Natl Acad Sci US, 55:* 1567, 1966.

54. Hollaender, A. (Ed.): *Chemical Mutagens.* New York, Plenum, 1971.

55. Epstein, S.S. (Ed.): *Drugs of Abuse: Their Genetic and Other Chronic Nonpsychiatric Hazards.* Cambridge, MIT Pr, 1971.

56. Vogel, F., and Röhrborn, G. (Eds.): *Chemical Mutagenesis in Mammals and Man.* New York, Springer-Verlag, 1971.

57. Jackson, L.G.: Genetics in neoplastic diseases. In Goodman, R.M. (Ed.): *Genetic Disorders of Man.* Boston, Little, 1970.

CHAPTER 3

IMMUNOLOGY, CANCER

AND GENETICS

Edward A. Chaperon

Historical Background— Animal Experiments

THE IDEA THAT the immune mechanism might play a role in the resistance of individuals to neoplastic disease is not new, since it dates back to the beginnings of scientific research in Bacteriology and Immunology.[1] The *infectious* nature of cancer was first suggested in the seventeenth century, and early efforts to inoculate fragments of malignant tumors into laboratory animals were motivated by a desire to isolate and identify, according to Koch's postulates, a suspected etiological agent. Although such transplanted tumors did not usually survive, there were significant exceptions.[2] In 1893, Morau studied the influence of age, sex, race, pregnancy, heredity and other factors on the survival of transplanted cylinder-cell epitheliomas in mice.[3] He found that although these tumors were inoculable into animals of the same species, heredity played a considerable role in the development of the neoplasms. Furthermore, he noted that the transplanted tumors not only possessed a variable virulence, but that they became progressively less inoculable upon successive transplantation into other hosts. A few years later Loeb,[4] upon noting that transplanted rat sarcomas frequently regressed and disappeared, suggested that an "individual predisposition or immunity" to transplanted tumors might exist in such animals.

Jensen, in 1903,[5] was the first to implicate a serological reaction in resistance to trans-planted tumors when he reported the regression and subsequent absorption of a tumor in a mouse preinjected with serum from a rabbit which had been inoculated with cells from the same tumor. During the next twenty years, cancer immunology went through a period of what Southam has called "naive enthusiasm."[6] The discovery that upon regression of a transplanted tumor, the host animal became resistant to reimplantation with the same kind of tumor, and the finding that immunity against transplanted tumor cells could be artificially induced in experimental animals by injecting living cells taken from either normal or neoplastic tissue, led investigators of that period to conclude that humoral antibodies, developing in the blood of resistant hosts, were responsible for tumor regression. The development of vaccines for effective serum therapy against cancer seemed inevitable.

This early enthusiasm proved, however, to be premature since the presence of humoral antibodies could not be demonstrated, with the techniques then available, in the blood of animals following their rejection of transplanted tumor cells. Furthermore, it was established by Rous, in 1910,[7] that the protective immunity observed in the early studies was directed against transplanted tumors as alien tissues, and that the antigens involved were not cancer specific. Such findings led to a period of scepticism, and Woglom, in 1929,[8] upon reviewing the literature, concluded that "a specific antibody has been sought for thirty years as tangible basis for immunity in cancer, but none has been discovered. Nothing can be hoped for in respect to a successful therapy in this direction."

The next major breakthrough came when highly inbred strains of mice became commercially available in the 1930's and 40's.[9] It was soon established that the Mendelian segregation of dominant genes, later designated as histocompatibility genes, governed the transplantability of both neoplastic and normal tissues. It became clearly evident that the "transplantable" tumors of the earlier reports, which *had* grown freely across genetic barriers, did so not because they lacked the relevant histocompatibility antigens, but because they somehow had avoided the host's immune response. This type of evidence contributed to a feeling that all tumor rejection responses were probably transplantation artifacts, having nothing to do with resistance to cancer in man.

Tumor Specific Antigens in Mice

A new era started when Gross, in 1943,[10] reported the active immunization of inbred mice to transplants of a tumor which had been induced with methylcholanthrene (MC) in a mouse of the same strain. Ten years passed, however, before these results were confirmed. In 1953, Foley[11] ligated isografted MC-induced sarcomas, thereby inducing tumor necrosis, and subsequently challenged these animals with more of the same sarcoma. He found that the pretreated animals frequently rejected these second grafts while similar grafts were readily accepted by the unsensitized control animals. The possibility that this rejection might have been due to residual heterozygosis within the strain of mice used in these experiments was considered unlikely since mammary carcinoma of spontaneous origin, derived from and carried in the strain, failed to show the same

difference between ligated and control groups. Prehn and Main[12] corroborated Foley's results and demonstrated that skin grafts could readily be exchanged between different members of the same inbred strain of mice, whereas MC-induced sarcoma isografts were frequently rejected by hosts with ligated tumors. The final proof, definitely excluding the possibility that residual heterozygosis might account for the phenomenon, was obtained when the rejection of MC-induced sarcomas was demonstrated in the primary autochthonous host.[13] These findings were rapidly followed by other reports of rejection of tumors by syngeneic or autochthonous hosts.[14]

It was soon discovered that the tumor-specific transplantation antigens (TSTA) of these MC-induced sarcomas were unique for each tumor, even those which were morphologically similar[12,13,15] or produced in the same animal.[16] In addition, the immunogenicity of the antigens in different MC-induced tumors varied.[13,17] In some cases resistance could be built up against a relatively large inoculum of tumor cells, whereas with others resistance could only be demonstrated against a relatively small number of cells. Also, it was found that strongly immunogenic tumors tended to develop in methylcholanthrene treated mice after shorter latency periods than those seen for weakly immunogenic tumors.[17,18,19] It would appear from this that the hosts were capable of eliminating highly immunogenic tumors unless they grew fast enough to outrace the host's immune mechanism, and that slowly growing tumors survived only when their antigens were weak and not readily detected by the host.

In the 1960's, it was discovered that polyoma virus induced murine tumors contain a common antigen, irrespective of the histological type of the tumor or the strain of mice in which it was produced.[20,21,22] Furthermore, these tumors were antigenically distinct from those induced by other viral or nonviral agents.[23,24,25] Adult mice could be immunized against a transplanted polyoma induced tumor by preinoculation with either tumor cells or infective virus, but attenuated viruses had no protective effect. It was concluded that the new specificities of the tumor cells were induced by the virus, and that these were responsible for the rejection reaction. Of particular interest here is the report by Chang and Hildemann[26] that susceptibility to polyoma virus in mice appears to be controlled by a single autosomal gene, and that early and efficient maturation of the immune system is a major component of genetic resistance to malignant infection.

It was soon found that the occurrence of virally determined antigens is a general feature of all known virally induced tumors, but it was noted that nononcogenic viruses can also produce changes in the membranes of infected cells. Presumably innocuous viruses may be carried by and confer new antigenic specificities on infected cells for prolonged periods of time, thereby interfering with the search for etiological clues in tumors of unknown origin.

The one flaw which prevented acceptance of the above studies as proof that all tumors are antigenic, thereby permitting host reactivity against them, came from work on the so-called "spontaneously arising" tumors. *In vivo* studies with such tumors failed to demonstrate any tumor specific antigens, and it was suggested that these tumors either were not antigenic or that their antigens were too weak to be demonstrable by the techniques then available. However, it appeared likely to many investigators that more sensitive *in vitro* methods might be developed for the detection of TSTA, and a number of such assays were soon introduced.[27,28,29] With these methods, it has since been demonstrated

that the great majority, and probably all tumors, have tumor specific antigens.

Historical Background—Human Cancer

From the foregoing, it can be concluded that TSTA exist in experimental tumors, and that these antigens probably play a role in resistance to neoplasms. There are data suggesting that this is also true for human tumors, but a conclusive demonstration here is difficult due to the absence of pure human lines without histocompatibility barriers and the existence of ethical factors limiting human experimentation. Nevertheless, several lines of clinical evidence have accumulated which indicate that specific immunity plays a role in man's resistance to cancer.

In 1967, Everson[30] compiled an impressive list of documented spontaneous regressions in cases of human cancer. More than half of these cases were of four tumor types: hypernephroma, neuroblastoma, choriocarcinoma and malignant melanoma. In addition, Everson noted a high frequency of regressions in sarcomas of bone and soft tissue. Other investigators have since described spontaneous regressions in cases of Burkitt's lymphoma.[31]

Reports of tumor infiltration by lymphocytes and plasma cells, and the evidence of lymph node hyperplasia in cancer patients constitute further evidence that host immunity may be involved in spontaneous remissions. It was concluded, as long ago as 1920,[32] that survival of patients with gastric cancer was related to an infiltration of the tumor by lymphocytes, and there have since been a number of similar correlations in cases of breast cancer, squamous cell carcinoma of the esophagus, testicular seminoma, and other tumors.[33] That these infiltrating lymphocytes may actually represent a host reaction against the tumor is supported by the finding[34] that such patients also demonstrate a delayed hypersensitivity reaction following intradermal challenge with cellular extracts of their own tumors.

Tumor Specific Antigens in Man

Over the years, serologic techniques have been employed in attempts to demonstrate tumor immunity in cancer patients. In 1955, Graham and Graham[35] found complement-fixing antibodies, reactive against autologous tumor cells, in the sera from 12 of 48 women with gynecologic cancers. During the next few years, a number of investigators reported the presence of antitumor antibodies in the sera of cancer patients.[33] Unfortunately, most of the antigens used in these studies were prepared from sources other than the donors of the sera, and the results could easily have been due to isoantibodies against normal histocompatibility antigens. Recently, however, results from several laboratories have provided convincing evidence for the existence of four reasonably distinct systems of tumor associated antigens in man and the presence of circulating antibodies and sensitized lymphocytes against these antigens in the circulation of patients with a variety of neoplasms.

Burkitt's lymphoma, a malignant neoplasm of undifferentiated lymphoreticular cells, afflicting children of tropical central Africa, was first described and identified as a specific clinical syndrome in 1958.[36] This disease has created great interest because it appears to be transmitted by a viral agent. The Epstein-Barr virus (EBV) has been found in many isolates from Burkitt's lymphoma, and titers of circulating antibodies to EBV related antigens have frequently been found in the sera of patients with this disease.[37] It is of interest to note that antibody titers to EBV antigens have also been reported in patients with nasopharyngeal carcinoma, sarcoidosis and infectious mononuclcosis.

A second group, the sarcoma antigens, have been studied primarily in cultivated cell lines. Antibodies to these antigens, as in the case of the EBV antigens, are widespread throughout the human population.[38] In 1968, Morton and Malgren[39] noted a high incidence of antitumor antibodies in the sera of patients with osteosarcoma, each patient's serum reacting not only with his own tumor, but also with similar tumors from other patients. Moreover, antibodies to tumor antigens could also be found in sera from members of the immediate family and close associates of the patients, suggesting that this neoplasm may also be associated with an infective virus.

A third group of antigens associated with malignant cells was found in both fresh surgical specimens and in cultured melanoma cells.[38] Antibodies to two classes of antigens have been demonstrated in human sera, the first an intracellular antigen shared by all malignant melanomas and the second a cell-surface antigen distinct for each tumor.[40] A study of malignant melanoma patients by Lewis in 1967[41] resulted in the finding that although those with localized tumors often had cytotoxic antibodies against autologous tumor cells, such antibodies were not detectable in patients with disseminated disease.

The final group of tumor associated antigens are the fetal antigens, generally considered to be determined by host genes which are active during embryonic development but not during normal adult life. A neoplastic change presumably results in the reactivation of these genes, and their products reappear in the circulation of the cancer patient. Two major systems of fetal antigens are well established. The first is the carcinoembryonic antigen (CEA) first reported by Gold and Freedman in 1965.[28] This antigen is normally found in fetal gut, but it is also present in the circulation of patients with adenocarcinomas arising from entodermally derived digestive system epithelium including colon, rectum, stomach, esophagus, liver and pancreas.[42] The antigen has not been found in any other normal, diseased or neoplastic human tissues. A second similar fetal antigen is an alpha$_1$-fetoprotein which appears in the sera of patients with hepatoma and embryonal adenocarcinoma.[43,44] It would be of interest to know whether or not the expression of these fetal antigens in the adult is under genetic control. Unfortunately, no family studies have been reported which might answer this question.

The development in 1965[29] of a sensitive *in vitro* colony inhibition assay has resulted in the demonstration of both humoral and cellular immune reactions against specific antigens from a variety of tumors.[45,46,47] Antitumor antibodies have been found in the sera of patients with adenocarcinoma of the colon, neuroblastoma and soft tissue sarcomas. Also, specifically sensitized lymphocytes have been demonstrated in the blood of patients with adenocarcinoma of the colon, neuroblastoma, cancer of the breast and lung, Wilm's tumors, squamous cell carcinoma of the lip, carcinoma of the larynx and myosarcoma.

Possible Mechanisms for Tumor Survival

The question arises as to why, if tumor specific antigens exist to which the host can respond, do tumors grow out at all? Extreme advocates of an important role for immune surveillance in host resistance to cancer would say that tumors only develop when the immune system breaks down. Jerne has gone so far as to postulate that the immune system has evolved primarily to detect and eliminate incipient tumors.[48]

It is well known that the incidence of cancer is quite high in certain immunologic deficiency disorders in man (cf. Chapter 4), particularly those involving defects of the thymus. In addition, patients with transplanted kidneys, treated for prolonged periods with immunosuppressive agents, develop lymphoreticular neoplasms with higher incidence than one would expect. Also, the well known, increased incidence of neoplasms in older people correlates well with a decreased capacity to manifest cell-mediated immune functions during senescence. If, on the basis of such evidence, we accept the conclusion that the immune mechanism plays an important role in tumor prevention, it follows that the only way such tumors can develop in the otherwise immunologically competent host is by escaping early detection and later overwhelming the host's defenses. A number of different mechanisms have been proposed to account for this.

In 1962, Old *et al.*[17] observed that small numbers of cells from chemically induced antigenic tumors sometimes grew in syngeneic mice that were capable of inhibiting the growth of larger inocula of cells from the same tumor. Old[14] attributed this "sneaking through" phenomenon to a failure of the host to always respond quickly enough to weak or diluted tumor antigens, thereby permitting rapidly growing neoplastic cells bearing such antigens to proliferate until there were too many of them to be adequately handled. It was predicted that if the immune response of the host could be augmented by increasing the number of immune cells with the appropriate specific reactivity or by increasing the immunogenicity of the antigens, such tumors might be eliminated. Preliminary studies along these lines have been encouraging.[49]

It has been suggested that in some malignancies a state of tolerance might be induced so that tumor antigens are not recognized as such by the host. It is still not clear whether immunological tolerance involves a deletion of those cells capable of making a specific antibody or whether potentially responsive cells are inhibited by the continued presence of antigen.[50] The Hellströms and others[51] have demonstrated that lymphocytes from tumor bearing animals and patients with a variety of neoplastic diseases are generally reactive against the appropriate TSTA *in vitro,* and that sera from such individuals frequently contain circulating anti-tumor antibodies. This clearly indicates that the potential for an immune response against autochthonous tumors persists in such individuals and suggests that if tolerance is indeed involved, it is not mediated by the destruction of specifically responsive cells. Moreover, a mechanism involving the blockade of specific receptors on the lymphocytes by soluble antigen, as postulated by Nossal,[50] is supported by the numerous reports of tumor associated antigens in the sera of cancer patients (c.f. Alexander and Currie 52).

A third mechanism, not necessarily distinct from the above, by which experimental animals and cancer patients might become refractory against tumor antigens *in vivo,* even though their lymphocytes or sera may show anti-tumor activity *in vitro,* involves the phenomenon of immune enhancement.[53] Such an explanation proposes that blocking antibodies may interact with the TSTA, thereby protecting the tumor cells from recognition and elimination by the thymus dependent immune system. It is supported by the work of Biozzi[54] who separated mice into two lines by selectively breeding them for their ability to produce agglutinins against sheep erythrocytes. He found that although Sarcoma 180 cells grew rapidly when implanted subcutaneously into the "high responder" mice, cells from the same tumor, after initial growth, regressed and disappeared when implanted into "low responder" animals.

Attempts to overcome immune enhancement have been predicated on the existence of a state of equilibrium between the activities of thymus-dependent "T" cells, responsible for cellular immunity, and thymus-independent "B" cells, responsible for circulating antibodies (including blocking antibodies). Presumably, such an equilibrium is generally desirable, with the survival of malignant cells being a notable exception. Attempts have been made to provide a greater cellular response in such cases by adoptively transferring allogeneic immune lymphocytes or transfer factor from sensitized donors.[55,56] Also, augmentation of the host's own cellular immunity has been attempted by injecting such known stimulators of T cell activity as adjuvants, BCG, *Corynebacterium parvum* and bacterial toxins.[55,56] Results from animal experiments have been impressive, but data from treatment of cancer patients, although encouraging, are still in the preliminary stages.

Another hypothesis for the survival of antigen-bearing tumors has evolved from observations that cancer is often accompanied by an increase of normal and the appearance of new serum glycoproteins.[57] These glycoproteins become attached to the surface of tumor cells, and it has been proposed that they might constitute an inpenetrable electrochemical barrier to immunologically competent cells. Simmons and Rios[58] successfully produced remissions in MC-induced fibrosarcoma bearing mice by treating them with living tumor cells which had been treated with *Vibrio cholera* neuraminidase *in vitro,* and suggested that the enzyme treatment unmasked hidden antigens on the tumor cell surface. They were not, however, able to demonstrate an increased number of antigenic determinants on neuraminidase treated cells by *in vitro* absorption studies with specific antibody. Also, no infiltration by lymphocytes was seen in the regressing tumors. Other mechanisms for immunosuppression by glycoproteins have been proposed, and there is now considerable interest in the role of an alpha$_2$-macroglobulin as a possible humoral "immunoregulator."[59,60,61,62]

Role of Genetics in Susceptibility to Cancer

Sufficient evidence has accumulated in recent years to support the thesis that susceptibility to a number of different diseases, including cancer, may be influenced by genetic factors in the host. It is well known that genetically determined defects in general immune responsiveness such as hereditary agammaglobulinemia, ataxia telangiectasia, the Wiskott-Aldrich syndrome and a number of other similar conditions result in markedly increased susceptibility to infections and neoplastic diseases. Since 1952, over 2000 patients, with a variety of immunological deficiency disorders, have been studied,[63,64,65] and it has been well established that malignancy occurs far more frequently in man when his immune defenses are compromised genetically. The pattern of inheritance in cases of general immune insufficiency is usually described as that of an autosomal, sex-linked recessive, but the genetics in many cases is undoubtedly much more complex. There are many steps in the development of the immune system that could be blocked by mutations in structural genes coding for hormones, membrane proteins or immunoglobulin molecules, and intermediate defects are well known, ranging in severity from a complete absence of the reticuloendothelial system, as seen in patients with reticular dysgenesia, to dysgammaglobulinemias involving reduced levels of a single class of immunoglobulins.

The recent demonstration of genetic control in the immune response of mice and guinea pigs to certain purified or synthetic antigens suggests the existence of a more specific type of inherited susceptibility. In most of these studies, the ability of the animals to make antibodies was shown to be controlled by autosomal dominant immune response (*Ir*) genes, which are linked with genes for the major histocompatibility genes of the species (cf. Chapter 5).

The mechanism by which the presence of certain histocompatibility antigens might influence the immune response is unknown, but a number of explanations have been proposed. The simplest of these is based on the premise that histocompatibility antigens may possess determinants similar to those on the foreign agent. In such a model, an increased susceptibility to virally induced tumors could be attributed to the presence of virus-like determinants on the host cells, resulting in a state of "cross tolerance" and a failure of the host to respond to these antigens. This susceptibility would only be transmitted as a dominant trait unless genetics systems exist in which the responder parent and the F$_1$ hybrid lack an antigen which is present in the nonresponder parent. The increased susceptibility of mice carrying the Fv-2^s allele to the SFFV component of the Friend virus appears to be an example of this mode of transmission.

A second mechanism by which histocompatibility gene linked factors might alter susceptibility to diseases is one in which the immune response gene itself might limit the antigenic specificities to which an individual might respond. Such a pattern of inheritance would involve genes coding for specific antigen receptors on the surface of thymus derived T lymphocytes, and the ability to respond would be transmitted as a dominant. The H-2 linked control of susceptibility to Gross leukemogenesis (the Rgv-1 gene) might be explained by such a mechanism.

Evidence that such genetic defects involve T cell function comes primarily from the work of Benacerraf and his colleagues[66] who demonstrated that, in addition to differences in the production of circulating antibodies to DNP poly-L-lysine, responder and non-responder guinea pigs could be differentiated in terms of their ability to demonstrate delayed hypersensitivity reactions. Nonresponding animals immunized with DNP-PLL on a carrier failed to give positive skin tests to the hapten conjugate, although they made antibodies to DNP. McDevitt, *et al.*[67] corroborated Benacerraf's findings by showing that thymectomy of adult mice abolished the differences in antibody production against a synthetic polypeptide antigen in responder and nonresponder animals. McDevitt's group also reported data which suggest that T cells from responder strains can induce the production of antibody by nonresponder B cells in some allophenic (tetraparental) mice.

Another class of *Ir* genes, distinct from the above, since they segregate independently from the major histocompatibility genes, are presently being studied in several laboratories.[68] In this system, the ability of the animals to make good antibody responses to certain antigens is associated with the presence of specific immunoglobulin allotypes. The *Ir* gene thus appears to be linked to the structural genes for the immunoglobulin molecules themselves. Eichmann, *et al.*[69] showed that following stimulation of heterozygous rabbits (high responder × low responder) with streptococcal antigens, there was a selective increase in the production of immunoglobulin molecules bearing an allotypic marker derived from the responder parent. In the mouse, Blomberg, *et al.*[70] discovered that the structure of antibodies produced against the alpha 1-3 glucosyl linkage in a dextran antigen was due to a locus linked to the allotype marker on the constant region

of the heavy chain. These findings suggest that the antibody producing B cells in different strains may differ in their genes for the variable end of the peptide chains in the immunoglobulin molecule (V-region genes), and that some strains may lack certain combining sites, thereby restricting their ability to respond effectively to some antigenic determinants.

Summary

In this introductory chapter, we have presented a chronology of progress thus far in the application of immunological theory and techniques to the study of neoplastic diseases. Although a number of unanswered questions still exist, a pattern is beginning to emerge, and the enthusiasm of investigators in this area today is probably justified. It is now generally agreed that all tumors, at least at some time during their development, possess antigenic determinants which distinguish them from their hosts, and one is led to conclude that, were it not for the surveillance activities of the immune system, the incidence of malignant disease would be far greater than it actually is.

The data from animal experiments showing a genetic basis, which may or may not be linked to genes for histocompatibility antigens, in the ability of individuals to respond immunologically to certain antigens, is particularly exciting in view of the reports of a high incidence of some forms of cancer in certain kindreds[71] and the association of an increased frequency of certain HLA antigens in individuals with a variety of malignant diseases.[72] A further discussion of these ideas will be found in subsequent chapters of this book.

REFERENCES

1. Ewing, J.: Cancer problems. In *The Harvey Lectures*. Lippincott, Philadelphia, 1909, pp. 34–88.

2. Doutrelepont, J.: Versuche überdie Uebertragung der Carcinoma von Thier auf Thier. *Arch Pathol Anat Physiol, 45:*507, 1869.

3. Morau, H.: Recherches éxpérimentales sur la transmissibilite de certains neoplasmes (épithéliomas cylindriques). *Arch Med Exp, 16:* 677–705, 1894.

4. Loeb, L.: On transplantation of tumors. *J Med Res, 6:*28–38, 1901.

5. Jensen, C. O.: Experimentelle Untersuchungen über Krebs bei Maüsen. *Centralbl Bakteriol, Parasitenk Infektionskrankh, 34:*28–34, 122–143, 1903.

6. Southam, C.M.: Immunopathology of cancer. *Fed Proc, 24:*1007–1008, 1965.

7. Rous, P.: An experimental comparison of transplanted tumor and a transplanted normal tissue capable of growth. *J Exp Med, 12:*344–366, 1910.

8. Woglom, W.H.: Immunity to transplantable tumours. *Cancer Rev, 4:*129–214, 1929.

9. Staats, J.: The laboratory mouse. In Green, E.L., (Ed.): *Biology of the Laboratory Mouse*, New York, McGraw-Hill, 1965, pp. 1–5.

10. Gross, L.: Intradermal immunization of C3H mice against a sarcoma that originated in an animal of the same line. *Cancer Res, 3:* 326–333, 1943.

11. Foley, E.J.: Antigenic properties of methylcholanthrene-induced tumors in mice of the strain of origin. *Cancer Res, 13:*835–837, 1953.

12. Prehn, R.T., and Main, J.M.: Immunity to methylcholanthrene-induced sarcomas. *J Natl Cancer Inst, 18:*769–778, 1957.

13. Klein, G., Sjögren, H.O., Klein, E., and Hellström, K.E.: Demonstration of resistance against methylcholanthrene-induced sarcomas in the primary autochthonous host. *Cancer Res, 20:*1561–1572, 1960.

14. Old, L.J., and Boyse, E.A.: Immunology of experimental tumors. *Ann Rev Med, 15:* 167–186, 1964.

15. Revesz, L.: Detection of antigenic differences in isologous host-tumor systems by pretreatment with heavily irradiated tumor cells. *Cancer Res, 20:*443–451, 1960.

16. Rosenau, W., and Morton, D.L.: Tumor-specific inhibition of growth of methylcholanthrene-induced tumors *in vivo* and *in vitro* by sensitized isologous lymphoid cells. *J Natl Cancer Inst, 38:*825–836, 1966.

17. Old, L.J., Boyse, E.A., Clarke, D.A., and Carswell, E.A.: Antigenic properties of chemically induced tumors. *Ann NY Acad Sci, 101:*80–106, 1962.

18. Johnson, S.: The effect of thymectomy and of the dose of 3-methylcholanthrene on the induction and antigenic properties of sarcomas in C57B1 mice. *Br J Cancer, 22:*93–104, 1968.

19. Bartlett, G. L.: Effect of host immunity on the antigenic strength of primary tumors. *J Natl Cancer Inst, 49:*493–504, 1972.

20. Habel, K.: Resistance of polyoma virus immune animals to transplanted polyoma tumors. *Proc Soc Exp Biol Med, 106:*722–725, 1961.

21. Sjögren, H.O., Hellström, I., and Klein, G.: Transplantation of polyoma virus induced tumors in mice. *Cancer Res, 21:*329–337, 1961.

22. Hellström, I., and Sjögren, H.O.: Demonstration of common specific antigen(s) in mouse and hamster polyoma tumors. *Int J Cancer, 1:*481–489, 1966.

23. Sjögren, H.O.: Further studies on the induced resistance against isotransplantation of polyoma tumors. *Virology, 15:*214–219, 1961.

24. Habel, K.: Immunological determinants of polyoma virus oncogenesis. *J Exp Med, 115:*181–193, 1962.

25. Sjögren, H.O.: Studies on specific transplantation resistance to polyoma virus induced tumors. *J Natl Cancer Inst, 32:*361–374, 374–394, 645–649, 1064.

26. Chang, S., and Hildemann, W.H.: Inheritance of susceptibility to polyoma virus in mice. *J Natl Cancer Inst, 33:*303–313, 1964.

27. Klein, G., Clifford, P., Klein, E., and Stjern-sward, J.: Search for tumor specific immune reactions in Burkitt lymphoma patients by the membrane immunofluorescence reaction. *Proc Natl Acad Sci, 55:*1628–1635, 1966.

28. Gold, P., and Freedman, S.O.: Demonstration of tumor-specific antigens in human colonic carcinomata by immunological tolerance and absorption techniques. *J Exp Med, 121:* 439–461, 1965.

29. Hellström, I.: A colony inhibition (CI) technique for demonstration of tumor cell destruction by lymphoid cells *in vitro. Int J Cancer, 2:*65–68, 1967.

30. Everson, T.C.: Spontaneous regression of human tumors. In Ariel, I.M. (Ed.): *Progress in Clinical Cancer.* New York, Grune, 1967, Vol. III.

31. Burkitt, D.P., and Kyalwazi, S.K.: Spontaneous remission of African lymphoma. *Br J Cancer, 21:*14–16, 1967.

32. MacCarty, W.C., and Mahle, A.E.: Relation of differentiation and lymphocyte infiltration to postoperative longevity in gastric carcinoma. *J Lab Clin Med, 6:*473–480, 1920.

33. Fisher, B.: Present status of tumor immunology. *Adv Surg, 5:*189–254, 1971.

34. Stewart, T.H.: The presence of delayed hypersensitivity reactions in patients toward cellular extracts of their malignant tumors. *Cancer, 23:*1368–1379, 1380–1387, 1969.

35. Graham, J.B., and Graham, R.M.: Antibodies elicited by cancer in patients. *Cancer, 8:* 409–416, 1955.

36. Burkitt, D.P.: A sarcoma involving the jaws of African children. *Br J Surg, 46:*218–223, 1958.

37. Miller, G.: Human lymphoblastoid cell lines and Epstein-Barr: A review of their interrelationships and their relevance to the etiology of leukoproliferative states in man. *Yale J Biol Med, 43:*358–384, 1971.

38. Morton, D.L., Eilber, F.R., and Malmgren, R.A.: Immune factors in human cancer: Malignant melanomas, skeletal and soft tissue sarcomas. *Prog Exp Tumor Res, 14:* 25–42, 1971.

39. Morton, D.L., and Malmgren, R.A.: Human osteosarcomas: Immunologic evidence suggesting an associated infectious agent. *Science, 162:*1278, 1968.

40. Lewis, M.G., Idonopisov, R.L., Nairn, R.C., Phillips, T.M., Fairley, H.G., Badenham, D.C., and Alexander, P.: Tumor specific antibodies in human malignant melanoma and their relationship to the extent of the disease. *Br Med J, 1:*547–562, 1969.

41. Lewis, M.G.: Possible immunological factors in human malignant melanomas in Uganda. *Lancet, ii:*921, 1967.

42. Gold, P., and Freedman, S.O.: Cellular location of carcinoembryonic antigens of the human digestive system. *Cancer Res, 28:* 1331–1334, 1968.

43. Abelev, G.I.: Antigenic structure of chemically induced hepatomas. *Prog Exp Tumor Res,* 104–157, 1965.

44. Abelev, G.I.: Production of embryonal serum -globulin by hepatomas: A review of experimental and clinical data. *Cancer Res, 28:*1344–1350, 1968.

45. Hellström, K.E., and Hellström, I.: Some aspects of the immune defense against cancer. I. *In vitro* studies on animal tumors. *Cancer, 28:*1266–1268, 1971.

46. Hellström, K.E., and Hellström, I.: Some aspects of the immune defense against cancer. II. *In vitro* studies on human tumors. *Cancer, 28:*1269–1271, 1971.

47. Hellström, K.E., Hellström, I., Sjögren, H.O., and Warner, G.A.: Cell mediated immunity to human tumor antigens. In Amos, B. (Ed.): *Progress in Immunology.* New York, Acad Pr, 1971, pp. 939–949.

48. Jerne, N.K.: The somatic generation of immune recognition. *Eur J Immunol, 1:*1–9, 1971.

49. Sophocles, A.M.: Immunologic aspects of cancer. *Surg Gynecol Obstet, 133:*321–331, 1971.

50. Nossal, G.J.V.: Recent advances in immunological tolerance. In Amos, B., (Ed.): *Progress in Immunology.* New York, Acad Pr, 1971, pp. 666–677.

51. Hellström, K.E.: In Smith, R.T., and Landy,

M. (Eds.): *Immune Surveillance*. New York, Acad Pr, 1970, pp. 263–275.

52. Alexander, P., and Currie, G.A.: The role of circulating tumor-specific antigens in the tumor-host relationship. In *Immunological Aspects of Neoplasia*. 26th Annual Symp. on Fund. Cancer Res. Houston, M.D. Anderson Hospital and Tumor Institute, 1973.

53. Snell, G.D.: Immunologic enhancement. *Surg Gynecol Obstet, 130:*1109–1119, 1970.

54. Biozzi, G.: In McDevitt, H.O., and Landy, M. (Eds.): *Genetic Control of Immune Responsiveness*. New York, Acad Pr, 1972.

55. Smith, R.T.: Potentials for immunologic intervention in cancer. In Amos, B. (Ed.): *Progress in Immunology*. New York, Acad Pr, 1971, pp. 1115–1129.

56. *Immunological Aspects of Neoplasia*. 26th Annual Symp. on Fund. Cancer Res. Houston. M.D. Anderson Hospital and Tumor Institute, 1973.

57. Apffel, C.A., and Peters, J.H.: Tumors and serum glycoproteins. The 'symbodies'. *Prog Exp Tumor Res, 12:*1–54, 1969.

58. Simmons, R.L., and Rios, A.: Immunotherapy of cancer: Immunospecific rejection of tumors in recipients of neuraminidase-treated cells plus BCG. *Science, 174:*591–593, 1971.

59. Cooperband, S.R., Davis, R.C., Schmid, K., and Mannick, J.A.: Competitive blockade of lymphocyte stimulation by a serum immunoregulatory alpha globulin (IRA). *Transplant Proc, 1:*516–523, 1969.

60. Kamrin, B.B.: Role of alpha globulins in immunosuppression: Reactive site occlusion hypothesis. *Transplant Proc, 1:*506–510, 1969.

61. Ashikawa, K., Inoue, K., Shimizu, T., and Ishibashi, Y.: An increase of serum alpha-globulin in tumor-bearing hosts and its immunological significance. *Jap J Exp Med, 41:*339–355, 1971.

62. Chase, P.S.: The effects of human serum frac-

tions on phytohemagglutinin- and concanavalin A-stimulated human lymphocyte cultures. *Cell Immunol, 5:*544–554, 1972.

63. Good, R.A., Peterson, R.D.A., Perey, D.Y., Finstad, J., and Cooper, M.D.: The immunological deficiency diseases in man: Consideration of some questions asked by these patients with an attempt at classification. In Good, R.A., and Bergsma, D. (Eds.): *Immunologic Deficiency Diseases in Man* (Birth Defects Original Article Series). New York, The National Foundation, 1968, pp. 17–39.

64. Good, R.A.: In Smith, R.T., and Landy, M. (Eds.): *Immune Surveillance*. New York, Acad Pr, 1970, pp. 439–451.

65. Waldemann, T.A., Strober, W., and Blaese, R.M.: Immunodeficiency disease and malignancy. *Ann Intern Med, 77:*605–628, 1972.

66. Benacerraf, B.: The genetic control of specific immune responses. In *The Harvey Lectures*. New York, Acad Pr, 1973, pp. 109–141.

67. McDevitt, H.O.: Genetic control of the antibody response. *Hosp Practice, 8:*61–74, 1973.

68. McDevitt, H.O., and Landy, M. (Eds.): *Genetic Control of Immune Responsiveness*. New York, Acad Pr, 1972, pp. 143–203.

69. Eichmann, K., Braun, D.C., and Krause, R.M.: Influence of genetic factors on the magnitude and the heterogeneity of the immune response in the rabbit. *J Exp Med, 134:*48–65, 1971.

70. Blomberg, B., Geckeler, W.R., and Weigert, M.: Genetics of the antibody response to dextran in mice. *Science, 177:*178–180, 1972.

71. Lynch, H.T., Krush, A.J., and Kaplan, A.: Cancer frequency among and within families. *Acta Genet Med Gemellol* (Roma), *21:*53–65, 1972.

72. Possible relationships between HL-A system and susceptibility to cancer in man. *Transplant Proc, 3:*1273–1325, 1971.

OCCURRENCE OF MALIGNANCY IN

IMMUNODEFICIENCY DISEASE*

RICHARD A. GATTI AND ROBERT A. GOOD

EVER SINCE PREHN and Main[1] demonstrated the presence of tumor-specific antigens in the late fifties, the association of malignancy and immunity has grown steadily more plausible as a mechanism for understanding oncogenesis. Tumor-specific antigens have now been demonstrated in a number of human malignancies.[2-8] In addition, it can be shown in many animal models that as immunity wanes with aging, the incidence of malignant tumors increases.[9-12] Further, certain forms of malignancy can be shown to occur with dramatically increased frequency in immunodeficient neonatally thymectomized rodents.[13-16] There is also evidence to support a decreasing immunologic vigor with aging in man,[17-21] a time when the incidence of cancer is on the rise. By far, the most convincing evidence for an association between oncogenesis and immunity, however, remains the fact that the frequency of malignancy in some patients with primary immunodeficiencies is roughly 10,000 times greater than that of the general age-matched population. Within the past 10 years, much progress has been made toward understanding immunologic mechanisms and diseases so that it is now possible to distinguish clearly between certain primary forms of immunodeficiency disease.[23,24,25] Almost every one of the primary immunologic abnormalities is associated with distinctive constellations of malignancy which, although there is much overlapping, give support to speculations concerning oncogenetic mechanisms.

*Portions of this material reprinted through Courtesy of Editor of *Cancer*.

Table 4-I comprises a survey of the literature on cancer in patients with immunodeficiency diseases.

The patients with infantile X-linked agammaglobulinemia (Bruton-type) lack humoral immunity. They do not make antibodies in response to antigenic stimulae, such as immunizations with diphtheria, tetanus, or typhoid antigen. Isohemagglutinin titers are absent. Immunoglobulin levels are extremely low. On the other hand, these children reject skin grafts and manifest delayed hypersensitivity skin reactions in normal fashion. Cell-mediated immunity is intact. When their lymphocytes are stimulated *in vitro* with phytohemagglutinin (PHA) or with allogeneic cells, the responses are normal. These children suffer mainly from infections with high-grade encapsulated pyogenic organisms such as pneumococcus, Haemophilus influenzae, streptococcus, meningococcus, and Pseudomonas aeruginosa.

Five patients with X-linked agammaglobulinemia have developed malignancy.[26-28] In each of these, the malignancy has involved the hematopoietic lymphoid system. Two children presented with tumors of the thymus gland[27] somewhat reminiscent of Furth and McEndy's work with mice strains with high incidences of spontaneous leukemia.[29,30] When these workers removed the thymus of mice, they prevented the development of leukemia. They also were able to demonstrate that the very earliest clones of malignant cells were seen first in the thymus. Further, Gorer presented evidence long ago that humoral immune responses seem to be of

TABLE 4-I
A LITERATURE SURVEY ON CANCER IN PATIENTS WITH IMMUNODEFICIENCY DISEASES*

	Estimated incidence of malignancy (percent)
A. Infantile X-linked agammaglobulinemia	5
1. Acute lymphocytic leukemia (Page 1963)	
2. Malignant lymphoma (Page 1963)	
3. Chronic monomyelogenous leukemia (Reisman 1964)	
4. Thymoma with leukemia (Good)	
5. Lymphatic leukemia (Good)	
B. III-IB Pharyngeal Pouch Syndrome in DeGeorge	—
C. Severe Combined Immunodeficiency (Gold and Freeman, 1965b)	5
1. Acute leukemia (Kadowaki 1965)	
2. Lymphosarcoma (Lamvik 1969)	
3. Hodgkin's Disease (von Bernuth 1970)	
D. Wiskott-Aldrich	10
1. Malignant reticuloendotheliosis (Coleman 1961)	
2. Malignant reticuloendotheliosis (Kildeberg 1961)	
3. Reticulum cell sarcoma (CPC 1962)	
4. Astrocytoma of brain (Amiet 1963)	
5. Malignant lymphoma (Pearson 1966)	
6. Lymphoma (Preason 1966)	
7. Myelogenous leukemia (Ten Bensel 1966)	
8. Malignant reticuloendotheliosis 9 (Ten Bensel 1966)	
9. Reticular lymphosarcoma (Radl 1967)	
10. Malignant reticulosis (Huber 1968)	
11. Malignant reticulosis of brain (Brand 1969)	
12. Leiomyosarcoma, multiple (Rupprecht 1970)	
13. Acute leukemia (Oppenheim 1970)	
E. Common Variable Immunodeficiency	10
1–2. Chronic lymphatic leukemia—2 sibs (Brem 1955)	
3. Chronic lymphatic leukemia (Hudson 1960)	
4. Lymphoma (Fudenberg 1961)	
5. Adenocarcinoma of stomach (Huizenga 1961)	
6. Malignant reticulosis (Pelkonen 1963)	
7. Lymphosarcoma (Green 1966)	
8. Rectosigmoid carcinoma (Hermans 1966)	
9. Adenocarcinoma of stomach (Hermans 1966)	
10–11. Non-lymphoid 2/176 (Lancet 1969)	
12–17. Lymphoreticular 6/176 (Lancet 1969)	
18. Lymphosarcoma (Douglas 1970)	
19. Carcinoma of breast (Hart)	
20. Carcinoma of bladder (Gatti)	
F. Isolated IgA deficiency	10
1. Gastric adenocarcinoma (Fraser 1970)	
G. Ataxia-telangiectasia	
1. Reticulum cell sarcoma (Boder 1963)	
2. Hodgkin's disease (Boder 1963)	
3. Undifferentiated round cell sarcoma (Boder 1963)	
4–6. Malignant lymphoma—3 sibs (Szanto 1963)	
7. Glioma (Young 1964)	
8. Ovarian dysgerminoma (Dunn 1964)	
9. Reticulum cell hyperplasia (Peterson 1964)	
10. Small cell hyperplasia (Peterson 1964)	
11. Reticulum cell sarcoma (Murphy 1965)	
12. Lymphoma (Rosenthal 1965)	
13. Cerebellar medulloblastoma (Shuster 1966)	
14. Leukemia (Fois 1966)	
15. Lymphosarcomatosis (Fois 1966)	
16–17. Acute lymphocytic leukemia—2 sibs (Hecht 1966)	
18. Lymphosarcoma (Smeby 1966)	
19. Reticulum cell lymphoma (Miller 1967)	
20. Hodgkin's lymphoma (Dugois 1967)	
21. Lymphosarcoma and tuberous sclerosis (Gotoff 1967)	
22. Leukemia (Harley 1966)	
23. Malignant lymphoma (Harley 1966)	

TABLE 4-I (CONTINUED)

	Estimated incidence of malignancy (percent)
24. Malignant lymphoma (Landing 1967)	
25. Hodgkin's disease (Morgan 1968)	
26. Reticulum cell lymphoma (Aguilar 1968)	
27–28. Gastric adenocarcinoma—2 sibs (Haerer 1969)	
29–30. Acute lymphoblastic leukemia—2 sibs (Lampert 1969)	
31–32. Lymphosarcoma—2 sibs (Castaigne 1969)	
33. Acute lymphoblastic leukemia (Taleb 1969)	
34–35. Lymphosarcoma—2 sibs (Ammann 1969)	
36. Reticulum cell sarcoma (Feigen 1970)	
37. Lymphoma (Arey 1970)	
38. Lymphoma (Boder 1970)	

* Reference numbers are stated in text.

prime importance in the defense against certain forms of mouse leukemias, suggesting that leukemogenesis requires not only a proper organ for differentiation and perhaps expansion of malignant clones but also an impaired humoral immune response.[31] On the other hand, Dupuy, *et al.*,[32] have shown that thymectomy has little effect on the development of Friend virus-induced leukemia in DBA mice. Here again, however, inadequate humoral immune responses were closely linked with leukemogenesis. The patients with infantile, X-linked agammaglobulinemia lack plasma cells. Differentiation of this line of lymphoid cells in chickens is dependent upon traffic of lymphoid stem cells through the bursa of Fabricius (a lymphoid structure in the gastrointestinal tract just anterior to the cloaca) early in development and is independent of thymic influence since this differentiation takes place equally well in thymectomized animals.[33,34] Peterson, *et al.*, in our laboratories, demonstrated that in chickens, removal of the bursa of Fabricius prevents the development of RPL-12-induced avian leukosis.[35] Similarly to Furth's observations, Dent, *et al.*, showed that the earliest clones of malignant cells were found in the bursa.[36] Unfortunately, this line of investigation cannot be pursued much further until the bursa of Fabricius or its homologues are identified in other animal classes.

The immunologic antithesis of infantile, X-linked aggammaglobulinemia is the DiGeorge syndrome in which humoral immunity is intact while cell-mediated immunity is absent. Failure of embryonic development of the third and fourth pharyngeal pouches lead to extremely small or absent thymuses in such patients. Plasma cells are present in normal numbers while small lymphocytes are often completely absent. Skin homografts are not rejected, delayed hypersensitivity skin responses are absent, and peripheral lymphocytes do not respond to stimulation with PHA or allogeneic cells *in vitro*. These infants also lack parathyroid glands and suffer from neonatal tetany. They die very early in life either from hypoparathyroidism or from overwhelming viral or fungal infections. To date, no cases of malignancy have been described in such patients.

Patients suffering from severe combined immunodeficiency (formerly called lymphopenic agammaglobulinemia of the Swiss or X-linked types) lack both humoral and cell-mediated forms of immunity, and, consequently, they are plagued by bacterial, viral, fungal, and protozoal infections. They also die in early infancy, seldom surviving much beyond the first year of life without therapy. Recently, bone marrow transplantation has made immunologic reconstitution of both lymphoid systems a reality, guaranteeing these children a normal, healthy life.[37,38] In spite of the rarity of this disease and the early deaths from infection, three reports of associated malignancies have appeared in the literature. In the first case, karyotypes of bone marrow cells taken shortly before death resembled the abnormal metaphases of acute leukemia.[39] Neoplasia in the second infant, a lymphosarcoma, was serendipitously diagnosed at postmortem examination at 6 months of age.[40] The third patient, only recently described, died at 5 months of age. Reovirus type 3 was isolated from lung tissue, and a Hodgkin's lymphoma was found.[41]

Until now, we have described primarily lymphoreticular malignancies associated with immunologic deficiencies. Among the patients with Wiskott-Aldrich disease, several nonlymphoid tumors are also found; however, the majority of malignancies seen in such patients is again of lymphoreticular origin.[42–53] These children suffer from severe recurrent bacterial infections, eczema, and thrombocytopenia. They seldom live beyond the age of puberty. Immunologically, IgM levels are very low, IgG levels are usually normal, and IgA levels may be normal but are often quite high. Recent reports indicate that IgE levels are also very much above normal in some of these patients.[54] Cell-mediated immunity is intact early in the course of the disease, but, with time, these children become anergic to delayed hypersensitivity skin tests and the *in vitro* lymphocyte responses to phytohemagglutinin, antigens, and allogeneic cells are depressed. Antibody responses to many antigens are normal; however, poor or absent responses to polysaccharide antigens are a hallmark of this form of immunodeficiency. Isohemagglutinin titers are usually low or absent. Such patients meet an early death either from overwhelming infection, massive bleeding secondary to the thrombocytopenia or malignancy. Roughly one in ten of these children die with malignancy, and it is entirely possible that with improved general pediatric care this incidence will actually rise. Platelet function, size, and metabolism are also abnormal in many of these patients.

A striking feature of this disease is the marked lymphadenopathy which persists for years. Probably the most striking example of this persistent, unexplainable lymphadenopathy recorded in the literature is a CPC describing a 20-year-old male who had suffered from 2 years of age with eczema, pustules, deep ulcers of the skin, frequent bleeding episodes, and recurrent otitis media.[45] Although megakaryocytes were present in the bone marrow in adequate numbers, platelet counts were often as low as 4700/mm[42] before splenectomy. Isohemagglutinin titers were extremely low. Shortly after a bout of staphylococcal pneumonia which resolved with gamma globulin and antibiotic therapy, the patient had his first febrile response to what in retrospect seems to have been the gamma globulin injection. Five months later, after extensive diagnostic testing including antigenic challenges with DNP-labeled bovine globulin, typhoid-paratyphoid, mumps, and DPT vaccines and A and B substances, gamma globulin administration was resumed. During the next 24 hours he noted swelling of the lymph nodes in the cervical, axillary, and inquinal areas, as well as feverishness and malaise. Ten days later, a similar syndrome was observed following another injection of 10 ml gamma globulin. Shortly thereafter, biopsy of one of the enlarged tender lymph nodes revealed reticulum cell hyperplasia. An inguinal node biopsied 5 months before had appeared normal. Massive lymphadenopathy and tenderness persisted and became immediately worse after two subsequent injections of 1 ml gamma globulin. At postmortem examination several months later, reticulum cell sarcoma was found which involved lymph nodes, gastrointestinal tract, liver, kidneys, skin, and periadrenal tissue. One is tempted in such patients to biopsy these enlarged lymph nodes. In the few instances where we have biopsied such nodes, the histology suggested only chronic antigenic stimulation and showed no evidence of malignant changes. Eventually, however, a number of these children have developed lymphoreticular malignancies.

Chronic antigenic stimulation followed by frank malignancy is also seen in certain patients with the "common variable" form of immunodeficiency (formerly called "late-onset, acquired, sporadic hypo-or dysgammaglobulinemia").[55-65] In these patients, intestinal lymphadenopathy is often found in association with Giardia lamblia infections; a few of these patients have later developed carcinomas of the stomach or rectum.[61] Benign follicular lymphoma has also been a problem to some patients with this form of immunodeficiency.[55,66-70] In the family of one patient with the "common variant" form of immunodeficiency associated with chronic lymphoid hyperplasia, several members died of systemic lupus erythematosis (in an uncle a benign thymoma was discovered at postmortem examination), one died of Hodgkin's disease, two others had idiopathic thrombocytopenia, several members suffered with rheumatoid arthritis, regional ileitis, or erythema multiforme, and three members have had prolonged fevers of unknown origins. Three additional family members have been found to have different forms of so-called dysgammaglobulinemia.[69,70]

This group of patients with the "common variant" form of immunologic deficiency accounts for the largest number of immunodeficiency patients, hence, the new name.[23] However, the group is not a homogeneous one and probably includes a number of yet unsorted immunodeficiencies.[24] In general, immunoglobulin levels are very low, and

cell-mediated immune responses are usually intact until late in the course of the disease. Eventually, most of these patients lose their ability to manifest vigorous skin hypersensitivity responses, and lymphocyte responses to phytohemagglutinin and other *in vitro* stimuli also become depressed. It is at this stage that lymphoid hyperplasia is most frequently observed. As can be seen in Table 4-I, lymphoid malignancies again outnumber other types of malignancy in this form of immunodeficiency while the incidence of both lymphoid and nonlymphoid malignancies is far in excess of that in the general age-matched population.

Of further interest is the observation that selective deficiency of IgA has been associated in four instances with gastric adenocarcinoma. Two of these patients had generalized hypogammaglobulinemia,[61] one had ataxia-telangiectasia[71] with typically low IgA levels, and the fourth patient had an isolated IgA deficiency.[72] In a fifth patient with ataxiatelangiectasia associated with gastric adenocarcinoma, the IgA levels were not studied but were most likely low as is commonly found in this disease.[71] The patients with ataxia-telangiectasia were young adults, and, even more strikingly, they were siblings. In general, individuals with isolated IgA deficiency do not suffer from any particular maladies; indeed, the incidence of isolated IgA deficiency in the general population is approximately 1:700. When disease is present, however, it takes the form of sino-pulmonary infections, a sprue-like syndrome, or autoimmune disorders. The association of IgA deficiency and gastric carcinoma deserves further attention and may be related to the inability of IgA molecules to fix complement. Pernicious anemia and malfunction of the gastric intestinal mucosa have been frequently described in association with agammaglobulinemia and hypogammaglobulinemia.[61,73,74] Thus far, however, similar evidence of gastrointestinal malfunction preceding gastric or intestinal malignancy has not been described in association with isolated absence of IgA. Such a study would seem worthwhile.

Ataxia-telangiectasia is a neurologic disease of childhood which begins with ataxia sometimes as early as 6 months of age; telangiectasias over the ears and eyes often become apparent several years thereafter. Immunologically, these children usually have low IgA levels and varying inadequacies of their cell-mediated immunity. At postmortem examination, Hassall's corpuscles are not seen in the thymus of such patients suggesting that their deficient cell-mediated immune responses are an integral part of this disease. The incidence of cancer in these children is again remarkably high; at least 10 percent die with malignancy.[71,75-100] Probably the most provocative characteristic of this group of malignancies is that in six families more than one sibling with ataxia-telangiectasia has developed the same type of cancer.[71,76,80,88,89,98] We have already mentioned the occurrence of so rare a tumor as gastric adenocarcinoma in two Negro sisters, 19 and 21 years of age. In another family, 3 siblings developed malignant lymphoma over a period of less than 2 years. In none of these families did other siblings not affected with ataxia-telangiectasia develop malignancies of any kind.

Chromosomal breaks and other karyotypic abnormalities are fairly common in patients with ataxia-telangiectasia with or without malignancy and have also been observed in some patients with Wiskott-Aldrich disease and in a child with Bruton-type agammaglobulinemia associated with chronic monomyelogenous leukemia. On the other hand, karyotypes of a number of immunodeficiency patients with cancer have been normal. This relationship also deserves further study, however, since patients with Bloom's syndrome[101] and Fanconi's anemia, both diseases in which chromosomal breaks

are common, have a similarly high incidence of malignancy. Todaro, *et al.*[102] have described an increased susceptibility of the fibroblasts of such patients to *in vitro* malignant transformation with SV_{40} virus. By contrast, fibroblasts of patients with primary immunodeficiencies did not show such susceptibility to transformation with SV_{40} virus suggesting that the increased frequency of malignancy seen in these patients is related to an abnormality of host surveillance mechanisms.[103]

The role of immunity in oncogenesis seems even more plausible in light of the recent demonstration of a blocking effect of the serum of patients with neuroblastoma on the capability of sensitized lymphocytes to kill target neuroblastoma cells *in vitro*.[5] This blocking effect is no longer present after all immunoglobulins have been absorbed from the serum.[104] This work has now been extended, and the presence of blocking antibodies in a number of other solid tumors from patients as well as in methylcholanthrene-induced tumors in mice has been demonstrated.[105] The lymphocytes of patients with neuroblastoma appear to be quite capable of destroying the tumor cells in the absence of serum from patients with neuroblastoma. While blocking antibody now appears to play a major role in the oncogenesis of solid tumors, its role in the production of lymphoid tumors has not yet been demonstrated. The absence of cancers of epithelial origin in immunodeficiency patients who are incapable of antibody production in response to specific antigens, such as those with Bruton-type agammaglobulinemia and the severe combined immunodeficiencies, supports the hypothesis of Hellstrom, *et al.*[5,104] and further suggests that production of blocking antibodies may not be so important in the formation of leukemias. Indeed, as suggested earlier, antibodies may constitute the main defense mechanism against this form of cancer.

We have recently demonstrated an inhibitor of lymphocyte response to phytohemagglutinin in the plasma of 60 percent of patients with various types of solid tumors.[106] These studies were performed prior to any treatment. Similar plasma inhibitors of *in vitro* lymphocyte responses have been described in ataxia-telangiectasia[107] and in Hodgkin's disease,[108] as well as in tuberculosis,[109] syphilis,[110] multiple sclerosis,[111] and hepatitis.[112] Their role in oncogenesis remains unclear. Our studies on the plasma inhibitor of patients with solid tumors originated from a prior survey of lymphocyte responses to phytohemagglutinin (PHA) in these patients in which we found markedly depressed PHA responses in 70 of 104 patients, as compared to age-matched controls.[113,106] This finding was not surprising in light of many previous studies demonstrating deficiencies of allograft rejection capacity and delayed hypersensitivity skin responses in cancer patients.[114-118]

Another set of observations which deserves comment relates to the unusually high incidence of malignancy among renal transplant recipients who have been maintained on immunosuppressants for prolonged periods of time.[119] Approximately 40 of these patients have developed *de novo* malignancies; of these, 23 have been of epithelial origin while only 17 were lymphoreticular.[120,121] The most common tumor among this group of patients has been reticulum cell sarcoma; however, the majority of malignancies has been epithelial and not lymphoid as suggested by others.

In this same group of patients, a number of cancers have been inadvertently transplanted from the kidney donor.[122] These have included cancers of breast,[123] lung,[124,70] liver,[125] kidney,[126] thyroid,[127] and larynx.[128] The fascinating observation here has been that when immunosuppression was discontinued the cancers have regressed and have been conspicuously absent at postmortem examination in several cases. In only one instance has regression of a supposedly *de novo* malignancy occurred following discontinuance of immunosuppression; the patient received a kidney from an 8-year-old donor who had died following a fall from a bicycle.[18] The recipient later developed an ovarian dysgerminoma and when she discontinued her immunosuppression, unbeknown to her physicians, the transplanted kidney was rejected and the cancer disappeared. The kidney donor, however, was female so that one cannot be certain that this was truly a *de novo* malignancy. One also cannot exclude the possibility that the immunosuppressed patient could have been sufficiently reactive to a *de novo* tumor to have contributed immunologically to its elimination.

Recent experiences with anti-lymphocyte globulin (ALG) preparations have also added further evidence to an association of immune functions with oncogenesis. Allison and Law[13] have demonstrated a marked increase in the incidence of viral-induced tumors in mice treated with ALG as compared to untreated controls, while Deodhar, *et al.*[129] have reported the appearance of a reticulum cell sarcoma of the buttock at the site of 37 injections of ALG over a period of 8 weeks. Again, these findings are hardly surprising in light of many previous studies showing enhanced tumor development in neonatally thymectomized animals.[13-16]

Summary

The incidence of malignancy in some patients with primary immunodeficiencies is roughly 10,000 times that of the general age-matched population. It is apparent from this review of the literature that each type of immunodeficiency has a distinctive constellation of malignancies associated with it. In light of studies demonstrating both immunologically aggressive lymphocytes and the presence of blocking antibodies or antigen-antibody complexes in the blood of neuroblastoma patients, a major role for immunity in oncogenesis seems almost certain. However, the unusual preponderance of lymphoid malignancies among immunodeficient patients suggests that factors other than a faulty immunosurveillance mechanism are involved.

Addendum

To facilitate collection and analysis of data related to this problem, an Immunodeficiency-Cancer Registry was established in 1971 at the recommendation of the World Health Organization Committee on Primary Immunodeficiency Disease. Forms for communication of pertinent data will be sent upon request to physicians who know of cases of primary immunodeficiency and cancer. Write to: Dr. John Kersey, University of Minnesota, 184 M Jackson Hall, Minneapolis, Minn., 55455, or Dr. Robert A. Good, Sloan-Kettering Institute, 410 E. 68th Street, New York, N.Y. 10021.

REFERENCES

1. Prehn, R.T., and Main, J.M.: Immunity to methylcholanthrene-induced sarcomas, *J Natl Cancer Inst, 18:*769–778, 1957.

2. Gold, P., and Freedman, S.O.: Demonstration of tumor-specific antigens in human colonic carcinomata by immunological tolerance and absorption techniques. *J Exp Med 121:*439–462, 1965a.

3. Gold, P., and Freedman, S.O.: Specific carcinoembryonic antigens of the human digestive system. *J Exp Med, 122:*467–481, 1965b.

4. Helstrom, I., Hellstrom, K.E., Pierce, G.E., and Bill, A.H.: Demonstration of cell-bound and humoral immunity against neuroblastoma cells. *Proc Acad Sci USA, 60:*1231–1238, 1968.

5. Hellstrom, I., and Hellstrom, K.E., Pierce, G.E., and Yang, J.P.S.: Cellular and humoral immunity to different types of human neoplasma. *Nature, 220:*1352, 1968.

6. Henle, G., and Henle, W.: Immunofluorescence in cells derived from Burkitt's lymphoma. *J Bacteriol, 91:*1248, 1966.

7. Morton, D., and Malmgren, R.A.: Human osteosarcoma: Immunologic evidence suggesting an associate infectious agent. *Science, 162:*1279–1281, 1968.

8. Morton, D.L., Malmgren, R.A., and Holmes, E.C.: Demonstration of antibodies against human malignant melanoma by immunofluorescence. *Surgery, 64:*233–240, 1968.

9. Stjernswärd, J.: Age-dependent tumor-host barrier and effect of carcinogen-induced immunodepression on rejection of iso-grafted methylcholanthrene-induced sarcoma cells. *J Natl Cancer Inst, 37:*505–512, 1966.

10. Teller, M.N., Mikell, M., and Freeman, J.J.: Growth of human tumor H. Ep. #3 in nonconditioned Swiss mice. *Proc Amer Ass Cancer Res, 3:*273, 1961.

11. Teller, M.N., Stohr, G., Curlett, W., Kubisek, M.L., and Curtis, D.: Aging and cancerigenesis. I. Immunity to tumor and skin grafts. *J Natl Cancer Inst, 33:*649–656, 1964.

12. Wigzell, H., and Sternsward, J.: Age-dependent rise and fall of immunological reactivity in the CBA mouse. *J Natl Cancer Inst, 37:*513–517, 1966.

13. Allison, A.C., and Law, L.W.: Effects of anti-lymphocyte serum on virus oncogenesis. *Proc Soc Exp Biol Med, 127:*207–212, 1968.

14. Defendi, V.: Induction of tumors by polyoma in adult hamsters. *Nature, 188:*518, 1960.

15. Gaugas, J.M., Chesterman, F.C., Hvisch, M.S., Rees, R.J.W., Harvey, J.J., and Gilchrist, C.: Unexpected high incidence of tumours in thymectomized mice treated with anti-lymphocyte globulin and Mycobacterium leprae. *Nature, 221:*1033–1036, 1969.

16. Miller, J.F.A.P., Ting, R.C., and Law, L'.W.: Influence of thymectomy on tumor induction by polyoma virus in C57B1 mice. *Proc Soc Exp Biol Med, 116:*323–328, 1964.

17. Cammarata, R.J., Rodnan, G.P., and Fennell, R.H.: Serum anti-T-globulin and anti-nuclear factors in the aged. *JAMA, 199:* 455–458, 1967.

18. Gatti, R.A., and Good, R.A.: Aging, immunity, and malignancy. *Geriatrics, 25:*158–168, 1970.

19. Giannini, D., and Sloan, R.S.: A tuberculin survey of 1285 adults with special reference to the elderly. *Lancet, I:*525–527, 1957.

20. Litwin, S.D., and Singer, J.M.: Studies of the incidence and significance of anti-gamma-globulin factors in the aging. *Arthritis Rheum, 8:*538–550, 1965.

21. Pisciotta, A.V., Westring, D.W., DePrey, D., and Walsh, B.: Mitogenic effect of phyto-hemagglutinin at different ages. *Nature, 215:*193–194, 1967.

22. Gatti, R.A., and Good, R.A.: Immunological deficiency disease. In Meier, A.E., and Hotchkiss, D.J. (Eds.): *Medical Clinics of North America.* Philadelphia, Saunders, *54:*281–307, 1970.

23. Fudenberg, H.H., *et al:* Classification of the primary immune deficiencies: WHO recommendations. *Pediat, 47:*927, 1971.

24. Gatti, R.A., and Seligmann, M.: The primary immunodeficiency diseases: Classification, pathogenesis and treatment. *J Pediat, (Turkey) 15:*195–215, 1973.

25. Good, R.A., and Finstad, J.: The association of lymphoid malignancy and immuno-logic functions. In Zarafonetis, C. (Ed.): *Proc of the International Conference on Leukemia-Lymphoma.* Philadelphia, Lea and Febiger, 1968, pp. 175–197.

26. Good, R.A.: Unpublished observations.

27. Page, A.R., Hansen, A.E., and Good, R.A.: Occurrence of leukemia and lymphoma in patient with agammaglobulinemia. *Blood, 21:*197–206, 1963.

28. Reisman, L.E., Mitani, M., and Zuelzer, W.W.: Chromosome studies in leukemia. *New Engl J Med, 270:*591–597, 1964.

29. Furth, J., Kunii, A., Ioachim, H., Sanel, F.T., and Moy, P.: Parallel observations on the role of the thymus in leukogenesis, immunocompetence and lymphopoiesis, in The Thymus: Experimental and Clinical Studies. CIBA Foundation Symposium, G.E.W. Wolstenhome and R. Porter, Eds. Boston, Little, 1966, pp. 288–309.

30. McEndy, D.P., Boon, M.C., and Furth, J.: On the role of the thymus, spleen, and gonads in the development of leukemia in a high-leukemia stock of mice. *Cancer Res, 4:*377–383, 1944.

31. Gorer, P.A., and Amos, D.B.: Possible immunity in mice against C57B1 leukosis EL4 by means of isoimmune serum. *Cancer Res, 16:*388, 1956.

32. Dupuy, J.M., Stutman, O., and Good, R.A.: Unpublished observations.

33. Cooper, M.D., Peterson, R.D.A., and Good, R.A.: Delineation of the thymic and bursal lymphoid systems in the chicken. *Nature, 205:*142–146, 1965.

34. Cooper, M.D., Peterson, R.D.A., South, M.A., and Good, R.A.: Functions of the thymus system and the bursa system in the chicken. *J Exp Med, 123:*75–102, 1966.

35. Peterson, R.D.A., Burmester, B.R., Frederickson, T.M., Purchase, H.G., and Good, R.A.: The effect of bursectomy and thymectomy on the development of visceral lymphomatosis in the chicken. *J Natl Cancer Inst, 32:*1343, 1964.

36. Dent, P.B., Cooper, M.D., Payne, L.N., Solomon, J., Burmester, B.R., and Good, R.A.: The pathogenesis of avian lymphoid leukosis. II. Immunological reactivity during lymphomagenesis. *J Natl Cancer Inst, 41:*391–401, 1968.

37. Gatti, R.A., Meuwissen, H.J., Allen, H.D., Hong, R., and Good, R.A.: Immunologic reconstitution of sex-linked lymphopenic immunologic deficiency. *Lancet, 2:*1366–1369, 1968.

38. De Koning, J., Dooren, L.J., van Bekkum, D.W., van Rood, J.J., Dicke, K.A., and Radl, J.: Transplantation of bone marrow cells and foetal thymus in an infant with lymphopenic immunological deficiency. *Lancet, 1:*1223–1227, 1969.

39. Kadowaki, J.I., Thompson, R.I., Zuelzer, W.W., Woolley, P.V., Brough, A.J., and Gruber, D.: XX/XY lymphoid chimaerism in congenital immunological deficiency syndrome with thymic alymphopasia. *Lancet, 2:*1152–1156, 1965.

40. Lamvlk, J., and Moc, P.J.: Thymic dysplasia with immunological deficiency. *Acta Pathol Microbiol Scand, 76:*349–360, 1969.

41. Von Bermuth, G., Minielly, J.A., Logan, G.B., and Gleich, G.J.: Hodgkin's disease and thymic alymphoplasia in a 5-month-old infant. *Pediatrics, 45:*792–799, 1970.

42. Amiet, A.: Aldrich's syndrome: A report of two cases. *Ann Pediatr, 201:*315, 1963.

43. Brand, M.M., and Marinkovich, V.A.: Primary malignant reticulosis of the brain in Wiskott-Aldrich syndrome. Report of a case. *Arch Dis Child, 44:*536–542, 1969.

44. Chaptal, J., *et al.:* Syndrome de Wiskott-Aldrich avec Survie Prolongee (9 ans). *Arch Fr Pediatr, 23:*907–920, 1966.

45. Clinicopathological Conference: Rademacher's disease. *Am J Med, 32:*80–95, 1962.

46. Coleman, A., Leikin, S., and Guin, G.H.: Aldrich's syndrome. *Clin Proc Child Hosp* (Wash.), *17:*22–27, 1961.

47. Huber, J.: Experience with various immunologic deficiencies in Holland. In Immunologic Deficiency Diseases in Man, R.A. Good and D. Bergsma, Eds. *Birth Defects Original Article Series,* vol. 4, New York, *13:*200, 1960.

48. Kildeberg, P.: A case of Aldrich's syndrome. *Acta Paediatr. Suppl, 140:*120–121, 1961.

49. Oppenheim, J.J., Blaese, R.M., and Waldmann, T.A.: Defective lymphocyte transformation and delayed hypersensitivity in Wiskott-Aldrich syndrome. *J Immunol, 104:*835–844, 1970.

50. Pearson, H.A., Shulman, N.R., Oski, F.A., and Eitzman, D.V.: Platelet survival in Wiskott-Aldrich syndrome. *J Pediatr, 68:* 754–760, 1966.

51. Radl, J., Masopust, J., Houstek, J., and Hrodek, O.: Paraproteinanemia and unusual dys-gamma-globulinemia in a case of Wiskott-Aldrich syndrome. An immunochemical study. *Arch Dis Child, 42:*608–614, 1967.

52. Rupprecht, L., and Huff, D.: In preparation.

53. Ten Bensel, R.W., Stadlan, E.M., and Krivit, W.: The development of malignancy in the course of the Aldrich syndrome. *J Pediatr, 68:*761–767, 1966.

54. Polmar, S.H., Lischner, H.W., Huang, N.N., Waldmann, T.A., and Terry, W.D.: IgE levels in immunological deficiency states. *Clin Res, 18:*431, 1970 (Abstr.).

55. Brem, T.H., and Morton, M.E.: Defective serum gamma globulin formation. *Ann Intern Med, 43:*465–479, 1955.

56. Douglas, S.D., Goldberg, L.S., and Fudenberg, H.H.: Clinical, serologic, and leukocyte function studies on patients with idiopathic "acquired" agammaglobulinemia and their families. *Am J Med, 48:*48–53, 1970.

57. Fudenberg, H., and Solomon, A.: Acquired agammaglobulinemia in autoimmune hemolytic disease: Graft-vs-host reaction? *Vox Sang, 6:*68–79, 1961.

58. Gatti, and Good, R.A.: To be published.

59. Green, I., Litwin, S., Adlersberg, R., and Rubin, I.: Hypogammablobulinemia with late development of lymphosarcoma. *Arch Intern Med, 118:*592–602, 1966.

60. Hart, T., and Good, R.A.: To be published.

61. Hermans, P.E., Huizenga, K.A., Hoffman, H.N., Brown, A.J., and Markowitz, H.: Dysgammaglobulinemia associated with nodular lymphoid hyperplasia of small intestine. *Am J Med, 40:*78–89, 1966.

62. Hudson, R.P., and Wilson, S.J.: Hypogammaglobulinemia and chronic lymphatic leukemia. Cancer National Foundation Press. 1968, pp. 53–66.

63. Huizenga, D.A., Wollaeger, E.E., Green, P.A., and McKenzie, B.F.: Serum globulin deficiencies in nontrotical sprue, with report of two cases of acquired agammablobulinemia. *Am J Med, 31:*572, 1961.

64. Hypogammaglobulinemia in the United Kingdom. Summary Report of a Medical Research Council Working-Pary. *Lancet, 1:* 163–168, 1969.

65. Pelkonen, R., Siurala, M., and Vuopio, P.: Inherited agammaglobulinemia with malabsorption and marked alterations in the

gastrointestinal mucosa. *Acta Med Scand, 173:*549–555, 1963.

66. Latimer, E.O., Fitzsimmons, E.J., and Rhoads, P.S.: Hypogammaglobulinemia associated with a severe wound infection. *JAMA, 158:*1344–1347, 1955.

67. Martin, C.M., Gordon, R.S., and McCullough, D.B.: Acquired hypogammaglobulinemia in adult: report of case, with clinical and experimental studies. *New Engl J Med, 254:*449–456, 1956.

68. Van Gelder, D.W.: Clinical significance of alterations in gamma globulin levels. *South Med J, 50:*43–50, 1957.

69. Wolf, J.K.: Primary acquired agammaglobulinemia with a family history of collagen disease and hematologic disorders. *New Engl J Med, 266:*473–479, 1962.

70. Wolf, J.K., Gokcen, M., and Good, R.A.: Heredo-familial disease of the mesenchymal tissue: Clinical and laboratory study one family. *J Lab Clin Med, 61:*230–248, 1963.

71. Haerer, F., Jackson, J.F., and Evers, C.G.: Ataxia-telangiectasia with gastric adenocarcinoma. *JAMA, 210:*1884–1887, 1969.

72. Fraser, K.J., and Rankin, J.G.: Selective deficiency of IgA immunoglobulins associated with carcinoma of the stomach. *Aust Ann Med, 2:*165–167, 1970.

73. Twomey, J.J., Jordan, P.H., Jarrold, T., Trubowitz, S., Ritz, N.D., and Conn, H.O.: The syndrome of immunoglobulin deficiency and pernicious anemia. *Am J Med, 47:*340–350, 1969.

74. Twomey, J.J., Jordan, P.H., Laughter, A.H., Meuwissen, H.J., and Good, R.A.: The gastric disorder in immunoglobulin deficient patients. *Ann Intern Med, 72:*499–504, 1970.

75. Aguilar, M.J., Kamoshita, S., Landing, B.H., Boder, E., and Sedgwick, R.P.: Pathological observations in ataxia-telangiectasia. A report on 5 cases. *J Neuropathol Exp Neurol, 27:*659, 1968.

76. Ammann, A.J., Good, R.A., Bier, D., and Fudenberg, H.H.: Long-term plasma infusions in patients with ataxia-telangiectasia and deficient IgA and IgE. *Pediatrics, 44:*672–676, 1969.

77. Arey, J.B., and DiGeorge, A.: Person communication.

78. Boder, E.: In discussion following paper by Peterson, *et al., J Pediatr, 63:*702–703, 1963.

79. Boder, E., and Sedgwick, R.P.: Ataxia-telangiectasia. In: Handbook of Clinical Neurology. Eds. P.J. Vinken and G.W. Brayn. North-Holland Publ. Amsterdam, 1972. Vol. 13. Pp. 267–339.

80. Castaigne, P., Cambier, J., and Brunet, P.: Ataxia-telamgiectasies, desordres immutaires, lymphosarcomatose terminale chez deux freres. *La Presse Med, 77:*347, 1969.

81. Dugois, P., Ambilard, P., and Imbert, R.: Ataxie telangiectasie et maladie de Hodgkin (A propos d'une observation). *Bull Soc Fran Derm Syph, 74:*507, 1967.

82. Dunn, H.G., Meuwissen, H., Livingstone, C.S., and Pump, K.K.: Ataxia-telangiectasia. *Can Med Asso J, 91:*1106–1118, 1964.

83. Feigin, R.D., Vietti, T.J., Wyatt, R.G., Kaufman, D.G., and Smith, C.H.: Ataxia-telangiectasia with granulocytopenia. *J Pediatr, 77:*431–438, 1970.

84. Fois, A.: Resentazione di 4 casi di atassia telangiectasia. *Riv Clin Pediatr, 77:*250, 1966.

85. Gofoff, S.P., Amirmokri, E., and Liebner, E.J.: Ataxia-telangiectasia: neoplasia, untoward response to x-irradiation and tuberous sclerosis. *Am J Dis Child, 144:*617–619, 1967.

86. Harley, R.D., Baird, H.W., and Crawen, E.M.: Ataxia-telangiectasia. Report of 7 cases. *Arch Ophthalmol, 77:*582–592, 1957.

87. Harley, R.D., Baird, H.W., and Muffett, E.A.: Ataxia-telangiectasia. Report of 7 cases. Read before the Ophthalmology Section, A.M.A., Chicago, June, 1966.

88. Hecht, F., *et al.:* Leukemia and lymphocytes in ataxia-telangiectasia. *Lancet, 2:*1193, 1966.

89. Lampert, F.: Akute lymphoblastische Leukämie bei geschwistern mit progressiver Kleinhiruataxia (Louis-Bar Syndrome). *Dsch Med Wochenschr, 94:*217–220, 1969.

90. Landing, B.H.: Unpublished data.

91. Miller, D.G.: Association of immune disease

and malignant lymphoma. *Ann Intern Med,* *66:*511, 1967.

92. Morgan, J.L., Holcomb, T.M., and Morrissey, R.W.: Radiation reaction in ataxia-telangiectasia. *Am J Dis Child, 116:*557, 1968.

93. Murphy, M.L., and O'Neal, M.: Malformations observed in children's cancer population. Presented at Annual Meeting of the Teratology Society, San Francisco, California, May 27, 1965.

94. Peterson, R.D.A., Kelly, W.D., and Good, R.A.: Ataxia-telangiectasia, its association with defective thymus, immunologic deficiency disease and malignancy. *Lancet, 1:*1189–1193, 1964.

95. Rosenthal, I.M., Markowitz, A.S., and Medenis, R.: Immunologic incompetence in ataxia-telangiectasia. *Am J Dis Child, 110:* 69, 1965.

96. Shuster, J., Hart, Z., Stimson, C.W., Brough, A.J., and Poulik, M.D.: Ataxia-telangiectasia with cerebellar tumor. *Pediatrics, 37:* 776, 1966.

97. Smeby, B.: Ataxia-telangiectasia. *Acta Paediatr* (Stockholm), *55:*239–243, 1966.

98. Szanto, P.B.: Personal communication.

99. Taleb, N., Tohme, S., Chostine, S., Barmada, B., and Nahas, S.: Association d'une ataxie-telangiectasie avec une leucemie aigue lympho-blastique. *Presse Med, 77:* 345–346, 1969.

100. Young, R.R., Austen, K.F., and Moser, H.W.: Abnormalities of serum gamma-1-A globulin and ataxia telangiectasia, *Medicine, 43:*423–433, 1964.

101. Bloom, G.E., Warner, S., Gerald, P.S., and Diamond, L.K.: Chromosome abnormalities in constitutional aplastic anemia. *New Engl J Med, 274:*8–14, 1966.

102. Todaro, G.J., Green, H., and Swift, M.R.: Susceptibility of human diploid fibroblast strains to transformation by SV_{40} virus, *Science, 153:*1252–1253, 1966.

103. Kersey, J.H., Gatti, R.A., Good, R.A., Aaronson, S.A., and Todaro, G.J.: Susceptibility of cells from patients with primary immunodeficiency diseases to transformation by Simian virus 40. *Proc Nat Acad Sci (USA), 69:*980–982, 1972.

104. Hellstrom, I., Hellstrom, K.E., and Sjogren, H.O.: Serum mediated inhibition of cellular immunity to methylcholanthrene-induced murine sarcomas, *Cell Immunol, 1:*18–30, 1970.

105. Hellstrom, K.E., and Hellstrom, I.: Immunologic defenses against cancer. *Hosp Prac, 5.*45–61, 1970.

106. Gatti, R.A., Garrioch, D.B., and Good, R.A.: Depressed PHA responses in patients with non-lympoid malignancies. In Harris, J. (Ed.): Proc. of the Fifth Leukocyte Culture Conference. Acad Pr, New York, 1970, pp. 339–355.

107. McFarlin, D.E., and Oppenheim, J.J.: Impaired lymphocyte transformation in ataxia-telangiectasia in part due to a plasma inhibitory factor. *J Immunol, 103:* 1212, 1969.

108. Trubowittz, S., Masek, B., and Del Rosario, A.: Lymphocyte response to PHA in Hodgkin's disease, lymphatic leukemia and lymphosarcoma. *Cancer, 19:*2019, 1966.

109. Heilman, D.H., and Macfarland, W.: Inhibition of tuberculin-induced mitogenesis in cultures of lymphocytes from tuberculous donors. *Int Arch Allergy, 30:*58, 1966.

110. Levene, G.M., Turk, J.L., Wright, D.J.m., and Grimble, A.G.S.: Reduced lymphocyte transformation due to a plasma factor in patients with active syphilis. *Lancet, 2:*246, 1969.

111. Knowles, M., Hughes, D., Caspary, E.A., and Field, E.J.: Lymphocyte transformation in multiple sclerosis: inhibition of unstimulated thymidine uptake by a serum

112. Paronetto, F., and Popper, H.: Lymphocyte stimulation induced by halothan in patients with posthalothan hepatitis. *New Engl J Med, 283:*277–280, 1970

113. Garrioch, D.B., Good, R.A., and Gatti, R.A.: Lymphocyte response to PHA in patients with non-lymphoid tumours. *Lancet, 1:* 618, 1970.

114. Black, M.M.: Immunology of cancer. *Surg Gynec Obstet, 109:*105–106, 1959.

115. Black, M.M., Kerpe, S., and Speer, F.C.: Lymph node structure in patients with cancer of breast. *Am J Pathol, 29:*505–521, 1953.

116. Good, R.A., Kelly, W.D., Rotstein, J., and

Varco, R.L.: Immunological deficiency disease, agammaglobulinemia, hypogammaglobulinemia, Hodgkin's disease and sarcoidosis. In Kallos, P., and Waksman, B.H. (Eds.): *Progress In Allergy.* New York, Karger, 1962, pp. 187–319, vol. 6.

117. Grace, J.T., and Kondo, T.: Investigations of host resistance in cancer patients. *Ann Surg, 148:*633–641, 1958.

118. Logan, J.: The delayed type of allergic reaction in cancer: altered response to tuberculin and mumps virus. *NZ Med J, 55:*408, 1956.

119. McKhann, C.F.: Primary malignancy in patients undergoing immunosuppression for renal transplantation. *Transplantation, 8:* 209–212, 1969.

120. Penn, I., Halgrimson, C.G., and Starzl, T.E.: *De novo* malignant tumors in organ transplant recipients. *Transplantation Proc.*

121. Starzl, T.E., Penn, I., and Halgrimson, C.G.: Immunosuppression and malignant neoplasma. *New Engl J Med, 283:*934, 1970.

122. Wilson, R.E., Hager, E.B., Hampers, C.L., Corson, J.M., Merrill, J.P., and Murray, J.E.: Immunologic rejection of human carrier transplanted with a renal allograft, *New Engl J Med, 278:*479, 1968.

123. MacLean, L.D., Dossetor, J.B., Gault, M.H., Oliver, J.A., Inglis, F.G., and Mackinnon, K.J.: Renal homotransplantation using cadaver donors. *Arch Surg, 91:*288, 1965.

124. Martin, D.C., Rubini, M., and Rosen, V.J.: Cadaver in renal homotransplantation with inadvertent transplantation of carcinoma. *JAMA, 192:*752, 1965.

125. Zukoski, C.F., Killen, D.A., Ginn, E., Matter, B., Lucas, D.O., and Seigler, H.F.: Transplanted carcinoma in an immunosuppressed patient. *Transplantation, 9:*71–74, 1970.

126. Hume, D.M.: Progress in clinical renal homotransplantation. *Adv Surg, 2:*419, 1966.

127. Muiznieks, H.W., Berg, J.W., Lawrence, W., and Randall, H.T.: Suitability of donor kidneys from patients with cancer. *Surgery, 64:*871, 1968.

128. McPhaul, J.J., and McIntosh, D.A.: Tissue transplantation still vexes. *New Engl J Med, 272:*105, 1965.

129. Deodhar, S.D., Kuklinca, A.G., Vidt, D.G., Robertson, A.L., and Hazard, J.B.: Development of reticulum-cell sarcoma at the site of antilymphocyte injection in a patient with renal transplant. *New Engl J Med, 280:*1104–1106, 1969.

CHAPTER 5

HISTOCOMPATIBILITY

IN CANCER

MITSUO TAKASUGI, LAWRENCE KRAIN AND PAUL I. TERASAKI

Histocompatibility Antigens

HISTOCOMPATIBILITY HAD ITS beginnings in early cancer research.[1] Spontaneously arising tumors in experimental animals were transplanted to other animals of the same species when death of the primary host was imminent. The sporadic success of tumor passage from animal to animal soon led to the realization that host genetic factors were of direct importance in the acceptance or rejection of transplanted tumors. This eventually led to the genetic theory of transplantation[2] and the development of inbred strains of mice.[3] Through a brilliant series of studies by Gorer from 1937 to 1942, the importance of histocompatibility or transplantation antigens in tumor rejection was demonstrated.[4] He showed the importance of genetically determined alloantigens (isoantigens) controlled by the H-2 locus on both normal and tumor transplants and the presence of specific antibodies following graft rejection. The demonstration of antibodies supplied serological reagents which allowed Gorer, Snell,[5,6] and others to begin unraveling the complex relationship of antigens controlled by the H-2 locus in mice. The elucidative approach used was to detect antigens with antiserum prepared in inbred isogenic lines controlled for identity of histocompatibility antigens within each strain by tumor and skin grafts. Through absorption with cells in various strain combinations, at least 25 alloantigenic specificities[6] were known by the mid 1960's when the bulk of the work on histocompatibility antigens in man was carried out.

The approach to clarifying histocompatibility antigens in man differed from that of animal models due to obvious limitations; tests in isogeneic systems in man (identical twins) were more restricted as were actual transplantation studies. Antibodies against leukocyte antigens were first detected by Dausset using a leukoagglutination test with antisera from patients who had received multiple transfusions.[7] Dausset described the first leukocyte antigen "Mac" in 1958 using seven sera which reacted similarly against a panel of leukocytes. Leukocytes from the donor of these sera were negative against their own and other sera of this group. Also in 1958, Payne and Rolfs[8] and van Rood, Eernisse, and van Leeuwen,[9] independently demonstrated the presence of leukoagglutinins in the serum of mothers. These sources of specific antibody reagents opened the possibility for histocompatibility studies in man.

The problem of histocompatibility antigens in humans was reversed from the situation in animal models. For example, in mice histocompatibility differences defined by graft survival were exploited for the production of antibodies. Even congenic lines (strains which differed theoretically from each other by a single histocompatibility loci) were developed and used. In mice differences were emphasized with antiserum raised in strains across various combinations and by absorption of these sera. The results were antigenic differences divided into components showing differences between most strains of mice. In contrast, antisera for the serological analysis of human antigens were obtained primarily from women immunized through fetomaternal incompatibilities. Since no two sera were exactly parallel in reactivity, the approach was to find antisera which behaved alike. The result was a more simplified representation consisting of two closely linked allelic systems.[10-12] The two regions in the HL-A complex have been called the first and second segregant series. The first allelic series consists of HL-A antigens 1, 2, 3, 9, 10, 11, 28, W23, W24, W25, W26, W29, W30, W31, and W32 while the second series includes HL-A5, 7, 8, 12, 13, 14, 17, 27, W5, W10, W15, W16, W18, W21, W22, and W27. These antigens have been recognized by a WHO committee on nomenclature and in addition to these, several specificities have been proposed and are awaiting recognition. One must also consider the possibility of still unidentified antigens in each series. Thus, each chromosome controlling HL-A can be identified by two markers, an antigen from each of the segregant series. This is a haplotype.

Most animal models which have been studied appear to possess a single major genetic histocompatibility system. Besides HL-A, there is the H-2 locus in mice, Ag B in rats, H-1 in rabbits, DL-A in dogs, and locus B in chickens. Antigens controlled by these loci usually stand out as the strongest barrier to successful grafting among a number of genetically controlled transplantation antigens. The others constitute the minor histocompatibility systems. Since major systems have not been serologically detected or defined in man, comparisons and analogies in this review are limited to the H-2 and HL-A system of antigens.

Originally, antigens controlled by the H-2 locus were depicted as a series of specificities which differentiated mouse strains and were present or absent for different lines.[6] Crossover studies within the H-2 system, however, indicated that there are at least two or more regions within this complex.[13] The important regions in transplantation are the K and D regions of the H-2 complex. These are located on the ninth linkage group and together with other markers or known loci as presently viewed by Klein and Shreffler[14] are shown in Figure 5–1. H-2 specificities can be divided into two groups: private and public specificities. Private specificities are more individual, sharply defined, raise higher titers, and differentiate alleles from various strains while public antigens are frequently shared between strains and exhibit considerable cross-reactivity. Between the two regions, which are separated by 0.5 recombination units, are loci controlling the immune response to some defined antigens and the production of a serum protein. One of these, the IR-1 locus, will be discussed later.

Recent serological and biochemical studies emphasize the homologies between H-2 and

H–2 COMPLEX

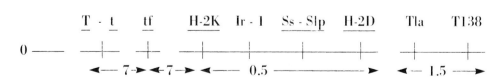

Figure 5–1. Linkage group IX of the mouse showing the H-2 complex. Genetic loci are shown above with recombination distance. (Taken from Klein and Shreffler, "Evidence Supporting a Two-gene Model for the H-2 Histocompatibility System of the Mouse," *Journal of Experimental Medicine,* 35:924–937 (1972).

HL-A as suggested by Thorsby[15] and further documented by Snell, *et al.*[16] Klein's and Shreffler's[17] results with tests of crossovers within the H-2 complex also strongly support a two-region rather than a multi-region interpretation of the H-2 locus. Using heterozygous crossovers and appropriate donors, they showed that graft rejection or survival depended only upon antigens of the K and D regions. The merging of the interpretations of the reactions for the two species and the realization of homologous systems for major histocompatibility systems have immediate implications for cancer.

Genetics of Resistance

The genetics of resistance and susceptibility to viral carcinogenesis in animals has been studied most adequately when genetically defined hosts were available. Understanding the mechanism of the host's genetic contribution to cancer induction requires identifying and locating of the gene or genes involved. With multi-gene effects and randomly bred populations as found in humans, the problem seems almost insurmountable. The homology between histocompatibility systems of man and mice might provide a basis on which studies in man can be designed.

Two general approaches are used to find allelic differences for a trait governing susceptibility and resistance to cancer in mice. A susceptible and a resistant parent strain with the F_1, F_2, and backcross generations are given virus challenges. Susceptibility was defined by the frequency of leukemia or some indication of virus take in the backcross and F_2 generations. If a single or limited number of genes is involved, the incidence of leukemia approaches 50 percent in the backcross and 25 or 75 percent in the F_2 generation depending upon dominance or recessiveness of the trait and the penetrance

of the gene. A second method is to test a number of congenic resistant strains of mice that differ from each other by a single H-2 allele. When differences are found, they can be analyzed further for association with H-2 by the methods just described. Several relationships between histocompatibility and disease susceptibility have been reported. Some examples where limited numbers of genes are involved are described.

The relationship of H-2 antigens and susceptibility to Gross virus-induced leukemia was first established by Lilly, *et al.*[18] when the H-2 genotype was associated with the incidence of leukemia. When challenged with Gross virus, C3H (*H-2k*) mice were observed to be susceptible while C57Bl (*H-2b*) mice were resistant. The F_1 hybrids showed an even lower incidence of leukemia than the C57Bl parent strain and it was concluded that resistance was dominant and also that a single or a group of closely linked genes (*Rgv-1*) was the major determinant for susceptibility to Gross virus leukemogenesis.

Further studies indicated that at least two and possibly more genes were involved in the susceptibility trait.[19] *Rgv-1* is believed to be within the *H-2* locus and, in recombination studies, *Rgv-1* was observed to be more closely associated with the K region. *Rgv-2* is yet to be mapped and was postulated only on statistical grounds.

Although *Rgv-1* was first identified in studies of susceptibility to Gross virus, it also influences host response to other leukemia viruses. Its influence appears to be an immunologic one and because of its location within the *H-2* locus, a relationship has been postulated with other IR genes which control the immune response to natural and synthetic antigens.

The host's relationship with Friend virus appears to be more complex than with Gross virus.[20] *H-2* is only peripherally involved through its linkage to *Rgv-1* which affects the splenomegalic phase of Friend virus leukemia and the recovery from splenomegaly. More closely involved, are two genes, *Fv-2* and *Fv-1*, which control the host relationship with two specific viruses in the Friend virus complex. It had been discovered that Friend virus really consisted of several viruses, the dominant ones being spleen focus-forming virus (SFFV), lymphatic leukemia virus (LLV), and lactose dehydrogenase-elevating virus (LDV). One of these, SFFV, is a defective virus, and needs the help of another in the complex, LLV, to complete its cycle. The susceptibility to SFFV is controlled by the *Fv-2* gene located in the second linkage group near the dilute gene and resistance is dominant over susceptibility.

On the other hand, *Fv-1* controls susceptibility to many murine leukemia viruses including the helper virus, LLV, in the Friend virus complex. In genetic studies of infectivity of cultured cells, these murine leukemia viruses were divisible into two N- and B-tropic groups depending upon the host range of the viruses. The cells and the strains they represent were N or B type depending upon this infectivity. This gene system, $Fv-1^n$ and $Fv-1^b$, appeared to be at a single locus and allelic, with susceptibility to both N- and B-tropic viruses recessive in the heterozygote. The helper LLV virus in the Friend virus complex was N-tropic and thus infectious in N type mice.

Three genes which affect the differentiation of erythropoietic elements were also found to influence susceptibility to spleen focus formation.[21] These are *W* which affects the progenitor cell, *Sl* which renders the environment nonconductive to spleen focus formation, and *F* which limits the proliferative capacity of erythropoietic precursor cells. The complexity of the leukemogenic activity of the Friend virus complex becomes more apparent and emphasizes the probability that equally complex mechanisms should be expected in human systems.

The second approach to determine the association of histocompatibility and susceptibility to the Balb/c Tennant leukemia was used by Tennant and Snell.[22] Strains which differ with a standard strain by a single locus have been developed through breeding and are called congenic strains. If this locus is a histocompatibility locus, the strains are referred to as congenic resistant (CR). The CR lines used in the study by Tennant and Snell all shared the C57B1/10ScSn (*H-2b*) background and were B10.A (*H-2a*), B10.Br (*H-2k*), and B10D2 (*H-2d*). Congenic strains differing at other than the *H-2* locus were also tested but no differences were observed. When CR lines with varying H-2 antigens were tested with dilutions of the virus, the increased susceptibility of mice carrying H-2d antigens was observed. This was of special interest since the Tennant leukemia virus is indigenous to Balb/c which carries H-2d. The *b* allele conferred a higher degree of resistance while mice carrying the *a* and *k* alleles exhibited intermediate susceptibility. Dominance of susceptibility or resistance was not clear in F_1 backcrosses indicating greater complexity in the mechanism of leukemogenesis.

Mühlboch and Dux[23] used the same approach with the Bittner C3H-MTV virus, which is transmitted through the mother's milk and causes a high percentage of mammary tumors. The virus was given to congenic resistant mice with a C57B1/10 background as a cell-free purified extract. The incidence of mammary tumors was higher in females with H-2a, H-2f, and H-2m, than the original strain with the H-2b loci. Substitution in non-H-2 loci again did not appear to make a difference. In contrast, G-R MTV transmitted through the sperm and ovum as well as the mother's milk in the G-R strain showed no significant differences in susceptibility among the congenic resistant strains.

The differences in resistance to the C3H mammary tissue observed by Muhlbock and Dux may be a response or resistance factor associated with the H-2 locus as Nandi[24] does not find strain specificity for the M-MTV form of the virus. M-MTV is associated with B particles and is transmitted by the mother's milk under a protected viral coat which resists digestion. In the new host, it has been postulated that MTV infects erythropoietic tissue and is carried by red blood cells (R-MTV) to reinfect mammary tissues, the site of M-MTV production. R-MTV was found to be highly strain specific with the existence of a relationship to H-2 compatibility. R-MTV from both C3H mice and Balb/c mice fostered on C3H mice (C+) demonstrated a clear preference for the homozygous parent strain of the virus origin to their own C3H or Balb/c strain. The susceptibility of the F_1 from both strains free of virus to each virus strain was again variable. The C3H R-MTV was more effective in inducing nodules in F_1, F_2, and backcrosses than the Balb/c virus suggesting other complicating factors. The mechanism for strain specificity for an artificial mode of transfer which was experimentally introduced is not understood. Both intact red cells and hemolyzed erythrocytes were used to transfer R-MTV so H-2 antigens on the red cells do not appear to be a significant factor.

Immunologic Responsiveness

The consistent association between histocompatibility antigens and susceptibility to cancer in mouse systems suggests important biological relationships with parallels to be sought in man. Mechanisms behind these relationships have been theorized but basically, the proposals fall into the two categories of 1) a gene-controlling responsiveness linked to histocompatibility and 2) unresponsiveness as a result of cross-reaction with one's own antigens. The concurrent works of McDevitt, *et al.* on the mouse and Benacerraf and his group working with guinea pigs have definitely established the genetic relationship

between histocompatibility antigens and responsiveness to some natural and synthetic antigens and have been reviewed recently.[25]

Two inbred strains of guinea pigs, 2 and 13, were observed to respond differentially to poly-L-lysine (PLL), poly-L-arginine, to a copolymer of L-glutamine and L-lysine, and to hapten conjugates of these polypeptides. A single gene designated the PLL gene in strain 2 guinea pigs controlled the response to those antigens and was absent in strain 13 guinea pigs. Two other genes, GA and GT, controlling responsiveness to a polymer of glutamine and alanine and of glutamine and tyrosine were also found. The genes were identified by the ability of animals to respond by cellular immunity (delayed hypersensitivity) and antibody levels. Strain 2 was able to respond to PLL and GA while strain 13 responded to GT. GA and PLL were linked in most Hartley guinea pigs but the existence of a few segregants indicated the distinctness of the two loci. The tendency of GT to segregate away from GA and PLL also indicated allelism or at least pseudoallelism between these genes. Strain 2 guinea pigs also responded to limited dosages of BSA and HSA with antibody production while strain 13 was unresponsive. The response to BSA and HSA appears to be controlled by a single locus linked to GA and PLL in strain 2 guinea pigs.

Benacerraf, *et al.* carried out a study with histocompatibility and responsiveness to PLL which provided an excellent model for similar studies among human populations.[26] They prepared an anti-strain 2 antiserum in strain 13 guinea pigs to detect strain 2 specificities. Seventy-eight random-bred Hartley guinea pigs were tested and 42 PLL responders and 36 nonresponders were found. Possession of the PLL gene was always associated with strain 2 specificities. Also, only PLL nonresponders were able to produce antibodies against strain 2 antigens.

In analogous studies in mice McDevitt,

TABLE 5-1

FREQUENCIES OF HL-A SPECIFICITIES AMONG NORMAL PERSONS AND PATIENTS WITH CANCER
THE FREQUENCIES ARE COMPARED TO THE TOTAL NORMALS BY CHI-SQUARES AND
THOSE WITH .002 < P < .05 ARE DENOTED BY AN ASTERISK

	No. Tested	1	2	3	9	10	11	W28	W32	W29	W30	5	7	8	12	13	W5	W22	W27	W14	W15	W17	W18	W10
Laboratory Normals	47	23	53	19	28	6	15	13	9	2	15	2	23	11	30	6	30	6	4	0	15	11	6	21
Parous Women	204	25*	48	16	26	8	12	16	6	6	16	13	21	16	25	5	22	9	8	7	10	8	9	14
Other Donors	300	29	47	26	21	13	8	11	9	8	9	13	25	23	22	6	21	3	10	10	5	6	10	14
Vol. blood donors	228	30	47	25	19	10	15	8	8	8	6	11	26	23	25	2	21	5	7	7	7	10	8	10
Kidney Donors	127	20	51	33	18	16	13	11	7	7	9	7	29	21	24	2	26	5	7	6	9	6	6	19
Total	906	27	48	24	21	11	12	12	8	7	10	11	25	21	24	4	22	5	8	7	8	8	9	14
Jewish Names (normals)	103	19	43	19	31	20	9	9	6	8	9	9	22	11	23	6	21	2	13	17	3	11	12	12
Mexican Names (normals)	277	15	47	15	28	12	15	21	4	5	18	18	10	9	17	4	34	4	7	9	6	5	13	13
Bladder	139	22	45	26	22	14	12	11	6	6	10	10	27	15	24	8	13*	6	9	12	7	9	10	9
Breast	384	32*	45	24	23	14	10	13	6	7	10	8	20	24	26	4	20	5	7	8	9	10	13	13
Prostate	214	21	51	20	19	14	14	14	5	8	13	10	24	14	24	6	24	6	12	9	11	9	12	10
Lung	250	28	51	23	19	11	7	8	8	9	14	10	24	22	25	5	16*	6	10	9	10	9	8	13
Colon	121	31	47	25	26	11	10	11	7	6	11	8	26	23	25	7	14*	4	10	6	12	12	8	12
Cervix	142	35*	39	28	15*	9	11	16	6	12	11	6	30	21	32*	2	24	4	8	5	6	8	13*	15
Hodgkin's	321	31	45	26	26	14	7	15	9	7	10	17*	19*	20	24	5	23	7	9	11	10	11	14*	12
Rectum	55	33	44	22	36*	13	7	9	4	7	5	13	22	15	33	5	24	7	9	11	11	9	9	5
Stomach	63	24	51	22	24	19	6	13	8	8	10	11	17	16	29	5	14	10	10	6	5	11	14	6
Endometrium	68	24	41	24	32	7	18	10	13	4	12	10	25	19	18	10	22	7	3	4	12	10	6	9
Lymphoma	51	22	51	27	25	20	14	6	6	12	8	12	31	12	24	6	35*	2	8	12	10	12	18	16
Lymphosarcoma	39	15	59	18	33	8	5	26*	8	8	5	10	18	18	28	3	13	3	13	15	5	13	10	13
Melanoma	50	26	54	22	16	6	16	6	6	6	10	14	26	16	30	8	18	4	12	2	4	10	10	16
Ovary	69	26	43	20	26	12	9	13	13	7	6	10	19	23	14	1	26	4	13	13	9	10	10	7
Total Cancers	1996	28	46	24	23	13	11	12	7	8	10	10	23	20	25	5	20	6	9	8	9	10	12	12

et al. used a branched multichain polypeptide, polyalanyl-polylysine, with sequences of tyrosine and glutamic acid on the ends of the side chains (T,G)-A-L. Substituting histidine and phenylalanine for tyrosine, they obtained (H,G)-A-L and (Phe,G)-A-L. When CBA and C57 mice were immunized with (T,G)-A-L, CBA mice responded poorly while C57 mice responded quite well. On the other hand, the animals responded in exactly the opposite manner with (H,G)-A-L. A single locus was indicated when response to both antigens was genetically dominant in the F_1 generation and the backcross to the unresponsive parent strain segregated on a 1:1 basis.

Linkage with the H-2 complex was first suspected when C3H.SW mice congenic to C3H/DnSn, a low responder to (T,G)-A-L, responded well. C3H.SW has the same background but carried *H-2b* antigens while the original C3H is *H-2k*. Similarly C57Bl/10 (*H-2b*) responded well while its congenic partner, B10.Br (*H-2k*), responded poorly. These results indicated that good response to (T,G)-A-L was linked to the *H-2b* allele while the response to (H,G)-A-L was linked to the *H-2k* allele. The genes controlling ability to respond to (T,G)-A-L, (H,G)-A-L, and (Phe,G)-A-L behave as alleles carried by different mouse strains and were designated the IR-1 locus. It has been mapped by recombination studies and lies within the H-2 complex between the K region and the Ss locus of the ninth mouse linkage group (Fig. 5–1).

Further studies have shown that the IR-1 gene is expressed on and can be transferred with immunocompetent cells. The difference between responder and nonresponder lies in the ability to produce a 7S secondary antibody response. The affected pathway appears to be an early recognition stage and is thymus dependent. The ability to form the specific antibody is not involved since nonresponders are capable of producing these same antibodies if the antigen is presented complexed to a charged foreign protein.

The studies just described deal with a genetic locus for responsiveness to a specific antigen and involves the functioning of an antibody-synthetic pathway by one strain. Its genetic control is not clearly understood. The ability to respond by some tetraparental mice from responder and nonresponder strains indicates that (T,G)-A-L does not mimic histocompatibility antigens of nonresponder mice.[27] This observation is limited to (T,G)-A-L, however, and does not rule out the possibility that viral or tumor antigens approximate histocompatibility antigens. Viruses and tumors present an antigen profile of greater complexity to the host with possibilities of cross-reactions. Theoretically, unresponsiveness to viral antigens through mimicry or identity with host histocompatibility antigens receives much support. Absence of host immune responses would give a definite advantage to microorganisms showing similarity in antigens to that of the host. It has been suggested that the polymorphism of histocompatibility antigens is the result of host counter defenses to circumvent parasitic infiltrations.

The motivation behind numerous studies of H-2 and susceptibility to cancer-inducing viruses including those of Nandi, *et al.* is related to the identity of host and parasite antigens. In the assembly of oncorna and other viruses at the cell membrane, a coat of host membrane with histocompatibility antigens may be formed as the virus buds from the cell. Aoki, *et al.*[28] have reported the absence of H-2 antigens on viruses from one leukemia (E ♂G2) and the presence on another (K-6). The role of histocompatibility antigens on viral membranes needs to be more clearly identified in relation to susceptibility or resistance.

Whether genetic control of unresponsiveness is due to linkage to the histocompatibility locus of a response gene or to tolerance from similarity with host antigens may be partially answered by testing offspring. If the inability to respond is due to tolerance to host antigens, the trait of susceptibility or unresponsiveness is dominant and F_1 animals should be found accordingly. The response in F_1 to the polypeptide antigens and gross-virus leukemogenesis indicates that genetic control is other than tolerance to one's own antigens. The control of responsiveness to other oncogenic viruses needs to be further clarified and single gene effects more clearly isolated before conclusions can be made.

Linkage of HL-A with Cancer Susceptibility

Genetic linkage of histocompatibility antigens to cancer in man is ideally studied in families with multiple cases of cancer. Linkage is demonstrated when members of the family with cancer are shown to have inherited the same HL-A identified chromosome while other members free of cancer have received alternate chromosomes. The difficulty in obtaining this data is that rela-

tives who have died from cancer are no longer available for typing while there is no way to predict who may eventually succumb to cancer among those who are currently alive. Aside from the family shown below, which was typed for Dr. Yonemoto of the City of Hope and the cancer families which we have been studying in collaboration with Dr. Lynch and Dr. Henderson of the USC Medical School, we are not aware of other studies using this approach. In the family shown in Figure 5-2, segregation of melanoma incidence is with the HL-A chromosome which is unfortunately *blank* or without known specificities. The mothers and three sons with melanoma all have this chromosome. In another family, susceptibility to breast cancer did not appear to be linked to HL-A. More families in both categories with or without evidence of linkage, and for all cancers, must be gathered to prove or disprove genetic relationships between cancer and HL-A.

Population studies attempting to find association between HL-A antigens and types of cancers are a simpler and therefore more popular approach toward gathering information on HL-A and cancer. The many pitfalls

MELANOMA FAMILY

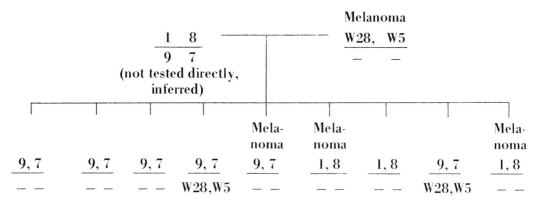

Figure 5–2. Incidence of melanoma in a family. The numbers represent HL-A antigens in haplotypes. - means the antigen was inferred from segregating haplotypes and were not detected serologically. Members of the family with melanoma are shown.

encountered utilizing such a method have been discussed fully.[29] Linkage between cancer and HL-A cannot be ruled out by the absence or failure to detect relationships. Only a strong positive association may suggest linkage disequilibrium. A weak association may be spurious, resulting from the selection of a high association sought for among many possible specificities. A simple, although perhaps overly conservative, method of correction is to multiply the P values by the number of specificities being compared.[29] A difficulty derived from this correction, however, is the concealment of genuine weak associations.

Several reports already in the literature demonstrate the problem of too small populations with associations which were not reproducible on retesting even by the same laboratory on another set of subjects. The ethnic composition of each sample must also be rigorously controlled. HL-A specificities are well known to vary widely in frequency among different races, and even within a given race.[30] An example is seen in Table 5-I. Among Caucasians in the United States, it was necessary to separate Jews from other Caucasians as differences in the HL-A frequency for the Jewish population were found.

The association between Hodgkin's disease and HL-A has been most frequently studied. As reviewed by Lawler in Chapter 6, the accumulated evidence indicates some association of antigens in the HL-A5, W5, W18, 4c complex with Hodgkin's disease. Our findings, given in Table 5-I, show that W18 and W5 are elevated in tests of 321 patients with Hodgkin's disease. Subdivision into the subclasses of lymphocytic predominance, mixed cellularity, nodular sclerosis, and lymphocyte depletion are now being investigated to sharpen associations, but most studies unfortunately still do not have sufficient numbers to draw meaningful conclusions. Although a clear disturbance in the frequency of HL-A antigens exists in Hodg-

kin's disease, the effect does not appear to be a striking one.

Studies performed on a variety of other types of cancer have all dealt with fewer than 40 patients each and no attempt will be made here to review them. Both Lawler (Chapter 6) and Walford[31] have exhaustively analyzed these reports.

Our laboratory has recently undertaken a large-scale study of different types of solid tumors with 50 to 384 patients in each group. As shown in Table 5-I, patients with cancer of the prostate, stomach, endometrium, ovary and with melanoma showed essentially identical HL-A frequencies as the control population. Patients with cancer of the bladder, breast, lung, colon, rectum, and patients with lymphomas and lymphosarcoma exhibited deviations from control levels for only one of the 23 specificities at a significant level ($P < 0.05$). Since a significant difference occurs by chance in one of 20 samples, and 23 specificities are concurrently being examined, the level of deviation may have occurred by chance alone. Any of these differences may be considered valid if encountered again in a second series.

Cancer of the cervix and Hodgkin's disease appear to be most promising areas of study. Three specificities were *significantly* different in frequency from normal populations suggesting that a genuine disturbance in HL-A frequency may exist in the patient population. Among patients with carcinoma of the cervix, HL-A1 was 35 percent and HL-A12 was 32 percent compared to 27 percent and 24 percent, respectively, in normals. One antigen was lower in frequency; HL-A9 was 15 percent compared to 21 percent in normals. An interesting observation is the finding that HL-A1 is low and HL-A9 is high among Jewish persons, a relationship which is the direct opposite of that found in cervix carcinoma patients. The low incidence of cervical carcinoma in Jewish women might possibly be related to this association.

In the present series of 321 patients with Hodgkin's disease, W5 and W18 were increased at the expense of HL-A7. Since both W18 and W5 were increased in studies by other laboratories, this finding is probably valid. As noted earlier, division of the broad categories of Hodgkin's disease must now be done to increase the degree of association found.

The current status of our knowledge of associations between HL-A and Hodgkin's disease illustrates the difficulties in advancing our understanding of the genetics of cancer. Even if W18 were significantly associated with Hodgkin's disease (Table 5-I), it must be remembered that the vast majority of persons with W18 do not develop Hodgkin's disease. Moreover, of 100 patients with disease only 14 carry W18 and 86 do not. Obviously W18 is not directly involved in the disease process and if a cross-reactivity exists between W18 and a possible Hodgkin's virus, the cross-reactivity is a weak one.

On the other hand the role of HL-A antigens may be simply as markers for a susceptibility gene found on the same chromosome. Although a population association can not be taken as evidence of linkage, it can be used to experimental advantage in postulating such a linkage. The existence of a similar situation in mice has already been cited. Employing this assumption and the simplest explanation of linkage between HL-A and a single susceptibility gene, the data might be interpreted as follows. The susceptibility gene is more frequently found in conjunction with W5 or W18 but may also segregate with any other HL-A haplotype. Not all persons possessing W5 or W18 need carry the linked susceptibility gene.

Complicating factors such as multigene effects and penetrance of the cancer susceptibility or resistance genes may obscure the fundamental relationships underlying the genetic relationships in cancer. These are dealt with in other chapters of this book. The potential value of HL-A as possible markers for these genes emerges best from family studies, many of which will have to be done across generations. As patients with cured cancer become more widely available, more family studies may become possible. Perhaps large-scale long-term prospective studies starting with current cancer patients can be initiated.

REFERENCES

1. Triolo, V.A.: Nineteenth century foundations of cancer research. Origins of experimental research. *Cancer Res, 24:*4–27, 1964.
2. Little, C.C., and Strong, L.C.: Genetic studies on the transplantation of two adenocarcinomata. *J Exp Zool, 41:*93–114, 1924.
3. Bittner, J.J.: A review of genetic studies on the transplantation of tumours. *J Genet, 31:* 471–487, 1935.
4. Gorer, P.A.: The genetics and antigenic basis for tumor transplantation. *J Pathol, 44:* 691–697, 1937.
5. Gorer, P.A., Lyman, S., and Snell, G.P.: Studies on the genetic and antigenic basis of tumor transplantation. Linkage between a histocompatibility gene and 'fused' in mice. *Proc R Soc Lond* (Biol), *135:*399–505, 1948.
6. Snell, G.D., and Stimpfling, J.H.: Genetics of tissue transplantation. In Green, E.L. (Ed.): *Biology of the Laboratory Mouse.* New York, McGraw, 1966.
7. Dausset, J.: Iso-leuco-anticorps. *Acta Haematol, 20:*156, 1958.
8. Payne, R., and Rolfs, M.R.: Fetomaternal leukocyte incompatibility. *J Clin Invest, 37:* 1756, 1958.
9. van Rood, J.J., Eernisse, J.G., and van Leeuwen, A.: Leukocyte antibodies in sera from pregnant women. *Nature,* (Lond), *181:* 1735, 1958.

10. Dausset, J., Ivanyi, P., and Ivanyi, D.: Tissue alloantigens in humans: Identification of a complex system (HU-1). In Balner, H., Cleton, F.J., and Eernisse, J.G., (Eds.): *Histocompatibility Testing 1965*. Baltimore, Williams & Wilkins, 1965, pp. 51–62.

11. Cepellini, R., Curtoni, E.S., Mattiuz, P.L., Miggiano, V.C., Scudeller, G., and Serra, A.: Genetics of leukocyte antigens. A family study of segregation and linkage. In Curtoni, E.S., Mattiuz, P.L., and Tosi, R.M. (Eds.): *Histocompatibility Testing 1967*. Baltimore, Williams & Wilkins, 1967, pp. 149–187.

12. Kissmeyer-Nielsen, F., Svejgaard, A., and Hauge, M.: Genetics of the human HL-A transplantation system. *Nature, 219:*1116, 1968.

13. Allen, S.L.: Linkage relations of the genes histocompatibility—2 and fused tail, brackyury and kinky tail in the mouse as determined by tumor transplantation. *Genetics, 40:*627–650.

14. Klein, J., and Shreffler, D.C.: The H-2 model for the major histocompatibility system. *Transplant Rev, 6:*3–29, 1971.

15. Thorsby, E.: A tentative new model for the organization of the mouse H-2 histocompatibility system: Two segregant series of antigens. *Eur J Immunol, 1:*57–59, 1971.

16. Snell, G.D., Cherry, M., and Demant, P.: Evidence that H-2 private specificities can be arranged in two mutually exclusive systems possibly homologous with two subsystems of HL-A. *Transplant Proc, 3:*183–186, 1971.

17. Klein, J., and Shreffler, D.C.: Evidence supporting a two-gene model for the H-2 histocompatibility system of the mouse. *J Exp Med, 135:*924–937, 1972.

18. Lilly, F., Boyse, E.A., and Old, L.J.: The genetic basis of susceptibility to viral leukemogenesis. *Lancet, 2:*1207–1209, 1964.

19. Lilly, F.: The influence of H-2 type on Gross virus leukemogenesis in mice. *Transplant Proc, 3:*1239–1241, 1971.

20. Lilly, F.: Mouse leukemia: A model of a multiple-gene disease. *J Nat Cancer Inst, 49:*927–934, 1972.

21. Steeves, R.A.: Genes other than H-2 determining susceptibility to Friend virus. *Transplant Proc, 3:*1237–1238, 1971.

22. Tennant, J.R., and Snell, G.D.: The H-2 locus and viral leukemogenesis as studied in congenic strains of mice. *J Natl Cancer Inst, 41:*597–604, 1968.

23. Mühlboch, O., and Dux, A.: Histocompatibility genes and susceptibility to mammary tumor virus (MTV) in mice. *Transplant Proc, 3:*1247–1250, 1971.

24. Nandi, S., Haslam, S., and Helmick, C.: Inheritance of susceptibility to erythrocyte-born Bittner virus in mice. *Transplant Proc, 3:*1251–1257.

25. McDevitt, H.O., and Benacerraf, B.: Genetic control of specific immune responses. *Adv Immunol, 11:*31–74, 1969.

26. Benacerraf, B., Bluestein, H.G., Green, I., and Ellman, L.: Specific immune response genes of guinea pigs. *Prog Immunol, 1:*486–494, 1971.

27. McDevitt, H.O., Bechtol, K.B., Grumet, F.C., Mitchell, G.F., and Wegman, T.G.: Genetic control of the immune response to branched synthetic polypeptidic antigens in inbred mice. *Prog Immunol, 1:*495–508, 1971.

28. Aoki, T.: Surface antigens of murine leukemia cells and murine leukemia virus. *Transplant Proc, 3:*1195–1198, 1971.

29. McDevitt, H.O., and Bodmer, W.: Histocompatibility antigens immune responsiveness and susceptibility to disease. *Am J Med, 1:*52, 1972.

30. White, S., Newcomer, V.D., Mickey, M.R., and Terasaki, P.I. Disturbance of HL-A in psoriasis. *New Engl J Med, 287:*740–743, 1972.

31. Walford, R.L., Smith, G.S., and Waters, H.: Histocompatibility systems and disease states with particular reference to cancer. *Transplant Rev, 7:*78–111, 1971.

CHAPTER 6

THE HL-A SYSTEM

AND NEOPLASIA

SYLVIA D. LAWLER

Definition of the HL-A Antigens

THE ANTIGENS BELONGING to the major human histocompatibility system, HL-A, are widely distributed throughout the tissues of the body. In the laboratory they are usually detected on lymphocytes by some form of microcytotoxicity test using antibodies raised in human subjects by isoimmunization. The antigens can also be identified on platelets by the use of a complement fixation assay.

The phenotype of an individual is expressed in terms of internationally recognized antigens. According to current dogma, a person may have up to four of these, but not more. Borrowing a term from poker schools, anyone in whom four different antigens can be recognized is said to carry a full-house.

Operationally the genetical control appears to be by two adjacent segregant series which are called the 1st or LA locus, and the 2nd or Four locus. The antigens have been defined at a series of International Workshops.[1,2,3,4] The results of the fifth such Workshop, which are still being analyzed, were discussed at Evian, France, in May of 1972. The antigens as they were defined at the conclusion of the Fourth International Workshop are listed in Tables 6-I (1st locus) and 6-II (2nd locus): the antigens identified as HL-A followed by a number are already well-defined, those antigens with the prefix W await final definition. W stands for Workshop Terasaki. After the Fifth International Workshop the World Health Organization Nomenclature Committee assigned some additional W Specificities. These are shown in Table 6-III.

The first description of a leucocyte antigen was made by Dausset[7] in France in 1958; the antigen is now defined as HL-A2 but at the time of discovery it was called Mac—an abbreviation of the name of the donor of the serum. It has become customary for new specificities either to be described by such an abbreviation of the name of the donor or of the Chief of the laboratory in which they are described—in which case a number or additional letters are also used. The HL-A1 and HL-A3 antigens were described by Payne[6,8] and her colleagues in California,

TABLE 6-I
ANTIGENS BELONGING TO THE
FIRST LOCUS (1971)

Definition	Previous Descriptions
HL-A1	LAI†
HL-A2	Mac‡ = LA2†
HL-A3	LA3
HL-A9	LC11
HL-A10	Da17
HL-A11	Da21, GE20, KN-1LN*, Te13, To26**
W19	<LI, LA-W, Thompson, Ge32**
W28	Ba*, Da15, LC17**

† R. Payne, et al., "A New Leukocyte Isoantigen System in Man," Cold Spring Harbor Symposia on Quantitative Biology, 29:285–295 (1964).

‡ J. Dausset, "Iso-leuco-anticorps," Acta Haematologica (Basel), 20:156–166 (1958).

W. Bodmer, et al., "Genetics of '4' and 'LA' human leucocyte groups," Annals of the New York Academy of Sciences, 129:473–489 (1966).

R. L. Walford, "Lc-11 as a mutually exclusive specificity to Lc-1, 2 and 3 in the main human leukocyte group," Vox Sanguinis (Basel), 15:338–344 (1968).

J. Dausset, et al., "The HL-A sub-loci and their importance in Transplantation," Transplantation Proceedings (New York), 1:331–338 (1969).

** Histocompatibility Testing 1970, Munksgaard, Copenhagen, 1970.

TABLE 6-II
ANTIGENS BELONGING TO THE
SECOND LOCUS (1971)

Definition	Previous Descriptions
HL-A5	To5*
HL-A7	7C†
HL-A8	To7* 7D†
HL-A12	Da4, KN-T12, Te9, To11, Sly1‡
HL-A13	Bt23, KN-HN, Te26, To21‡
W5	4c(R), To25, Da20‡
W10	BB
W14	MaKi
W15	LND
W17	MaPi, Te17‡
W18	Te18‡
W22	AA, Bt22‡
W27	FJH

* R. Ceppellini, *et al.*, "Genetics of Leukocyte Antigens: A Family Study of Segregation and Linkage in Histocompatibility Testing, 1967," Munksgaard, Copenhagen 1967.

† J.J. Rood, *et al.*, "Leukocyte groups, the Normal Lymphocyte Transfer Test and Homograft Sensitivity," Munksgaard, Copenhagen, 1967.

‡ Histocompatibility Testing 1970, Munksgaard, Copenhagen, 1970.
A. Svejgaard, *et al.*, "Genetics of the HL-A System. A Population and Family Study," *Vox Sanguinis*, 18: 97–133 (1970).
W.R. Mayr, "A New Leucocyte Antigen. Preliminary Report," *Vox Sanguinis*, 18:180–182 (1970).
E. Thorsby, and F. Kissmeyer-Nielsen, "New HL-A Alleles. Identification by Planned Immunization," *Vox Sanguinis*, 18:134–148 (1970).

TABLE 6-III
NEW W SPECIFICITIES ASSIGNED BY WHO
NOMENCLATURE COMMITTEE, EVIAN 1972

W16	U18
W21	ET Da24
W23	HL-A9.1
W24	HL-A9.2
W25	HL-A10.1
W26	HL-A10.2
W29	W19.1
W30	W19.3
W31	W19.4
W32	W19.5

From: Histocompatibility Testing, 1972, Munksgaard, Copenhagen.

HL-A9, described by Walfords'[9] group also has a Californian origin. HL-A7 antigen was first defined by Van Rood, *et al.*[12] in Holland, using a leucoagglutinating antibody. Other antigens identified in Dausset's laboratory include HL-A10,[10] HL-A11,[4] W28[4] and HL-A12.[4] As the international collaboration progressed, antibodies with similar specificities were recognized at about the same time in different laboratories, for example, HL-A13 by Batchelor[4] in the United Kingdom, Kissmeyer-Nielsen[4] in Denmark, Terasaki[4] in California and Ceppellini[4] in Italy.

Indubitably all possible antigens in this extremely polymorphic system have not yet been defined, therefore if only one antigen is detected, at either locus, the implication cannot necessarily be made that the individual is homozygous for that antigen. It is not possible to distinguish between single or double doses of the antigens serologically by the standard methods.

Genetics of the HL-A System

A person inherits one paternal and one maternal antigen belonging to each locus. The term haplotype is used to describe the HL-A combination contributed by a single parent. It is conventional to represent the chromosomes of the parents by letters, 'a,' 'b' for paternal and 'c,' 'd' for maternal (or vice versa). When families are studied the HL-A constitution of each child can usually be described as 'ac,' 'ad,' 'bc' or 'bd.' Sib pairs with the same paternal haplotypes are said to be identical. The assignment of haplotypes is demonstrated in Table 6-IV; the family was one of a series in which there was a child with leukemia.[16] The fact that the father is homozygous for HL-A2 could only be determined by studying the family. The letter X indicated an undetermined specificity at the second locus. It can be seen that the father is not homozygous for the HL-A5 because some of the children have inherited from him HL-A2 not accompanied by HL-A5.

It has been estimated that the frequency of recombination between the two loci is of the order of 1 percent.[17] Therefore, in

TABLE 6-IV
SEGREGATION OF HAPLOTYPES

	HL-A genotypes	*Chromosomes*
Father	2, X/2, 5	a/b
Mother	W28, W10/3, 7	c/d
Child	2, 5/W28, W10	b/c
Child 2	2, X/3, 7	a/d
Child 3	2, X/W28, W10	a/c
Child 4	2, X/3, 7	a/d
Child 5	2, X/W28, W10	a/c
Child 6	2, 5/W28, W10	b/c
Child 7	2, X/W28, W10	a/c

Family 58, Lawler *et al.,* "The HL-A System In Lymphoblastic Leukaemia," *British Journal of Haematology,* 21:595–605 (1971).

X indicates an undetermined specificity.

about one family in a hundred a child has a 1st locus antigen of one of the parental chromosomes and a 2nd locus antigen from the other chromosome. For example, in a family studied in my laboratory,[18] a father with genotype HL-A1,8/2,12(a/b) had one child with a 2,8 paternal haplotype. Thus the first locus antigen HL-A2 came from the parental 'b' chromosome and the HL-A8 antigen from the 'a' chromosome.

Histocompatibility and Leukemia

In mice, there is evidence that susceptibility to leukemia induced by the Gross virus is influenced by the H2 system.[19] In the case of murine leukemia induced by the Friend virus, survival rather than susceptibility is related to the H2 system.[20] In man viral aetiology of leukemia is as yet nonproven. Recently evidence of association between influenza in pregnancy and subsequent development of leukemia has been recorded by Fredrick and Alberman[21] in a longitudinal study. Infants born in the first week of March 1958 to mothers who were reported to have influenza during pregnancy showed a four-fold increase in incidence of leukemia and other neoplasms of lymphatic and haemopoietic tissue as compared with children born to mothers who did not have influenza. This work suggests that virus infection *in utero* could be a factor of importance in the development of leukemia in childhood. The searches for an association between histocompatibility and leukemia in man have been inspired by the observations in the mouse, and are further encouraged by the possibility of viral factors operating in human leukemia.

In 1968, Kourilsky *et al.*[22] looked for phenotypic associations between the HL-A system and leukemia in two diagnostically defined categories—acute lymphoblastic (102 cases) and acute myeloblastic (14 cases). They concluded that the antigens for which they tested had a similar distribution in the patients as in normal controls. Walford and colleagues[23,24] have stressed the importance of looking for associations on the basis of genotypic as well as of phenotypic data. They suggested[23] but did not confirm[24] a statistically significant increase in the 2,12 haplotype in acute lymphoblastic leukemia. In a recent analysis of the cases recorded in the literature Walford, *et al.*[25] concluded that a numerical increase in either HL-A2 or HL-A12, usually both, had been found in most studies of acute lymphoblastic leukemia, but that the overall result on 214 patients was not statistically significant when the probability value was corrected for the number of comparisons of antigenic frequencies between patients and controls that had been made. In most studies at least twenty different specificities were defined, so that a probability value for the deviation of the observed frequency distribution of any one antigen between a series of patients and a control group would have to be multiplied by 20. Then, for example, a *P* value of 0.005 (result obtainable only once in two hundred times by chance) would become 0.1 (result obtainable once in ten times by chance) and this result would no longer be regarded as statistically significant.

Family Study in Acute Lymphoblastic Leukemia

In a study of 58 Caucasian patients attending the Hospital for Sick Children in London, England,[16] the available close relatives were also typed for the antigens of the HL-A system. No gross disturbance in the frequency distribution of any internationally defined antigens except W27 (corrected *P* value < .018) was found in the patients or their families. When using family data a comparison of the frequency distributions must be made with a normal control group when phenotypic associations are being assessed. This is because a low or high frequency of a particular antigen amongst the patients is bound to be reflected in the frequency distribution amongst the parents. For example, the W27 antigen had a frequency of 17 percent amongst the patients and 13 percent in both mothers and fathers. Our normal control panel has a lower frequency, 3 percent of the W27 antigen, than most other Caucasian panels in which the frequency varies between 2 and 16 percent. At the time of the study the ten patients with the W27 antigen included three out of the five patients who had already lived for four years since the diagnosis was made. This indicated a possible association of the W27 antigen with long term survival. The data was reassessed in March 1972 as shown in Table 6-V. Information was available on 55 of the patients and the association between a survival of more than four years and the

TABLE 6-V
THE W27 ANTIGEN IN CHILDREN WITH
ACUTE LYMPHOBLASTIC LEUKAEMIA

	Survival		
	More than 4 years	*Less than 4 years*	
W27 +	4	6	10
W27 −	7	38	45
Total	11	44	55

0.10 > *P* > 0.05

presence of the W27 antigen was found not to be statistically significant at the 1 in 20 level.

By typing families it is possible to look for disturbances in segregation patterns when comparing the leukemic children with their normal sibs. In the London family study[16] there were 68 sibs in whom it was possible to trace the segregation of parental haplotypes. In Table 6-VI the parental haplotypes

TABLE 6-VI
THE SEGREGATION OF THE HL-A
HAPLOTYPES AMONGST SIBS OF
LEUKAEMIC PATIENTS

	Patients	*Like sibs*	*Unlike sibs*		
Haplotypes	*ac*	*ac*	*ad*	*bc*	*bd*
No obs.	38	19	19	13	17
No exp.	38	17	17	17	17

have been assigned on the basis of the abcd convention. The chromosomes of the parents were allocated so that the leukemic children in each family had the 'ac' haplotypes. As can be seen from Table 6-VI there is a random distribution of parental haplotypes amongst the sibs and the leukemic children had an HL-A identical sib as often as would be expected.

Another advantage of examining families is that it is possible to deduce the frequency of the different haplotypes amongst the patients and their relatives. This is important because some combinations of antigens of the 1st and 2nd locus occur more frequently in any population than would be expected on the basis of chance coupling. Thus certain haplotypes occur more frequently in a given population and other combinations are rare. As shown in Table 6-VII the three commonest haplotypes in the patients and their relatives were 1,8; 3,7; and 2,12. These are the commonest combinations amongst Caucasians.

Thus the investigation of families did not reveal any disturbance in segregation pat-

TABLE 6-VII
PERCENTAGES OF THE COMMONEST
HAPLOTYPES IN FAMILIES WITH A
LEUKAEMIC CHILD

Haplotype	Patients	Fathers	Mothers	Sibs
1,8	11	10	6	12
3,7	8	5	6	8
2,12	6	7	3	5

terns and for genetical studies these families can be regarded as normal and so they have been used for linkage studies.[26]

Chronic Leukemias

The data on a chronic myeloid leukemic are somewhat sparse: in a study of 47 cases an increase in HL-A3 and decrease in HL-A12 has been recorded.[27]

The combined results of Jeannet and Magnin[28] and Walford, *et al.*[25] do not show any gross disturbance in the distribution of HL-A antigens in patients with chronic lymphocytic leukemia. Typing these patients is complicated by the fact that some HL-A typing sera show increased reactivity with their lymphocytes which cannot be ascribed to HL-A specificities. Similarly, additional serological reactions have been observed by Dick, *et al.*[29] when using HL-A typing sera to characterize cultured peripheral lymphoblastoid cells from various sources.

In general, the lymphocytes of unrelated individuals and non-HL-A identical sibs when mixed together *in vivo* stimulate each other to undergo metabolic changes, DNA synthesis and ultimately mitosis. The reaction is termed MLR—mixed lymphocyte reaction. The genetical control of this system is apparently closely linked to the loci of the HL-A system. Although the lymphocytes of HL-A identical sibs usually do not stimulate each other in the MLR test, such like pairs may rarely be found to have

mutually stimulatory cells.[30] This finding, together with the observations that the lymphocytes of unrelated HL-A identical individuals nearly always stimulate each other in the MLR test,[31,32] and occasionally HL-A nonidentical do not[33] mitigate against the genetic identity of the HL-A and MLR loci. Evidence from families in which an HL-A recombinant has been detected suggests that the MLR locus is sited closer to the second than to the first HL-A locus.[34]

Pentycross[35] has studied the lymphocytes of patients with chronic lymphocytic leukemia in the MLR test using both the two-way (both populations viable) and the one-way (one population viable) systems. The lymphocytes of the patients were as capable as normal cells of invoking a response to HL-A nonidentical normal lymphocytes. Conversely barely any response was produced when the lymphocytes of the patients were stimulated by nonviable foreign lymphocytes. The failure of the leukemic lymphocytes to respond in the MLR test is correlated with a poor response to mitogenic stimulants. However, the cells from these patients do respond when challenged with specific bacterial or viral antigens. The fact that the cells of these patients can stimulate but do not respond in the MLR accords with the view of Yunis and Amos[30] that the stimulatory factor and the response mechanism may be separable genetic entities.

Hodgkins Disease

In 1967 Amiel[36] reported that among 41 patients typed for five specificities, 51 percent were positive for an antigen then called 4c, whilst among normal controls there were only 27 percent of positive reactions. The 4c antigen is now known to include HL-A5, W5, W18 and CM*, a specificity that is probably the same as W18 recognized by Kissmeyer-Nielsen *et al.*[37] The published

TABLE 6-VIII
HL-A ANTIGENS AND HODGKINS DISEASE

No. of Patients	Geographical Location	Significant Conclusions		References
27	United Kingdom	HL-A5	↑	Zervas, et al. 1970
127	Australia	4c (W5)	↑	Morris and Forbes 1971
		HL-A11	↑	
40	France	4c	↑	Amiel 1971
78	Canada	HL-A5	↑	Thorsby, et al. 1971
		W-28	↑	
39	Norway	HL-A11	↓	Thorsby, et al. 1971
98	Holland	W5	↑	Van Rood and Van Leeuwen 1971
50	Denmark	HL-A1	↑	Kissmeyer-Nielsen, et al. 1971
		HL-A8	↑	
		W18 (CM*)	↑	
44	U.S.A.	HL-A2	↑	Coukell, et al. 1971
		HL-A3	↓	
		W15	↑	
33	Switzerland	W10	↓	Jeannet and Magnin 1971
		W15	↑	
82	West Germany	W18	↑	Bertrams, et al. 1971

↑ Statistically significant increase in frequency.
↓ Statistically significant decrease in frequency.

findings to date are summarized in Table 6-VIII. Each group of patients has been compared with a normal control population typed at the same center. Only those deviations which can be regarded as statistically significant have been included. It should be noted that seven out of the ten investigations show an increase in frequency of an antigen belonging to the 4c complex. Morris and Forbes[38] studied the families, either parents or children of 40 patients and were able to show that the W5 antigen in some of the patients was a heritable characteristic, thereby excluding the very real possibility of serological artifacts. This work supports the contention that the presence of an antigen of the 4c region is associated with an increased susceptibility to the disease.

During the Fifth Histocompatibility Workshop, teams from all over the world typed patients with Hodgkins Disease. Particular attention was paid to the histological diagnosis and sufficient data should be available to make an analysis according to histological type. These data were still being analyzed at the time of writing. The international collaborative effort should enable the associa-

tion between the disease and antigens related to 4c to be firmly substantiated.

Trophoblastic Neoplasia

Study of Families

During gestation in mammals a normal fetus may be regarded as a homograft. It is widely believed that immunological rejection of the fetus is prevented because of a deficiency in the expression of the allo-antigens of the trophoblast.[46] On the other hand there is experimental evidence in mice which suggests that a fetus may be favored by being maternally incompatible for histocompatibility antigens. In matings involving different inbred strains of mice fetuses that were unlike the mother were found to be larger than compatible ones, the larger sized fetuses have a better chance of survival.[47]

Human tumors arising from trophoblastic tissue are also foreign to the maternal hsot through a hemizygous set of paternal genes. As in the case of the normal fetus, even though the genetic information for antigenic foreigness may be present it does not necessarily follow that this antigenicity will be adequately expressed.

It is difficult to obtain material from trophoblastic tumors in a form that is suitable for direct examination. It is therefore necessary to resort to indirect methods in order to study the role of the histocompatibility antigens in trophoblastic neoplasia. In about one third of cases choriocarcinoma is preceded by a normal term birth. In such cases it is reasonable to assume that the antecedent child carries the same genetic information as the malignancy. By typing the patient, her husband, antecedent child and sibs when available, it can be seen whether the antecedent children are more compatible with the mothers than would be expected. Thus it is possible to ascertain whether choriocarcinomas are always, sometimes or never HL-A compatible with the host. During the last few years 19 such Caucasian families have been tested for the HL-A antigens which could be defined at the time of testing.[48]

In this group of families there was no gross disturbance in the mating patterns. Since a child must have one maternal haplotype, any child has the chance of being incompatible with the mother for two paternally derived antigens, one belonging to each HL-A locus. In these 19 families, considering only the child antecedent to the tumor, 14 were incompatible for an antigen belonging to each locus, 4 children were compatible only for a 1st locus antigen, namely, HL-A1, HL-A9 and two examples of HL-A2 compatibility. One child was completely antigenically compatible with the mother, HL-A2, HL-A12. In comparable single child families in the United Kingdom, 24 percent of families would be expected to have a child who inherited from the father an antigen present in the mother, 2 percent of children would be expected to be antigenically compatible with the mother. So these children whose

gestation was associated with the subsequent development of choriocarcinoma were neither more nor less compatible with the patients than the children of healthy mothers. Furthermore, there were examples of incompatibility for the antigens, HL-A1, HL-A2, HL-A3, HL-A5, HL-A7, HL-A8, HL-A12, W18 and W27. In a similar study of 15 such families Lewis and Terasaki,[49] found two children who were HL-A compatible with the mother. Thus the development of choriocarcinoma is not preferentially associated with maternally HL-A compatible conceptuses, and the incompatible conceptuses can differ from the mother over the whole range of HL-A specificities.

Mating Patterns

The patients in whom choriocarcinoma was preceded by a live-term birth form a special group in which the indirect approach, through studying the antecedent child, can give information about the antigenic relationship between the tumor and the host. However, when neoplasia follows an abortion, still-birth, or molar pregnancy the only way to find out about potential antigenic differences between the patient and the tumor is to make deductions from the phenotypes of the husband. If the HL-A system plays a role in immunological surveillance against these tumors then some disturbance in the distribution of the HL-A antigens between the patients and their husbands might be expected.

Between March 1969 and December 1971, 75 Caucasian patients and their husbands were typed for the HL-A system.[50] The study included 41 cases of confirmed choriocarcinoma, 20 following live-term birth, 8 following nonmolar abortion or still-birth and 13 following a pregnancy with a hydatidiform mole. The remaining 34 cases required treatment for trophoblastic neo-

TABLE 6-IX
HL-A MATINGS—PATIENTS WITH TROPHOBLASTIC NEOPLASIA

	1st. Locus X^2_7							
	1	2	3	9	10	11	W19	X
Husbands	2.59	0.86	6.19	3.92	18.21*	3.27	8.03	4.52
Patients	4.67	2.07	3.85	1.91	25.99**	2.68	4.23	2.19

* $0.05 > P > 0.01$.
** $P > 0.01$.

plasia following hydatidiform mole, but it had not been possible to define the leison histologically.

The mating patterns were analyzed on the basis of phenotypes, not haplotypes, and the statistical analysis was confined to the antigens, HL-A1,2,3,9,10,11 and W19 at the 1st locus and 5,7,8,12 and 13 at the 2nd locus. If only one specificity was detected serologically at a locus then the unspecified antigen was scored as an X antigen. This means that the possibilities of homozygosity or, remotely, the existence of silent alleles in the HL-A system were ignored. For each locus each husband/wife pair was scored four times. For example, suppose the results of the HL-A typing were:

Husband HL-A1,X,HL-A5,HL-A8

Patient HL-A1,HL-A2,HL-A8,X.

This pair was scored thus:

1st locus Husband X Wife 1 × 1,
1 × 2, X × 1, X × 2

2nd locus Husband X Wife 5 × 8,
5 × X, 8 × 8, 8 × X.

The observed number of matings for each category was compared with the number that would be expected. The expected number of matings were estimated by using the actual reaction frequencies of antigens amongst the husbands and the patients. An X^2 value was then calculated for each mating type. The sums of these X^2 values are given in Table 6-IX for 1st locus and Table 6-X for the 2nd. The X^2 values are statistically

TABLE 6-X
HL-A MATINGS—PATIENTS WITH
TROPHOBLASTIC NEOPLASIA

	2nd. Locus X^2_5					
	5	7	8	12	13	X
Husbands	5.02	3.38	6.60	1.68	3.94	1.69
Patients	7.44	6.15	1.75	0.98	1.51	4.48

insignificant for all the antigens except HL-A10. The mating analysis of a polymorphic system like HL-A is difficult when the number of observations is relatively small. The statistically significant X^2 value for the sum of matings involving HL-A10 can be explained by the low reaction frequency of the HL-A10 antigen, for example one mating HL-A10 × HL-A10 was observed whilst the expectation was less than one.

Taking an overall view the analysis of these husband/wife pairs showed that HL-A mating was at random for both 1st and 2nd loci. For example, there was no assortment leading to a tendency for like to mate with like. These observations indicate that the risk of a woman getting a trophoblastic neoplasm is not influenced by her choice of mate as far as the HL-A system is concerned.

These negative findings in the HL-A system are in marked contrast to the observations as far as the ABO system is concerned.[51] The risk of choriocarcinoma developing after any form of pregnancy is critically related to the ABO groups of both the woman and her spouse. Women of Group A with Group O husbands were found to be most at risk, whereas women of Group A married to Group A males had the least risk: the relative risk for these two groups was estimated to be 10.4/1. Both these types of matings can result only in conceptions which are ABO compatible with the mother, so that the mechanics of the ABO effect cannot be simply by maternal compatibility with the conception. The authors considered the possibility of the foreigness of the maternal tissue acting as a stimulus to trophoblastic proliferation. However, when they considered the group of patients in whom choriocarcinoma had followed a term delivery, they found that amongst 13 couples, patient Group A, husband Group O, the occurrence of a tumor had been associated with an antecedent child of Group A in 7 families and with a Group O child in 6 families. This distribution fits normal segregation ratios. Thus direct examination of the antigenity of the mother to the conception antecedent to choriocarcinoma precluded maternal ABO incompatibility as a major factor. For the present the explanation of the ABO effect must remain an enigma.

Prognosis

Even though the choice of mate with regard to the HL-A system may not influence the chance of a woman getting a trophoblastic tumor, once the tumor has developed the prognosis could be affected by the degree of foreigness of the tumor. To investigate this problem the extent of histocompatibility differences between husband and wife can be scored.[52] A simple way of scoring is to divide the patient/husband pairs into those in which the wife has no antigens in common with the husband and those in which one or more antigens are common to husband and wife. Amongst 73 patients who had completed treatment there were 4 deaths among 30 who had no antigens in common with their husbands and 8 deaths amongst

43 having one or two antigens in common with the husband. So the chance of survival does not appear to be influenced by the degree of compatibility between husband and wife. Furthermore, no obvious correlation could be found between the degree of compatibility and the duration of therapy necessary to obtain a remission in the survivors, or the extent of metases. Nevertheless, immune mechanisms may make some contribution to the killing of tumor cells. For example, it has been claimed that patients with choriocarcinoma have a better prognosis when the histology shows a well-marked mononuclear cell reaction in the vicinity of the tumor.[53]

Analysis of the data revealed that a most important influence on the chance of survival was the length of time that elapsed between the pregnancy preceding the development of the tumor and the commencement of therapy. The mean value of this time interval for the patients who had died was fourteen months, but for the survivors the interval was only six months. Thus the effect of all other factors has to be viewed against the background of the extreme importance of early diagnosis and treatment in prognosis.

Antibodies

HL-A antibodies can be stimulated by normal pregnancies, transfusions and deliberate immunization with skingrafts or leucocytes. The combination of pregnancy and transfusion sometimes results in the formation of particularly potent antibodies. This has been found to be the case in some of the patients with trophoblastic neoplasia. Sera from 97 of these patients have been screened for antibodies,[54] 53 cases of choriocarcinoma and 44 from patients who required treatment for a trophoblastic neoplasia, the nature of which was not defined histologically. There was no difference in the frequency of occurrence of antibodies in the two groups of patients both having lympho-cytotoxic antibodies in 45 percent of cases. Most of the antibodies reacted with HL-A antigens present on the lymphocytes of the husbands, but occasionally antibodies were found that reacted only with cells of the normal donor panel, but not with those of the husband. This could be attributed to response limited to the allogeneic transfused lymphocytes.

Many of the antibodies were multispecific, but monospecific sera were also found. A most interesting feature was the way in which the specificity and titre of the antibody changed during the time the patient was being treated. This was observed by examin-ing a series of samples of sera from each pa-tient. With the passage of time, as treatment proceeded, the titres of the antibodies de-creased and concomitantly they became more specific as the weaker ones disappeared. There was a tendency for even the specific antibodies eventually to disappear. Although antibodies were found as long as two years after the disease had been cured, in order to assess the frequency of antibodies the screen-ing should be done whilst the patient is still hospitalized. Some of the patients in the present series were tested when the disease was no longer active, so it is likely that the frequency of 45 percent quoted above is an underestimate.

As far as can be judged at present, the presence of antibodies does not bear a sim-ple correlation with prognosis. Antibodies have been found in patients who have been cured and in those who have died. Although the antibody is detected by a cytotoxic test *in vitro*, it does not necessarily follow that the antibody would have a cytotoxic effect on allogeneic cells *in vivo*. On the contrary, it could even be that the antibodies could under certain circumstances, have an en-hancing effect and promote the growth of the tumor.

Hydatidiform Moles

The question whether transplantation anti-gens are present on murine or human tropho-blast is controversial.[46] Evidence suggesting the presence of HL-A antigens on cells cultured from normal placenta has been obtained by Loke, *et al.*[55] As far as hydati-diform moles are concerned there is no direct evidence of the expression of HL-A antiges. However, as early as 1964, Máthe, *et al*,[56] found leucoglutinins, of undetermined speci-ficity, which reacted with the husbands' leucocytes, in a patient who had only a single pregnancy with a hydatidiform mole.

If the husbands and children of patients with trophoblastic neoplasia are typed for the HL-A antigens and the serum of the mother is tested for specific HL-A antibodies, then it is possible to find out whether these antibodies can be stimulated by a molar pregnancy. Amongst the 97 patients studied in the present series, there were three in whom evidence suggesting stimulation by molar pregnancy was obtained. One of the patients has the haplotypes 9,12/W19,5 and her hus-band's are 11,12/2,W27. A normal child was born in 1965 having the haplotypes 11,12/ 9,12. Following a molar pregnancy in 1968 the patient required treatment from March to May of that year for persistent tropho-blastic disease. On investigation in February 1969, her serum had been found to contain a mixture of anti-Hl-A2 and anti-W27; in May 1969 a monospecific serum containing anti-W27 was found, but by June 1970 both the antibodies had disappeared. The patient had had some transfusions in December of 1968 and it is, of course, possible that the anti-HL-A2 component could have been stimu-lated by the transfusion since this antigen is so common in Caucasians. An attempt was made to trace the donors of the blood and the only one who could be found had neither the HL-A2 or W27 antigens. The presence of the anti-W27 antibody is more significant since the chance of a random Caucasian donor having this antigen is only about one in twenty-five. It seemed most likely that both the antibodies had been stimulated by the molar pregnancy, and that these antibodies disappeared when trophoblastic tissue was no longer present. The conclusion could be reached that the paternal haplotype of the mole, HL-A2,W27 had been determined by detecting the antibodies raised in the mother by this conceptus.

A second patient had had only one pregnancy with a hydatidiform mole and while she was under treatment for persistant trophoblastic disease, an anti-W22 antibody was detected in her serum. The husband had the W22 antigen which was lacked by the wife. There had been some previous history of transfusion, but again it must be regarded as significant that an antibody was formed against such a rare antigen (the frequency of W22 in Caucasians is of the order of 7%).

The most convincing evidence was obtained in the case of a patient who had not been transfused, who had had only one pregnancy with a mole, whose husband was HL-A8 positive and who formed a monospecific HL-A8 antibody which disappeared after successful treatment had been completed.

Thus it may be concluded that a pregnancy with a hydatidiform mole can be immunogenic to the mother for the antigens of the HL-A system.

Summary

The HL-A system is of major importance in histocompatibility reactions in man. The antigens belonging to the system are widely distributed throughout the body. The genetic control is by two linked loci which are sited adjacent to a separate locus that controls the mixed lymphocyte reaction.

Due to the relationship between the H2 system and virus induced leukemia in mice, attempts have been made to find similar associations in man. Up till now the evidence of suggested phenotypic associations in leukemia have not been adequately confirmed. However, the world-wide data on Hodgkins Disease suggest a positive correlation with the presence of the W5 and related antigens.

Gestational choriocarcinoma is a malignant allograft, foreign to the patient through the genetic contribution of the husband. By typing children antecedent to choriocarcinoma in those cases in which the tumor was preceded by a live term birth, it is possible to obtain information about the HL-A constitution of the tumor. Evidence has thus been obtained that choriocarcinoma is not preferentially associated with HL-A compatible conceptions and that such conceptions differ from the mother over the whole range of HL-A specificities. It would also appear that the risk of a woman suffering from trophoblastic neoplasia following live-term birth, abortion or pregnancy with a hydatidiform mole is not directly related to the choice of mate as far as the HL-A system is concerned.

Acknowledgments

I thank Dr. K. D. Bagshawe, Professor R. M. Hardisty and Dr. Mouvenna Till for up-to-date information about their patients.

REFERENCES

1. Histocompatibility Testing—Publication 1229 National Academy of Sciences—National Research Council, Washington, D.C. 1965.
2. Histocompatibility Testing 1965, Munksgaard, Copenhagen, 1965.
3. Histocompatibility Testing 1967, Munksgaard, Copenhagen, 1967.
4. Histocompatibility Testing 1970, Munksgaard, Copenhagen, 1970.
5. Histocompatibility Testing 1972, Munksgaard, Copenhagen, 1973.
6. Payne, R., Tripp, M., Weigle, J., Bodmer, W., and Bodmer, J: A new leukocyte isoantigen system in man. *Cold Spring Harbor Symp Quant Biol, 29:*285–295, 1964.
7. Dausset, J: Iso-leuco-anticorps. *Acta Haematol (Basel), 20:*156–166, 1958.
8. Bodmer, W., Bodmer, J., Adler, S., Payne, R., and Bialek, J.: Genetics of '4' and 'LA' human leucocyte groups. *Ann NY Acad Sci, 129,* 473–489, 1966.
9. Walford, R.L., Wallace, O., Shanbrom, E., and Troup, G.N.: Lc-11 as a mutually exclusive specificity to Lc-1, 2 and 3 in the main human leukocyte group. *Vox Sang, 15:*338–344, 1968.
10. Dausset, J., Walford, R.L., Colombani, J., Legrand, L., Feingold, N., and Rapaport, F.T.: The HL-A sub-loci and their importance in Transplantation. *Transplant Proc, 1:*331–338, 1969.
11. Ceppellini, R., Curtoni, E.S., Mattiuz, P.L., Miggiano, V., Scudeller, G., and Serra, A.: Genetics of leukocyte antigens: a family study of segregation and linkage. In Histocompatibility Testing, 1967, pp. 149–185.
12. Rood, J.J., van., Leeuwan, A., van., Schippers, A.M.J., Vooys, W.H., Frederiks, E., Balner, H., and Eernisse, J.G.: Leukocyte groups, the normal lymphocyte transfer test and homograft sensitivity. In normal lymphocyte transfer test and homograft sensitivity. In Histocompatibility Testing 1965, pp. 37-50.
13. Svejgaard, A., Thorsby, E., Hauge, M., and Kissmeyer-Nielsen, F.: Genetics of the HL-A system. A population and family study. *Vox Sang, 18:*97–133, 1970.
14. Mayr, W.R.: MaKi, a new leucocyte antigen. Preliminary report. *Vox Sang, 18:*180–182, 1970.
15. Thorsby, E., and Kissmeyer-Nielsen, F.: New HL-A alleles. Identification by planned immunization. *Vox Sang, 18:*134–148, 1970.
16. Lawler, S.D., Klouda, P.T., Hardisty, R.M., and Till, M.M.: The HL-A system in lymphoblastic leukaemia. A study of patients and their families. *Br J Haematol, 21:*595–605, 1971.
17. Bodmer, W.F., Bodmer, J.G., and Tripp, M.: Recombination between the LA and 4 loci of the HL-A system. In Histocompatibility Testing, 1970, pp. 187–191.
18. Klouda, P.T., and Lawler, S.D.: Another recombination within the HL-A system. *Vox Sang, 22:*85–88, 1972.
19. Lilly, F., Boyse, E.A., and Old, L.J.: Genetic basis of susceptibility to viral leukaemogenesis. *Lancet, ii:*1207–1209, 1964.
20. Lilly, F.: Genetic determination of susceptibility to Friend virus in mice. Proceedings of the American Association for Cancer Research, *8:*41, 1967.
21. Fedrick, J., and Alberman, E.D.: Reported influenza in pregnancy and subsequent cancer in the child. *Br Med J, 2:*485–488.
22. Kourilsky, F.M., Dausset, J., Feingold, N., Dupuy, J.M., and Bernard, J.: Etude de la répartition des antigènes leucocytaires chez les malades atteints de leucemie aigue en rémission. Advance in Transplantation, p. 515–522. Munksgaard, Copenhagen, 1968.
23. Walford, R.L., Finkelstein, S., Neerhaut, R., Konrad, P., and Shanbrom, E.: Acute childhood leukaemic relation to the HL-A human Transplantation genes. *Nature* (Lond), *225:*461–462, 1970.
24. Walford, R.L., Zeller, E., Combs, L., and Konrad, P.: HL-A specificities in acute and chronic lymphatic leukaemia. *Transplant Proc, 3:*1297–1300, 1971.
25. Walford, R.L., Smith, G.S., and Waters, H.: Histocompatibility systems and disease states with particular reference to cancer. *Transplant Rev, 7:*78–11, 1971.
26. Hardisty, R.M., Till, M.M., Lawler, S.D.,

Klouda, P.T., Batchelor, J.R., Edwards, J.H., Stuart, J., Cook, P.J.L., and Robson, E.B.: Data on the linkage relationships of the HL-A and α-haptoglobin loci in man. *Ann Hum Genet, 35:*161–166, 1971.

27. Degos, L., Drolet, Y., and Dausset, J.: HL-A antigens in chronic myeloid leukaemia (CML) and chronic lymphoid leukaemia (CLL). *Transplant Proc, 3:*1309–1310, 1971.

28. Jeannet, M., and Magnin, C.: HL-A antigens in haematological malignant diseases. *Transplant Proc, 3:*1301–1303, 1971.

29. Dick, H.M., Steel, C.M., and Crichton, W.B.: HL-A typing of cultured peripheral lymphoblastoid cells. *Tissue Antigens, 2:*85–93, 1972.

30. Yunis, E.J., and Amos, D.B.: Three closely linked genetic systems relevant to Transplantation. *Proc U.S. Natl Acad Sci, 68:* 3031–3035, 1971.

31. Johnston, J.M., and Bashir, H.V.: Response of HL-A Identical Individuals in the mixed lymphocyte culture test. *Brit Med J, 4:*581–584, 1971.

32. Koch, C.T., Eysvoogel, V.P., Frederiks, E., and van Rood, J.J.: Mixed-lymphocyte—culture and Skin-graft data in unrelated HL-A identical individuals. *Lancet, ii:*1334–1336, 1971.

33. Pentycross, C.R., Klouda, P.T., and Lawler, S.D.: The HL-A system and the mixed lymphocyte reaction. *Lancet, i:*95, 1972.

34. Dupont, B., Nielsen, L.S., and Svejgaard, A.: Relative importance of four and LA loci in determining mixed-lymphocyte reaction. *Lancet, ii:*1336–1340, 1971.

35. Pentycross, C.R., Chronic lymphocytic leukaemic and the mixed lymphocyte reaction. *Lymphology, 7:*7–12, 1972.

36. Amiel, J.L.: Study of the leucocyte phenotypes in Hodgkins Disease. In Histocompatibility Testing, 1967, p. 79.

37. Kissmeyer-Nielsen, F., Jensen, K.B., Ferrara, G.B., Kjerbye, K.E., and Svejgaard, A.: HL-A phenotypes in Hodgkins Disease. Preliminary Report. *Transplant Proc, 3:* 1287–1289, 1971.

38. Morris, P.J., and Forbes, J.F.: HL-A and Hodgkins Disease. *Transplant Proc, 3:* 1275–1277, 1971.

39. Zervas, J.D., Delamore, J.W., and Israels, M.C.O.: Leucocyte phenotypes in Hodgkins Disease. *Lancet, ii:*634–635, 1970.

40. Amiel, J.L.: In Discussion. Relationships between tumor antigens and histocompatility systems. *Transplant Proc, 3:*1279–1281, 1971.

41. Thorsby, E., Falk, J., Engeset, A., and Osoba, D.: HL-A antigens in Hodgkins Disease. *Transplant Proc, 3:*1279–1281, 1971.

42. Rood, J.J. van, and Leeuwen, A. van: HL-A and the group five system in Hodgkins Disease. *Transplant Proc 3:*1283–1286, 1971.

43. Coukell, A., Bodmer, J.G., and Bodmer, W.F.: HL-A Types of forty four Hodgkins patients. *Transplant Proc, 3:*1291–1293, 1971.

44. Jeannet, M., and Magnin, C.: HL-A antigens in haematological malignant diseases. *Eur J Clin Invest, 2:*39–42. 1971.

45. Bertrams, J., Kuwert, E., Böhme, U., Reis, H.E., Gallmeier, W.M., Wetter, O., and Schmidt, C.G.: HL-A antigens in Hodgkins Disease and multiple myeloma. Increased frequency of W18 in both diseases. *Tissue Antigens, 2:*41–46, 1971.

46. Beer, A.E., and Billingham, R.E.: Immunobiology of mammalian reproduction. *Adv Immunol, 14:*1–83, 1971.

47. Clarke, B., and Kirby, D.R.S.: Maintenance of histocompatibility polymorphisms. *Nature, Lond, 211:*999–1000, 1966.

48. Lawler, S.D.: The HL-A system and choriocarcinoma. Proceedings of II International symposium on immunology of reproduction. *Sofia, Bulg Acad Sci, 193:*567–569.

49. Lewis, J.L., and Terasaki, P.I.: HL-A leukocyte antigen studies in women with gestational trophoblastic neoplasms. *Am J Obstet Gynecol, 111:*547–552, 1971.

50. Klouda, P.T., Lawler, S.D., and Bagshawe, K.D.: HL-A matings in trophoblastic neoplasia. *Tissue Antigens. 2:*280–284, 1972.

51. Bagshawe, K.D., Rawlins, G., Pike, M.C., and Lawler, S.D.: ABO blood-groups in trophoblastic neoplasia. *Lancet, i:*553–557, 1971.

52. Lawler, S.D., Klouda, P.T., and Bagshawe, K.D.: The HL-A system in trophoblastic neoplasia. *Lancet, ii:*834–837, 1971.

Cancer Genetics

53. Elston, C.E.: Cellular Reaction to Choriocarcinoma. *J Pathol, 97:*261–268, 1969.

54. Klouda, P.T., Lawler, S.D., and Bagshawe, K.D.: HL-A antibodies in patients with trophoblastic neoplasia I General Survey. Symposia series in immunological standardization. New York, Kaiger, Basel. *18:*268–271, 1973.

55. Loke, Y.W., Joysey, V.C., and Borland, R: HL-A antigens in human trophoblast cells. *Nature* (Lond), *232:*403–405, 1971.

56. Mathe, G., Dausset, J., Hervet, E., Amiel, J.L., Colambani, J., and Brule, G.: Immunological studies in patients with placental choriocarcinoma. *J Natl Cancer Inst, 33:* 193–208, 1964.

CHAPTER 7

VIRUSES, GENES, AND CANCER

HARVEY DOSIK AND GEORGE J. TODARO

ALTHOUGH THE CAUSES OF leukemia and cancer are unknown, the combination of epidemiologic research, chromosome studies, immunologic testing, and tumor viral transformation studies have helped to identify susceptible groups and individuals. This presentation is concerned with summarizing the contributions and interrelationships of these techniques.

The epidemiologic method has been used to identify genetic influences in cancer, especially leukemia. The initial studies of Krivit and Good[1,2] revealed an increase in acute leukemia in children with Down's syndrome. This association was noted prior to the discovery that patients with Down's syndrome had an extra G group chromosome in all their cells[3] (Fig. 7–1). The increased incidence of leukemia in Down's syndrome was subsequently found to be between 18 and 30 times greater than the expected rate.[4–6] Although the increased incidence of other tumors does not appear to be as marked as the increased incidence of acute leukemia, one study has reported that the incidence of other cancers was 2.6 times greater than expected.

The relationship of Down's syndrome to leukemia extends beyond their occurrence in the same patient. In a study involving 1,000 siblings of leukemic children, Miller[7] found five with Down's syndrome compared with an expected rate of 1.4; this is statistically significant at the 5 percent level. Another feature that both leukemia and Down's syndrome have in common is their increased occurrence with relation to maternal age.

It is well known that the risk of Mongolism markedly increases with the mother's age at the birth of her child.[8] A similar phenomenon is found in childhood leukemia.[9,10] In fact, leukemia has been found to be 40 percent more common in children whose mothers' were over 40 years of age than those under 20 years of age. The possibility exists that chromosomal nondisjunction, which causes Down's syndrome, may also play a role in the etiology of childhood leukemia.[11]

The incidence of leukemia and cancer in other trisomic conditions is not clear. There would appear to be an increase of leukemia in D Trisomy. Since D Trisomy is a rare condition where patients die shortly after birth, the finding of any cases at all would be unusual; two cases have been reported.[12,13] There are a number of case reports of leukemia in Klinefelter's syndrome, but no conclusive evidence of a relationship between the two conditions.[14]

An increase in leukemia and cancer is not limited to chromosomal aneuploidy and is probably more common in conditions where unstable chromosomal anomalies predominate. Fanconi's anemia is an autosomal recessive disorder characterized by multiple congenital abnormalities, chromosome anomalies and irreversible aplastic anemia. Chromosome anomalies consist of chromosome and chromatid breaks, exchange figures, endoreduplications and translocations[15] (Fig. 7–2). Patients with Fanconi's anemia demonstrate a marked increase in leukemia and other tumors.[16,17] A similar, but lower, increase in malignancy has been

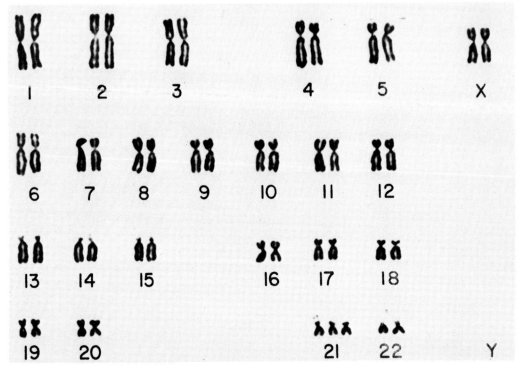

Figure 7–1. Karyotype from a patient with Down's syndrome showing an extra G group chromosome.

postulated for Fanconi heterozygotes,[18] and this finding has been recently confirmed.[19]

Bloom's syndrome, which is also inherited as an autosomal recessive disorder, is characterized by photosensitive telangiectasia and the same type of unstable chromosome anomalies found in Fanconi's anemia. Sawitsky, *et al.*[20] reported three cases of acute leukemia among 23 persons with this syndrome.

The relationship of unstable chromosome anomalies to an increased risk of malignancy is further emphasized by the increased incidence of leukemia in populations exposed to ionizing radiation. Chromosome studies performed after exposure to ionizing radiation reveal chromosome breaks, translocations, exchanges and fragments; all these findings are similar to the abnormalities present in patients with an inherited tendency to chromosomal breakage. Gradually, the less stable anomalies disappear, but translocations and aneuploidy remain many years later.[21] An increased incidence of leukemia has been linked with total body radiation[22] as well as partial body exposure.[23] The peak incidence occurs about six years after exposure,[24] but an increase is still detected more than twenty years later.[22]

Recently, it has become clear that genetic disorders other than those in which chromosome abnormalities are present may have a higher incidence of malignancy. Patients with primary immunodeficiency disorders, for instance, have an incidence 10,000 times that of an age-matched population.[25] These disorders include infantile x-linked agammaglobulinemia, Wiskott-Aldrich disease, Ataxia-telangiectasia, etc. In addition, individuals who have been treated with immunosup-

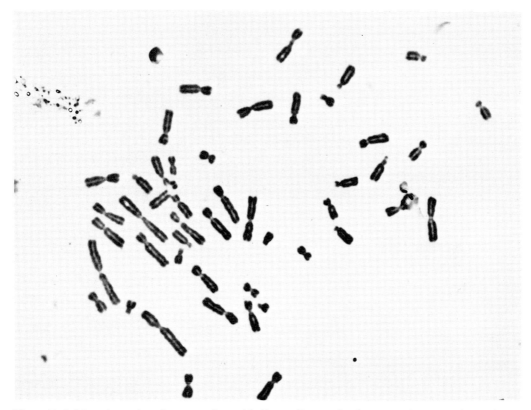

Figure 7–2. Metaphase plate from a patient with Fanconi's anemia, demonstrating an exchange figure.

pressive agents for prolonged periods, i.e. renal transplant recipients, have an unusually high incidence of malignancy.[26]

A genetic influence on leukemia occurrence is confirmed by studies in twins and siblings of patients with leukemia without congenital defects.[27] McMahon and Levy,[28] using birth and death certificates, uncovered seventy-two twin pairs in which at least one twin had developed leukemia; there were five instances in which both twins developed leukemia. Of the seventy-two twins, forty-seven were of identical sex. One would expect twenty-two out of forty-seven to be monozygous; all five twin pairs with leukemia appeared to be monozygous. This would indicate that between 20 to 25 percent of the monozygous twins of patients with leukemia would also be expected to develop leukemia. Further suggestive evidence for a genetic factor is the finding that siblings of leukemic children have a greater incidence of leukemia than the expected rate. Miller[7] estimates this to be four times greater than normal, but data accumulated thus far are not conclusive enough (four cases versus one expected case) to determine an exact incidence.

Both RNA and DNA containing viruses have been shown to produce tumors in animals and to transform cells in culture. In addition, they frequently produce extensive chromosomal damage in the cells they infect and transform. Recently, studies in a variety of systems have shown that tumor viruses can be carried as part of the genetic information of cells in an unexpressed form for long periods, only to become activated by a variety of extrinsic and intrinsic factors. Although there is no evidence implicating virus specific genetic material in the etiology of human tumors, the discovery that many animal tumors are virus induced has led to the assumption that viruses also play a role in human malignancy. Growth of both animal and human cells in tissue culture have enabled evaluation of the effect of various tumor viruses on them. The effect on cultured cells varies with the type of virus employed.[29] We will concern ourselves only with the effects of one of the nonenveloped DNA tumor viruses, Simian Virus SV40.

Several systems for studying the *in vitro* transformation of cells in tissue culture by oncogenic viruses have previously been described.[30,31] After inoculation of fibroblast cultures with SV40, about 20 percent of the cells are killed. Others become infected with virus, but only a small percentage go on to multiply until they form transformed colo-

nies. These colonies can be easily identified against the background of untransformed cells by their dense and disordered pattern of growth. Approximately three weeks after infection, staining with 1 percent hematoxylin identifies the transformed colonies as darkly stained areas[32] (Fig. 7 3). The colonies can be isolated and the cells transferred and serially propagated. When grown in mass culture, the cells are capable of producing virus. Characteristics of transformed colonies include loss of contact inhibition of cell division, increase in growth density, chromosome anomalies (aneuploidy), morphologic alterations and the ability to propagate indefinitely.[29] On the other hand, normal cells in culture have only a finite lifetime.[33] Thus, transformed cells in culture may be considered as, in some respects, counterparts of tumor cells *in vitro*.

Koprowski *et al.*[34] and Shein and Enders[35] showed that SV40 was capable of transforming human fibroblast cultures. Such transformed human cells acquire new antigens

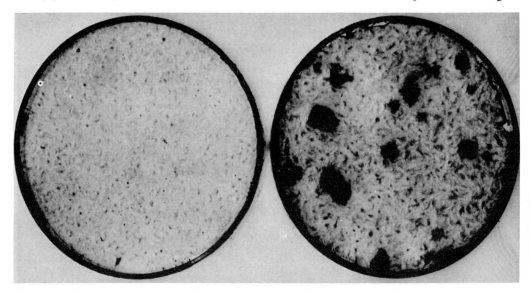

Figure 7 3. Photograph of two petri dishes. The one on the left shows a control culture not infected with SV40. The one on the right shows a culture three weeks after infection with SV40. Both have been fixed with formalin and stained with 1% hematoxylin. Each of the large dark staining areas is a transformed colony produced by SV40.

not present in the virus itself. One of these antigens, the T antigen, is located in the cell nucleus. It can be identified by staining with fluorescent antibody.[36] Though an early marker of virus infection, the T antigen does not require either virus replication or DNA synthesis for its presence. T antigen can be identified in about 1 percent of infected cells, and only about 1 in 250 T antigen positive cells become transformed colonies (a transformation rate of 1 in 25,000).[37] Transformation of human cells with SV40 is, thus, an inefficient system.

In 1966, Todaro *et al.*[32] described a method for quantitating transformation in human diploid fibroblasts. By using a fixed reproducible number of virus particles, a constant number of transformed colonies could be obtained from a given cell strain. This enabled one to look for differences between cultures from various disease states. Because of the length of time necessary to perform the transformation assay by this method, a more rapid one was needed. A technique utilizing the presence of SV40 T antigen was found to correlate well with transformation. The percentage of cells containing T antigen at seventy-two hours was directly proportional to the number of transformed colonies formed after three weeks.[37,38]

Initially, the transformation assay was performed on patients with Fanconi's anemia and their parents. These studies showed a markedly increased number of transformed colonies in the homozygotes compared to normal controls. The heterozygotes also formed increased numbers of colonies[16,32,39,40] (Table 7-I). This increased susceptibility to transformation for patients with Fanconi's anemia has been confirmed in other laboratories,[41,42] though one laboratory did not find increased transformation in Fanconi heterozygotes.[41] Todaro, *et al.* have also shown an increased susceptibility to SV40 in patients with Down's syndrome

TABLE 7-I
TRANSFORMATION FREQUENCY OF
VIRUS-INFECTED HUMAN CELL LINES
(Values are means, $\pm$ standard errors, of 2–6 separate experiments, in each of which a total of at least 2×10^5 infected cells were plated.)†

Cell strain	$\dfrac{Transformed\ colonies}{cells\ plated} \times 10^4$	
	SV40*	E46**
Normal adults		
A	4.4 ± 1.1	0.8 ± 0.3
PB	1.6 ± 0.2	
JW	4.3 ± 0.6	0.5 ± 0.2
LG	5.1 ± 0.6	0.4 ± 0.3
HG	2.6 ± 0.7	0.4 ± 0.2
LK	3.0 ± 0.5	
RT	3.7 ± 0.6	
Fanconi's anemia, homozygous		
AM	79.7 ± 18.1	16.3 ± 3.4
JV	41.4 ± 12.5	
Fanconi's anemia, heterozygous		
TM	20.1 ± 3.2	
CV	28.2 ± 8.7	

† Reprinted from *Science*, 153:1252–1254, 1966.
* Infected with $10^{8.0}$ TCID/ml.
** Infected with $10^{8.2}$ CID/ml.

(Table 7-II),[39,40,43] a finding confirmed in other laboratories,[42,44] and these observations have been extended to other chromosome abnormalities. Single patients with D Trisomy and Klinefelter's syndrome were found to have an increased susceptibility to

TABLE 7-II
TRANSFORMATION OF NORMAL AND
TRISOMIC HUMAN SKIN FIBROBLAST
CULTURES BY SV40*

Cell Strain		Transformed Colonies/10^4 Cells				
		Exp 1	Exp 2	Exp 3	Exp 4	Avg.
Normal	GULB	2.6	2.2	—	—	2.4
	MART	1.9	2.8	1.5	2.2	2.1
	DEYM	3.0	1.6	—	—	2.3
	TAYL	—	—	3.1	3.1	3.1
Trisomy 21–22	HOWA	7.2	9.3	—	—	8.2
	AUBE	9.2	4.3	—	—	6.8
	RICE	10.6	10.5	—	—	10.6
	LAVI	—	—	6.6	7.6	7.1
	MEYE	—	—	4.6	8.3	6.4
Trisomy 18	GALV	—	—	14.2	15.5	14.8

* Reprinted from *Proceedings of the Society for Experimental Biology and Medicine.* 124:1232–1236, 1967.

SV40.[43,45] However, Payne and Schmickel[42] found that triploid cells (69XXY) had a normal susceptibility to SV40, although cells of patients with Down's syndrome and Fanconi's anemia were more susceptible, as expected. This would seem to indicate that aneuploidy alone is not enough to predispose to susceptibility to viral transformation.

Increased susceptibility to SV40 is not limited to disorders with chromosome abnormalities. It has been found in a number of *cancer families*[39,46] and in a patient with xeroderma pigmentosum[47] (a hereditary disease manifested by a high skin sensitivity to ultraviolet light and an increased incidence of skin tumors). Radiation-treated cells also demonstrate an increase in the number of transformed colonies when exposed to SV40.[48] Susceptibility was increased as the radiation dose was increased (Table 7-III).

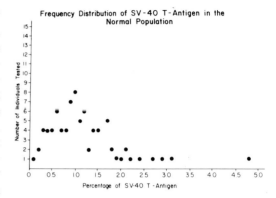

Figure 7–4.

TABLE 7-III
TRANSFORMATION FREQUENCY IN 3T3,
IRRADIATED BEFORE INFECTION WITH
SV40 ($10^{7.0}$ TCID.ml.)*

Radiation Dose (Rads)	CFA (Percent)	Transformed Colonies Cells Plated ($\times 10^{-4}$)	Total Colonies ($\times 10^{-3}$)
0	50.4	5.4	1.1
75	46.2	4.0	0.9
150	50.3	31.5	6.3
300	46.0	14.0	3.0
500	28.3	28.5	10.1
900	3.3	10.2	30.9

*Reprinted from *Nature*, 219:520–521, 1968.
Each value represents data obtained from at least 6 plates, each inoculated with at least 5×10^3 cells.

Recently, a *control* population has been studied to determine the number of normals with increased susceptibility to SV40 and to look for possible differences in transformation associated with age, sex, and race. The population was selected to eliminate those who had a strong family history of malignancy, and consisted of *normal* nonhospitalized volunteers, many of whom were workers at two Brooklyn hospitals. Eighty-four individuals were studied. T antigen percentage

was used as a measure of SV40 transformation. The mean for T antigen was 1.1 ± 0.7 percent, and all values above 2.5 percent were considered abnormal (Fig. 7–4). There was no difference in percentage related to race or sex. People over 50 years of age had a mean value that was slightly lower than the overall population (Table 7-IV). However, this may represent an insufficient number of tested individuals. Chromosome studies were performed on peripheral blood lymphocytes of the *normal* population to determine if minor abnormalities could be linked to increased transformation. There was no correlation of increased susceptibility to SV40 of these controls with an increase in chromosome abnormalities.

Studies on the normal population have provided a reference to compare patient

TABLE 7-IV
T ANTIGEN MEANS AND STANDARD ERRORS
FOR VARIOUS AGE GROUPS

Age	No. Tested	Mean	S.E.	T Value	P Value
1–10	6	1.143	0.207	0.208	>0.45
11–20	14	1.477	0.223	1.668	<0.05
21–30	13	1.051	0.109	0.309	<0.35
31–40	13	1.007	0.151	0.554	>0.35
41–50	14	1.442	0.286	1.174	<0.10
51–60	15	0.686	0.100	3.377	>0.005
61–70	9	0.941	0.181	0.817	>0.20
51–70	24	0.782	0.467	2.68	>0.01
Overall values	84	1.098	0.714		

groups and individuals. It will enable the identification of groups where susceptibility to transformation is present in some, but not all the individuals. For example, preliminary results indicate that untreated patients with acute myeloblastic leukemia and their first-degree relatives have an increased susceptibility to SV40. (Mean T antigen was 2.41% in a group of 30 patients and 2.3% in 14 relatives.) In this group of patients, individuals with both normal and markedly elevated values were found. Patients with inherited disorders of immunodeficiency who have a greatly increased risk of developing cancer do not have an increased susceptibility to SV40.[49]

In an attempt to identify populations with an increased susceptibility to SV40, a number of relatively inbred human population groups have been studied. Studies are also in progress to determine the susceptibility to SV40 in the following groups:

1. Patients with leukemia and their family members.
2. *Cancer* families.
3. Family members of patients and normals with a high susceptibility to SV40.

4. Patients with leukemias or solid tumors prior to and after therapy.

RNA tumor viruses are also capable of transforming human cell cultures, and quantitative systems to estimate susceptibility to these viruses have been reported.[50] Again, marked variations in susceptibility of cells from different individuals have been noted. The association with clinical risk has not been adequately explored with the RNA tumor virus system.

Table 7-V summarizes data available on SV40 susceptibility and its relationship to malignancy in various patient groups. It would appear that the virus transformation assay detects one group of patients with an increased risk of malignancy. This group would seem to include patients in which an inherited or acquired genetic cellular defect is present. Another group of patients with a high risk of malignancy are those with disorders of immunodeficiency. Screening of normals and various patient groups for immunologic defects may detect yet another group of susceptible individuals who have normal SV40 susceptibility.

A more thorough knowledge of who will

TABLE 7-V
SUMMARY OF SUSCEPTIBILITY TO SV40 OF VARIOUS PATIENT GROUPS

Patient Group	Risk of Malignancy	SV40 Susceptibility
Fanconi's anemia	Homozygotes and heterozygotes have an increased risk.	Increased greatly in homozygotes and somewhat in heterozygotes.
Down's syndrome	20 to 30-fold increase in acute leukemia. Questionable increase in other tumors.	Increased.
Other trisomies	Questionable.	Increased.
Radiation treated	Increased in atom bomb survivors, polycythemia treated with P32 and radiotherapy and ankylosing spondylitis treated with radiotherapy.	Increased in cells previously treated. Dose related.
Identical twins of children with leukemia	Incidence of leukemia in the second twin is 1 in 5.	Not adequately tested.
Siblings of leukemic children	Four-fold increase in leukemia.	Appears increased in acute myeloblastic leukemia. Results not complete with acute lymphoblastic leukemia.
Xeroderma pigmentosum	Increase in skin cancer.	Increasrd in one study; normal in another.
Cancer families	Familial increase in specific or all malignancies.	Not adequately tested. Increased in one AML prone family (46).
Primary immuno-deficiency syndromes	Marked increase.	Not increased.

develop cancer and why they develop it may aid in the prevention and early discovery of malignancy. Virus transformation of cells in tissue culture might provide a valuable screening procedure for detecting susceptible individuals, and, perhaps, ultimately, for getting at the cellular defects that allow a normal cell to transform into a cancer cell.

REFERENCES

1. Krivit, W., and Good, R.A.: The simultaneous occurrence of leukemia and Mongolism. *Am J Dis Child, 91:*218–222, 1956.

2. Kirivit, W., and Good, R.A.: Simultaneous occurrence of Mongolism and leukemia. Report of nationwide survey. *Am J Dis Child, 94:*289–293, 1957.

3. Leujeune, J., Gautier, M., and Turpin, R.: Les chromosomes humains en culture des tissus. *CR Acad Sci* (Paris), *248:*602, 1959.

4. Wald, N., Borges, W.H., Li, C.C., Turner, J.H., and Harnois, M.C.: Leukemia associated with Mongolism. *Lancet, 1:*1228, 1961.

5. Hollan, R., Doll, R., and Carter, C.O.: The mortality from leukemia and other cancers among patients with Down's syndrome (Mongols) and among their parents. *Br J Cancer, 16:*177–186, 1962.

6. Barber, R., and Spiers, P.: Oxford survey of childhood cancer. Progress report 11. *Monthly Bull Minst Health* (London), *23:*46–52, 1964.

7. Miller, R.W.: Down's syndrome (Mongolism), other congenital malformations and cancers among the sibs of leukemic children. *New Engl J Med, 268:*393–401, 1963.

8. Shuttleworth, G.E.: Mongolism imbecility. *Br Med J, 2:*1097–1099, 1962.

9. Stewart, A., Webb, J., and Hewitt, D.: Survey of childhood malignancies. *Br Med J, 1:*1495–1508, 1958.

10. MacMahon, B., and Newill, V.A.: Birth characteristics of children dying of malignant neoplasms. *J Natl Cancer Inst, 28:*231–244, 1962.

11. Miller, R.W.: Radiation, chromosomes and viruses in the etiology of leukemia. Evidence from epidemiologic research. *New Engl J Med, 271:*30–36, 1964.

12. Schade, H., Schoeller, L., and Schultze, K.W.: D-trisomie (Patausyndrom) mit kongeni-taler myeloischer leukamie. *Med Welt, 50:*2690–2692, 1962.

13. Zuelzer, W.W., Thompson, R.I., and Mastrangelo, R.: Chromatid exchange and breakage in the pedigree of a child with leukemia and partial D-trisomy: Evidence for a genetic factor in leukemogenesis and congenital malformations. *Blood, 28:*10008, 1966 (Abs.)

14. Fraumeni, J.F., and Miller, R.W.: Epidemiology of human leukemia: Recent observations. *J Natl Cancer Inst, 38:*593–605, 1966.

15. Bloom, G.E., Warner, S., Gerald, P.S., and Diamond, K.K.: Chromosome abnormalities in constitutional aplastic anemia. *New Engl J Med, 274:*8–14, 1966.

16. Dosik, H., Hsu, L.Y., Todaro, G.J., Lee, S.L., Hirschhorn, K., Selirio, E.S., and Alter, A.A.: Leukemia in Fanconi's anemia. Cytogenetic and tumor virus susceptibility studies. *Blood, 36:*341–352, 1970.

17. Swift, M.R., and Hirschhorn, K.: Fanconi's anemia. Inherited susceptibility to chromosome breakage in various tissues. *Ann Intern Med, 65:*496–503, 1966.

18. Garriga, S., and Crosby, W.H.: The incidence of leukemia in families of patients with hypoplasia of the marrow. *Blood, 14:*1008–1014, 1959.

19. Swift, M.: Fanconi's anemia in the genetics of neoplasia. *Nature, 230:*370–373, 1971.

20. Sawitsky, A., Bloom, D., and German, J.: Chromosomal breakage and acute leukemia in congenital telangiectatic erythema and stunted growth. *Ann Intern Med, 65:*487–495, 1966.

21. Court Brown, W.M., Buckton, K.E., and McLean, A.S.: Quantitative studies of chromosome aberrations in man following acute and chronic exposure to x-rays and gamma rays. *Lancet, 1:*1239–1241, 1965.

22. Bizzozero, O.J., Johnson, K.G., and Ciocco, A.: Radiation related leukemia in Hiroshima and Nagasaki. 1. Distribution, incidence, and appearance time. *New Engl J Med, 274:*1095–1101, 1966.

23. Court Brown, W.M., and Doll, R.: Mortality from cancer and other causes after radiotherapy for ankylosing spondylitis. *Br Med J, 2:*1327–1332, 1965.

24. Miller, R.W.: Persons with exceptionally high risk of leukemia. *Cancer Res, 27:*2420–2423, 1967.

25. Gatti, R.A., and Good, R.A.: Occurrence of malignancy in immunodeficiency diseases. *Cancer, 28:*89–98, 1971.

26. McKhann, C.F.: Primary malignancy in patients undergoing immunosuppression for renal transplantation. *Transplantation, 8:* 209–212, 1969.

27. Miller, R.W.: Etiology of childhood leukemia. Epidemiologic evidence. *Pediatr Clin North Am, 13:*267–277, 1966.

28. MacMahon, B., and Levy, M.A.: Prenatal origin of childhood leukemia evidence from twins. *New Engl J Med, 270:*1082–1085, 1964.

29. Macpherson, I.: The characteristics of animal cells transformed *in vitro. Adv Cancer Res, 13:*169–215, 1970.

30. Temin, H.M., and Rubin, H.: Characteristics of an assay for Rous sarcoma virus and Rous sarcoma cells in tissue culture. *Virology, 6:*669–688, 1958.

31. Todaro, G.J., and Green, H.: An assay for cellular transformation by SV40. *Virology, 23:*117–119, 1964.

32. Todaro, G.J., Green, H., and Swift, M.R.: Susceptibility of human diploid fibroblast strains to transformation by SV40 virus. *Science, 153:*1252–1254, 1966.

33. Hayflick, L.: The limited *in vitro* lifetime of human diploid cell strains. *Exp Cell Res, 37:*614–636, 1965.

34. Koprowski, H., Ponten, J.R., Jensen, F., Ravdin, R.H., Moorehead, P.S., and Saksela, E.: Transformation of cultures of human tissue infected with Simian Virus 40. *J Cell Comp Physiol, 58:*281–292, 1962.

35. Shein, H.M., and Enders, J.F.: Transformation induced by Simian Virus 40 in human renal cell cultures. 1. Morphology and growth characteristics. *Proc Natl Acad Sci USA, 48:*1164–1172, 1962.

36. Pope, J.H., and Rowe, W.R.: Detection of specific antigen in SV40 transformed cells by immunofluorescence. *J Exp Med, 120:*124–128, 1964.

37. Aaronson, S.A., and Todaro, G.J.: SV40 T antigen induction and transformation in human fibroblast cell strains. *Virology, 36:* 254–261, 1968.

38. Potter, C.W., Potter, A.M., and Oxford, J.S.: Comparison of transformation and T antigen induction in human cell lines. *J Virol, 5:*293–298, 1970.

39. Todaro, G.J.: Variable susceptibility of human cell strains to SV40 transformation. *Natl Cancer Inst Monogr, 29:*271–273, 1968.

40. Miller, R.W., and Todaro, G.J.: Viral transformation of cells from persons at high risk of cancer. *Lancet, 1:*81–82, 1969.

41. Young, D.: SV40 transformation of cells from patients with Fanconi's anemia. *Lancet, 1:* 294–295, 1971.

42. Payne, F.E., and Schmickel, R.D.: Susceptibility of trisomic and of triploid human fibroblasts to Simian Virus 40 (SV40). *Nature* [New Biol], *230:*190, 1971.

43. Todaro, G.J., and Martin, G.M.: Down's syndrome. Increased sensitivity of fibroblast in cell culture to transformation by an oncogenic virus. *Proc Soc Exp Biol Med, 124:* 1232–1236, 1967.

44. Young, D.: The susceptibility to SV40 virus transformation of fibroblasts obtained from patients with Down's syndrome. *Eur J Cancer, 7:*337–339, 1971.

45. Mukerjee, D., Bowen, J., and Anderson, D.E.: Simian papovavirus 40. Transformation of cells from cancer patient with XY/XXY mosaic Klinefelter's syndrome. *Cancer Res, 30:*1769–1772, 1970.

46. Snyder, A.L., Li, R.P., Henderson, E.S., and Todaro, G.J.: Possible inherited factors in familial acute myelogenous leukemia. *Lancet, 1:*586–589, 1970.

47. Veldhuisen, G., and Pouwels, P.H.: Transformation of xeroderma pigmentosum cells by SV40. *Lancet, 2:*529–530, 1970.

48. Pollock, E.J., and Todaro, G.J.: Radiation enhancement of SV40 transformation in 3T3 and human cells. *Nature, 219*:520–521, 1968.

49. Kersey, J.H., Gatti, R.A., Good, R.A., Aaronson, S.A., and Todaro, G.J.: Susceptibility of cells from patients with primary immuno-deficiency diseases to SV40 transformation. *Proc Natl Acad Sci USA, 69*:980–982, 1972.

50. Klement, V., Freedman, M.H., McAllister, R.M., Nelson-Rees, W.A., and Heubner, R.J.: Differences in susceptibility of human cells to mouse sarcoma virus. *J Natl Cancer Inst, 47*:65–73, 1971.

CHAPTER 8

XERODERMA PIGMENTOSUM, DNA REPAIR

AND CARCINOGENESIS

James E. Cleaver

An extremely wide range of factors, both inherited and environmental, are involved in carcinogenesis. Amongst the environmental factors radiation has been known to be carcinogenic for many decades; the permissible doses set for occupational and medical exposures to X rays have been determined to a large extent by the carcinogenic risk involved. Similar considerations enter into problems of human exposure to many chemicals. Whether or not cancer will eventually be recognized as a predominantly viral disease, in the manner that much current research envisages, we must still take into account the major role played by factors such as radiation in stimulating the processes which produce malignant cells. In addition to environmental factors a variety of genetic factors also determine the frequency with which cancer occurs in man and other animals. Various strains of mice and rats with characteristic incidences of specific kinds of cancers are well known in the laboratory, as well as human families with abnormally high incidences of specific types[1-3] of cancer.

A unique human disease which shows remarkable association of environmental and genetic carcinogenic factors is the skin disease xeroderma pigmentosum (XP).[4-6]

Xeroderma Pigmentosum—Symptoms of the Disease

Xeroderma pigmentosum (Fig. 8–1) is a rare human hereditary disease in which the skin is extremely sensitive to radiation of the short wavelength end of the sun's spectrum (below 3100 Å approximately).[5] Sunlight produces skin cancers of both ectodermal and mesodermal origin (basal cell carcinomas, squamous cell carcinomas, melanomas, angiosarcomas, fibrosarcomas, and keratoacanthomas). The cancers develop on the sun-exposed areas during the first years of life and continually recur. When skin from an unexposed area is transplanted to the face, the typical progression on the transplanted skin consists of increased pigmentation, keratoses and then malignancy. Death often occurs in early life from metastases, unless careful palliative and preventative treatment is given. Hebra and Kaposi first identified the disease in 1874;[4] they accurately described the malignancies and suggested that the disease might be hereditary in view of its appearance in early childhood. In a minority of cases there are additional severe neurological complications including microcephaly with mental deficiency, premature closing of the epiphyses and cranial sutures, cerebellar ataxis, retarded development, and adrenal and pituitary decline; this form—the de Sanctis Cacchione syndrome—is named after those who first described it.[7] These two forms have never been described within the same family.

Two other conditions deserve mention. An XP variant has been described in several families in which the symptoms are indistinguishable from the common form of XP, but the biochemistry appears to be

Work performed under the auspices of the U.S. Atomic Energy Commission.

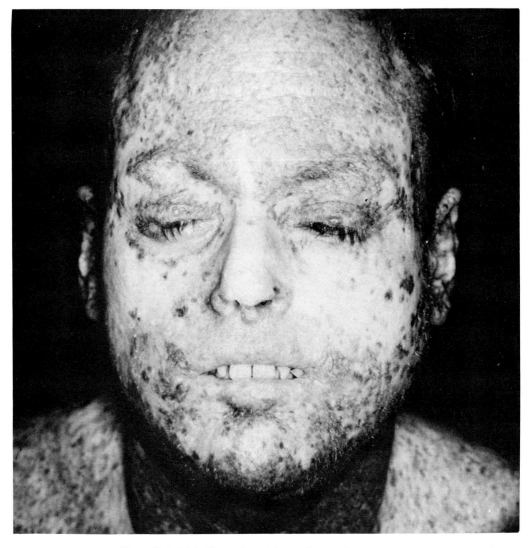

Figure 8–1. Male Caucasian with xeroderma pigmentosum.

quite different.[8,9] A disease with mild actinic skin sensitivity appearing in middle to late age has been described by Jung (1970) and named "pigmented xerodermoid"[10] but at present it has not been proven that this is a disease distinct from chronic sun-damaged skin in a normal person. Except where explicitly mentioned, all that is said about XP applies equally to the common and the de Sanctis Cacchione forms.

The disease is usually inherited as an autosomal recessive gene(s) without any obvious chromosomal abnormalities, although one family is known with apparently dominant inheritance. In one case of XP German[11] has identified a very small proportion of cells in fibroblast cultures (2 to 3%) which have a balanced translocation (between groups 1 and D, or within group C). The general significance of this as a possible characteristic of XP remains to be established with other cases. The chromosomal rearrangement is, however, considerably smaller than that seen in other hereditary diseases associated with malignancy in which the biochemistry of DNA repair is apparently normal e.g. Blooms syndrome, Fanconi's anemia, and Louis-Barr syndrome or ataxia telangiectasia.[11] Cells from patients with XP also have normal sensitivity to transformation with SV40 virus,[12] although some reports claim either abnormally high or abnormally low transformation rates. These results distinguish XP cells from a few other diseases in which high levels of malignancy, e.g. Fanconi's anemia, Down's syndrome and "high-sarcoma" families are correlated with high transformation rates *in vitro*.[13,14] Cultured XP cells have normal lifetimes *in vitro* and show no features of premature aging.[15]

XP as a Defect in the Biochemistry of Repair of Radiation Damage

In 1968[16-18] it was first recognized that XP has features in common with certain classes of radiation, i.e. ultraviolet light, (UV) sensitive bacteria. These classes of bacteria carry mutations that affect the enzymes by which radiation damage to the genetic material of the chromosome (DNA) is repaired.[19] To appreciate this similarity it is necessary to understand some of the mechanisms by which radiation damages DNA, the manner in which damage is repaired, and the biochemical defect in XP. Then, it is possible to speculate on the kind of carcinogenesis seen in this disease.

Major Classes of DNA Damage and Repair Mechanisms

Most kinds of damage (Fig. 8–2) to DNA involve only one strand of the molecule,

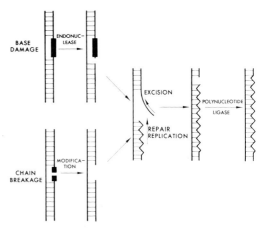

Figure 8.2. Heuristic scheme for the operational steps in excision repair of damaged bases, e.g. pyrimidine dimers and broken strands, e.g. ionizing radiation damage by a common pathway. Initial step for each kind of damage has some unique features.

either a broken phosphodiester chain (caused by X rays and certain mutagenic and carcinogenic chemicals) or an altered base, e.g. cyclobutane pyrimidine dimer, (induced by sunlight, UV light and certain mutagenic and carcinogenic chemicals). Even chemically induced crosslinks between strands rarely involve both bases of a hydrogen bonded base pair. The redundancy of information in the complementary strands of DNA is thus a guarantee against the irretrievable loss of genetic information induced by radiations or chemical agents.

Most repair systems consist of biochemical pathways by which an intact double-stranded region of DNA is reconstructed from a region containing a damaged site on one of the strands. There are three major classes of repair systems in bacteria[19] photoreactivation, host cell reactivation (excision repair), and recombination (Table 8-I). Photoreactivation, a one enzyme system which uses visible light as an activating agent, is specific for repair of the pyrimidine dimer but is completely absent from placental mammals and will concern us no further

TABLE 8-I
MAIN CLASSES OF DNA REPAIR SYSTEMS

	Mechanism	Sensitive Agents
Photoreactivation (PHR)	Direct reversal	
Excision repair (UVR, HCR)	Removal and resynthesis	UV, 4NQO, 8MOP, MIT-C
Recombination (REC) or post replication repair	Synthesis around damage	UV, 4NQO, MIT-C, XRays, MMS, EMS, NTG

UV, ultraviolet light; 4NQO, 4-nitroquinoline-1-oxide; 8MOP-methoxypsoralen; MIT-C, mitomycin C; MMS, methyl methanesulfonate; NTG, N-methyl-N'-nitro-nitrosoguanidine; EMS, ethyl methanesulfonate.

here.[19] Host cell reactivation (excision repair) involves the removal of damaged bases from DNA and synthesis of replacement regions; a model for this repair system has been derived from bacteria and mammalian cells (Fig. 8–2). Recombinational repair involves repair of DNA strand breaks, semiconservative synthesis on damaged templates and possible strand exchange between parental and newly synthesized strands.

XP is a human mutation which is an analog of the excision repair mutants designated UVR*A, B, C[9,16–18,20–24] although a close parallel between the human disease and the three distinct loci in *Escherichia coli* cannot yet be made. Jung[10] has claimed that the pigmented xerodermoid condition is an analog of the REC-mutants, but the evidence thus far adduced is not sufficient to prove the claim.

Excision Repair—Biochemical Steps and the XP Defect

The biochemical steps in excision repair and the defect in XP can be illustrated by various experimental tests:

(a) How sensitive are individual cells of XP genotype to UV light?[15,20]

*Capitalized nomenclature denotes the phenotype of the mutants; lower case denotes genotype.

(b) How well do XP fibroblasts support the growth of UV-damaged viruses?[12,26]

(c) Are thymine dimers formed and removed from DNA?[22,23,27]

(d) Are single strand gaps made and joined during excision?[23,28,29]

(e) Are short regions of new bases inserted into DNA to replace excised dimers?[16–18,20,24,25]

(f) Are short regions of new bases inserted to repair single strand breaks?[17,21]

Sensitivity of Xeroderma Pigmentosum Cells

The clinical symptom of XP patients is a high incidence of UV-induced skin cancers, but this could be due to various systemic factors other than the inherent properties of individual cells. It is important to demonstrate that the XP genotype has a phenotypic expression in individual cells, and it appears that XP fibroblasts are in general much more sensitive to UV than normal cells[15,20] (Fig. 8–3). Certain XP cases have been identified, however, with normal UV sensitivity[9] (Fig. 8–3) and normal levels of excision repair.

Although most experimental work with UV light is done with wavelengths of 2537 Å., because of the ease by which this wavelength is obtained, results are equivalent in most respects to those obtained with sunlight. The lethal effect[30] and the dimer formation[31] of direct sunlight is equivalent to a dose of 1 to 2 ergs/mm^2/min of UV at 2537 Å. Comparison of this dose rate with the survival curves for normal cells indicates that sunlight is potentially very deleterious to unprotected cells (30 min exposure can kill 90% of unprotected cells). This sensitivity illustrates the importance of the variety of protective mechanisms in the skin for survival.

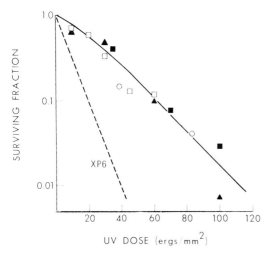

Figure 8.3. Survival curve for human fibroblasts irradiated with UV light. Normal cells ▲, ■; XP variants with normal repair □, ○; XP cells with low excision repair ----.

Host Cell Reactivation (Excision Repair) of UV-Damaged Viruses

Some classes of UV-sensitive bacteria have a reduced ability to support the reproduction of UV-damaged phage, presumably because the same enzyme system repairs host DNA and infecting phage DNA. Experiments which illustrate this phenomenon in human cells have been done with herpes[26] and SV40 virus[12] (Fig. 8–4) and XP fibroblasts appear to be analogs of bacteria which are defective in host cell reactivation.

Excision of Pyrimidine Dimers from Human Cells

The number of dimers formed in the DNA of human cells increases linearly with UV

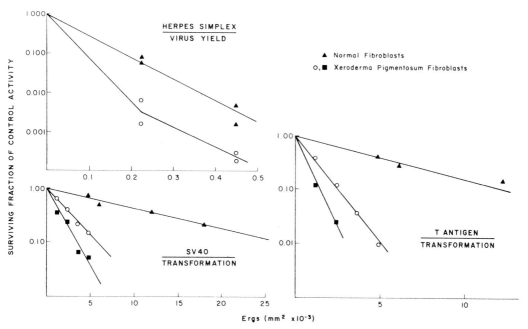

Figure 8–4. Percentage remaining virus activity of irradiated viruses grown in normal or XP cells. Top, survival of herpes virus (A.S. Rabson, *et al., Proceedings for the Society of Experimental Biology and Medicine,* 132:802, 1969); bottom, T antigen induction by SV40, Aronson and Lytle, *Nature,* 228:359, 1970); right, transformation frequency by SV40, (Ibid). Data redrawn from cited publications.

dose if the cells are fixed immediately after irradiation. When cells are allowed to grow for a time after irradiation before fixation and measurement, normal cells excise some of the dimers from their DNA, whereas xeroderma pigmentosum cells apparently do not[23,27] (Fig. 8–5).

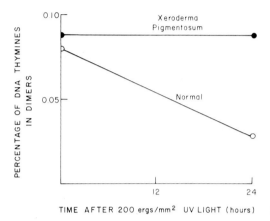

Figure 8.5. Percentage of thymine containing dimers in DNA of normal and XP cells after irradiation with UV light.

Formation and Sealing of Single Strand Breaks during Dimer Excision

The detection of small numbers of DNA strand breaks in animal cells is undoubtedly one of the most difficult technical problems in studies of DNA repair. If there were no *a priori* concept of the sort of results expected on the basis of dimer excision and repair replication experiments, few of the studies of strand breaks during excision repair would be believable.[23,28,29] The problem is that the number of breaks made during excision repair is small, and similar numbers of breaks are made by technical procedures. The UV-induced enzymatic breaks then produce only a small change in the size of single strands that can be isolated from mammalian cells by alkaline sucrose gradient techniques.

From studies made in human cells,[28,29] we can fairly confidently say that excision repair appears to involve a relatively small number of strand breaks at any one time in relation to the number of dimers (about 10^4 breaks per cell in contrast to about 10^6 dimers per cell at 100 ergs/mm²). One can therefore envisage repair proceeding by means of complex associations of enzymes which operate on a small proportion of the total number of lesions and move on sequentially from one lesion to another. The number of breaks is a measure of the number of lesions being repaired at any one time and may indicate the order of magnitude of enzyme complexes in a cell i.e. 10^4.

Insertion of New Bases to Repair DNA

Replacement of excised dimer-containing regions requires synthesis of very small amounts of DNA in short regions, "repair replication." This has to be detected in the presence of the relatively large amounts of semiconservative DNA replication that occur during the cell cycle. Various methods are available to study repair replication: 1) auto-radiographic detection of small amounts of radioactive thymidine (^{3}HTdR) incorporated into cells when they are not engaged in semi-conservative replication ("unscheduled synthesis,"[16–18,24,25,28] Fig. 8–6, 8–7); 2) iso-pycnic gradient centrifugation to separate DNA labeled with a density analog ^{3}H bromodeoxyuridine (^{3}HBrUdR) by semi-conservative replication, from DNA labeled by repair replication;[16,18,19,20,21] 3) selective disruption of repaired regions of DNA containing BrU by illumination with 313 nm wavelength light.[32] Proof that repair replication really involved small patches in DNA was established by the second method of isopycnic gradient centrifugation, and estimates of the size of the patch (less than 100 to 200 bases) are obtained more accurately from the third method though all the

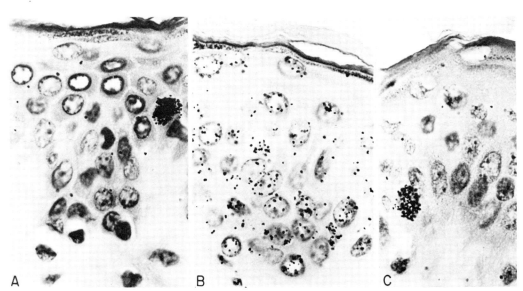

Figure 8–6. (A) Normal human epidermis not subjected to UV irradiation. There is dense labeling of one basal cell in normal S phase DNA synthesis. (B) Normal human epidermis irradiated with 13.6×10^4 ergs/mm^2 UV light. There is sparse labeling of cells throughout the epidermis. (C) Epidermis of an XP patient irradiated with 13.6×10^4 ergs/mm^2 UV light. There is one densely labeled basal cell but no sparse labeling. All skin injected with ^{3}HTdr (10 μCi/ml, 11 Ci/m mole) intradermally and biopsies taken 1 hour later. (Photographs reproduced from J.H. Epstein *et al.*, *Science*, 168:1477, 1970.)

methods do allow patch size estimates to be made.

Repair can be detected in the form of unscheduled synthesis in tissue cultures of skin fibroblasts (Fig. 8–7) and *in vivo* in the skin (Fig. 8–6). In these experiments normal skin cells are capable of repair and XP cells show reduced or negligible amounts or repair (Fig. 8–6, 8–7). Most XP fibroblasts from donors in North America have residual repair capacity that is below 55 percent of normal.[16,17,18,22,37] Higher levels have been found in some Dutch cases in which a correlation has also been established between the severity of the disease and the reduction in unscheduled synthesis.[24] Most heterozygotes show normal repair levels although a few have been identified in which reduced excision repair levels have been detected at moderate UV doses (greater than about 100 ergs/mm^2).[9,20,22] Repair replication starts immediately after irradiation and most of the incorporation of new bases is complete within 3 to 5 hours in cultured cells, although some repair replication can still be detected 24 hours after irradiation (15 to 20 percent of initial rate).

From hybridization experiments in tissue culture it has been shown that cells from patients with the common form of XP and the de Sanctis Cacchione form can complement one another.[33] In hybrid binucleate cells with one nucleus from each form of XP the level of unscheduled synthesis is indistinguishable from that in normal cells. This would suggest that the two forms of the disease represent different mutations that can complement one another either inter- or intra-genically. Subsequent hybridization experiments indicate that there are at least 4 genetically distinct complementation groups in XP,[37] and there will probably be more.

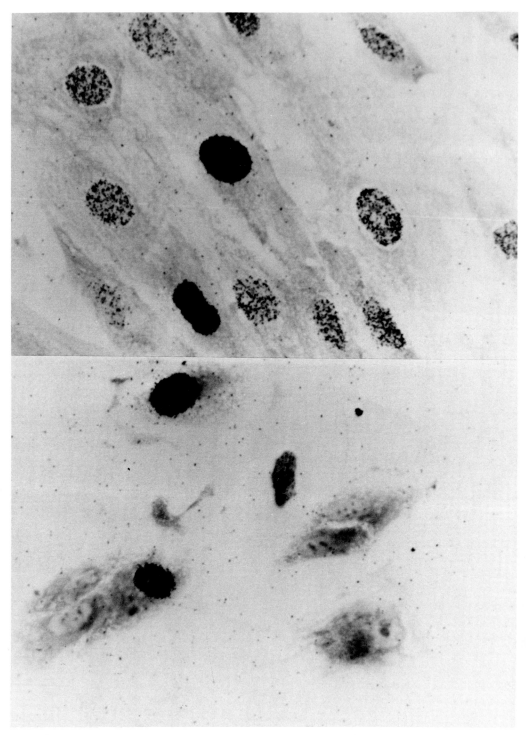

Figure 8–7. Human fibroblasts in culture irradiated with 220 ergs/mm² uv light and labeled for 2 hr. in ³HTdR (10 μCi/ml, 18 Ci/m mole). Top: normal cells showing heavy labeling from normal DNA synthesis and light labeling from repair synthesis. Bottom: XP cells showing heavy labeling from normal DNA synthesis but no repair synthesis.

Xeroderma Pigmentosum—Summary of Characteristics

The accumulated evidence of the biochemical features of XP cells indicates that this cell type is very similar to the bacterial strains that are designated UVR$^-$ HCR$^-$. Both XP cells and these bacterial mutants are UV-sensitive and X-ray-resistant, have reduced abilities to excise UV photoproducts and perform repair replication, but repair damage associated with DNA breaks at normal efficiency. Damage which is repaired to normal extents includes that from X-rays, methylmethane sulfonate and N-methyl-N'-nitro-nitrosoguanidine.[17,21,38] Thus, it is probable that the biochemical defect in XP is in an enzyme associated with dimer excision such as an endonuclease. The detection of at least four mutually complementing defects in XP (the common form and the de Sanctis Cachione syndrome) implies that either the enzyme in XP is a multiunit enzyme with subunits that have different functions, or that there are several enzymes involved. There are useful analogies to be made with bacteria in which at least three distinct genetic loci (UVRA, B, C) are associated with excision.

DNA Repair and Carcinogens

The detection of new bases incorporated during repair provides an easy, rapid technique, especially using autoradiographic procedures, to detect the effect of agents which cause damage to DNA. Correlations can be made[34] between the amount of unscheduled synthesis produced by derivatives of the carcinogen 4-nitroquinoline-1-oxide and the carcinogenic activity of these derivatives. 4NQO acts by binding to guanine bases and producing a lesion in DNA which is repaired in a similar manner to pyrimidine dimers. Thus, in this family of derivatives which presumably have qualitatively similar modes of action the amount of unscheduled synthesis induced is indicative of the amount of DNA damage caused by each derivative. The damage is thus correlated with the carcinogenic activity. If this observation on chemical carcinogenesis is compared with the radiation carcinogenesis in XP, then in both situations the carcinogenic potential is correlated with the amount of damage to DNA. In the one case the amount of unscheduled synthesis indicates the amount of chemical damage, of which only a portion may be repaired; in the other the amount of unscheduled synthesis indicates the amount of initial damage that has been repaired.

When a variety of chemically different potential carcinogens are investigated there is, however, no guarantee that there will be any correlation between unscheduled synthesis and carcinogenic activity. In fact there are good reasons why one should not even expect such correlations. The amount of unscheduled synthesis that one observes following treatment with any agent will depend not only on the amount of damage to DNA but on its chemical nature and stability and on the manner in which it is repaired. Some kinds of damage involve the insertion of large numbers of bases whereas other kinds involve insertion of relatively few. Such contrasts are readily seen in a comparison between the effects of X-rays and UV light (Table 8-II). At the same levels of killing and mutagenesis there are extremely large dif-

TABLE 8-II
LESIONS, MUTATIONS AND UNSCHEDULED
SYNTHESIS IN HUMAN CELLS

	X-Rays	UV Light
D_0	100R	30 ergs/mm^2
Lesions	600 s.s. breaks 60 d.s. breaks 400 bases	2.5×10^5 dimers
Mutation rate	2×10^{-4}	3×10^{-4}
Unscheduled synthesis	180 (1 base/break)	4×10^6 (100 bases/excised dimer)

ferences between the amounts of unscheduled synthesis; this difference is due to the small number of bases that are involved in repairing X-ray damage in contrast to UV damage. If mutation rate is any indication of the carcinogenic activity of an agent, then there is no correlation between unscheduled synthesis and mutation (or carcinogenic) rates from UV and X-rays. Thus, any comparison that is made between chemically disparate compounds in an attempt to predict carcinogenic activity on the basis of unscheduled synthesis is likely to be misleading.[38]

Xeroderma Pigmentosum, DNA Repair and Carcinogenesis

The most important aspect of XP—its outstanding clinical symptom of carcinogenesis—has received little attention experimentally. Experimental definition of the biochemical features of the disease has taken priority; the implications of these features for carcinogenesis are something for speculation and future experiments. XP is, so far, a unique disease in its association between defective repair and carcinogenesis. Other malignant cells and diseases which have been studied with DNA repair in mind have shown normal DNA repair levels.[18] If XP is unique, how does the disease fit into the general picture of carcinogenesis that is beginning to take shape? Is it a special case which conveys no general message, or is it a pregnant example with much yet to produce?

The first question to be decided is whether the DNA repair defect is likely to have anything to do with the aetiology of the disease. All XP cases now appear to involve some repair defect: either excision repair or, for the variant, postreplication (REC) repair.[39] If we conclude that DNA repair has some relevance to the disease, we have

at least a working hypothesis. Several lines of argument make this reasonable: the defective pathway is involved intimately with a major biological effect of the carcinogenic agent, there is correlation between the severity of the disease and the extent of the biochemical defect, and two clinical forms of the disease have different mutually complementing biochemical defects in repair.

Assuming, therefore, that defective DNA repair is somehow involved with UV carcinogenesis in XP, some possibilities can be rapidly dismissed, such as radiation damage increasing the permeability of the cell membrane to oncogenic viruses. Unrepaired lesions in the human cell DNA which thereby alter the cell's genetic information potentiate the chances of carcinogenesis in XP. The possible implication of this is illustrated by some of the properties of UVR⁻ strains of *E. coli*. In response to UV damage these strains show an elevated mutation rate in many loci and also a reduction in the dose needed for induction of lysogenic phage.[35] Both phenomena might occur also in XP cells, which gives two alternatives to consider in relation to carcinogenesis. In addition there are several reports which indicate that irradiation of animal cells causes an increase in their transformation rate by oncogenic viruses, although with UV light the increase is only relative to cell survival; there is a decrease in the absolute number of transformed cells.[36]

There are then at least three alternatives, not necessarily mutually exclusive, by which we can consider the mechanism of carcinogenesis in XP: 1) increased mutation rate (which can also include rates of chromosome aberration production by UV), 2) induction of oncogenic viruses by low UV doses, 3) increased malignant transformation of UV-damaged cells by oncogenic viruses. Ironically, with the precedents set by information from *E. coli* and tumor virus work, all three of these alternatives may prove experimentally demonstrable, though none have yet been described for XP. XP may provide a tool to understand some of the mechanisms which result in expression of altered genetic information in a cancer cell.

REFERENCES

1. Lynch, H.T., Shaw, M.W., Magnuson, C.W., Larsen, A.L., and Krusch, A.J.: *Arch Intern Med, 117:*206, 1966.
2. Lynch, H.T.: *Cancer, 24:*277, 1969.
3. Lynch, H.T., and Krusch, A.J., *Am J Med Sci, 254:*322, 1967.
4. Hebra, F., and Kaposi, M.: *On Diseases of the Skin Including the Exanthemata.* London, New Sydenham Society, 1874, Vol. III, p. 252.
5. Rook, A., Wilkinson, D.S., and Ebling, F.J.: *Textbook of Dermatology.* Oxford and Edinburgh, Blackwell, 1968, Vol. I, p. 62.
6. El-Hefnawi, H., Smith, S.M., and Penrose, L.S.: *Ann Hum Genet, 28:*273, 1965.
7. De Sanctis, C., and Cacchione, A.: *Riv Sper Freniat, 56:*269, 1932.
8. Burk, P.G., Lutzner, M.A., Clark, D.D., and Robbins, J.H.: *J Lab Clin Med, 77:*759, 1971.
9. Cleaver, J.E.: *J Invest Dermatol, 58:*124, 1972.
10. Jung, E.G.: *Nature, 228:*361, 1970.
11. German, J.: Proceedings, Symposium on Biology of Skin. *J Invest Derm, 60:* , 1973.
12. Aaronson, S.A., and Lytle, C.D.: *Nature, 228:*359, 1970.
13. Todaro, G.J., Green, H., and Swift, M.R.: *Science, 153:*1252, 1968.
14. Aaronson, S.A., and Todaro, G.J.: *Virology, 36:*254, 1968.
15. Goldstein, S.: *Proc Soc Exp Biol Med, 137:*730, 1971.
16. Cleaver, J.E.: *Nature, 218:*652, 1968.
17. Cleaver, J.E.: *Proc Natl Acad Sci, 63:*428, 1969.
18. Cleaver, J.E.: *J Invest Dermatol, 54:*8, 1970.
19. Smith, K.C., and Hanawalt, P.C.: *Molecular Photobiology.* New York, Acad Pr, 1969.
20. Cleaver, J.E.: *Int J Radiat Biol, 18:*557, 1970.
21. Cleaver, J.E.: *Mutat Res, 12:*453, 1971.
22. Cleaver, J.E.: Nucleic acid-protein interactions-nucleic acid synthesis in viral infection, I. (Ribbons, D.W., Woessner, J.F., Schultz, J. (Eds.): Amsterdam, North-Holland, 1971, p. 87.
23. Setlow, R.B., Regan, J.D., German, J., and Carrier, W.L.: *Proc Natl Acad Sci, 64:*1035, 1969.
24. Bootsma, D., Mulder, M.P., Pot, F., and Cohen, J.A.: *Mutat Res, 9:*507, 1970.
25. Epstein, J.H., Fukuyama, K., Reed, W.B., and Epstein, W.L.: *Science, 168:*1477, 1970.
26. Rabson, A.S., Tyrell, S.A., and Legallais, F.Y.: *Proc Soc Exp Biol Med, 132:*802, 1969.
27. Cleaver, J.E., and Trosko, J.E.: *Photochem Photobiol, 11:*547, 1970.
28. Cleaver, J.E.: *Radiat Res, 57:*207, 1974.
29. Ben-Hur, E., and Ben-Ishai, R.: *Photochem Photobiol, 13:*337, 1971.
30. Harm, W.: *Radiat Res, 40:*63, 1969.
31. Trosko, J.E., Krause, D., and Isoun, M.: *Nature, 228:*358, 1970.
32. Regan, J.D., Setlow, R.B., and Ley, R.D.: *Proc Natl Acad Sci, 68:*708, 1971.
33. De Weerd-Kastelein, E.A., Keijzer, W., and Bootsma, D.: *Nature, 238:*80, 1973.
34. Stich, H.G., San, R.H.C., and Kawazoe, Y.: *Nature, 229:*416, 1971.
35. Kondo, S., Ichikawa, H., Iwo, K., and Kato, T., *Genetics, 66:*187, 1970.
36. Lytle, C.D., Hellman, K.B., and Telles, N.C.: *Int J Radiat Biol, 18:*297, 1970.
37. Robbins, J.H., Kraemer, K.H., Lutzner, M.A., Festoff, M.D., and Coon, H.G., *Ann Int Med, 80:*221, 1974.
38. Cleaver, J.E., *Cancer Res, 33:*362, 1973.
39. Lehman, A.R., in press (1974).

CHAPTER 9

THE ROLE OF CHROMOSOMAL STUDIES IN

CANCER EPIDEMIOLOGY

Avery A. Sandberg and Masaharu Sakurai

THIS CHAPTER WILL concern itself primarily with *visibly recognizable* chromosomal changes and how studies of these changes may contribute to our knowledge of the epidemiology of human cancer and leukemia. Thus, it is beyond the scope of this paper to analyze those chromosomal alterations which are submicroscopic and, hence, not detectable with presently available techniques and instrumentation and those which are even more subtle in nature, e.g. changes at the gene level which manifest themselves as enzymatic and other metabolic abnormalities in specific cells or in the body, in general. It is possible that in the future the study of the latter group of changes, i.e. those secondary to chromosomal alterations, may be more fruitful in cancer epidemiology than the data obtained by direct examination of the chromosomal number and morphology in human cells.

To date, the contributions emanating from the chromosomal studies to the epidemiology of human neoplasia have been relatively restricted and meager. Nevertheless, it is hoped that recently developed techniques for karyotypic analysis and even more informative methods, which undoubtedly will become available in the future, will greatly expand the armamentarium of cytogeneticists and epidemiologists interested in human cancer and leukemia. In the present paper an attempt will be made to analyze and discuss existing cytogenetic findings in human

The studies from our laboratory presented or alluded to in this chapter have been supported in part by a grant from the American Cancer Society, Inc. (VC-91 L).

diseases, including neoplastic ones, which may be of value in the epidemiology of cancer and to point out some possible future approaches in this area.

The contribution of chromosomal studies to the epidemiology of human cancer should consist, *ideally,* of the detection of susceptibility to a specific cancer or leukemia at the earliest possible time in the life of an individual and, *minimally,* of definite indications of imminent development of such neoplasia. Unfortunately, at our present stage of knowledge about human chromosomes and with the techniques presently available for their study, neither the ideal nor the minimal requirements for the detection of chromosomal abnormalities in evaluating the epidemiology of cancer have been met. For, as it will be discussed later, the picture is further complicated by the fact that when cancer or leukemia appears in humans, the chromosomal changes, when present, are with only rare exceptions confined to the cells or tissues involved by the neoplastic process. Thus, at present, the contributions of cytogenetic studies to the epidemiology of human cancer must rely primarily on a correlation between congenital and hereditary chromosomal anomalies and the incidence of neoplasia in such subjects; the development of malignant disease following exposure to carcinogenic agents and the nature of cytogenetic changes present in such patients; and a correlation of karyotypic abnormalities in diagnosed tumors or leukemia with clinical, therapeutic, and other parameters. These correlations probably have generally no direct bearing on the epidemiology of human cancer and leukemia, though this is the best information available to us at the moment. Quite possibly these studies may point the way to more direct and meaningful approaches in cancer epidemiology and to the development of more sensitive and informative techniques related to this area of medicine.

The cytogenetic findings in the human, in relation to their possible role in cancer epidemiology, will be discussed under four major headings. Even though these subdivisions are somewhat arbitrary, it will become apparent that they do represent fairly homogeneous groups of chromosomal changes, in terms of the number and kind of cells affected by the karyotypic deviations. Thus, the four major categories of cytogenetics to be discussed are:

Congenital and/or Hereditary Chromosomal Abnormalities

The salient features of this group of subjects with cytogenetic abnormalities is the involvement of almost all the cells in the body by the chromosomal abnormalities and their presence at the earliest embryonic stage.

Acquired Karyotypic Changes, Primarily Due to Physical, Biological or Chemical Agents

The outstanding feature of these cytogenetic abnormalities is that they usually affect only a portion of the cells in the body, some of the agents having specificity for the cell type they affect, and the relatively transient nature of these cytogenetic changes.

Cytogenetic Anomalies in Preneoplastic and Neoplastic Cells

These anomalies almost invariably are confined to the affected tissues and persist in the tumor for the duration of the neoplastic process.

Future Approaches in Cancer Epidemiology

This will require more refined techniques for chromosome visualization at a more detailed level than afforded by present techniques and a correlation between the cytogenetic findings and cancer epidemiology (Fig. 9–1 and Fig. 9–2).

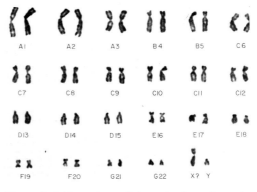

Figure 9–2. Karyotype of the metaphase shown in Figure 9–1, in which the chromosomes have been grouped into 22 pairs of autosomes and one pair of sex chromosomes (gonosomes).

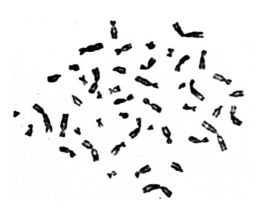

Figure 9–1. Bone marrow metaphase of a normal male cell containing 46 chromosomes.

Each one of these subjects will be presented in some detail and the application of the findings in the various groups to cancer epidemiology will be stressed. No attempt will be made, however, to review the very extensive literature on human cytogenetics, or even that on human cancer and leukemia, for which the reader may wish to consult several recent publications and reviews.[1-3] The appropriate literature will only be cited as it bears cogently on the subjects being discussed, for even a review of the very specific areas to be presented is beyond the scope and intent of this chapter.

Congenital and/or Hereditary Chromosomal Abnormalities

Autosomal Anomalies

Most of the patients with these anomalies do not live sufficiently long enough to develop cancer or leukemia. In all probability the preponderant number of cases with autosomal aberrations die *in utero* or shortly after birth, with the exception of a few trisomies.

Down's syndrome (due to trisomy of chromosome #21). This is the most common autosomal anomaly in man and compatible with a relatively long survival.[4] In about 95 to 98 percent of the cases the anomaly is manifested by trisomy of chromosome G21 and in the remaining 2.5 percent by translocation of the extra chromosome onto an autosome in group G or D.

The high incidence of acute leukemia in subjects with Down's syndrome is well established and is of particular interest.[4-6] The role played by the extra autosome in the development of the acute leukemic state is uncertain, since only a small percentage of the patients with Down's syndrome develop acute leukemia, even though the incidence among these subjects is much higher

than in a comparable population with a diploid chromosome constitution. The acute leukemia in Down's syndrome may be either myeloblastic or lymphoblastic (Table 9-I) and the leukemic chromosomal changes,

TABLE 9-I
SUMMARY OF MORPHOLOGIC TYPES OF ACUTE LEUKEMIA IN DOWN'S SYNDROME

	Acute Myeloblastic Leukemia (%)	Acute Lymphoblastic Leukemia (%)
From the literature		
Children with Down's syndrome	30.9	69.1
Newborns with Down's syndrome	57.9	42.1
Recent experience in U.S.A.		
Children with Down's syndrome	30.2	69.8
Newborns with Down's syndrome	80.0	20.0

All patients with *transient* leukemia have been eliminated from this analysis.

when present, are similar to those found in the leukemic cells of patients without the trisomy. It should be mentioned that the G-group trisomy persists in the marrow cells, even when aneuploidy related to the various forms of leukemia appears (see below).

The association of Ph[1]-positive chronic myelocytic leukemia (CML) with Down's syndrome has not been convincingly described to our knowledge. In a recent review of leukemia and Down's syndrome, the authors felt that in *none* of the 8 reported cases of Down's syndrome with either the Ph[1]-chromosome or morphologic evidence of CML could the diagnosis of this form of leukemia be substantiated.[6] The presence or lack of such an association would be of great interest, since it would supply considerable information on the susceptibility of the G-group trisomy to the formation of the Ph[1]-chromosome (see below). Even though the incidence of acute leukemia is undoubtedly higher in Down's syndrome, it is probably not as high as reported by some, since leukemoid reactions may occur in these subjects and be mistaken for one form of leukemia or another.[6] The incidence of leukemia in Down's syndrome with translocation trisomy (G-G or G-D) has not been established satisfactorily.

The relationship of the extra G-21 chromosome to the control of leukopoeisis, in general, and to the development of acute leukemia, in particular, remains unclear. For example, for some years it was thought that the Ph^1-chromosome (see below) in CML was an abbreviated G-21 and, thus, more emphasis was placed on this chromosome in relation to the leukemogenesis than it probably deserved. However, it has been recently shown with fluorescent techniques that the Ph^1-chromosome is more likely a G-22 autosome than a G-21.[7] Nevertheless, the G-group of chromosomes continues to be implicated in leukemogenesis, e.g. the Ch^1-chromosome[8] in chronic lymphocytic leukemia (CLL) and the statistically frequent involvement of the G-chromosomes in acute leukemia observed by some workers.[9] In all probability, this one group of chromosomes will receive special attention in the future when still more refined methods become available for chromosomal analysis.

Since the development of the stigmata of Down's syndrome requires the invariable presence of trisomy of chromosome #21, there must be other factors, possibly including genetic (chromosomal?), aside from the trisomy, which play an important role in the genesis of the acute leukemia in this disease. So far, these factors are totally unknown and the search for them should constitute one of the major aims of those interested in the epidemiology of acute leukemia.

Except for the definitely higher incidence of acute leukemia in Down's syndrome, a convincingly higher incidence of any other neoplastic process has not been reported in

these patients with trisomy of chromosome #21.[9,10]

Other autosomal trisomies (monosomies are probably not compatible with survival). These conditions primarily involve chromosomes in groups D, E, and F. Even though usually resulting in severe multiple congenital anomalies, they are compatible with survival following birth, though generally for less than one year. Hence, these subjects do not live sufficiently long enough to develop cancer or leukemia and the number of cases in which these abnormal states develop must be extremely small, judging by the paucity of publications dealing with the association of the above trisomies and neoplasia. Even though sporadic cases of trisomy with leukemia or cancer[11] may be reported, the exact incidence of neoplasia in these cytogenetically abnormal conditions is difficult to ascertain, since no reports have appeared on a relatively large group of cases.

Other autosomal anomalies. Included in this group is a host of chromosomal anomalies, ranging from such conditions as partial deletions of group-B chromosomes (Cri-du-chat syndrome), transformation of normal autosomes into ring chromosomes, extra chromosomes in group C, partial deletion of a number of other chromosomes besides group B and many other abnormal chromosomal conditions. The number of cases with each one of these syndromes is rather small and, hence, we do not know the exact role the karyotypic changes would play in neoplasia, were the affected subjects to live long enough to develop cancer or leukemia.

It is an intriguing fact, that even though the cytogenetic anomalies discussed in this section and in the following one are probably present from the time of fertilization of the ovum or very shortly thereafter, the presence of these chromosomal aberrations throughout the period of gestation, i.e. during the most crucial embryologic changes and growth, does not lead, as far as is known, to a higher incidence of neoplasia in these subjects at birth.

Sex Chromosome Anomalies

Almost all of these syndromes are characterized by abnormal gonadal anatomy and function, though they may be accompanied by other phenotypic abnormalities unrelated to the sex organs. Neoplasia in these subjects tends to involve the gonads and related organs. However, it is not certain whether the development of such neoplasia is due primarily to genetic factors or to a radically modified hormonal environment in such subjects, as a result of abnormal gonadal development and physiology.

XO karyotype and its variations. Gonadal dysgenesis, including Turner's syndrome—incidence is about 1 in 1000 to 1500.

Germ cell tumors are extremely rare in pure Turner's syndrome (XO gonadal dysgenesis).[12-15] Hence, the phenotypic picture of these subjects appears to have little relationship to the possible development of gonadal germ cell tumors, which tend to occur at a much higher frequency in subjects with gonadal dysgenesis associated with the presence of a Y chromosome[12-15] (XO/XY, XO/XYY, XY), though it has been reported in XO, subjects with XO/XX with fragments or iso-X chromosome constitution. Gonadoblastoma tends to occur most frequently in patients with female phenotypes showing primary amenorrhea, signs of masculinization and usually negative sex chromatin pattern. It is of interest that the pure XO syndrome has not been found frequently among patients with cancer or leukemia,[16,17] but some patients with XO/XX mosaicism and these diseases have been described.

XXY and its variations (Klinefelter's syndrome). Incidence is 1 in 500 to 750. Even though patients with Klinefelter's syndrome have been described to develop various forms of leukemia and lymphoma, the exact incidence of these neoplastic diseases in this syndrome is still unknown. On firmer ground

is the distinct probability that cancer of the breast is much more common in these male subjects with Klinefelter's syndrome than in other males.[18,19] To establish this contention more securely,[20] it is imperative that a survey be made of as many patients with Klinefelter's syndrome as possible and of the exact incidence of cancer of the breast in these subjects and in other males. Only through an evaluation of large groups of such subjects will the exact incidence of cancer of the breast be established in this condition.

XXX syndrome. As in the case of the XXY syndrome, occasional cases of XXX with cancer or leukemia are encountered,[21] but the exact incidence of neoplastic disease in this condition is unknown. Since this chromosomal abnormality is not uncommon (1 in 1,000–1,500) and the patients are not easily detected because of lack of characteristic phenotypic manifestations, a survey of these cases may yield appropriate information regarding cancer and leukemia in these females.

Gonadal dysgenesis without chromosomal changes. This group of patients has been discussed under the section on Turner's syndrome and includes those female subjects with an XY or, rarely XX, chromosome constitution and gonadal dysgenesis. The high incidence of gonadoblastomas in these subjects has been established.[22] Thus, it is incumbent upon the physician to establish the cytogenetic nature of the gonadal dysgenesis in these patients, particularly those with female phenotype and an XY sex chromatin complement, and submit these patients to surgical exploration and the removal of the abnormal gonads.

Survey of Cancer Patients for Chromosomal Anomalies

Even though the approaches in establishing constitutional chromosomal aberrations in the cells, usually blood lymphocytes, of patients with cancer, lymphoma and leukemia vary from laboratory to laboratory and involve facets which may affect the interpretation or even the results themselves, it was thought advisable to pool data on large groups of patients[21,23-26] (Table 9-II),

TABLE 9-II
INCIDENCE OF CONSTITUTIONAL
CHROMOSOMAL ANOMALIES IN CANCER
AND LEUKEMIA PATIENTS

34 anomalies in 4543 patients—0.75%	*Reference*
1149 cancer patients—8 anomalies	Harnden, *et al.*, 1969
356 cancer and leukemia patients —6 anomalies	Berger, 1971
100 leukemia and lymphoma patients—2 patients	Prigogina, *et al.*, 1970
1919 cancer patients—12 patients	Harnden, quoted by Koller, 1972
1019 cancer patients—6 patients	present study, 1972

in order to obtain an inkling regarding this parameter, i.e. the incidence of constitutional chromosomal anomalies in patients with neoplasia.

The autosomal and gonosomal anomalies in patients with neoplastic disease are summariezed in Table 9-III. The frequency of

TABLE 9-III
TYPE OF CONSTITUTIONAL CHROMOSOMAL
ANOMALIES IN CANCER PATIENTS

6 (?8)	—Sex chromosome aberrations
10	—Autosomal translocations (6 D-D)
3	—Marker chromosomes
1	—Autosomal deletion
1	—Autosomal inversion

these anomalies is, in some respects, slightly higher than would be expected (Table 9-IV), but the figures are so small and the variations between individual surveys so great that it would not be wise to attach too much significance to these observations at present. But, it does suggest that a continuation of these surveys is necessary. Thus, it has been shown that in 228 women with breast cancer only 4 abnormal chromosomal constitutions were found,[21] only 1 (XXY) in 50 patients with testicular tumors, and 9 in 730 patients

TABLE 9-IV
INCIDENCE OF AUTOSOMAL
ABNORMALITIES IN CONTROL
AND CANCER SUBJECTS

Groups studied	*Incidence of abnormalities %*	*Total number of subjects studied*
Incidence of autosomal aberrations (exclusive of trisomies) in control population	0.4	3045
Incidence of autosomal aberrations (exclusive of trisomies) in cancer patients	0.6	2624
D-D translocation in control population	0.13	3045
D-D translocation in cancer patients	0.11	2624

with leukemia or lymphoma. The frequency of variants of normal chromosomes (elongated short arms of chromosomes in groups G or D, long Y, large chromosome #1 or #16) appears to be not much different in patients with cancer or leukemia than that found in surveys of general populations.

The reporting of single cases of patients with constitutional chromosomal defects and with either cancer or leukemia tends to distort the actual coincidence of these conditions, as borne out by the above cited surveys. Nevertheless, more data are necessary on the possible protective or enhancing effect autosomal or sex chromosomal anomalies have on the development or progression of neoplasia in man. The presence of certain cytogenetic abnormalities in families (translocations) with high incidence of cancer or leukemia[27-29] may or may not play a role in the genesis of the neoplasia, since familial predisposition to cancer occurs without any familial karyotypic abnormalities; but, they do afford an opportunity to evaluate the role of chromosomal changes in the development of cancer and leukemia.

The Missing Y in the Marrow of Elderly Males

The loss of sex chromosomes with advancing age in cultured blood lymphocytes has been reported by several groups.[30-33] However, a much higher incidence of a missing Y has been reported in marrow cells of males with the frequency increasing with the age of the males. In the most extensive study to-date, 45 males out of 210 (normal male subjects, patients with myeloproliferative disorders, and subjects with nonhematopoietic diseases) were found to have a missing Y in their marrow cells.[34] That this is an age associated phenomenon is indicated by the finding that the number of males exhibiting Y chromosome loss increases with age. Incidentally, the frequency of X chromosome loss in marrows of 140 females studied in parallel with the males was very low. In 2 other studies 5 males with a missing Y in their marrow were found in 55 males studied.[32,33]

These findings have an important bearing on several parameters related to leukemia. Since the cytogenetic picture in human leukemia is most reliably established by examining marrow cells, it is not surprising that a number of patients with leukemia and a missing Y has been described. Whether the incidence of a missing Y in marrow cells is more or less frequent in leukemia and other myeloproliferative disorders[35] is not clear at the moment. What is interesting is the observation that subjects with CML and a missing Y appear to respond more readily to therapy and have a more favorable course than those patients with CML who do have a Y-chromosome in their cells.

We wish to advance the hypothesis that the missing Y may prevent the affected subjects from developing acute leukemia or the blastic phase of CML, even though exceptions may occur. Thus, the better prognosis of CML patients with a missing Y may be related to the possibility that these subjects do not transform into the blastic phase as readily as those patients who have a Y in their marrow cells. We have examined our material on over 200 males with acute

leukemia and we cannot find one patient with a missing-Y. Of interest is our observation that in 50 male patients over the age of 62 with multiple myeloma, only one subject with a missing Y was found in the marrows of these subjects, all of the marrows containing varying percentages of aneuploid metaphases. At least 5 males with a missing Y should have been found, on the basis of available data. On the other hand, when we examined the marrow of 30 male patients over the age of 62 with various cancers and lymphoma admitted to our Institute, we found at least 5 patients with a missing-Y in their apparently normal marrows (Table 9-V). Thus, it is possible that the missing-Y may confer resistance to the marrow cells in developing acute leukemia. To our knowledge, no Ph[1]-positive cases of CML in female patients with a missing sex chromosome have been described and the incidence of acute leukemia in female subjects with XO chromosome constitution is probably extremely low.[16,17] All of these facets raise the distinct possibility that the Y-chromosome plays a crucial role in leukemogenesis and this subject deserves further attention of investigators.

The missing-Y in the marrow cells raises the possibility that other tissues in the male may lack this chromosome. Since the marrow cells are considered a rapidly dividing tissue, it will be of interest to determine the incidence of a missing-Y in other tissues which are also characterized by rapid turnover of their cells, e.g. the intestinal tract.

It is possible that the higher incidence of missing-Y chromosomes in relatively young male patients with CML and allied disorders may be related to the same factors which lead to the missing Y in elderly males without hematopoietic disorders. It is possible that the mechanism resulting in the loss of the Y in the marrow cells of elderly males[30-33] may also be operative in the marrow of patients with CML but at a somewhat

TABLE 9-V
INCIDENCE OF MISSING-Y IN MALES WITH VARIOUS DISEASES

Disease	Age	No. of Patients	No. of Patients with Missing Y	% of Patients with Missing Y
Cancer	Under 60	3	0	0%
	Over 60	22	5	23%
	Total	25	5	20%
Hematological disorders other than leukemia	Under 60	5	0	0%
	Over 60	16	2	13%
	Total	21	2	10%
CML	Under 60	24	3	13%
	Over 60	6	0	0%
	Total	30	3	10%
Lymphomas	Under 60	28	1	4%
	Over 60	20	2	10%
	Total	48	3	6%
Multiple Myeloma	Under 60	2	0	0%
	Over 60	4	0	0%
	Total	6	0	0%

accelerated stage, as indicated by the fact that patients with CML tend to have a missing-Y at a much lower age than observed in the nonleukemic male population.

Chromosomal Breakage Syndromes

In this group of diseases, which are associated with a higher incidence of leukemia and cancer than in the general population, the cytogenetic findings consist of a fragile chromosomal morphology of cells (lymphocytes, fibroblasts) grown *in vitro* (Table 9-VI) and occasionally of cells of the marrow examined without culture.[36] The chromosomal instability is manifested by breaks and rearrangements in metaphase figures, lagging and bridged chromatin in anaphase and telophase and distorted nuclei and formation of micronuclei at telophase and interphase. Apparently, these karyotypic abnormalities represent a phenotypic expression on the part of chromosomes of an underlying gene defect, possibly responsible for the diseases *and* subsequent development of neoplasia. Not all of the conditions to be mentioned are characterized by the quantitative and qualitative chromosomal changes and

TABLE 9-VI
CHROMOSOMAL BREAKAGE SYNDROMES

Name of Syndrome	Major Phenotypic Manifestations	Complicating Neoplasia	Outstanding Chromosomal Aberrations
Bloom's syndrome	a. Small body size b. Sun-sensitive telangiectatic skin lesions over face	Acute leukemia; cancer	Quadriradial formation
Fanconi's anemia	a. Pancytopenia with depressed bone marrow b. Anatomic defects—multiple	Acute leukemia	Chromosomal breaks and gaps
Ataxia Telangiectasia (the Louis-Bar syndrome)	a. Cerebellar ataxia b. Telangiectasia c. Stunted growth and hypogonadism	Cancer and lymphoma	Chromosomal breaks and rearrangements
Xeroderma Pigmentosum	a. Severe skin lesions b. Other defects	Skin cancer	Chromosomal rearrangements

not all cases with these diseases have been shown to have these karyotypic abnormalities. Interestingly, heterozygous members of the families of affected subjects have been shown to have to some degree some of the chromosomal changes just described, in particular families of subjects with Bloom's syndrome or Fanconi's anemia.

Since some of the conditions are associated with abnormal immunologic responses, it is possible that the chromosomal changes observed may be a reflection of the immunologic abnormality.[36] There is no evidence that the chromosomal changes are related to the genesis of neoplasia in these subjects. Furthermore, the karyotypic changes observed are not characteristic of either leukemia or cancer. Nevertheless, since in some of these conditions the heterozygous members of the family and possibly others have a tendency to develop cancer, the karyotypic changes described deserve the attention of both the cytogeneticist and epidemiologist.

Acquired Karyotypic Changes

Effects of X-ray and Other Forms of Irradiation

The immediate effect of ionizing radiation is the production of a number of different types of damages to the chromosomal set. These changes consist of rearrangements, ring chromosome formation, deletions, dicentrics, acentric fragments, and many other morphologic abnormalities of the chromosomes. The incidence, persistence and nature of the chromosomal changes induced by ionizing radiation are dependent on the type of tissue being examined, the nature of the irradiation, source, dosage and duration of exposure,[37] the length of time between the exposure and the cytogenetic examination,[38] and the method utilized for the karyotypic observations.

Apparently, the cytogenetic abnormalities may persist for a very long time (more than 20 yrs.) in the lymphocytes of blood,[38] when these are cultured *in vitro* with PHA. On the other hand, the changes in marrow cells may be rapidly eliminated and may not be found after an interval of days or weeks following exposure to the irradiation, though persistence of some karyotypic changes of the stable type in the marrow have been described in individuals exposed to an H-bomb explosion.[39] Since the most common neoplastic process resulting from ionizing irradiation is one form of leukemia or another,[40-42] it would seem that the modification of chromosomal function occurs at a level below the resolution of visual microscopy and may, in fact, have little to do with the chromosomal changes observed in cultured lymphocytes. Nevertheless, there is the distinct possibility that chromosomal damage and changes produced by the initial ionizing insult may lead to permanent (usually structural rather than numerical) changes in the karyotypes of some hematopoietic cells. These changes may be dormant and submicroscopic and lead to the genesis of leukemia many years after exposure to the irradiation.[40-42] Thus, the persistence of chromosomal aberrations in cells of patients exposed to dangerous dosages of ionizing radiation behooves us to follow these subjects closely and carefully in order to ascertain the incidence of neoplasia in these subjects and the possibility of preventing it in the future by one means or another.

The relation of ionizing radiation to the development of leukemia is further illustrated by a recent rash of publications on leukemia complicating Hodgkin's disease and other lymphomas.[43-45] In all cases so far described, X-ray therapy was given a few years before the appearance of the leukemia. In our experience the application of radiotherapy to the abdomen appeared to be essential for the development of leukemia and an analysis of cases published in the literature revealed that almost all of them had received abdominal irradiation for one condition or another. The chromosomal picture present in the cases of leukemia complicating Hodgkin's disease or other lymphomas does not differ qualitatively from that observed in other leukemias, including the presence of a Ph[1]-chromosome in CML complicating Hodgkin's disease.[43] It will be of interest to establish whether patients with diseases other than Hodgkin's and lymphoma develop leukemia when given the same amount of X-ray therapy to the abdomen and other areas of the body. Of course, there is always a possibility that the ionizing radiation further modifies an agent or activates one in the patients with Hodgkin's disease or lymphoma leading to the development of leukemia.

That ionizing radiation leads to the development of leukemia and other neoplastic processes in a significant portion of an exposed population is most cogently illustrated by the high incidence of such diseases in individuals exposed to the A-bomb explosions at Hiroshima and Nagasaki.[40-42] For many years it was known that exposure to ionizing radiation by radiologists,[46] patients receiving X-ray therapy for ankylosing spondylitis or other diseases, was associated with a high incidence of leukemia in these subjects.[9,47,48]

Since at least 50 percent of the patients with acute leukemia have no demonstrable cytogenetic changes in their leukemic cells,[49-51] it will be of interest to establish with time the incidence of chromosomal changes in patients developing leukemia following irradiation, since to-date almost all of them (though this is based on a small number of cases) have had karyotypic changes in their leukemic cells.[43]

Noxious effects on chromosomes have been shown to be produced by *mild* ionizing radiation, such as radium used by luminous dial painters,[52] in whom the incidence of karyotypic abnormalities appeared to be related to the body content of radium, in patients receiving isotope therapy for thyroid disease, and even following diagnostic X-ray.[9]

Irradiation induced neoplasia remains an area in which chromosomal analysis could be of considerable help in heralding the susceptibility of affected individuals to the development of cancer or leukemia. Unfortunately, the cytogenetic criteria remain to be clearly and more definitely delineated.

Effects of Chemical Agents

A host of chemical substances, ranging from inorganic ions to organic drugs, to which man is either exposed accidentally or through daily use has been shown to produce chromosomal damage *in vitro* and *in vivo*[53] (Fig. 9–3). Most of the time the results are based on the effects on cultured lymphocytes, but some of the agents produce chromosomal damage in marrow cells, when these are examined without any *in vitro* procedures. A number of these substances has been shown to be carcinogenic or leukemogenic in man, some in animals, and others have

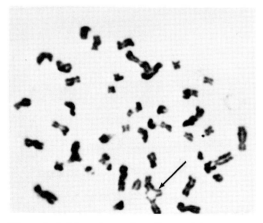

Figure 9–3. Metaphase of a cell containing severely damaged chromosomes and the formation of an abnormal chromosome (arrow) as a result of exposure to a noxious agent.

been considered as potentially carcinogenic hazards.

Benzene toxicity and its possible role in leukemogenesis. Among the definitely carcinogenic substances shown to cause chromosomal damage is benzene.[54] In some of the subjects exposed to benzene chromosomal aberrations in cultured lymphocytes can be found some time before the development of leukemia, particularly during the period of severe anemia preceding the leukemia. When leukemia develops, the cytogenetic changes are not different from those observed either in acute myeloblastic or lymphoblastic leukemia, though AML tends to be more frequent in these subjects than ALL. Again, as in the case of irradiation induced chromosomal changes, we do not know the exact significance of the karyotypic changes in the cultured lymphocytes, for not all subjects that have these changes in their lymphocytes develop leukemia and neither do all the patients who succumb to acute leukemia have necessarily the chromosomal changes in their cultured lymphocytes.

Arsenic and other chemicals toxicity. As mentioned previously, an extremely large number of chemicals has been shown to produce chromosomal changes *in vitro,* usually in cultured blood lymphocytes.[53,55,56] How these karyotypic changes affect the possibility of neoplastic development is an area which needs more intensive work and analysis. For example, it has been shown that arsenic and other compounds produce changes similar to those observed following benzene poisoning. Since some of these chemicals have been implicated in the genesis of cancer and leukemia, they may deserve the special attention of cytogeneticists and epidemiologists.

Generally, toxic agents, be they physical or chemical, which lead to the development of leukemia usually cause an initial severe depression of bone marrow function, following which the proliferative stage sets in with the possibility of a leukemic picture. There is little doubt that our natural development has undergone and is continuing to undergo rapid change, including the exposure of populations to a remarkable variety of chemical substances, drugs, industrial products, food additives, and radiation of one type or another, all of which bring new problems in their wake. Not infrequently has it been found that such substances are linked with specific or nonspecific dangers to health, including cytogenetic effects. Karyotypic analysis of cells for chromosomal changes could possibly indicate the carcinogenic potentiality of these substances.

Effects of toxic chemotherapeutic agents. Many, if not all, chemotherapeutic agents used in cancer or leukemia have been shown to produce chromosomal damage either *in vitro* or *in vivo.*[48] It is probable that some of the clinical effects of these drugs are mediated through such chromosomal changes and, hence, their significance in this regard is of a different quality than those karyotypic changes taken up in previous sections of this paper. Even though the untoward effects of chemotherapeutic agents are best determined on cultured lymphocytes, in which cells such aberrations may persist for a long period of time (years), we have seen similar changes in marrow cells, which, however, are short-lived and disappear after a relatively short period of time (weeks?). It is possible that in the future we will have to become concerned about the long-term effect of chemotherapeutic agents on chromosomal integrity, but at the moment there are more pressing facets connected with these agents than their effects on chromosomes. Possibly, this also applies to various forms of radiotherapy.

Effects of Viruses

Obviously, space and other limitations do not afford justice to be done to the large field of cytogenetics and viruses. The reader may wish to consult other more comprehensive and extensive publications in this area. Besides the possibility that viruses may play a role in the genesis of human neoplasia, as they appear to do so in some animals (chickens, rabbits, mice, rats, guinea pigs), and their capability to produce a number of chromosomal changes, including breakage of chromosomes, total pulverization of the chromosomal set (to be differentiated from so-called "chromosome pulverization" in *fused* cells, which is not chromosomally damaged at all but a premature induction of prophase (Fig. 9–4) by a metaphase cell in an interphase nucleus present in a fused cell), possibly numerical changes in the chromosome number, and, more importantly, specific alterations in certain chromosomes. An example of the latter is association of a heterochromatic region in a group C autosome (possibly chromosome #10) with the presence of a virus associated with Burkitt's syndrome (Epstein-Barr virus).[60,61] It should be pointed out, however, that not all of the materials examined have been found to contain this karyotypic anomaly in Burkitt's lymphoma[62] and, thus, it does not appear to be an essential prerequisite for the genesis of Burkitt's lymphoma. As a matter of fact, most of the cases with this disease are accompanied by a

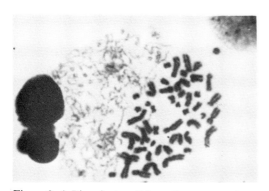

Figure 9–4. Binucleate cell from the marrow showing so-called chromosome pulverization of one nucleus. In fact, it has been shown that this pulverization is merely the induction of premature prophasing by the metaphase nucleus in the interphase one.

diploid chromosomal picture in the tumors and no consistent karyotypic anomaly has been established for this disease.

Infections with measles, chicken pox, infectious mononucleosis and other viruses have been shown to result in the presence and persistence of chromosomal anomalies (primarily breaks, gaps, deletions, pulverizations) in cultured lymphocytes. These changes may persist for relatively long periods of time. Since there is some evidence that some oncogenic viruses may, in fact, become incorporated into the genome of the host, and produce relatively specific chromosomal changes, future studies will have to demonstrate the reproducibility and specificity of such changes and more intensive work is called for in this area of oncology and cytogenetics.

Some of the changes observed in cultured lymphocytes as a result of exposure to viruses may be seen in cervical lesions of the uterus.[63,64] Since no definitive evidence exists as to whether virus resident within the cervical tissue plays a role in the development of cervical neoplasia, it is difficult, at present, to evaluate the significance of the association, even if the virus were responsible for some of the cytogenetic changes observed in cervical cells.

Until the exact relationship between viruses and the genesis of human cancer and leukemia is established, it is premature to ascribe any basic significance to chromosomal changes produced by these agents, however specific they may be. Even when such a relationship will be ascertained, the various karyotypic changes produced by viruses will have to be more specifically and clearly defined and the changes resulting from immunologic parameters separated from those due to the virion per se. In addition, the cytogenetic changes induced by viruses leading to neoplasia will have to be clearly separated from those due to viruses not implicated in cancer and leukemia.

All the conditions discussed under the

heading of "acquired karyotypic changes," be they directly or inferentially accepted as possible causes of human neoplasia, have not been shown, to our satisfaction, to cause the type of chromosomal changes usually associated with either cancer or leukemia. It is possible that if these agents do cause neoplasia, then they do so by a change in the genetic material at a submicroscopic level, the chromosomal changes preceding, and even those succeeding the appearance of the neoplasia, being merely an expression of a metabolic condition resulting in a phenotypic change in the karyotype.

If the Philadelphia (Ph¹) Chromosome Is an Acquired Cytogenetic Anomaly, What Is Its Significance In Leukemogenesis?

There is little doubt that the Ph[1] is an acquired cytogenetic abnormality in the marrow cells and is attested to by the fact that the unaffected member of identical twins does not contain the Ph[1] in the marrow cells, whereas the member with CML does have the Ph[1] in his cells.[65] To-date, the Ph[1] has been seen only in those cases in which some evidence, e.g. cytologic, clinical, or laboratory, of the existence of CML is present. Hence, we are still in the dark as to the role the Ph[1] plays in the genesis of CML. Nevertheless, the distinct possibility exists that whatever is the cause for the formation of the Ph[1] (apparently an abbreviated G22 autosome), it may also cause CML independently of the Ph[1] or through the intervention of this abnormal chromosome. No other karyotypic abnormality with the specificity of the Ph[1] for CML has been found in human karyology.[66] Though some other allied conditions, e.g. AML, erythroleukemia and polycythemia vera, may rarely be associated with a Ph[1], the description of this chromosome in CML[66] continues to be a true milestone in human cytogenetics and

calls for a search for methodologies which will uncover and reveal karyotypic anomalies characteristic for other human neoplasias similar to the Ph[1] in CML.

The cause of the Ph[1] remains unknown. It has been found in CML apparently caused by radiation, it is present in patients of both sexes and CML of childhood, it is confined to the marrow cells, and does not disappear during remission of the disease and response to chemotherapy. Deciphering the cause of the Ph[1] could go a long way toward elucidating the cause of CML and possibly other human neoplastic conditions.

Reversible (Acquired) Karyotypic Changes

Deficiency states, e.g. vitamin B_{12} deficiency, may lead to remarkable chromosomal changes in cells.[9] In pernicious anemia the marrow cells may not only show structural aberrations but also numerical ones. Generally, these cytogenetic changes disappear with appropriate therapy which corrects the deficiency. Since the association of neoplasia with some of the deficiency conditions may be more than fortuitous, it is possible that some of the karyotypic changes produced may be of cogent significance to the genesis of tumors or leukemia in these subjects. This is based on the finding in those cases in which chromosomal changes appear to persist following the correction of the deficiency state.

Chromosomal Changes in Human Neoplastic Disease

Chromosomal Changes in Non-Neoplastic Cells in Patients with Cancer and Their Families

This area has been discussed previously in

this paper. Studies on non-neoplastic cells (usually cultured lymphocytes) in patients with cancer and their families have, with a few exceptions, not yielded much positive information. One of the possible exceptions is the Ch^1-chromosome (apparently a G22 chromosome with missing short arms) found to be present in the blood lymphocytes of a family with CLL in New Zealand. Apparently, the presence of this abnormal chromosome predisposes the individual to CLL, since in addition to the two original cases found in a family, a third member recently developed the disease.[67] Abnormalities of A-group chromosomes, apparently associated with a high incidence of cancer (breast), has been described.[68] In all of these conditions the karyotypic abnormalities are present in all the cells of the body, indicating their hereditary nature.

The significance of these findings is still in doubt. Ch^1-chromosome is extremely rare in other patients with CLL and may be present in subjects without this disease. Furthermore, familial CLL without the Ch^1 has been described.[1] In a study of several families with a high incidence of cancer of the breast or cancer of the colon at our Institute, we have been unable to find any consistent chromosomal changes either in the marrow cells or blood lymphocytes. In addition, chromosomal changes similar to those described in families with predisposition to neoplasia have been found in other families without a high incidence of cancer or leukemia. Thus, it is possible that the occurrence of familial cytogenetic changes may be coincidental and a fortuitous event and not necessarily related to the development of cancer or leukemia. The latter and the chromosomal changes possibly may be an expression of a single genetic defect at the gene level. Nevertheless, studies along these lines should be continued, if only to clarify the significance of finding abnormal chromosomal pictures in families with familial predisposition to cancer or leukemia.

Cytogenetic Abnormalities in Preneoplastic States

This is an area of oncologic epidemiology worthy of further work and investment. The application of cytogenetic findings to the other cytologic, clinical and laboratory data should prove very useful in the diagnosis and prevention of neoplastic diseases in human subjects.[69]

The salient shortcoming is the unavailability of the preneoplastic tissue or cells for examination. An exception is cervical lesions of the uterus and some hematologic disorders. It is possible that we are deluding ourselves in calling lesions preneoplastic, when, in fact, they may be already neoplastic when cytogenetic changes are present. Nevertheless, such lesions may represent an early stage of neoplasia and be more amenable to therapy. Certainly, the cytogenetic findings should be of definite help to the pathologist and clinician in evaluating early neoplasia or preneoplasia. To the epidemiologist it presents a possible approach in screening populations for certain cancers.

Cervical lesions of the uterus. The accessibility of obtaining tissue from the cervix for examination has afforded the most complete cytogenetic picture for a human neoplasm obtained to-date.[63,64,70] The karyotypic picture has been obtained in dysplasia, seemingly the earliest lesion, through the development of invasive carcinoma. It appears that the early lesions of the cervix are primarily diploid and that an evolution from minor morphologic and numerical chromosomal alterations through high chromosomal numbers to a more stable, aneuploid picture emerges for invasive cancer.[71] It should not be assumed that a characteristic or specific karyotypic picture has been established for lesions of the cervix, for the cytogenetic findings in established cancer of the cervix do not differ materially from those of other cancers. However, much more work is necessary in ascertaining the relation of the response to therapy and the biology of cervical cancer with the particular cytogenetic picture, e.g. presence of marker chromosomes, hypo- vs. hyperdiploidy, etc.

Preleukemia and other related hematopoietic disorders. In most of these conditions, in our opinion, hematopoietic disease exists at the time of examination and, hence, it is probably not appropriate to think of these states as preleukemic.[72] The presence of aplastic anemia, polycythemia vera, myeloid metaplasia and other hematologic abnormalities, are all considered to be preleukemic states and the chromosomal reports deal with such states. In essence, the causation and genesis of these disorders may not differ basically from that of leukemia and the finding of chromosomal abnormalities is, thus, not surprising. It is doubtful whether the examination of the chromosome constitution with presently available methodology will reveal a preleukemic condition in human subjects. In other words, it is our opinion that by the time chromosomal changes are observed in the cells of the marrow that the leukemic state is already in progress and it behooves us to look for other cytogenetic parameters which may give us more information regarding the so-called preleukemic state.

Meningiomas, neurinomas, and pituitary tumors. On a histologic and clinical basis most of these tumors have been considered to be *benign*, particularly when based on their microscopic appearance and infrequency of metastases. Recently, however, chromosomal changes, particularly in meningiomas, similar to those observed in frank neoplastic tissues have been described.[9,47] This raises the possibility that definition of *benign* vs. *malignant* neoplastic lesions may have to be re-evaluated in light of these cytogenetic findings. The fact that meningiomas may assume a sarcomatous character is a known biologic behavior of this particular tumor and the finding of remarkable karyo-

typic changes in meningiomas presents a puzzle in the definition of neoplasia by the pathologist, oncologist, cytogeneticist and biologist. A similar dilemma seems to be concerned with the chromosomal changes described in neurinomas and pituitary tumors.[9,47] This area is further complicated by the fact that one of the G-group chromosomes appears to be very frequently involved (missing) in meningiomas and, since such a finding is more than a coincidental one, it may have a significant bearing on the causation, progression and behavior of these particular tumors. We think that the cytogenetic findings in meningioma pose a very important challenge and question as to the significance of chromosomal changes in neoplasia and whether such changes may not constitute the most cogent and direct evidence for a neoplastic process, as compared to other presently well established criteria, such as cytology, biochemical changes, etc.

Karyotypic Changes in Cancer and Leukemia and the Relation of These Changes to the Causation and/or Progression of These Diseases

This area of cytogenetics has been adequately reviewed in several recent publications[1–3,73] and only the outstanding features will be listed. It should be stressed, again, that the karyotypic changes, when present, are confined solely to the cancerous or leukemic cells. Generally, when a cytogenetic picture is established in a neoplasia, such a picture remains stable throughout the course of the disease. This would indicate that each tumor selects a karyotype that endows it with definite growth potential and advantages. The extremely variable cytogenetic picture in human neoplasia, in which no two tumors of the same organ have identical or similar karyotypic pictures, indicates to us that it is probably due to the seemingly infinite variations among the human genomes, with the chromosomal changes (except for conditions like the Ph^1 chromosome) reflecting a phenotypic chromosomal response to a more basic disturbance leading to neoplasia.

Acute leukemia. No more than 50 percent of the patients with acute leukemia, either lymphoblastic or myeloblastic (Fig. 9–5), have chromosomal changes in the leukemic cells and no characteristic cytogenetic anomaly has been found in these diseases[48,74] (Table 9-VII). We continue to believe that hypodiploidy is very rare, if it occurs at all, in ALL.

Chronic leukemia. Over 80 percent of the patients with CML have the Ph^1 (Fig. 9–6) chromosome in their leukemic cells. The Ph^1-negative cases have a much poorer prognosis, since they are more resistant to therapy and develop the blastic phase earlier and more readily. Often patients with CML, either Ph^1-positive or negative, develop the blastic phase; the ensuing chromosomal changes may vary from one patient to another, similar to the pictures seen in AML. The cytogenetic findings in CLL are not

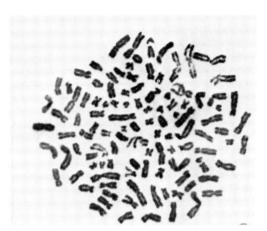

Figure 9.5. Bone marrow cell from a patient with acute lymphoblastic leukemia containing a large number of chromosomes.

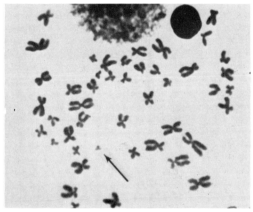

Figure 9–6. Metaphase from the bone marrow of a patient with chronic myelocytic leukemia and containing a very characteristic Philadelphia chromosome (arrow).

TABLE 9-VII
DISTRIBUTION OF MODAL CHROMOSOME NUMBER IN 427 CASES
OF ACUTE LEUKEMIA AT RPMI
(The difference between the number of patients with ALL and AML is solely due to special studies conducted by us)

	Modal Chromosome Number						
	41–45	46*	46	47–50	51–55	52–62	>80	Total Cases
AML	35	10	147†	47	12	7		257
ALL		3	99††	34	22	14	8	170

* Pseudodiploid cells.
† Includes 32 cases with some aneuploid cells in a preponderantly diploid population.
†† Includes 17 cases with some aneuploid cells in a preponderantly diploid population.

clear and will remain so until better ways of analyzing the leukemic cells in this condition become available.

Solid tumors and their metastases. Even though almost all human cancers examined to-date are associated with cytogenetic changes, no consistent or characteristic chromosomal picture has emerged for any tumor[75-80] (Table 9-VIII). The tremendous

TABLE 9-VIII
DISTRIBUTION OF MODAL NUMBER OF
CHROMOSOMES IN 139 CASES OF HUMAN
PRIMARY CANCERS AND IN 202 CANCEROUS
EFFUSIONS REPORTED IN THE LITERATURE

	Range of Model Chromosomal Number	% of Cases	
		Primary Cancers	Cancerous Effusions
Diploid	35–57	62	47
Triploid	58–80	29	40
Tetraploid	81–133	9	13

variability of the karyotypes from one case to another may be a reflection of the variability of the human genotype in its response to the cancerous state (Fig. 9–7).

In general, the metastatic lesions have karyotypes which reflect those of the original tumor, though the metastatic cells tend to have a higher ploidy and more variability in the chromosome number than the primary tumor.

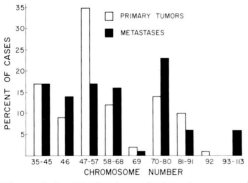

Figure 9–7. Distribution of the chromosome number in primary and metastiatic tumors.

Marker chromosomes are present in about one third of the cancers, but their exact significance continues to remain in doubt. In our opinion, there are no marker chromosomes which characterize one tumor or another. The similarity of certain markers in tumors[81] may only be an indication of the limited capacity of the human chromosomal set in the genesis of marker chromosomes.

Lymphomas (including Hodgkin's disease and Burkitt's lymphoma), paraproteinemias, and multiple myeloma. The changes described in these conditions do not differ materially from those in other cancers.[1,76,82] Since these conditions are often accompanied by abnormalities of the immunologic picture, it is possible that some of the chromosomal anomalies described, particularly those established on cultured cells, may be a reflection of karyotypic deviations induced or aggravated by immunologic changes affecting the cells *in vitro* and *in vivo*.

We have subscribed to the view that the chromosomal changes just summarized do not play a direct role in the causation of cancer or leukemia, though they may have an important bearing on the progression of the neoplasia, including metastatic spread, response to therapy, and other therapeutic and clinical parameters. The presence of a diploid chromosome constitution in over 50 percent of patients with acute leukemia, studies in induced and spontaneous tumors in animals caused by a variety of agents, observations on cervical neoplasia, and lack of characteristic karyotypic pictures in human cancer, all point to the chromosomal changes as being secondary epiphenomena to the underlying causation of human neoplasia. The latter must operate at a level of the genes, though cytoplasmic participation in the neoplastic process has not been ruled out completely.

Possible Future Approaches to Chromosome Studies in Human Cancer Epidemiology

Population Surveys for Karyotypic Changes

Generally, such surveys, though revealing important information regarding certain frequencies of chromosome changes in various populations, have not proven of much practical value in predicting cancer and leukemia.[83,84] The older methods of chromosome analysis, even though affording cytogeneticists remarkable strides in the deciphering, diagnosis and understanding of many abnormal human conditions, are not sensitive enough to reveal those genomic characteristics which underlie the genesis of neoplasia in human subjects. The newer techniques of fluorescent staining of human chromosomes and the *banding* patterns revealed by a number of different techniques relying on enzymatic and/or chemical modification of chromosomal structure, possibly may find application in cancer epidemiology.[85,86] Until we know more about the meaning and significance of *banding* in chromosomes, their distribution and consistency among various tissues, and their relationship to human disease, the benefit these new cytogenetic techniques bring to cancer epidemiology is still uncertain. Undoubtedly, newer techniques will be developed which will supply us with even more refined information of chromosomal substructure and the data obtained then would further help cytogeneticists and epidemiologists in applying the findings to human cancer and leukemia. If, in fact, human neoplasia turns out to be based on an oncogene which is an integral part of our genome[87,88] and whose malfunction (or awakening of func-

tion?) leads to the neoplastic state, the ultimate aim is to visualize these oncogenes as part of one chromosome or another and the ability to tell a functioning one from a nonfunctioning oncogene on morphologic basis. At the moment, this may be only a cytogeneticist's dream, but so were many of the methods now regularly utilized for chromosomal analysis.

Studies on Cancer and Leukemic Patients and Their Families

It is possible that the application of new techniques to an analysis of chromosomal substructure in patients with known cancer or leukemia and to their families may yield information regarding correlation of certain definite cytogenetic features with the neoplastic state. Such studies in the affected patients should be done in both neoplastic (tumor) and non-neoplastic tissues (lymphocytes). For example, what will be the pattern observed in the diploid leukemic cells of the marrow in acute leukemia when compared to that of cultured lymphocytes or fibroblasts? Only through such studies will we gain an insight into a possible correlation between chromosomal features and the tendency of individuals to develop cancer or leukemia or to predict the neoplastic state sooner than we can now.

Often chromosomal defects are more adequately realized following culture *in vitro* of lymphocytes or other cells of affected individuals or their families than afforded by other approaches. It is possible that a combination of *in vitro* techniques and newer methods for visualization of chromosomal substructure may yield more cogent information regarding cancer and leukemia than is presently available, particularly if these could be combined with some of the techniques to be discussed below.

Susceptibility of Cultured Cells to Chromosomal Changes upon Exposure to X-ray or to Transformation by Certain Viruses

The above mentioned methods may be but a few which can be used as a test of susceptibility of certain cells (and the individuals from whom they originated?) to undergo transformation into neoplastic ones upon exposure to oncogenic viruses[89-91] or to the development of chromosomal abnormalities in excess of those shown by normal cells after exposure to X-ray *in vitro*.[92-95] Thus, it has been shown that cells from patients and their heterozygous relatives with conditions in which the development of neoplasia is more frequent than in the general populations, e.g. Down's syndrome, Fanconi's anemia, show a much higher frequency of cell transformation *in vitro* when exposed to SV-40 virus (Table 9-IX). In addition, cells from a subject

TABLE 9-IX
FREQUENCY OF CELL TRANSFORMATION
IN VITRO BY SV-40

Source of Cells	Number of Transformed Colonies[a]
Controls (7)	1.6 – 5.1
Fanconi's anaemia	
Homozygotes:	
AM	79.7 ± 18.1
JV	41.1 ± 12.1
Heterozygotes:	
TM	20.1 ± 3.2
CV	28.2 ± 8.7

[a] 10,000 cells plated.

with an extra X-chromosome (Klinefelter's syndrome with XXY constitution) was shown to undergo a marked malignant transformation by SV-40 virus when compared to normal XY cells or to the XY cells present in the tissues of the affected individual (Table 9-X).

The findings with SV-40 transformation and with cells in Bloom's syndrome and Fanconi's anemia suggest that chromosomal

TABLE 9-X
TRANSFORMATION FREQUENCY OF
FIBROBLASTS BY SV 40 IN CONTROLS AND
PATIENT WITH KLINEFELTER'S SYNDROME

Cell-strains	Karyotypes	Transformation Frequence per 10^4 Cells	No. of Foci per 8×15^5 Cells
Control males	44 + XY	2.7 ± 0.10	199
Control females	44 + XX	3.0 ± 0.15	244
Cell-strains	44 + XY	9.7 ± 0.30	780
in patient	44 ± XXY	28.5 ± 4.30	2282

anomalies observed *in vitro* may be one of the heralding signals of abnormal cellular behavior, which can predispose to malignant transformation. Hence, it may be possible to utilize a karyotypic aberration which occurs in the cells of persons from higher susceptibility families or those exposed to environmental agents as indicators of the carcinogenic hazards to these individuals.

A simple, though possibly less reliable approach, in ascertaining the susceptibility of individuals to neoplasia is to study certain chromosomal aberrations following exposure of cells to X-ray *in vitro*.[92-95] A number of studies has appeared indicating that what

TABLE 9-XI
CHROMOSOMAL CHANGES (DICENTRICS,
RINGS, ACENTRICS) INDUCED BY X-RAY
IN CULTURED CELLS

Chromosome Constitution of Subjects	Amount of Change*
XX or XY†‡ §	+
XXY†‡	+ + +
XXX†	+ + +
XYY†	+ +
G-trisomy†‡§	+ + + +
D-trisomy‡§	+ + + +
F-trisomy†‡	+ + + +
XO‡	+
Deletions (B, E)‡§	+
	+ + +

*The changes shown represent deviations from the findings with control (nonirradiated) cells.
†A.A. Sandburg, unpublished observations.
‡M.S. Sasaki, *et al.*, "Chromosome Constitution and its Bearing on the Chromosomal Radio-Sensitivity in Man," *Mutation Research*, 10:617 (1970).
§M. Higurashi, and P.E. Conen, "*In vitro* chromosomal radiosensitivity in patients and in carriers with abnormal non-Down's syndrome karyotypes," *Pediatrics Research*, 6:514 (1972).

was found with SV-40 virus transformation is pretty much paralleled by the findings in cells following exposure to X-ray. Thus, the number of chromosomal aberrations in the cells of subjects with Down's syndrome, Fanconi's anemia, Bloom's syndrome and others, is much higher than that in control cells. We have investigated the frequency of such chromosomal changes in the irradiated cells of subjects with sex chromosome anomalies, since the data with SV-40 virus transformation indicated that an *unbalanced* chromosome constitution increases the cellular susceptibility to transformation. The results of our studies are shown in Table 9-XI.

Concluding Remarks

The relatively pessimistic and disappointed tenor in the introduction to this paper probably springs from the disappointment of cytogeneticists, interested in human neoplasia, in their inability to establish characteristic and specific cytogenetic pictures for human cancer and leukemia (their singular exception being the Ph^1 chromosome in CML). Nevertheless, this disappointment is tempered by the availability to the cytogeneticist of an ever-increasing number of new methodologies for examing chromosomal substructure and chromosomal susceptibility to changes *in vitro* and *in vivo* and the appearance of new cytogenetic approaches when a seeming impasse has been reached. There is little doubt that new and extremely refined techniques for karyotypic analysis will become available in the future, dissolving the pessimism and disappointment of those who are interested in deciphering the complicated riddle of human cancer and leukemia and how best to prevent and/or diagnose them for the benefit of the large number of human subjects afflicted with these diseases. There is little doubt that the interest of the oncologic epidemiologist in these developments is no less than that of the cytogeneticist.

REFERENCES

1. Sandberg, A.A., and Hossfeld, D.K.: Chromosomal abnormalities in human neoplasia. *Ann Rev Med, 21:*379, 1970.
2. Sandberg, A.A.: The chromosomes and causation of human cancer and leukemia. *Cancer Res, 26:*2064, 1966.
3. Koller, P.C.: *The Role of Chromosomes in Cancer Biology.* New York, Springer-Verlag, 1972.
4. Miller, R.W.: Neoplasia and Down's syndrome. *Ann NY Acad Sci 171:*637, 1970.
5. Miller, R.W.: Persons with exceptionally high risk of leukemia. *Cancer Res 27:*2420, 1967.
6. Rosner, F., and Lee, S.L.: Down's syndrome and acute leukemia: Myeloblastic or lymphoblastic? *Am J Med 53:*203, 1972.
7. O'Riordan, M.L., Robinson, J.A., Buckton, K.E., and Evans, H.J.: Distinguishing between the chromosomes involved in Down's syndrome (Trisomy-21) and chronic myeloid leukaemia (Ph¹) by fluorescence. *Nature, 230:*167, 1971.
8. Gunz, F.W., Fitzgerald, P.H., and Adams, A.: An abnormal chromosome in chronic lymphocytic leukaemia. *Br Med J, 2:*1097, 1962.
9. Sandberg, A.A., and Hossfeld, D.K.: Chromosomes in the pathogenesis of human cancer and leukemia. In Holland, J.F., and Frei E. (Eds.): *Cancer Medicine.* Philadelphia, Lea and Febiger.
10. Miller, R.W.: Relation between cancer and congenital defects in man. *New Engl J Med 275:*87, 1966.
11. Nevin, N.C., Dodge, J.A., and Allen, I.V.: Case Report. Two cases of trisomy D associated with adrenal tumours. *J Med Genet 9:*119, 1972.
12. McDonough, P.G.: Gonadal dysgenesis and its variants. *Pediatr Clin North Am, 19:*631, 1972.

13. Schellhas H.F., Trujillo, J.M., Rutledge, F.N., and Cork, A.: Germ cell tumors associated with XY gonadal dysgenesis. *Am J Obstet Gynecol, 109:*1197, 1971.

14. Sune, M.V., Centeno, J.V., and Salzano, F.M.: Case report: Gonadoblastoma in a phenotypic female with 45,X/47,XYY mosaicism. *J Med Genet 7:*410, 1970.

15. Teter, J., and Boczkowski, K.: Occurrence of tumors in dysgenetic gonads. *Cancer, 20:* 1301, 1967.

16. Wertelecki, W., and Shapiro, J. R.: 45,XO Turner's syndrome and leukaemia. *Lancet 1:*789, 1970.

17. Pawliger, D.F., Barrow, M., and Noyes, W.D.: Acute leukemia and Turner's syndrome. *Lancet, 1:*1345, 1970.

18. Jackson, A.W., Muldal, S., Ockey, C.H., and O'Connor, P.J.: Carcinoma of male breast in association with the Klinefelter syndrome. *Br Med J, 1:*223, 1965.

19. Robson, M.C., Santiago, Q., and Huang, T.W.: Bilateral carcinoma of the breast in a patient with Klinefelter's syndrome. *J Clin Endocrinol, 28:*897, 1968.

20. Nadel, M., and Koss, L.G.: Klinefelter's syndrome and male breast cancer. *Lancet, 2:*366, 1967.

21. Harnden, D.G., Langlands, A.O., McBeath, S., O'Riordan, M., and Faed, M.J.W.: The frequency of constitutional chromosome abnormalities in patients with malignant disease. *Eur J Cancer, 5:*605, 1969.

22. Ferrier, P.E., Ferrier, S.A., Scharer, K.O., Genton, N., Hedinger, C., and Klein, D.J.: Disturbed gonadal differentiation in a child with XO/XY/XYY mosaicism; relationship with gonadoblastoma. *Helv Paediatr Acta, 22:*479, 1967.

23. Berger, R.: Anomalies chromosomiques constitutionnelles et neoplasies. *Pres Med, 15:* 1107, 1971.

24. Prigogina, E.L., Stavrovskaja, A.A., Kakpakova, E.S., Streljuchina, N.V., Zakharov, A.F., Lelikova, G.P., Chudina, A.P., and Pogosianz, E.E.: Congenital chromosome abnormalities and leukaemia. *Lancet, 2:* 524, 1970.

25. Harnden, D.G.; quoted by Koller, P.C.

26. Sandberg, A.A.: Unpublished observations.

27. Zuelzer, W.W., and Cox, D.E.: Genetic aspects of leukemia. *Semin Hematol, 6:*228, 1969.

28. Lynch, H.T., Anderson, D.E., and Krush, A.J.: Heredity and carcinoma. *Ann NY Acad Sci, 155:*793, 1968.

29. Snyder, A.L., Li, F.P., Henderson, E.S., and Todaro, G.J.: Possible inherited leukaemogenic factors in familial acute myelogenous leukaemia. *Lancet, 1:*586, 1970.

30. Pierre, R.V., and Hoagland, H.C.: 45,X cell lines in adult men: Loss of chromosome, a normal aging phenomenon? *Mayo Clin Proc, 46:*52, 1971.

31. Pierre, R.V., and Hoagland, H.C.: Age-associated aneuploidy: Loss of Y chromosome from human bone marrow cells with aging. *Cancer, 30:*889, 1972.

32. Secker Walker, L.M.: The chromosomes of bone-marrow cells of haematologically normal men and women. *Br J Haematol, 21:*455, 1971.

33. O'Riordan, M.L., Berry, E.W., and Tough, I.M.: Chromosome studies on bone marrow from a male control population. *Br J Haematol, 19:*83, 1970.

34. Pierre, R.V., and Hoagland, H.C.: Sex chromosome loss from human bone marrow cells: an age-associated phenomenon. Program of the Am Soc Human Genet, 1972, p. 12.

35. Rowley, J.D.: Loss of the Y chromosome in myelodysplasia: A report of three cases studied with quinacrine fluorescence. *Br J Haematol, 21:*717, 1971.

36. German, J.: Genes which increase chromosomal instability in somatic cells and predispose to cancer. *Prog Med Genet, 8:*61, 1972.

37. Heddle, J.A.: Radiation-induced chromosome aberrations in man: A possible biological dosimeter. *Fed Proc, 28:*1790, 1969.

38. Awa, A., and Bloom, A.D.: Cytogenetics at the atomic bomb casualty commission: Report of a symposium. *Jap J Hum Genet, 12:*69, 1967.

39. Ishihara, T., and Kumuturi, T.: Chromosome studies on Japanese exposed to radiation resulting from nuclear bomb explosion, In Evans, H.J., Court-Brown, W.M., and McLean, A.S., (Eds.): *Human Radiation*

Cytogenetics. Amsterdam, North Holland Publishing Co., 1967, p. 144.

40. Brill, A.B., Tomonaga, M., and Heyssel, R.M.: Leukemia in man following exposure to ionizing radiation. A summary of the findings in Hiroshima and Nagasaki, and a comparison with other human experience. *Ann Intern Med, 56:*590, 1962.

41. Watanabe, S.: Present status of somatic effects in atomic bomb survivors living in Hiroshima. *Acta Haematol Jap, 27:*121, 1964.

42. Tomonaga, M., Ichimaru, M., Danno, H., Inove, A., Okabe, N., Kinoshita, K., Matsumoto, Y., Nonaka, M., Takahashi, Y., Tomiyasu, T., Toyomasu, S., Tamari, K., and Kawamoto, M.: Leukemia in atomic bomb survivors from 1946–1965 and some aspects of epidemiology of leukemia in Japan. *J. Kyush u Hematol Soc, 17:*1097, 1969.

43. Ezdinli, E.Z., Sokal, J.E., Aungst, C.W., Kim, U., and Sandberg, A.A.: Myeloid leukemia in Hodgkin's disease. Chromosomal abnormalities. *Ann Intern Med, 71:*1097, 1969.

44. Steinberg, M.H., Geary, C.G., and Crosby, W.H.: Acute granulocytic leukemia complicating Hodgkin's disease. *Arch Intern Med, 125:*496, 1970.

45. Burns, C.P., Stjernholm, R.L., and Kellermeyer, R.W.: Hodgkin's disease terminating in acute lymphosarcoma cell leukemia. A metabolic study. *Cancer, 27:*806, 1971.

46. Lewis, E.B.: Leukemia, multiple myeloma, and aplastic anemia in American radiologists. *Science, 142:*1492, 1963.

47. Sandberg, A.A.: Chromosome changes in human malignant tumors: An evaluation. In *Recent Results in Cancer Research.* New York, Springer-Verlag, Berlin-Heidelberg, 1972.

48. Sandberg, A.A.: The chromosomes and causation of human cancer and leukemia. *Cancer Res, 26:*2064, 1966.

49. Sandberg, A.A., Ishihara, T., Miwa, T., and Hauschka, T.S.: The *in vivo* chromosome constitution of marrow from 34 human leukemias and 60 nonleukemic controls. *Cancer Res, 21:*678, 1961.

50. Sandberg, A.A., Ishihara, T., Kikuchi, Y., and Crosswhite, L.H.: Chromosomal differences among the acute leukemias. *Ann NY Acad Sci, 113:*663, 1964.

51. Sandberg, A.A., Takagi, N., and Sofuni, T.: Chromosomes and causation of human cancer and leukemia. V. Karyotypic aspects of acute leukemia. *Cancer, 22:*1268, 1968.

52. Boyd, J.T., Court-Brown, W.M., Vennart, J., and Woodcock, G.E.: Chromosome studies on women formerly employed as luminous dial painters. *Br Med J, 1:*377, 1966.

53. Shaw, M.W.: Human chromosome damage by chemical agents. *Ann Rev Med, 21:*419, 1970.

54. Forni, A., and Moroe, L.: Cytogenetic studies in a case of benzene leukaemia. *Eur J Cancer, 3:*251, 1967.

55. Skerfving, S., Hansson, K., and Lindsten, J.: Chromosome breakage in humans exposed to methyl mercury through fish consumption. *Arch Environ Health, 21:*133, 1970.

56. Schwanitz, G., Lehnert, G., and Gebhart, E.: Chromosomenschäden bei beruflicher bleibelastung. *Dtsch Med Wochenschr, 95:*1636, 1970.

57. Gerber, P., Whang-Peng, J., and Monroe, J.H.: Transformation and chromosome changes induced by Epstein-Barr virus in normal human leukocyte cultures. *Proc Natl Acad Sci, 63:*740, 1969.

58. Miller, R.W., and Todaro, G.J.: Viral transformation of cells from persons with high risk of cancer. *Lancet, 1:*81, 1969.

59. Aaronson, S.A., and Todaro, G.J.: Transformation and virus growth by murine sarcoma viruses in human cells. *Nature, 225:*458, 1970.

60. Kohn, G., Mellman, W.J., Moorhead, P.S., Loftus, J., and Henle, G.: Involvement of C-group chromosomes in five Burkitt lymphoma cell lines. *J Natl Cancer Inst, 38:*209, 1967.

61. Epstein, M.A., Achong, B.G., and Barr, Y.M.: Virus particles in cultured lymphoblasts from Burkitt's lymphoma. *Lancet, 1:*702, 1964.

62. Huang, C.C., Minowada, J., Smith, R.T., and Osunkoya, B.O.: Reevaluation of relationship between C chromosome marker and Epstein-Barr virus: chromosome and immunofluorescence analyses of 16 human

hematopoietic cell lines. *J Natl Cancer Inst, 45:*815, 1970.

63. Auersberg, N., Corey, M.J., and Worth, A.: Chromosomes of preinvasive lesions of the human uterine cervix. *Cancer Res, 27:*1399, 1967.

64. Boddington, M.M., Spriggs, A.I., and Wolfendane, M.R.: Cytogenetic abnormalities in carcinoma *in situ* and dysplasias of the uterine cervix. *Br Med J, 1:*154, 1965.

65. Goh, K., and Swisher, S.N.: Identical twins and chronic myelocytic leukemia. *Arch Intern Med, 115:*475, 1965.

66. Nowell, P.C., and Hungerford, D.A.: A minute chromosome in human chronic granulocytic leukemia. *Science, 132:*1197, 1960.

67. Fitzgerald, P.H., and Hamer, J.W.: Third case of chronic lymphocytic leukaemia in a carrier of the inherited Ch^1 chromosome. *Br Med J, 3:*752, 1969.

68. Merz, T., El-Mahdi, A.M., and Prempree, T.: Unusual chromosomes and malignant disease. *Lancet, 1:*337, 1968.

69. Enterline, H.T., and Arvan, D.A.: Chromosome constitution of adenoma and adenocarcinoma of the colon. *Cancer, 20:*1746, 1967.

70. Cellier, K.M., Kirkland, J.A., and Stanley, M.A.: Statistical analysis of cytogenetic data in cervical neoplasia. *J Natl Cancer Inst, 44:*1221, 1970.

71. Wakonig-Vaartaga, R., and Hughes, D.T.: Chromosomal anomalies in dysplasia, carcinoma *in situ* and carcinoma of the cervix uteri. *Lancet, 2:*756, 1965.

72. Nowell, P.C.: Marrow chromosome studies in "Preleukemia". Further correlation with clinical course. *Cancer, 28:*513, 1971.

73. Hsu, T.C.: Chromosomal evolution in cell populations. *Int Rev Cytol, 12:*69, 1961.

74. Sandberg, A.A., Koepf, G.F., Crosswhite, L.H., and Hauschka, T.S.: The chromosome constitution of human marrow in various developmental and blood disorders. *Am J Human Genet, 12:*231, 1960.

75. Sandberg, A.A., Yamada, K., Kikuchi, Y., and Takagi, N.: The chromosomes and causation of human cancer and leukemia. III. Karyotypes of cancerous effusions. *Cancer, 20:*1099, 1967.

76. Sandberg, A.A., Ishihara, T., Kikuchi, Y., and Crosswhite, L.H.: Chromosomes of lymphosarcoma and cancer cells in bone marrow. *Cancer, 17:*738, 1964.

77. Yamada, K., Takagi, N., and Sandberg, A.A.: The chromosomes and causation of human cancer and leukemia. II. Karyotypes of human solid tumors. *Cancer, 19:*1879, 1966.

78. Makino, S., Ishihara, T., and Tonomura, A.: Cytological studies of tumors XXVII. The chromosomes of thirty human tumors. *Z Krebsforsch, 63:*184, 1959.

79. Makino, S., Sasaki, M.S., and Tonomura, A.: Cytological studies of tumors XL. Chromosome studies in fifty-two human tumors. *J Natl Cancer Inst, 32:*741, 1964.

80. Ishihara, T., Moore, G.E., and Sandberg, A.A.: Chromosome constitution of cells in effusions of cancer patients. *J Natl Cancer Inst, 27:*893, 1966.

81. Martineau, M.: A similar marker chromosome in testicular tumours. *Lancet, 1:*836, 1966.

82. Spiers, A.S.D., and Baikie, A.G.: Cytogenetic studies in the malignant lymphomas and related neoplasms. *Cancer, 22:*193, 1968.

83. Sandberg, A.A., Cohen, M.M., Rimm, A.A., and Levin, M.L.: Aneuploidy and age in a population survey. *Am J Hum Genet, 19:*633, 1967.

84. Carr, D.H.: Chromosome studies in abortuses and stillborn infants. *Lancet, 2:*603, 1963.

85. Caspersson, T., Zech, L., Johansson, C., and Modest, E.J.: Identification of human chromosomes by DNA-binding fluorescent agents. *Chromosoma, 30:*215, 1970.

86. Engel, E., McGee, B.J., Hartmann, R.C., and Engel de Montmollin, M.: Two leukaemic peripheral blood stemlines during acute transformation of chronic myelogenous leukemias in a D/D translocation carrier. *Cytogenetics, 4:*157, 1965.

87. Temin, H.M., and Mizutani, S.: RNA-dependant DNA-polymerase in virions of Rous sarcoma virus. *Nature, 226:*1211, 1970.

88. Scolnick, E.M., Aaronson, S.A., Todaro, Y.J., and Park, W.P.: RNA-dependant DNA-polymerase activity in mammalian cells. *Nature, 229:*318, 1971.

89. Todaro, G.J., and Martin, G.M.: Increased susceptibility of Down's syndrome fibroblasts to transformation by SV-40. *Proc Soc Exp Biol Med, 124:*1232, 1967.

90. Mukerjee, D., Trujillo, J.M., Cork, A., and Bowen, J.M.: Genetic susceptibility of human cells to transformation by oncogenic viruses. *Med Intern Cong, 233:*128, 1971.

91. Todaro, G.J., Green, H., and Swift, M.R.: Human diploid fibroblasts transformed with SV-40 a hybrid Adeno-7XSV-40. *Science, 153:*1252, 1966.

92. Sasaki, M.S., and Tonomura, A.: Chromosomal radiosensitivity in Down's syndrome. *Jap J Human Genet, 14:*81, 1969.

93. Sasaki, M.S., Tonomura, A., and Matsubara, S.: Chromosome constitution and its bearing on the chromosomal radiosensitivity in man' *Mut Res, 10:*617, 1970.

94. Higurashi, M., and Cohen, P.E.: *In vitro* chromosomal radiosensitivity in Fanconi's anemia. *Blood, 38:*336, 1971.

95. Higurashi, M., and Cohen, P.E.: *In vitro* chromosomal radiosensitivity in patients and in carriers with abnormal non-Down's syndrome karyotypes. *Pediatr Res, 6:*514, 1972.

96. Sakurai, M.: Chromosome studies in hematological disorders. III. Chromosome findings in "preleukemia" and related diseases. *Acta Haematol Jap, 33:*127, 1970.

CHAPTER 10

CYTOGENETICS WITH REFERENCE TO

GONADOBLASTOMAS AND TO GONOCYTOMAS

J. TETER

Introduction—Definition

THIS CHAPTER DEALS with special gonadal tumors occurring in intersexual patients with a negative sex-chromatin pattern and well defined sex-chromosome anomalies in apparently phenotypic females with male karyotype 46,XY.

The most characteristic neoplasm occurring in intersexes is the germ-cell tumor which may be formed solely of gonocytes (gonocytoma-dysgerminoma) or mixed with smaller, dark or oval cells of the granulosa-Sertoli type and may be classified as gonadoblastoma,[1] dysgenetic gonadoma,[2] or gonocytoma II or III.[3]

These two cellular components of the tumor form characteristic nests in a microfollicular pattern and are surrounded by Leydig cells occurring within fibrous stroma. Calcified concretions are another feature of these tumors.

Historical Review

These special gonadal tumors were first described in 1900, when Neugebauer,[4] a gynecologist from Warsaw, published nineteen cases of benign and malignant genital tumors in hermaphrodites in one of his numerous studies on hermaphroditism and genetic disturbances.

In 1931, Robert Meyer[5] described two women with dysgerminoma of one ovary and a rudimentary gonad on the contralateral side. In another patient he noted gonadal aplasia on one side and "a tumor composed of epitheliod cells" on the other side.

A typical case of intersexuality with features of male pseudohermaphroditism and dysgerminoma was described in 1941 by Long, et al.[6] It is noteworthy that these investigators stated that any large pelvic mass in patients with features of intersexuality should suggest the presence of dysgerminoma.[6]

In a comprehensive review of malignant testicular tumors occurring in maldeveloped testes in male pseudohermaphrodites, Gilbert[7,8] found two malignant tumors in scrotal testes, eight in inguinal testes and 48 in abdominally retained testes. These findings indicate that an increased risk for neoplasia occurs in abdominally situated gonads. A higher temperature in the abdomen is considered an important factor in neoplastic transformation.

Among sixty testicular tumors occurring in pseudohermaphrodites, Gilbert[7,8] found that 38 cases or 62 percent were malignant germ-cell tumors (classified as seminoma).

In 1953, Scully[1] described two patients with abnormal sexual development and gonadal tumors; he introduced the term "gonadoblastoma" to designate a steroid hormone-secreting gonadal tumor composed of germ cells and sex cord derivatives resembling immature granulosa and Sertoli cells, with stromal elements indistinguishable from lutein or Leydig cells. He emphasized that such neoplasms appear to recapitulate gonadal development more completely than any other type of tumor.

Spielman and Motyloff[9] concluded from their study on dysgerminoma occurring in pseudohermaphrodites that this tumor developed from primitive cells retained from the early undifferentiated gonad. They were of the opinion that the chief component cells of the tumors were not "germ cells" or "sex cells," but rather were cells derived from coelomic epithelium and for that reason they objected to the terms "dysgerminoma" and "seminoma" which imply a germ cell origin. Instead, they proposed that these neoplasms be called "neuter cell" tumors.

In Sohval's[10-14] series of gonadal dysgenesis and testicular malformations, a precise classification of the type of gonadal dysgenesis in patients having a dysgenetic tumor was given. According to Sohval, the peculiar type of gonads can be determined only by histopathologic study of the gonad with cytogenetic determination of the chromosomal pattern. He stressed the importance of the relationship between gonadal neoplasms and the types of gonadal dysgenesis. In "mixed gonadal dysgenesis" when one of the gonads is an intraabdominal testis, situated in the place normally occupied by the ovary, associated tumors should be anticipated.

Patients with congenital somato-sexual ambiguities, mixed gonadal dysgenesis, and XO/XY mosaicism have a tendency to develop gonadal neoplasms.

In 1957, Stange[15] described four patients in whom tumors had been found at laparotomy among a group of fifteen persons with gonadal dysgenesis. In one case, he found a Brenner tumor; in two cases, hilus cell tumors; and in the fourth case, an overabundance of rete testis elements. Shortly thereafter in 1959, Melicow and Uson[2] reported two instances of germ cell tumors classified as "dysgenetic gonadomas" in phenotypic males, in one of whom the tumor was demonstrated to have arisen in an abdominal testis.

The histological pattern of gonadal tumors is discussed in Melicow's series[16] of dysgenetic gonadal tumors in intersexes. According to Melicow, the histological pattern of gonadal tumors in intersexes differs from that in individuals with relatively normal sexual development whose gonads, otherwise "normal," became neoplastic. He pointed to the importance of accurate diagnosis of "dysgenetic gonadomas" in the early stage of their development. It would then be possible to accumulate sufficient data which should aid in understanding their pathological nature and in arriving at a proper classification for this bizzare group of gonadal tumors in intersexes.

One year later, in 1960, Teter[17] presented the clinico-pathologic features in a series of germ-cell tumors and demonstrated their relation to intersexuality and chromosomal anomalies. He pointed to the uniformity of the clinico-pathological features of the germ-cell tumors occurring in intersexes, thus permitting their early diagnosis. In general all of these patients have rudimentary testes or testicular remnants in dysgenetic gonads and differ from patients with testicular feminization by having müllerian derivatives (uterus and Fallopian tubes). The most characteristic finding is the presence of a negative sex chromatin pattern and the presence of the Y chromosome in the karyotype, in contrast to the normal feminine genitalia pattern.

Pathology of Germ Cell Tumors Occurring in Intersexes

Histogenesis—Pathogenesis

In experimental oncology it is generally assumed that hormonal imbalance, i.e. excessive amounts of gonadotrophin, plays a major role in the development of ovarian tumors.[18,19] However, the correlation be-

tween hormonal imbalance (high gonadotrophins and low estrogens) and other factors
(foci of gonadal malformation, genetics) has
not been conclusively established as yet.[20]

In analyzing dysgenetic gonadal tumors,
associated characteristic factors can be found
in almost every case as follows:

1. An excess of gonadotrophins and low
   estrogens.
2. Negative sex chromatin pattern and
   the presence of the Y chromosome in
   patients having a female genital tract
   (uterus and vagina).[21-24]
3. Gonadal malformations, i.e. foci of
   germ cells and granulosa-Sertoli type
   cells (sex-cord cells) within underdeveloped, undernourished environmental
   tissue.[3]

It is clear that the gonadoblastoma pattern
can arise from testicular tissue as is evidenced
in several cases described by Hughesdon[25]
in which the intra-tubular location and
nearby presence of seminoma *in situ* suggest
that small areas of germ cell neoplasia within
tubules are the primary source of tumor
development (Figs. 10–1 and 10–2).

In a literature review of a series of 33 cases
of gonocytoma III (gonadoblastoma) the
testicular tissue was found to be present in
15 cases, 13 on the same side as the tumor,
two on the opposite side, and seven on
both sides. In five cases it was the only
gonadal tissue reported[2,26,27] and in four
cases the tumor was continuous with proliferating germinal and Sertoli cells of the
associated testis tubules. This could mean
either an origin directly in such tubules or
an origin in dysgenetic "tubules" of already
abnormal pattern which had continuity with
less affected ones.[25]

Sohval[11,14] concluded from his study on
26 seminomas and 16 malignant teratomas
of the testicle that an inherent imperfection
of the testicle may predispose it to neoplasia.
Tubular immaturity in an adult's testis represents, according to Sohval, an anatomical

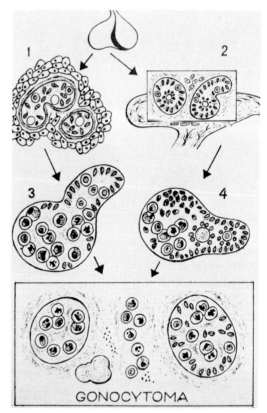

Figure 10–1. Diagrammatic scheme of some possible aspects of pathogenetic mechanisms in tumorigenesis relevant to germ cells. A permanent pituitary trophic hyperactivity. An excess of gonadotrophins favors the growth of the neoplastic cells.
(1) In intersexual subject with dysgenetic testes, a
germ cell tumor (gonocytoma) arises from atrophic,
disorganized tubular epithelium. (2) In cases of
gonadal dysgenesis, gonocytoma arises from persistent primordial germ cells in dystrophic background (testicular remanants in medullary zone of
fibrous streak gonad). (3) and (4) Preneoplastic
changes.

expression of such a defect. Data collected
suggest that an association between testicular maldevelopment and neoplasm is impressive enough to indicate that the relationship is more than coincidental (Figs.
10–3–10–5).

The histopathologic study of cryptorchid testes[10,11] revealed that testicular maldevelopment is of etiologic significance in some cases. It is suggested that the same congenital defect which contributes to the undescended testicles may also render them more susceptible to tumor development. This would account, in part, for the greater incidence of testicular neoplasms in undescended than in scrotal testes.[11]

Such findings and the prevalence of a Y chromosome in these cases have usually suggested that the tumor always arises in pre-formed testicular tissue.[22] Therefore, it is believed that the presence of testicular tissue in man is dependent upon the presence of the Y chromosome and that the presence of the Y chromosome in cases with gonadoblastoma is important evidence that the structures seen in the tumor are of testicular origin.[24]

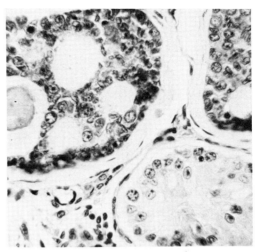

Figure 10–3. Gonadoblastoma *in situ*. A case with uterus, a rudimentary fibrous streak gonad on one side, and a testis on the other. Right testicular gonad: seminiferous tubule containing proliferating Sertoli-granulosa and germ cells with microfolliculoid spaces and laminated, calcified concretions (on the left). The tubules are expanded by an overgrowth of germ cells with an intermingling of undifferentiated Sertoli cells. An immature seminiferous tubule is visible at the bottom. There is no sharp dividing line between the typical testicular tissue and the neoplastic nests.

Microscopic Pathology

Recognition of an clinicopathological classification of these tumors based on histogenesis, morphology, and biological behavior was performed by Teter[3] in 1960, in order to formulate a more precise approach to grouping these closely related varieties of germ-cell tumors which may be mixed and, at times, difficult to distinguish from each other.

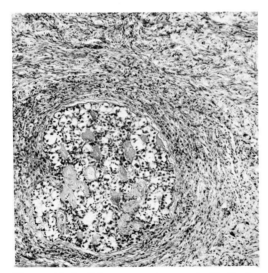

Figure 10–2. Fibrous streak gonad. Testicular remnants within medullary zone. Turner's syndrome with clitoral enlargement and XO/XY karyotype. Bizarre nest containing germ cell with an intermingling of Sertoli-granulosa type cells. Note the microfolliculoid pattern and interstitial Leydig-like cells surrounding the epithelial nest.

Gonocytoma I

This homogenous type of tumor is formed solely of germ cells (dysgerminoma, seminoma). In all of our 5 cases, as well as in the others reported in literature,[30] instances of

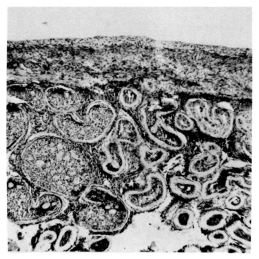

Figure 10–4. The same case as in Figure 10–3—Gonadoblastoma *in situ*. Cortical part resembling ovarian-like stroma is visible. Some tubules, showing gonadoblastomatous pattern are expanded. Note the small seminiferous tubules without lumens and thickened tubular wall in uninvolved fragment of testicle (on the right).

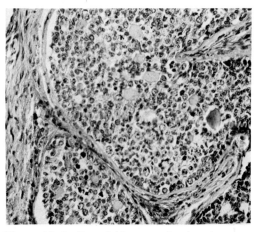

Figure 10–5. Gonadoblastoma *in situ,* the same case as in Figures 3 and 4. Typical nest of gonadoblastoma within tubule. Folliculoid arrangement of Sertoli-granulosa type cells and single germ cells scattered among them. Cellular anaplasia with variations in size and shape of the nucleus and hyperchromatism are visible. Malignant features occur both in germ cells and Sertoli-granulosa like cells.

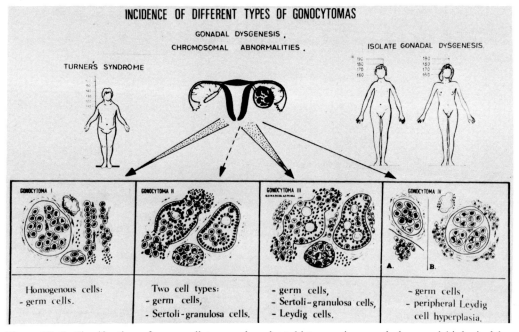

Figure 10–6. Classification of germ cell tumors based on histogenesis, morphology and biological behavior. Schematic drawing illustrating the incidence of different types of gonocytomas occurring in intersexual patients having gonadal dysgenesis.

typical nests of germ cells separated by connective tissue strands with lymphocytic infiltrations were noted. In two cases, multinucleated giant cells occurring in areas of tumor necrosis were seen and the presence of histiocytic cells was noted. In one tumor small nests of syncytiotrophoblast cells were present. Pathological peculiarities consist of psammoma-like calcifications and irregular calcific masses which are never found in cases of dysgerminoma (seminoma) in patients with normal somatosexual development (Figs. 10–7–10–9).

Gonocytoma II

This is a mixed form consisting of two types of cells—germ cells and a granulosa-Sertoli type cell—occurring in the embryonic gonad. Typical neoplastic nests are composed of single germ cells scattered inside the nests of granulosa-Sertoli cells. The latter form single files along the periphery of neoplastic nests or encircled individual germ cells and also are arranged in a folliculoid pattern (Fig. 10–10).

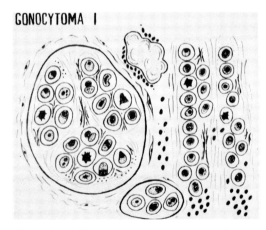

Figure 10–7. Homogeneous type of tumor formed solely of germ cells. From dysgerminomas (seminomas) occurring in normal women. This tumor differs by the presence of laminated calcific concretions or irregular calcific masses (schematic drawing).

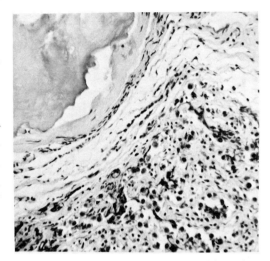

Figure 10–8. Gonocytoma I discovered in patient with primary amenorrhea, eunuchoidal habitus and male 46,XY karyotype. Note characteristic calcifications.

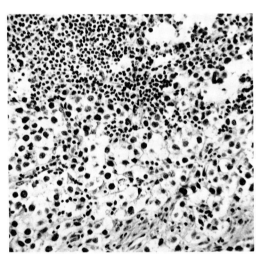

Figure 10–9. Another example of gonocytoma I discovered in a patient with clinicopathological features of gonadal dysgenesis.

Unlike the gonadoblastoma (gonocytoma III), the connective tissue bands separating the neoplastic nests and stroma do not contain Leydig cells. Small calcified concretions are seen. In some areas the germ cells penetrate outside the confines of typical neo-

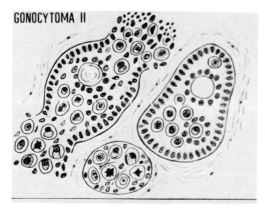

Figure 10–10. A schematic drawing of mixed form consisting of germ cell and Sertoli-granulosa type cells. Note the area overgrown by pure gonocytoma (bottom).

plastic nests into the stroma to form an invasive pure gonocytoma (dysgerminoma) in malignant fashion with marked lymphocytic infiltrations. With this special mixed germ cell tumor, classified as gonocytoma II, the main difficulty is that the tumors are few in number, variable in form, and often briefly described.[25]

Gonocytoma II occurs:

1. In young girls with normal somatosexual development, with symptoms of precocious puberty, which is due to feminizing activity of the tumor.[25,31]

2. In patients with somatosexual disturbances, primary amenorrhea, and a discrepancy between their male chromosomal sex pattern and their female type of genitals.

According to Hughesdon[25] there are 10 provisionally acceptable cases of gonocytoma II—eight ovarian and two testicular. Both testicular cases and one ovarian case showed calcified concretions.

In patients with gonadal dysgenesis and 46,XY karyotype, Guinet and Eyraud[30] described the tumor as containing typical islands of mixed germinal and granulosa-Sertoli cells. The connective tissue bands which separated the cellular nests contained only a few spindle-shaped cells resembling fibroblasts. Unlike the situation in gonadoblastoma, no Leydig cells could be found. This patient who was examined because of primary amenorrhea presented features of female phenotype, eunuchoidal body proportions, and infantile external genitalia.

In our Department in Warsaw, the gonocytoma II was revealed in a patient, age 20, examined because of primary amenorrhea and a failure to develop female secondary characteristics. Clinical examination revealed signs of slight estrogenic activity which consisted of partial development of breast and a fatty tissue topography consistent with the female type (Fig. 10–11). Cytologic examina-

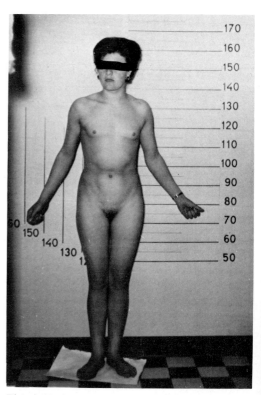

Figure 10–11. Gonocytoma II discovered in a patient with primary amenorrhea, high urinary gonadotrophin level, eunuchoidal habitus and male 46,XY karyotype. The clinical signs of slight estrogenic activity consisted of partial development of breast, and a fatty tissue topography developing toward the female type. Note the scanty pubic hair.

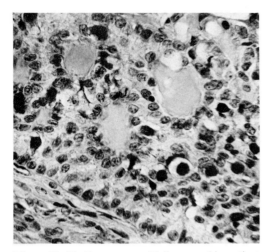

Figure 10–12. Gonocytoma II discovered in patient presented in Figure 10–11. Microscopic picture shows two distinct components of the tumor: (a) single germ cells scattered inside the nests of Sertoli-granulosa cells, and (b) microfollicular pattern of Sertoli-granulosa cells.

tion of a vaginal smear revealed the absence of estrogenic activity (Maturation Index: 10–90–0) and in consecutive cytosmears, slight estrogenic function (MI: 0–95–5) was noted. Repeated gynecological examinations showed no pelvic pathology. Cytogenetic examination revealed negative sex chromatin

pattern and male 46,XY Karyotype. Urinary gonadotrophin level was elevated (−59.2 and 121.4 M.U.). The normal limits for healthy women are 20 to 30 M.U. These findings pointed to the danger of gonadal neoplasia and the need for exploratory laparotomy.

Laparotomy disclosed an infantile uterus and Fallopian tubes. No gonad could be found on the right. On the left, in the place normally occupied by the ovary, a tumor covered by a grey-yellowish, smooth, glistening capsule measuring 4.5 × 6 × 4 cm was found. Unilateral left adnexectomy was performed. Microscopic examination revealed two structural patterns:

1. Neoplastic nests composed of germinal cells scattered among granulosa-Sertoli cells, the latter arranged in microfollicular pattern.

2. Typical pattern of pure gonocytoma (dysgerminoma) containing an aggregation of germ cells with solid or alveolar arrangements incompletely separated by delicate fibrous septums. Areas of a confusing admixture of germ-cells and sex-cord cell in malignant fashion were also found (Figs. 10–12–10–14). Scanty connective tissue bands separat-

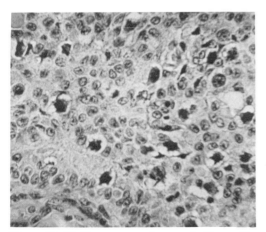

Figure 10–13. The same specimen as in Figure 10–12. Area consists of a confusing admixture of germ cells and sex-cord cells in malignant fashion. No Leydig cells are found.

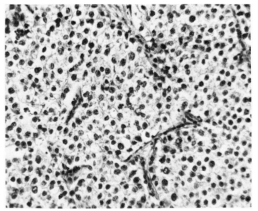

Figure 10–14. Gonocytoma II. The same case as in Figures 10–11 to 10–13. A large nest of germ cells similar to "pure dysgerminoma." Malignant feature of this tumor is indisputable.

ing neoplastic nests contained only fibroblast-like cells and no Leydig cells could be detected.

Gonocytoma III

This tumor was first described in 1953, by Scully[1] as gonadoblastoma. He recognized it as being distinct from a dysgerminoma and therefore classified it as a separate entity. The tumor is characterized histologically by the presence of distinctive neoplastic nests composed of germ cells scattered among granulosa-Sertoli cells (Fig. 10–15). The latter are arranged in the three typical patterns described by Scully: 1) in "coronal" fashion around germinal cells; 2) in peripheral single file along the base of the pseudo-tubules; and 3) in a folliculoid pattern (Figs. 10–15–10–17). Groups of Leydig cells are found between the nests, often in a hyalinized stroma which contains calcified concretions (Fig. 10–18).

In all our observed cases of gonocytoma III the area of overgrowth by germ cells was often found to be indistinguishable from pure dysgerminoma or seminoma (Figs.

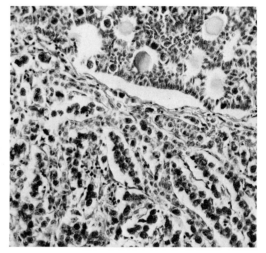

Figure 10–16. Gonocytoma III. Characteristic microscopic pattern with gonadoblastomatous nest visible at the top. The germ cells are organized in solid columns separated by delicate trabeculae or bands of connective tissue (bottom).

10–19–10–21). Sometimes peculiar granulomas with syncytial giant cells of the Langhans type are present (Figs. 10–22–10–23). Peculiar tubule-like structures, similar to the immature dysgenetic seminiferous tubules, are sometimes visible (Fig. 10–24).

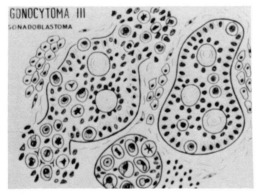

Figure 10–15. Gonocytoma III. Schematic drawing. Germ cells are scattered among Sertoli-granulosa cells. Note characteristic arrangement of Sertoli-granulosa cells: (a) in "coronal fashion" around individual germ cells; (b) in peripheral single file along the base of pseudotubule; and (c) in a folliculoid pattern.

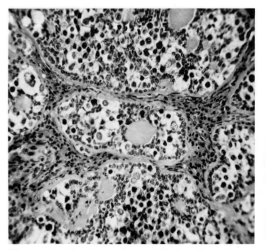

Figure 10–17. Gonocytoma III. Leydig cells are present between tumoral nests with epithelial nest showing more benign aspect—typical gonadoblastomatous pattern.

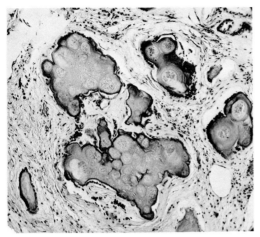

Figure 10–18. Gonocytoma III. Laminated calcific concretions within the gonadoblastoma nests which often replace the tumor elements.

A third type of cell, namely Leydig cells, represents only a kind of interstitial reaction (similar to the thecal reaction in certain ovarian carcinomas) of the specific rudimentary testicular tissue. Leydig cells are not real components of the tumor. However, they should be mentioned as a characteristic type of cell whose presence indicates

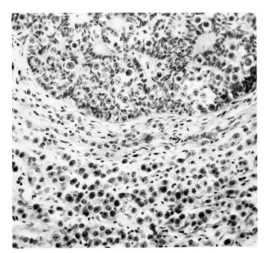

Figure 10–19. Gonocytoma III. The basic pattern of gonadoblastoma (top) is altered by overgrowth of the germ cell elements to form a pure gonocytoma-dysgerminoma (bottom).

gonocytoma III (gonadoblastoma). The Leydig cells never have neoplastic characteristics.

Numerous laminated, hyaline-like bodies that impart a psammomatous appearance and various irregular calcific masses may be considered as the specific features of gonadoblastoma. This tumor may have masculinizing and/or feminizing properties. In all reported cases, a wide variety of androgenic manifestations were observed including clitoral enlargement, deepening of the voice, acne, hirsutism and androidal body features. In many cases the labia majora has a scrotal appearance. Such findings reflect the androgenic activity of the interstitial Leydig-cell elements. In most of the reported cases of gonadoblastoma the above-mentioned androgenic features were present.[16,22,23,25,28,30,32–45]

In some patients estrogenic manifestations were also observed such as breast development, vaginal development, ability to have sexual intercourse, spontaneous episodes of uterine bleeding, withdrawal bleeding after gonadectomy (removal of the gonadal tumor), and climacteric-like symptoms following the operation. In our two patients the estrogenic manifestations were characterized by typical withdrawal bleeding after removal of the gonadal tumor (Table 10-I).

Of the 35 cases of gonadoblastoma reported by Hughesdon[25] from the literature, three assumed a male gender role, 30 were female, and two changed from female to male at puberty. Of the 30 who assumed a female role, 18 were virilized in some degree, and this occurred between the ages of 10 and 16. Nine of the 18 virilized cases had testicular tissue present also and 16 showed interstitial Leydig-like or lutein cells either in the tumor or in the associated gonad. Slight breast development occurred in 12 individuals and more marked estrogenic effects in seven others in the form of well-marked breast development. Three of the latter seven had testicular tissue (Figs. 10–27–

TABLE 10-I
ENDOCRINE MANIFESTATIONS AND THEIR MORPHOLOGY BASED ON
FIVE PATIENTS WITH GONOCYTOMA III (GONADOBLASTOMA)

	Pt. 1 (Age: 19)	Pt. 2 (Age: 21)	Pt. 3 (Age: 19)	Pt. 4 (Age: 19)	Pt. 5 (Age: 22)
Endogenous Estrogen Production					
Breast development	Pubertal	Pubertal	Absent	Absent	Developed Hypoplastic
Vaginal development	Rather poor	Good	Good	Poor	Good
Spontaneous episodes of uterine bleeding	No	Two episodes	No	No	One episode
Withdrawal bleeding after removal of tumor	Yes	Yes	No	No	No
Climacteric symptoms following operation	Present	Present	Present	No	Present
Endogenous Androgen Production					
Enlarged clitoris	Prominent	Present	Present	Prominent	Present
Labia majora	Scrotal-like	Female	Female	Scrotal-like	Female
Tendency to hirsutism	Present	Present	Discrete	Prominent	No
Skin	Pale, oily	Pale, oily	Female	Acne, oily	Female
Cells Capable of Hormone Production					
Sertoli-granulosa cells	Present	Present	Present in abundance	Present	Present
Leydig-like cells	Large group adenoma-like formations	Singular or small clumps	Small clumps	Large groups	Adenoma-like formations

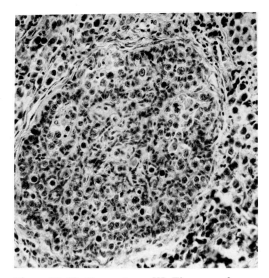

Figure 10–20. Gonocytoma III. The area of overgrowth by germ cells which is often indistinguishable from pure gonocytoma or seminoma. Note at the center, the admixture of germ cells and Sertoli-granulosa cells. The malignant pattern is evident.

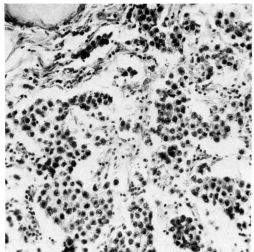

Figure 10–21. Gonocytoma III. An area of overgrowth of germ cell elements similar to "pure dysgerminoma."

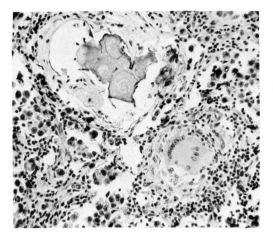

Figure 10–22. Gonocytoma III. The area of overgrowth by pure gonocytoma (seminoma), containing granulomas with giant syncytial cells, showing characteristic lymphocytic infiltration. Note the laminated calcific concretion at the top.

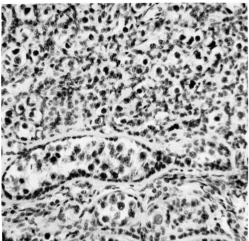

Figure 10–24. Gonocytoma III. The nest of germ cells scattered among Sertoli-granulosa type cells. Peculiar tubule-like structure is visible.

ulate a more intensive search for viable sex-cord (Sertoli-granulosa) elements. Scully believes that possibly all gonocytomas arising in dysgenetic gonads are germ-cell overgrowths of gonadoblastomas. It is very likely that some of these tumors have been wrongly identified as pure dysgerminomas.

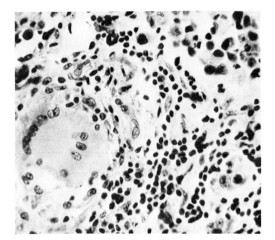

Figure 10–23. Gonocytoma III. Tubercle-like granuloma with epithelioid cells and isolated giant cells of the Langhans type.

10–28) and six had interstitial lutein or Leydig-like cells (Fig. 10–26).

According to Scully,[41] the type of gonadoblastoma that is most easily overlooked on microscopic examination is one overgrown by a pure gonocytoma (dysgerminoma). In such a case the presence of characteristic psammoma-like calcifications should stim-

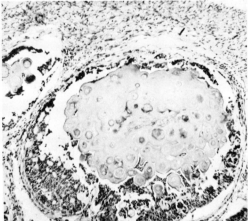

Figure 10–25. Gonocytoma III. Calcification replacing some of the masses of neoplastic cells. The surrounding stroma is fibrous and hyaline. Fibrocalcific masses dominate in such areas and visible neoplastic cells are compressed and sparse.

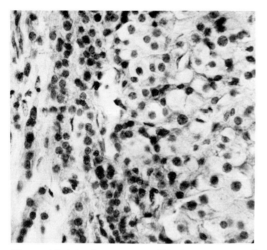

Figure 10–26. Gonocytoma III. Large nests of Leydig cells represent only a kind of interstitial reaction (analogous to thecal reaction in certain ovarian carcinomas) of the specific rudimentary testicular tissue.

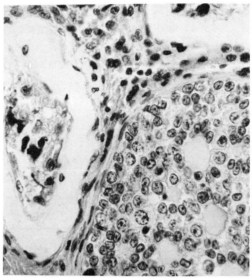

Figure 10–28. Immature seminiferous tubules at the periphery of gonocytoma III, without lumen and with thickened tubular wall.

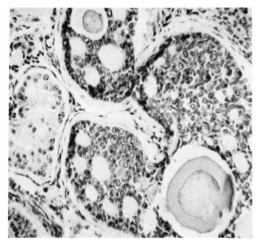

Figure 10–27. Dysgenetic germ cell tumor arising from testicular tissue. A case with primary amenorrhea, eunuchoidal habitus, XY karyotype, prominent enlarged clitoris, scrotal appearance of labia majora, uterus and Fallopian tubes, and complete vagina. A tumoral gonad was discovered on the one side and a testis on the other. Microscopic picture shows immature seminiferous tubules in nontumoral portion of testicle (on the left).

Most probably, the tumors reported by Ber,[46] Plate,[47] and Blocksma,[48] in Scully's opinion, belong to the group of gonadoblastomas.

A gonadoblastomatous pattern was found in embryonal carcinoma.[49] Scully[41] found 13 cases in which another type of tumor was found in the dysgenetic gonad harboring the gonadoblastoma (mucinous cystadenoma, teratoma, endodermal embryonal carcinoma, etc.).

Gonocytoma IV

This is a special form of a pure germ cell tumor with clinical symptoms of virilism caused by an overgrowth of androgenic interstitial cells (hilus Leydig cells) adjacent to the germ cell tumor or occurring in the contralateral uninvolved gonad (Fig. 10–29).

In 1963, Sohval described a case of gonocytoma IV in a chromatin-negative female with a streak gonad on the left and the tumor replacing the right gonad. The patient

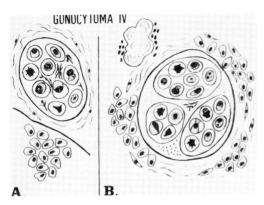

Figure 10–29. Schematic drawing of gonocytoma IV. Basically gonocytoma I, but with Leydig or Lutein-like cells present in the gonad outside the tumor analogous to interstitial or thecal reaction. Sometimes large nests of interstitial cells are present in the contralateral noninvolved gonad.

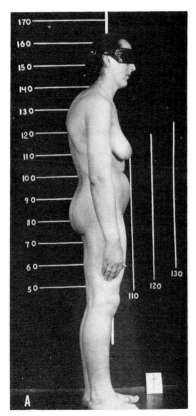

had female genitalia with an enlarged clitoris, a uterus, Fallopian tubes and a complete vagina.[50]

In 1957, we observed and treated a patient, age 33, who was referred because of primary amenorrhea, delayed puberty, and eunuchoidism. The patient had an enlarged but normal clitoris and underdeveloped female genitalia with a uterus and a complete vagina. Moderate enlargement of her breasts with large areolae of pubertal type was also noted (Fig. 10–30a & 10–30b). Initially, sex chromatin was erroneously assessed as slightly positive. A few years later, the sex chromatin was established as negative and cytogenetic examination was begun but the patient was subsequently lost from the study. Laparotomy revealed a typical fibrous streak on the left side and a knob-like tumor on the right measuring 4 × 1.5 cm. Bilateral gonadectomy was performed. Microscopic examination of the left gonad revealed an ovarian-like stroma and large nests of interstitial, Leydig-like cells. The right gonad contained typical nests of germ-cells arranged in solid columns

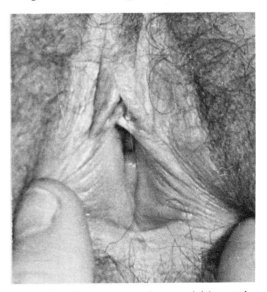

Figure 10–30. Gonocytoma IV. A eunuchoidal patient (a) with primary amenorrhea, partial breast development, pubic hair and enlargement of clitoris (b).

separated by delicate trabeculae or bands of connective tissue showing 9 varying degrees of lymphocytic infiltration (Fig. 10–31). Characteristic features consisted of: 1) laminated calcific concretions and 2) peripheral overgrowth of interstitial Leydig-like cells adjacent to the germ-cell tumor (Figs. 10–32, 10–33). As large aggregates of cal-

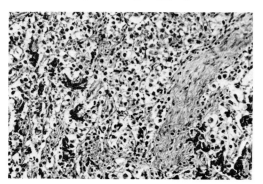

Figure 10–31. Gonocytoma IV. The same patient as in Figure 10–30. Malignant part of tumor. The distinct monocellular pattern with strands and nests of uniform germ cells. The neoplastic cells are vesicular, round, or polygonal in shape. Strands or nests of germ cells are separated by fibrous septa with lymphocytic infiltration.

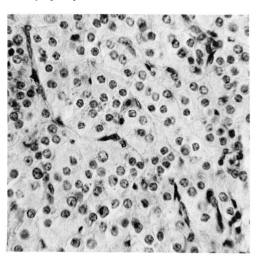

Figure 10–32. Gonocytoma IV. Peripheral overgrowth of androgenic interstitial cells adjacent to the germ cell tumor.

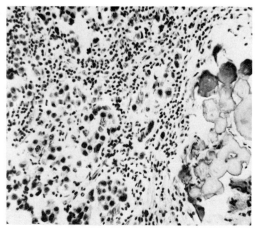

Figure 10–33. Gonocytoma IV. Area of calcific concretions in the fibrous, hyalinized stroma adjacent to neoplastic nests.

cium replaced the tumor cells, the surrounding stroma became fibrous and often hyaline, resulting in the formation of fibrocalcific masses in which viable tumor cells were sparse or absent (Fig. 10–33).

Conclusion

Classification and recognition of the different types of germ-cell tumors that occur in dysgenetic gonads would facilitate more precise pathologic diagnosis. Teter's gonocytoma I, II, III and IV classification is based on the most important characteristic of this type of tumor—an area of germ cells exhibiting typical malignant features. Even if these cells form a confused admixture with Sertoli-granulosa cells, the pattern is still malignant (Figs. 10–6 & 10–20).

The most conspicuous feature of these special germ-cell tumors is the presence of calcified concretions in the parenchyma. They occur in various forms from psammoma-like calcifications to irregular calcified masses, replacing the tumor.

Gross Appearance—Localization

In all our cases an infantile uterus and long, thin Fallopian tubes were found at exploratory laparotomy. The tumor is usually knob-like and is located in the place normally occupied by ovaries. It is difficult to palpate preoperatively because of a narrow and inelastic vagina.

In our 12 cases of dysgenetic germ-cell tumors, the neoplasm was limited to one gonad in 10 cases. The unilateral germ-cell tumors showed a predilection for the right gonad. In only two cases were both gonads involved with no evidence of gross metastases (Fig. 10–34).

The tumor varied from microscopically undetectable to that of 8 to 10 cm in greatest diameter. This obviously means that they were in the initial phase of neoplastic development. In only two patients were the tumors irregularly bosselated but not roughened. No adhesions between the gonadal masses and adjacent structures were noted.

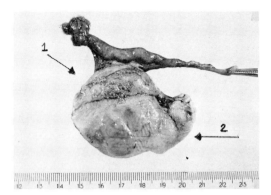

Figure 10–35. The cut surface of dysgenetic germ cell tumor classified as gonocytoma III shows chondroid-like nodules corresponding to gonadoblastomatous pattern with psammona-like calcifications and the areas of irregular calcific masses within hyalinized fibrotic stroma (arrow 1). Arrow 2 shows large soft area corresponding to pure gonocytoma and a malignant admixture of germ cells and Sertoli-granulosa cells. Note Fallopian tube at the top.

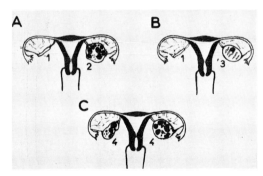

Figure 10–34. Tumor localization. A. Typical situation—the unilateral germ cell tumor shows a predilection for the right gonad (2), and on the other side a fibrous streak gonad is visible (1); B. In the mixed gonadal dysgenesis (often with XO/XY karyotype) dysgenetic germ cell tumor arises in and from dysgenetic or rudimentary testes (3); C. In some patients both gonads are completely destroyed by the neoplastic process (4).

The consistency of all of the germ-cell tumors was extremely firm and chondroid-like nodules were noted in five cases.

The cut surface of a dysgenetic gonadal tumor shows chondroid-like nodules corresponding to a gonadoblastomatous pattern with psammoma-like calcifications, with large aggregates of calcium in fibrous stroma. A soft area corresponds to pure gonocytoma and to malignant admixture of germ cells and Sertoli-granulosa cells (Fig. 10–35).

The most conspicuous feature of this special germ cell tumor is the presence of a uterus and Fallopian tubes which were observed in all patients with female habitus. Moreover, in phenotypic males with gonadoblastoma, a definite or questionable uterus was found in all patients whose abdomens were explored.[41] Among 11 such patients, six had bilateral Fallopian tubes and in the remaining five, a tube was present on one side.

Contralateral Gonadal Pathology

Histopathologic classification of the contralateral, uninvolved gonad is of great importance because the original gonadal tissue may elucidate the origin of the tumor. In many cases the tumor-involved gonad is completely destroyed by the neoplastic process and it is impossible to establish the type of original gonadal tissue.

The analysis of our own cases and others included slides of the gonads. These and a review of cases reported in the literature show the following pathologic changes in the contralateral uninvolved gonad:

1. Residual streak gonad composed of scanty fibrotic tissue without any active cellular elements (Fig. 10–36).
2. Well-developed cortical part resembling ovarian stroma, and in the medullary zone, ambiguous germinal and granulosal clusters with microfolliculoid pattern. Sometimes, testicular remnants consisting of bizarre seminiferous tubules with peculiar structures are described as laminated eosinophilic intratubular bodies and referred to as intratubular pseudo-ovocytes.[26,51–55] Such intratubular pseudo-ovocytes are

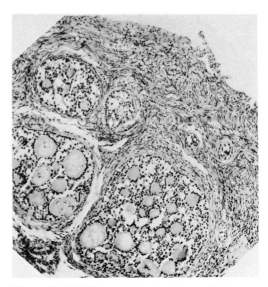

Figure 10–37. Histopathologic picture of the contralateral uninvolved gonad. Well-developed cortical part with multiple intratubular bodies in medullary zone and germ cells scattered among Sertoli-granulosa cells.

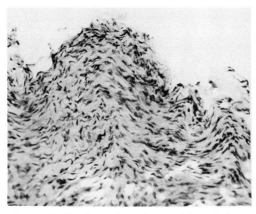

Figure 10–36. Contralateral gonadal pathology. Fibrous streak without any active cellular elements.

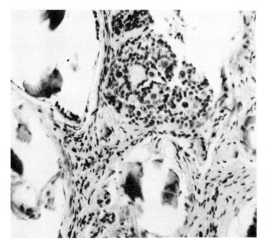

Figure 10–38. Histopathologic picture of the contralateral noninvolved gonad. Degenerative changes of bi-sexual formations. Germ cells and Sertoli-granulosa cells are compressed by laminated calcific concretions with empty spaces and fibrotic and hyalinized stroma.

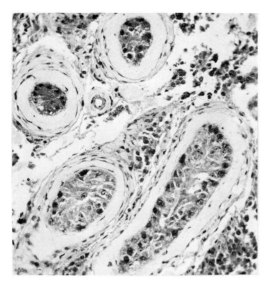

Figure 10–39. Histopathologic picture of contra-lateral uninvolved gonad. Testicular pattern. Semi-niferous tubules are immature with signs of degen-eration.

encircled by the inner layer of Sertoli-granulosa cells resembling corona radiata (Fig. 10–37). Laminated calcific concretions with advancing degenera-tion of these structures are often seen. Sometimes, irregular calcific masses re-placed the epithelial contents of the tubules (or nests); the surrounding stroma became fibrous and hyaline; and Sertoli-granulosa cells were com-pressed, sparse, or even completely absent (Fig. 10–38).

3. Testis—Seminiferous tubules are always immature with various signs of degen-eration (Fig. 10–39).

Nongerminal Tumors

Among the neoplasms of dysgenetic go-nads, several nongerminal tumors were de-scribed. In our material two benign non-germinal tumors were found.

In a patient with pure gonadal dysgenesis, a Brenner's tumor with the gross appearance of a slightly enlarged fibrous streak was discovered within the right gonad. Cells were present which resembled thecal cells in some areas proximal to the neoplastic epithelial cells which is analogous to the "thecal reaction" observed in ovarian carcinoma. A similar tumor was reported by Stange[15] in 1957.

In our amenorrheic patient classified as having Turner's syndrome with masculiniz-ation, a small tumor in the hilar area was detected and classified as an interstitial Leydig-cell tumor. Similar cases have been reported by others also.[56,57]

Several other cases of nongerminal tumor were described in the literature—Hauser, *et al.*,[58] described granulosa-thecal tumor and Goldberg and Scully[59] reported malignant papillary pseudo-mucinuous cystadenoma in a patient with Turner's syndrome.

Other cases not classified as gonocytoma or dysgerminoma (seminoma) but belonging to the group of germ-cell tumors are rare—an embryonal carcinoma of testicular type was reported by Ober;[60] teratocarcinoma by Melicow and Uson;[2] and embryonal carcinoma by Peyron, *et al.*,[61] Pinkerton,[62] and Santesson and Marrubini.[49]

Premalignant Changes in Dysgenetic Gonads

In some of our cases classified as pure gonadal dysgenesis or mixed gonadal dys-genesis (fibrous streak on the one side and maldeveloped testis on the other), peculiar structures were found which we labeled "bi-sexual formations" because the germ cells and Sertoli-granulosa cells are arranged in a pattern resembling both seminiferous tubules and an ovarian follicle (Fig. 10–40). Similar or identical structures were found at

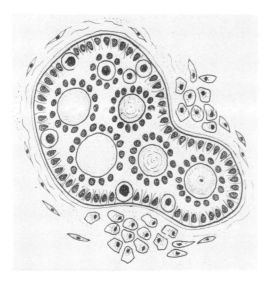

Figure 10–40. Schematic drawing of nontumoral nests of germ cells with an intermingling of Sertoli-granulosa cells showing microfolliculoid pattern. Such tubular areas are sometimes mistaken for a gonadoblastoma. Such peculiar structures occurring in medullary zone of dysgenetic gonad are termed "bi-sexual formations."

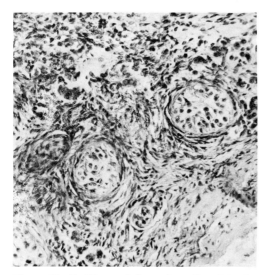

Figure 10–41. Bi-sexual formations found in the contralateral fibrous streak in the case of gonadoblastoma.

the periphery of a definite neoplastic gonad (Fig. 10–41).

The majority of individuals with gonadoblastoma were between the ages of 10 and 25 years. The youngest patient with gonadoblastoma was eight years of age. It is doubtful that patients from the ages of six months to five years who were initially given the diagnosis of gonadoblastoma actually had this diagnosis. Instead, it is possible that they had benign or premalignant changes, or perhaps it may be an example of overdiagnosis. Woodruff[63] noted that in the early embryonic gonad a peculiar pattern occurs which is suggestive of tumor formation. In many embryonic gonads investigated by Woodruff prior to encapsulation of the germ cell, which is usually complete by about five months, there are nests of germ cells with an intermingling of undifferentiated stromal and mesothelial cells which accurately simulate dysgerminoma. Similarly, in dysgenetic gonads of adults, the tubular areas with the unencapsulated germ cells of the rudimentary seminiferous tubules are in apposition to the characteristic primordial follicles. Such a confusing pattern may be mistaken for a gonadoblastoma.

It seems that malformed seminiferous tubules with multiple pseudo-ovocytes and proliferating Sertoli and germ cell expanding tubules may be considered as premalignant changes.[51–54]

Cytogenetic Approach to the Dysgenetic Gonadal Tumor

Cytogenetic studies are necessary for the diagnosis and clinical management of patients with malformed gonads who are suspected of having a germ cell tumor.

It is clear that tumors arise frequently in dysgenetic gonads of individuals with sex chromosome abnormalities. The review of gonadoblastomas published by Scully[41] showed that 89 percent of the patients were chromatin negative; the most common karyotypes were 46,XY and 45,X/46,XY. A Y chromosome was definitely identified in all but three cases with recorded karyotypes. Unfortunately, no karyotypes of the chromatin positive patients were performed.

Because of the high incidence of gonadal tumors, exploratory laparotomy is indicated in every case of primary amenorrhea in which a negative sex chromatin pattern and the presence of a Y chromosome are found.[23,45,50,54,64–66]

As can be seen from Table 10-II, among 43 recorded karyotypes of patients with dysgenetic germ cell tumors, a Y chromosome was definitely identified in 38 (88%)

and the recorded karyotypes were 46,XY in 24 patients (56%).

A review of the reported karyotypes also showed a relatively high incidence of XO/XY mosaicism (10 patients, 88%, had this mosaicism). As Van Campenhout has reviewed from the literature,[67] among 51 cases of XO/XY mosaicism with identification of both gonads, nine (17.6%) had a neoplasm. It is of interest to note that all of these patients were phenotypic females but presented signs of masculinization (hypertrophy of the clitoris, scrotal appearance of the labia majora, etc.). From the available data, it is clear that laparotomy with bilateral gonadectomy should be performed in all XO/XY mosaic individuals, particularly if

TABLE 10-II
CYTOGENETIC ANALYSIS OF THE GONOCYTOMA OCCURRING IN GONADAL DYSGENESIS

Karyotype	No. of Cases	Gonocytoma I	No. of Cases	Gonocytoma II	No. of Cases	Gonocytoma III (gonadoblastoma)	No. of Cases
XY	24	Carpentier, et al.	1	Guinet and Eyraud	1	Herve, et al.	1
		Brogger and Strand	1	Michalkiewicz, et al.	1	Netter, et al.	1
		Baron, et al.	1	Warsaw	1	Siebenmann	1
		Warsaw	1			Frazier, et al.	1
						Freeman, et al.	1
						Strumpf	1
						Bieger, et al.	1
						Taylor, et al.	1
						Teter, et al.	1
						Teter, et al.	1
						Teter, et al.	1
						Cohen and Shaw (sisters)	2
						Warsaw	2
XY/XO	10	Lewis, et al.	1			Hughesdon and Kamaramasy	1
		Miller, et al.	1			Gagnon and Cadotte	1
		Goodlin	1			Borghi, et al.	1
						Robinson	1
						Netter, et al.	1
						Boczkowski, et al.	1
						Philip and Teter	1
XO/X fragment	1					McDonough and Greenblatt	1
XO/XYq-	1					Desjeux, et al.	1
XX/XY	1					Overzier	1
XX/XY/XO	1					Sadasivan	1
XO/XX/XY	1					Schuster	1
XO/XM	1					Miller	1
XO	2	Rochet, et al.	1				
		Dominguez and Greenblatt	1				
XX	1					Salet, et al.	1

some symptoms of masculinization are noted.

Desjuex, et al.,[68] in reviewing the literature, found that the phenotype of XO/XY individuals is variable, but two principal features are: 1) a varying degree of masculinization (XY): and 2) stigmata of Turner's syndrome (XO). Our patient with gonadoblastoma and XO/XY mosaicism had typical stigmata of Turner's syndrome with clitoral enlargement and other signs of masculinization.[24,43]

In 41 cases reviewed by Desjeux, et al.,[68] three seminomas (gonocytoma I) and 12 gonadoblastomas (gonocytoma III) were found. This important statistic should be considered in the therapeutic approach.

The presence of the Y chromosome suggests that malformed dysgenetic gonads were intended to develop into testes. It is generally believed that the presence of testicular tissue in man is dependent upon the presence of Y-chromosome and that the presence of Y-chromosome in cases with gonadoblastoma is important evidence that the structures seen in the tumor have testicular origin.

In 51 cases of XO/XY mosaicism with bilateral gonadal identification, 36 had testicular tissue, whereas ovarian follicles have been clearly demonstrated in only one case. Individuals with fibrous streak gonads and XO/XY mosaicism are relatively rare.[66] On the other hand, it is known that the presence of a Y chromosome in the gonadal cells is not sufficient in itself to guarantee the differentiation of testicular tissue. Several patients with XY karyotype classified as pure gonadal dysgenesis had a rudimentary fibrous streak without testicular elements.[52,69]

All patients phenotypically female with XY or XO/XY chromosomal pattern and some testicular tissue exhibited some virilization, usually incomplete however, and the majority had differentiated Mullerian ducts which indicated that these testes were functionally abnormal during embryonic and fetal life. It seems that among the eunuchoidal patients with XY karyotype and total absence of sexual development (lack of pubic hair, absence of enlarged clitoris) in which pure gonadal dysgenesis is suspected, the risk of malignancy is not so high as in the same type of patient with signs of masculinization.

As can be seen from Table 10-II, germinal tumors are extremely rare in patients with gonadal dysgenesis and the absence of a Y chromosome. Only four such cases were found in the literature among 40 patients. However, three of them had a negative sex chromatin pattern, namely, the cases reported by Miller,[50] Dominguez and Greenblatt,[70] and Rochet, et al.[71] (also, additional references in Table 10-II).

An exceptional case of gonadoblastoma in a patient with a positive sex chromatin pattern and 46,XX karyotype was described by Salet, et al.[72] Another case of nongerminal feminizing granulosa-thecal cell tumor in an XX female with gonadal dysgenesis was reported by Hauser, et al.[58] Both of these cases indicated that attention should not be restricted to the chromatin negative group.

Incidence of Gonadal Neoplasia in Patients having a Uterus and Malformed Gonads

Because of the more frequent use of exploratory laparotomy and histologic examination of the gonads removed from patients with primary amenorrhea and congenital somatosexual disturbances, the special gonadal tumors occurring in intersexes have been reported recently with an increasing frequency. Between 1955 and 1970, laparotomy was performed on 80 patients with primary amenorrhea and malformed gonads. All of these patients were referred to the Departments of Gynecology or Clinical

Endocrinology because of primary amenorrhea and retardation of sexual development with high urinary gonadotrophin levels. In 16 of these cases (20%), tumors were discovered or confirmed during exploratory laparotomy (Table 10-III).

TABLE 10-III
RESULTS OF EXPLORATORY LAPAROTOMY
PERFORMED IN PATIENTS WITH PRIMARY
AMENORRHEA, UTERUS, FALLOPIAN TUBES
AND MALDEVELOPED GONADS
Department of Clinical Endocrinology, Medical
Academy, Warsaw Period 1955–1970

Diagnosis Classification	Number of Patients	Germ-cell Tumor	Benign Non-germinal Tumor
Turner's Syndrome	26	1	1
Isolated Gonadal Dysgenesis	40	13	1
Ovarian Dysplasia	14	0	—
Total	80	14	2

The frequency of dysgenetic gonadal tumors among patients with primary amenorrhea and sexual abnormalities is not known at this time. Evaluation of the frequency of gonadal tumors in various forms of congenital somatosexual disturbances with various cytogenetic patterns should be considered in any discussion of the occurrence of tumors in dysgenetic gonads. It is obvious that the incidence of neoplasia in maldeveloped or underdeveloped gonads varies among the types of gonadal dysgenesis and cytogenetic findings.

Turner's Syndrome

No gonadal tumors were detected in 21 patients with the classical form of Turner's syndrome (without signs of masculinization) with 45,X karyotype or with 45,X/46,XX mosaicism (Fig. 10–42). From the cytogenetic and oncologic point of view, in patients with Turner's syndrome showing 45,X karyotype, it may be concluded from

these findings that exploratory laparotomy is not necessary because gonadal tumors are almost never found. The extremely low incidence of gonadal neoplasia in classical Turner's syndrome (without signs of masculinization) is easily explainable in that the residual gonadal streak presents only a vestigial remnant composed of whorls of fibrotic tissue with no active cellular elements or germ cells (Fig. 10–43). This residual gonadal streak provides no material for neoplastic transformation.

From a clinical point of view, classical Turner's syndrome is characterized by short stature and other malformations, e.g. webbing of the neck, cubitus valgus, etc., whose streak gonads are found to consist of undifferentiated embryonic stroma. Radiological studies of 32 cases of gonadal dysgenesis in our department revealed that the most pronounced skeletal abnormalities, including osteoporosis and abnormalities in the hands and knees, were present in patients with Turner's syndrome. There were less marked findings in cases classified as pure gonadal dysgenesis or mixed dysgenesis.

Cytogenetic studies performed in 32 patients with Turner's syndrome showed an absence of sex chromosome Y. The chromosomal complements were as follows:

45,X	16 cases
45,X/46,XX	11 cases
45,X/47,XXX	1 case
46,XX	4 cases

No tumors were revealed in exploratory laparotomies performed on 21 patients in this group.

**Turner's Syndrome with
Clitoral Enlargement**

These patients were of the usual short stature with other stigmata of Turner's syndrome such as webbing of the neck, barrel-shaped chest, and cubitus valgus. In contrast to classical Turner's syndrome, gynecological examination showed that the pubic hair resembled that of a normal adult female (Fig. 10–44). In our five cases the pubic hair spread to the medial surface of the thighs but not up the linea alba. The clitoris was enlarged and was usually covered by a large prepubital fold with smegma (Fig. 10–45). The labia majora was hypertrophied with a scrotal appearance. The vagina was narrow, its walls smooth. The uterine cervix was of the thickness of a pencil and the fundus uteri was hypoplastic.

Radiological examination showed typical skeletal abnormalities as observed in classical Turner's syndrome; only osteoporosis seemed to be less pronounced. Cytogenetic studies in three cases investigated exhibited 45,X/46,XY mosaicism.

Exploratory laparotomy performed in all five cases revealed two tumors—gonadoblastoma (gonocytoma III) in one case and an interstitial hilar cell tumor in another case. In both cases of gonadal tumors, histologic examination of the contralateral noninvolved gonad revealed a well-developed cortical part containing connective tissue fibers resembling the stroma of the ovary in its whorled arrangement (Figs. 10–38 & 10–40).

A medullary part contained small nests of malformed rudimentary seminiferous tubules in which germ cells were scattered among Sertoli-granulosa cells, identifying a microfollicular pattern. Such peculiar structures are termed "bi-sexual formations" because the germ cells and Sertoli-granulosa cells are arranged in a pattern resembling

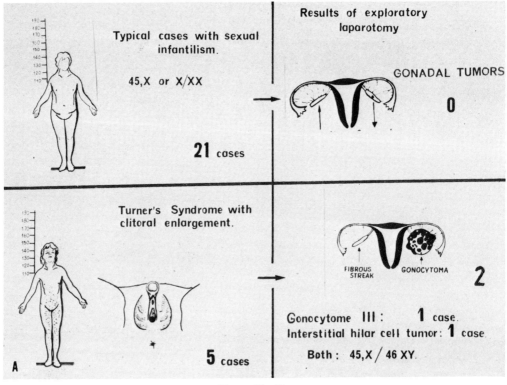

Figure 10–42a.

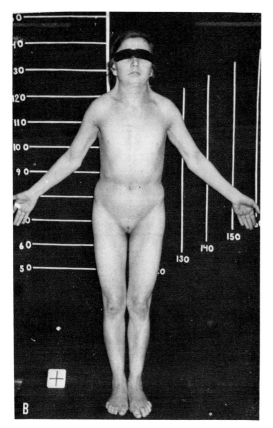

Figure 10–42. Classic form of Turner's syndrome in patient aged 20. Anterior view showing barrel shaped chest, webbed neck, complete lack of breast development, no pubic hair, and infantile external genitalia. Figure 10–42a illustrates the incidence of gonadal tumors among the patients classified as Turner's syndrome.

both seminiferous tubules and ovarian follicles.

In the three remaining cases, typical bilateral fibrous streaks were found and in two of the cases, microscopic examination revealed small "bi-sexual formations" in one gonad. The medullary part contained small foci of Leydig-like cells and meso-nephric remnants were visible in all three cases. These findings proved that the incidence of gonadal neoplasia among patients with Turner's syndrome (clitoral enlarge-

ment and the presence of sex chromosome Y) is high in contrast to the classical Turner's syndrome patients without sex chromosome Y (usually with XO sex complements) in whom the incidence of malignancy in the gonads is extremely low (only two cases reported in the literature, see Table 10-II).

A completely different situation exists among individuals with Turner's syndrome showing clitoral enlargement and other signs of masculinization such as those exhibiting 45,X/46,XY mosaicism or other chromosomal complements with the presence of sex chromosome Y. Among five of these cases, two gonadal tumors were discovered. Extrapolation suggests that all patients with Turner's syndrome exhibiting the Y

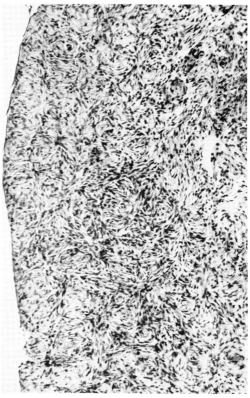

Figure 10–43. Turner's syndrome. Residual gonadal streak showing fibrotic tissue with no active cellular elements or germ cells.

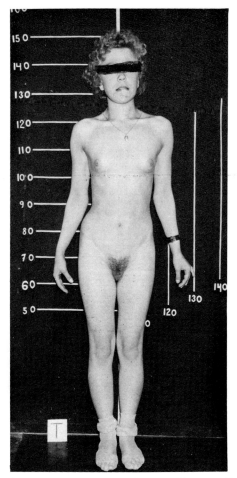

Figure 10–44. Turner's syndrome with masculinization. A patient with negative sex chromatin pattern and XO/XY karyotype, uterus, Fallopian tubes and complete vagina. Exploratory laparotomy revealed a gonadoblastoma on the right and on the left, fibrous streak (microscopically in medullary zone several bi-sexual formations were found).

chromosome should undergo exploratory laparotomy.

Isolated Gonadal Dysgenesis

Most cases of dysgenetic gonadal tumors reported in the literature were discovered

in patients with primary amenorrhea and average or above average height. Such patients are characterized by poor development of breasts, scanty or absent pubic and axillary hair, eunuchoidal body proportions (with no somatic malformations), and a high level of urinary gonadotrophins, which indicate most probably a congenital gonadal defect (Fig. 10–46). However, the incidence of neoplasia is variable in particular types of isolated gonadal dysgenesis. For this reason, precise classification based on cytogenetic study and exploratory laparotomy with pathologic study of the gonads is essential (Table 10-IV).

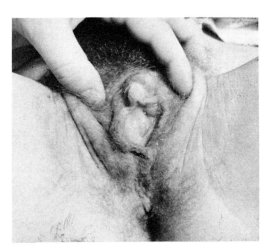

Figure 10–45. The same patient as in Figure 10–44. Note hypertrophied clitoris covered by a large preputial fold with smegma. The labia majora are hypertrophied with a scrotal appearance.

TABLE 10-IV
INCIDENCE OF NEOPLASIA IN PATIENTS WITH PRIMARY AMENORRHEA
AND VARIOUS FORMS OF MALDEVELOPED GONADS

Classification Chromosomal Pattern	No. of Cases	Gonadal Histology	No. of Cases	Classification of Tumors	No. of Cases
Classic Turner's syndrome XO; XO/XX; X/XXX; XX	21	Rudimentary fibrous streak	0		—
Turner's syndrome with clitoral enlargement XO/XY	5	Bi-sexual formations, Foci of Leydig-like cells	2	Gonocytoma III (gonadoblastoma) Interstitial hilar cell tumor	1
Pure gonadal dysgenesis with positive sex chromatin pattern XX; XO/XX	15	Fibrous streak	0		—
Isolated gonadal dysgenesis with negative sex chromatin pattern	25		14	Gonocytomas I, II, III (gonadoblastomas) Gonocytoma IV Brenner's tumor	13
					1
1) Pure gonadal dysgenesis		Fibrous streak. Bi-sexual formations			
b) Mixed gonadal dysgenesis		Testicular pattern and fibrous streak			
c) Syndrome of rudimentary testes XY/XYY		Malformed testicular tubules			
Ovarian dysplasia XX; XO/XX	14	Fibrotic stromal hypoplasia. Deficient follicles. Defective ova.	0		
Total	80		16		16

Pure Gonadal Dysgenesis with Positive Sex Chromatin Pattern and XX Karyotype

Eunuchoidal patients with a positive sex chromatin pattern, 46,XX karyotype and high urinary gonadotrophin levels may be classified as having "pure gonadal dysgenesis" or ovarian dysplasia according to the gonadal pathology. In patients with "pure gonadal dysgenesis," exploratory laparotomy usually revealed fetal uteri and bilateral rudimentary fibrous streaks in place of the gonads and no tumors were found in the tissues from 15 patients investigated at the Department of Clinical Endocrinology in Warsaw.

The residual gonadal streak presenting only a vestigial remnant composed of fibrotic tissue with no active cellular elements and no germ cells provides no material for neoplastic transformation. I believe that germ cells are of fundamental importance in the development of tumors.

In 1970, Scully[41] stated that "the conclusion that gonadoblastoma cannot develop in a patient with 46,XX karyotype may be premature." As a matter of fact, only one case has been reported so far supporting this view.

In 1960, Salet, et al.,[72] published a case of gonadoblastoma in a patient with primary amenorrhea and a normal female karyotype 46,XX. Clinically, this case was classified as pure gonadal dysgenesis. A karyotype 46,XX was established in 1000 cells studied. The patient was 18 years old and was admitted because of primary amenorrhea and sexual infantilism. Urinary gonadotrophin levels were from 25 I.U. to 45 I.U. Exploratory laparotomy showed a hypoplastic uterus, normal Fallopian tubes and bilateral gonads, macroscopically classified as small ovaries 3 mm/1.5 mm. Both gonads were biopsied and microscopic examination revealed gonadoblastoma. Two years later a second laparotomy was performed and bilateral adnexectomy carried out. The left gonad was larger than the right one. The histologic examination revealed a gonadoblastoma within the left gonad and remnants of the cortical part composed of fibrotic ovarian-like stroma was found in the right. This case could be classified as asymmetric gonadal dysgenesis.

A similar case is reported by Hauser, et al.,[58] who found a feminizing granulosa-theca cell tumor in a patient with gonadal dysgenesis and female XX karyotype.

These exceptionally rare cases indicate that attention should be focused not only on the chromatin-negative patients but to chromatin positive patients as well.[50] It is well proven that in dysgenetic testicular remnants found in male pseudohermaphrodites one can find only XX cells with intra-abdominal testes.[50] Therefore, one may not exclude gonadal neoplasia in patients with primary amenorrhea and XX karyotype.

It is worthy stressing once again that gonadoblastoma among patients with primary amenorrhea and 46,XX karyotype is extremely rare. Although one cannot exclude the possibility that more frequently conducted exploratory laparotomies may uncover gonadal malformations or tumors, to date it is proven that a high risk of neoplasia exists only in patients with negative sex chromatin patterns and the presence of a Y sex chromosome.

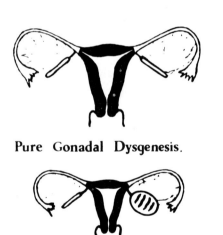

Pure Gonadal Dysgenesis.

Mixed (asymetric) Gonadal Dysgenesis

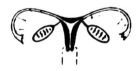

Syndrome of rudimentary testes.

A   total **40**

Eunuchoidal habitus without somatic malformations.

TUMORS

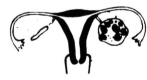

GONOCYTOMA I II III and IV	cases: **13**
BENIGN TUMORS	cases: **1**

Warsaw 1971.

Figure 10–46a.

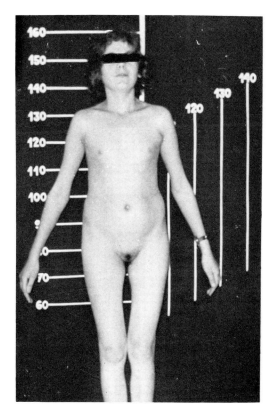

Figure 10–46. Isolated gonadal dysgenesis. Anterior view showing eunuchoidal body proportions, normal height, and an absence of breast development. Figure 10–46a illustrates the incidence of gonadal tumor among eunuchoidal patients with dysgenetic gonads.

Isolated Gonadal Dysgenesis with a Negative Sex Chromatin Pattern and a Male 46, XY Karyotype

According to histologic examination of removed gonads, three groups may be classified as follows:

Pure Gonadal Dysgenesis with Normal Male 46,XY Karyotype

Bilateral fibrotic streak gonads are present. Morphologically, the gonads appear as undif-ferentiated embryonic stroma without germinal elements, consisting mainly of a cortical portion. In rare cases, tubules with the unencapsulated germ cells of the rudimentary seminiferous tubules in apposition to the characteristic primordial follicles (bi-sexual formations) can be seen in the medullary zone. Laminated calcific concretions or empty spaces with remnants of sex-cord cells are visible at times (Fig. 10–38). More often, foci of interstitial-Leydig-like cells occur.

Mixed Gonadal Dysgenesis

One finds a fetal uterus and a rudimentary streak gonad on the one side and a testicle on the other, both in the position normally occupied by the ovaries.[45] One very early case of gonadoblastoma in a 46,XX patient having mixed gonadal dysgenesis was detected in our department in 1963.

Case Study: Patient K.J., aged 19, was admitted because of primary amenorrhea, retardation of sexual development and virilization. Physical examination revealed a eunuchoidal body build with masculine features. There was no breast development. Gynecological examination showed pubic hair of male type spreading toward the inguinal regions and internal part of the thighs. The external genitals were feminine except for an enlarged clitoris giving it a penis-like appearance. The labia minora were rather rudimentary and the labia majora were swollen and covered by wrinkled skin of scrotal appearance. Laparotomy disclosed an infantile uterus and Fallopian tubes. On the left, a typical dysgenetic whitish streak was found in the place normally occupied by the ovary. On the right, also in the location normally occupied by the ovary, a gonad resembling a testis was found. Typical gonadoblastomatic nests were found containing a mixture of germ cells and Sertoli-granulosa cells with characteristic psammoma-like calcifications. These neo-plastic changes occupied a very small area. On the basis of the histological features it may be assumed that gonadoblastoma arises in and from dysgenetic or rudimentary testes.

Syndrome of Rudimentary Testes

One finds an infantile uterus and bilateral rudimentary testicles situated in the place normally occupied by the ovaries. The con-tralateral noninvolved gonad, situated in the ovarian position near the uterus, may be determined as testis but if, on the other hand, the gonocytoma arises in and from malformed testicles, it certainly falls into the category of the syndrome of rudimentary testes (or male pseudohermaphroditism). Hughesdon[25] indicates that in seven of 33 gonocytoma III cases, testicular tissue was found to be present on both sides. Our recently observed case had testicular tissue on both sides. Microscopic examination re-vealed a testicular pattern at the periphery of a gonadoblastoma; immature seminif-erous tubules with signs of degeneration were found in the contralateral uninvolved gonad (Figs. 10–27 & 10–39). As can be seen from Table 10-IV, the incidence of gonadal tumors in this group of patients is extremely high. The risk for tumor in ab-normal dysgenetic gonads exists primarily in patients with female phenotype or a eunuchoidal habitus with a female genital tract who have primary amenorrhea and the presence of a negative sex chromatin pattern and a Y chromosome. These data demon-strate that through the cytogenetic approach one may predict the danger of neoplasia not only because of primary amenorrhea with high urinary gonadotrophin levels, but also because of the female phenotype with sexual infantilism.

Exploratory laparotomy with bilateral go-nadectomy should be performed in all XO/XY mosaicism individuals as well as in all phenotypic females with sexual infan-tilism and a 46,XY karyotype.[54,65,67]

Incidence of Gonadal Neoplasia among Amenorrhoeic Patients with Positive Sex Chromatin Pattern and 46, XX Karyotype Classified as "Ovarian Dysplasia"

Other groups of patients with primary amenorrhea and underdeveloped or poor secondary female sexual characteristics, with high-normal gonadotrophin excretion and normal female karyotype 46,XX, have re-vealed a hypoplastic uterus with small elon-gated ovaries at exploratory laparotomy. These patients are classified as "syndrome of ovarian dysplasia." Histologically, poorly developed stroma with deficient follicles and defective ova were found in biopsied ma-terial. In a few patients, retardation of sexual development and complete anosmia since early childhood were the main features. In all of these patients belonging to the group of "ovarian dysplasia," no tumors were found.

Incidence of Gonadal Neoplasia in Intersexual Patients having Testicular Dysgenesis with Uterus

Male Pseudohermaphroditism

A review of the literature shows a rela-tively small number of gonadal neoplasms among patients with male pseudohermaph-roditism. Lafferty[73] described testicular car-cinoma and Long[6] reported a case of dysgerminoma. Halley[74] published a case classified as seminoma.

It seems that the incidence of gonadal neoplasia in male pseudohermaphroditism is no greater than in cryptorchidism.

Our observations and findings from the literature suggest that a high risk for neoplasia occurs in phenotypic female patients with 46,XY karyotype (or XY/X mosaicism) having a uterus, Fallopian tubes, a complete vagina, and malformed gonads which are situated in the place normally occupied by the ovaries (Table 10-V).

In individuals with testicular dysgenesis without uterus, the incidence of malignancy in the gonads is relatively low. In our clinical practice the first gynecological procedure in patients with congenital somato-sexual malformations consists of determining whether the uterus is present. Very often a narrowed hypoplastic vagina hinders palpation and such a gynecological examination is of doubtful efficacy. Therefore, gynecological endocrine roentgenology should be employed in such cases.[37] In several of our cases vaginography disclosed the uterus and even Fallopian tubes which, together with negative sex-chromatin pattern and the presence of sex chromosome Y, were factors necessitating exploratory laparotomy.

Incidence of Malignant Neoplasia in Testicular Feminization Syndrome

The incidence of neoplasia among patients with testicular feminization has not been exhaustively explored. In 1953, Morris[75] collected data from the world literature on 92 cases of female pseudohermaphroditism in the form of a testicular feminization syndrome; in seven of these cases he demonstrated the existence of malignant tumors in underdeveloped male gonads. All recorded cases of neoplastic changes were from very old reports (1881, 1905, 1919, 1922, etc.) and, therefore, are not well documented.

It is generally believed that the risk for neoplasia is connected with abdominally located gonads. The high temperature in the abdomen is considered a factor in neoplastic malformation. However, it seems that this aspect is not as important as one might suspect. On the other hand, it is important to recognize and define the particular type of maldeveloped gonad in order to better evaluate the incidence and types of neoplasms associated with aberrant gonadal development.[22,23,43–45,64]

It is generally accepted that cryptorchidism carries with it an increased likelihood for the development of testicular neoplasia. More important is the relationship between gonadal neoplasms and the type of gonadal malformation. In the material from the Department of Clinical Endocrinology in Warsaw, among 24 cases classified as "testicular feminization," no malignant changes were found in the gonads (Table 10-V). The so-called "Pick's Tubular Adenomas" often observed within such testes cannot be considered as true neoplastic changes and are not an indication for early removal of these organs.[58,75–78] In recent well-documented re-

TABLE 10-V
INCIDENCE OF GONADAL NEOPLASIA IN INTERSEXUAL PATIENTS
WITH OR *WITHOUT* UTERUS

Diagnosis Classification	Mullerian Elements (uterus, Fallopian tubes) and Complete Vagina	No. of Cases	Malignant Germ-cell Tumor	Nongerminal Benign Tumor	Premalignant Formations
Gonadal Dysgenesis (including Turner's syndrome)	Well developed	66	14	Interstitioma Brenner's tumor 2 Pick's adenoma	3
Testicular Feminization	Total absence	24	0	6	0
Male pseudohermaphroditism	Total absence	9	0	0	0

TABLE 10-VI
RISK OF MALIGNANCY IN THE TESTES OF
PATIENTS WITH TESTICULAR FEMINIZATION
(ANDROGEN INTENSIVITY)

Authors	No. of Patients	Malignant Tumors	Material Source
Morris and	50 (age: over 50 years)	11 (22%)	Collected from literature
Hauser	128	10 (8%)	Review of literature
Dewhurst	82	0	Collected in Britain
Teter	24	0	Personal cases

ports about testicular feminization, a negligible number of malignant tumors were found. It seems that the incidence of malignant changes in this syndrome is no greater than in intra-abdominal testes or simple cryptorchidism. A recent report of Dewhurst[76] shows no malignant neoplasia among 82 patients in a British series of patients. An explanation for the relatively low incidence of malignancy in this syndrome may rest in the morphologic pattern of testes which are quite well-formed and show a regular tubular structure. Formations such as "intratubular bodies" or multiple pseudo-ovocytes are very rarely found in this syndrome. In our 24 cases, singular intratubular bodies were observed in only two instances.

The above observations suggest that malignant degeneration reflects a congenitally defective structure of the gonads and that the abdominal location is not the major factor in tumor development. The special predisposition to malignancy may occur only in malformed gonads with testicular remnants situated in an ovarian location in patients having well-developed Müllerian structures, i.e. uterus and Fallopian tubes, and with the presence of sex chromosome Y.

Familial Gonadal Dysgenesis with Gonocytoma

Many years ago familial male pseudohermaphroditism was thoroughly studied by Neugebauer,[4] a Warsaw gynecologist, who investigated a substantial number of such cases. He noted wide variations in this syndrome ranging from patients with predominantly masculine phenotype with hypospadia, bifid scrotum and a small vaginal opening, to cases with a vagina and uterus but with android body build, or with female habitus. The familial aspect of male pseudohermaphroditism has been studied mainly in cases of the testicular feminizations syndrome.[13,75-77,79-82]

The concurrence in a sibship of a male pseudohermaphrodite and an XY pure gonadal dysgenesis was recorded by Bar, *et al.*[83] While the concurrence of these rare abnormalities in the same sibship may be pure chance, evidence suggests that these abnormalities have some etiologic factor in common.[83] Scully,[41] in his review, mentioned that five patients of the 55 reported cases of gonadoblastoma had a family history suggestive or diagnostic of a gonadal disorder. Gonadoblastoma (gonocytoma III) was described by Cohen and Shaw[84] in two XY siblings with gonadal dysgenesis and female phenotype. Frasier, *et al.,*[34] reported gonadoblastoma associated with pure gonadal dysgenesis in monozygous twins.

Case Study: Two cases of primary amenorrhea, eunuchoidal body proportions, male karyotype 46,XY, and gonocytoma I (included in our series) occurring in two sisters at the age of 18 and 20 years were observed in the Department of Clinical Endocrinology in Warsaw, in 1970 to 1971.

One sibling, age 20, underwent surgery in a county hospital for an ovarian tumor. She had primary amenorrhea, eunuchoidal body proportions with absence of breast development and infantile external female genitalia. Microscopic examination of the tumoral gonad revealed a typical gonocytoma I (dysgerminoma). At laparotomy an infantile uterus and a fibrous rudimentary streak on the other side were observed. Cytogenetic examination revealed a negative sex chromatin pattern and a male 46,XY karyotype.

The second sibling, age 18, was admitted to our Department with the identical symptoms as the sibling above. A negative sex chromatin pattern and an infantile uterus, long and thin Fallopian tubes, a fibrous streak gonad on the left side, and, on the right side, a tumor measuring 9 × 8 × 4 cm. Bilateral adnexectomy was performed and microscopic examination revealed gonocytoma I histologically similar to the tumor found in the older sibling (Figs. 10–47 & 10–48).

A sister, age 14, menstruating for one year, had a normal female habitus. A brother, age 17, had a normal male habitus and no apparent abnormalities.

Another individual (not included in our series) received consultation in our Department and was investigated cytogenetically. Patient G.G., age 16, underwent surgery for primary amenorrhea, a negative sex chromatin pattern and signs of masculinization. This virilized phenotypic female had a uterus and, on the right side, a Fallopian tube and a tumoral knob-like gonad displacing the

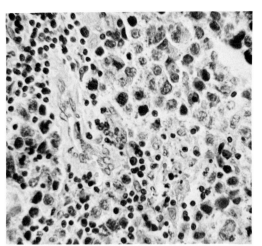

Figure 10–48. Familial gonadal dysgenesis with gonocytoma I. Specimen of the tumoral gonad from a patient aged 20 (older sister of patient in Figure 10–47). Histological pattern is similar to the picture presented in Figure 10–47—gonocytoma I.

right ovary. The left gonad was situated in the inguinal canal. Both gonads were removed. The inguinal gonad was identified as testis with immature, degenerative seminiferous tubules. Microscopic examination of the removed tumoral intra-abdominal gonad revealed a gonadoblastomatous pattern. The neoplasm arose in a testicular gonad because, at the edge of the gonadoblastoma, a few testicular tubules were identified in the peripheral region. The patient had two sisters age 13 and 20 years. The oldest was examined in the gynecological clinic in Gdańsk in 1968, because of primary amenorrhea and an absence of sexual development. She underwent surgery for an "ovarian tumor" which was classified as dysgerminoma. Cytogenetic examination in both patients revealed a negative sex chromatin pattern and a male 46,XY karyotype.

Detection and Early Preoperative Diagnosis

The present material and available data from the literature prove that uniformity of

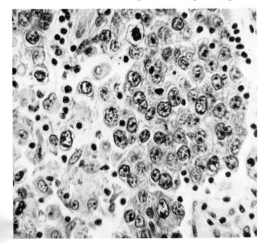

Figure 10–47. Familial gonadal dysgenesis with gonocytoma I. Specimen of the tumoral gonad from a patient aged 18 showing the typical pattern of gonocytoma I.

the clinico-pathological features of germ-cell tumors occurring in intersexes exists, thereby permitting early diagnosis. In general, these tumors occur in phenotypic females with:

1. Abnormal somatosexual development in patients reared as women with primary amenorrhea and some signs of masculinization.[2,14,16,25,30,32,36,41,45,50,64-68,85]

2. A negative sex chromatin pattern and the presence of a Y chromosome in the karyotype, contrasting with the feminine genitalia usually in the form of normal male 46,XY karyotype, or XO/XY mosaicism.

3. A high urinary gonadotrophin titer despite clinical signs of sex hormone activity.

4. Descoid foci of calcification on pelvix X-ray films.[2,16,21,33,44,86,87]

5. A knob-like tumor of unusual consistency replacing ovaries.

Proper diagnosis of germ-cell tumors (gonocytomas, gonadoblastomas) occurring in dysgenetic gonads is based on a clear histologic distinction between a frankly malignant germ-cell tumor and an early premalignant lesion.[88,89] It would seem that the classification and recognition of different types of germ-cell tumors that occur in dysgenetic gonads would facilitate more precise pathologic diagnosis. Teter's Gonocytoma I, II, III, and IV classifications are based on the most important characteristics of this type of tumor—an area of germ cells exhibiting typical malignant features.[3,21,31] Even if these cells form a confused admixture with Sertoli-granulosa cells, the pattern is still malignant.

In assessing the malignancy and prognosis of germ-cell tumors in dysgenetic gonads, the following point is extremely important:

Avoid overdiagnosing gonadoblastoma (gonocytoma) by applying the correct, precise diagnosis based on the original criteria for the diagnosis of malignant tumors, and the distinction between frankly malignant germ-cell tumors and early premalignant lesions (Fig. 10–49).

Management, Malignancy, and Prognosis

Postoperative prognosis in patients with gonocytomas occurring in gonads with dysgenesis is not simple. A relatively small number of cases has been reported in the literature; quite often the clinicopathological data are incomplete. The management of intersexes with gonadal tumors depends upon the pathological type and the developmental state. The prognosis is definitely better if the tumors are small, located only in one gonad, and if histologic examination reveals large foci of calcification. Various forms of psammoma-like calcifications or irregular calcified masses replacing the tumor indicate a limited degree of growth capacity and even a tendency toward spontaneous regression. Large areas of germ cells disposed in malignant fashion (pure dysgerminoma) will affect the prognosis adversely.

The malignancy of germ-cell tumors (gonocytomas, gonadoblastomas) has been questioned in spite of the fact that histological examination shows large areas of germ cells disposed in malignant fashion.[1,30,32]

Under continuous observation and control since 1953, we have had 14 patients with germ-cell tumors who had had primary amenorrhias and somatosexual disturbances. Seven patients have survived from six to 18 years without evidence of recurrence or metastases. The remaining seven patients have survived without recurrence for one to two years. Bilateral gonadectomy or unilateral removal of the tumor was the primary treatment in 12 patients with the tumor confined to one gonad. The remaining two

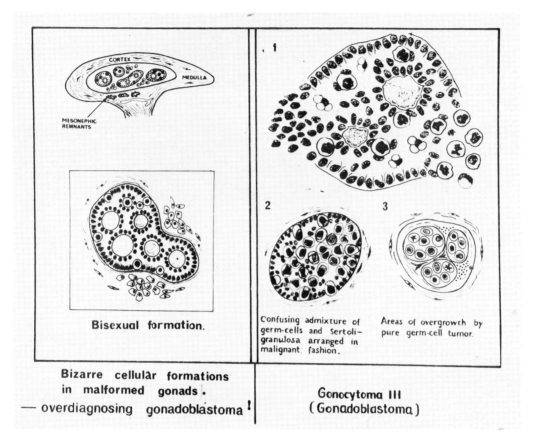

Figure 10–49. Schematic drawing of the nontumoral formations seen in dysgenetic gonad and frank malignant gonadoblastoma (gonocytoma III).

patients had bilateral gonadectomy with total hysterectomy. Postoperative irradiation was used in only one patient with bilateral gonadoblastoma. In all instances the tumor was localized to one or both gonads. None of our patients' tumors extended beyond the gonad.

The exceptional case (in a boy with X/XY karyotype) of recurrence and metastases of gonadoblastoma was due to the incomplete removal of the gonad at the time of the first operation and surgical dissemination during a second operation for incarcerated inguinal hernia containing a gonadal tumor. Micro-

scopic examination of biopsied metastatic nodules showed gonocytoma (malignant germ-cell tumor) pattern. The patient died during radiotherapy.

In a recent paper by Asadourian and Taylor,[90] the 10-year postoperative rate was very good for patients treated by unilateral oophorectomy alone (88%). In the past, reported mortality rates for patients with ovarian dysgerminoma have varied from 27 to 75 percent.[56,91,92] The results of Asadourian and Taylor[90] are considerably better than those reported in previous studies which show a poorer survival rate because at that time many tumors were discovered only at a late stage of development and when early diagnosis was less possible.

The largest tumor reported in our series was 10 cm in diameter. Whereas, in the paper of Pedowitz, *et al.,*[91] in which 17 cases of dysgerminoma of the ovary were reported, the *smallest* tumor was 11 cm in diameter. This fact points out that pre-operative diagnosis is now made earlier. In all our tumors which were macroscopically detectable, the median diameter was only 6 cm. At the time of exploratory laparotomy the gonadal tumors were small with capsule intact and no adhesions between the gonadal tissue and adjacent structures. These factors are decisive for producing a favorable prognosis.

The biological behavior of germ-cell tumors occurring in dysgenetic gonads seems to be less important for malignant transformation than their congenitally defective structure. According to our view, a conservative surgical approach (unilateral removal or bilateral adnexectomy) is recommended as the procedure of choice for gonocytoma (pure or mixed form) regardless of the patient's age and histological pattern.

REFERENCES

1. Scully, R.E.: Gonadoblastoma: a gonadal tumor related to the dysgerminoma (seminoma) and capable of sex-hormone production. *Cancer, 6:*455–463, 1953.

2. Melicow, M.M., and Uson, A.C.: Dysgenetic gonadomas and other gonadal neoplasm in intersexes. *Cancer, 12:*552–572, 1959.

3. Teter, J.: A new concept of classification of gonadal tumors arising from germ cells (gonocytoma) and their histogenesis. *Gynaecologia* (Basel), *150:*84–102, 1960.

4. Neugebauer, F.: 19 Fälle von Koincidenz von Gut-oder Bösartigen Neubildungen Vorcherrschend der Geschlectsorgane mit Scheinwitterthum. *Zbl Gynaek, 18:*466, 1900.

5. Meyer, R.: The pathology of some special ovarian tumors and their relation to sex characteristics. *Am J Obstet Gynecol, 22:*697–713, 1931.

6. Long, C.H., Ziskind, J., and Storck, A.H.: Dysgerminoma occurring in a pseudohermaphrodite. *Surg Gynecol Obstet, 73:*811–818, 1941.

7. Gilbert, J.B., and Hamilton, J.B.: Studies in malignant testis tumors: III. Incidence and nature of tumors in ectopic testes. *Surg Gynecol Obstet, 71:*731–743, 1940.

8. Gilbert, J.B.: Studies in malignant testis tumors: VIII tumors in pseudohermaphrodites: review of 60 cases and case report. *J Urol, 48:*665–672, 1942.

9. Spielman, F., and Motyloff, L.: Hermaphroditism and dysgerminoma (neuter cell tumor). *NY J Med, 55:*2168–2178, 1955.

10. Sohvall, A.R.: Testicular dysgenesis as an etiologic factor in cryptorchidism. *J Urol, 72:*693–702, 1954.

11. Sohval, A.R.: Testicular dysgenesis in relation to neoplasm of the testicle. *J Urol, 75:*285–291, 1956.

12. Sohval, A.R.: "Mixed" gonadal dysgenesis: A variety of hermaphroditism. *Am J Hum Genet, 15:*155–158, 1963.

13. Sohval, A.R.: Chromosomes and sex chromatin in normal and anomalous sexual development. *Physiol Rev, 43:*306–356, 1963.

14. Sohval, A.R.: Hermaphroditism with "atypical" or "mixed" gonadal dysgenesis: relationship to gonadal neoplasm. *Am J Med, 36:*281–292, 1964.

15. Stange, H.: Uber Fehlbildungen der Gonaden und ihre Beziehungen zur Geschwulstbildung. *Geburtshilfe Frauenheilkd, 1:*63–72, 1957.

16. Melicow, M.M.: Tumors of dysgenetic gonads in intersexes: case reports and dis-

cussion regarding their place in gonadal oncology. *Bull NY Acad Med, 42:*3–20, 1966.

17. Teter, J., and Tarlowski, R.: Tumors of the gonads in cases of gonadal dysgenesis and male pseudohermaphroditism. *Am J Obstet Gynecol, 79:*321–329, 1960.

18. Gardner, W.U.: Hormone production in endocrine tumors, *Ciba Foundation Colloq on Endocr, 12:*153–170, 1958.

19. Furth, J.: Hormone production in endocrine tumors. *Ciba Foundation Colloq on Endocr, 12:*170–171, 1958.

20. Gillman, J.: The development of the gonads in man with a consideration of the role of fetal endocrines and the histogenesis of ovarian tumors. *Contributions to Embryology, Carnegie Institution of Washington, 32:*81–85, 1948.

21. Teter, J.: The mixed germ cell tumours with hormonal activity. *Acta Pathol Microbiol Scand, 58:*306–320, 1963.

22. Teter, J., Philip, J., and Wecewicz, G.: "Mixed" gonadal dysgenesis with gonadoblastoma *in situ. Am J Obstet Gynecol, 90:*929–935, 1964.

23. Teter, J., Philip, J., Wecewicz, B., and Potocki, J.: A masculinizing mixed germ cell tumor (Gonocytoma III). *Acta Endocrinol, 46:* 1–11, 1964.

24. Philip, J., and Teter, J.: Significance of chromosomal investigation of somatic cells to determine the genetic origin of gonadoblastoma (Gonocytoma III). *Acta Pathol Microbiol Scand, 61:*543–550, 1964.

25. Hughesdon, P.E., and Kumarsamy, T.: Mixed germ cell tumours (gonadoblastomas) in normal and dysgenetic gonads. Case reports and review. *Virchows Arch (Pathol Anat), 349:*258–280, 1970.

26. Overzier, C.: Ein XX/XY-Hermaphrodit mit Einem "Intratubulären Ei" und Einem Gonadoblastom (Gonocytom 3). *Klin Wochenschr, 42:*1052–1060, 1964.

27. Robinson, A., Priest, R.E., and Bigler, P.C.: Male pseudohermaphrodite with XY/XO mosaicism and bilateral gonadoblastomas. *Lancet, 1:*111–112, 1964.

28. Siebenmann, R.E.: Male pseudohermaphroroditism with gonadoblastoma: unusual

intersex form. *Pathol Microbiol,* (Basel) *24:*233–238, 1961.

29. Naidu, P.N., Ramaswamy, S., and Rao, K.S.: Gonadoblastoma arising from testicular dysplasia in an intersexual individual. *J Obstet Gynaecol Br Commonw, 72:*437–443, 1965.

30. Guinet, P., and Eyraud, M.T.: Les Dysgenesies Gonadiques Avec Gonocytome. *Revue Lyon Med, 17:*975–994, 1968.

31. Teter, J.: A mixed form of feminizing germ cell tumor (gonocytoma II), *Am J Obstet Gynecol, 84:*722–730, 1962.

32. Blanc, B.: Les Gonadoblastomes. Revue generale. *Rev Fr Endocrinol Clin, 11:*529–537, 1970.

33. Copperman, L.R., Hamlin, J., and Elmer, N.: Gonadoblastoma: a rare ovarian tumor related to the dysgerminoma with characteristic roentgen appearance. *Radiology, 90:*322–324, 1968.

34. Fine, G., Mellinger, R.C., and Canton, J.N.: Gonadoblastoma occurring in a patient with familial gonadal dysgenesis. *Am J Clin Pathol, 38:*615–629, 1962.

35. Freeman, M.V.R., and Miller, O.J.: XY gonadal dysgenesis and gonadoblastoma, *Obstet Gynecol, 34:*478–483, 1969.

36. Hervé, R., Laveille, H., Ancla, M., de Brux, J., and de Grouchy, J.: Observation de Gonadoblastome. *Gynecol Obstet* (Paris), *66:*429–440, 1967.

37. Josso, N., Nezelof, C., Picon, R., de Grouchy, J., Dray, F., and Rappaport, R.: Gonadoblastoma in gonadal dysgenesis. a report of two cases with 46,XY/45,X mosaicism. *J Pediatr, 74:*425–437, 1969.

38. McDonough, P.G., Greenblatt, R.B., Byrd, J.R., and Hastings, E.V.: Gonadoblastoma (Gonocytoma III). Report of a case. *Obstet Gynecol, 29:*54–58, 1967.

39. Netter, A., Musset, R., Pelissier, C., Millet, D., Yaneva, H., and Sebacum, M.: Un Nouveau Cas de Gonadoblastome. *Gynecol Obstet* (Paris), *66:*385–394, 1967.

40. Przybora, L.: Gonadoblastoma. *Endokrynol Pol, 11:*63–68, 1960.

41. Scully, R.E.: Gonadoblastoma: a review of 74 cases. *Cancer, 25:*1340–1356, 1970.

42. Strumpf, I.J.: Gonadoblastoma in a patient

with gonadal dysgenesis. *Am J Obstet Gynecol, 92:*992–995, 1965.

43. Teter, J.: An unusual gonadal tumor (Gonadoblastoma) in a male pseudohermaphrodite with testicular dysgenesis. *J Obstet Gynecol Br Commonw, 67:*238–242, 1960.

44. Teter, J., Wecewicz, G., Marzinek, K., Przezdziecki, Z., and Groniowski, J.: [An Hormonally Active Mixed Germ Cell Tumor (Gonadoblastoma)]. *Rev Fr Endocrinol Clin, 3:*421–433, 1962. (Fr.)

45. Teter, J.: Les Dysgenesies Gonadiques Mixtes. Actualities Endocrinologiques, Journees Endocrinologiques de la Pitie, Paris, 1966, Expansion Scientifique Francaise, Paris, 1966, p. 13–22.

46. Ber, A.: A case of dysgerminoma ovarii tested hormonally. *Acta Obstet Gynecol Scand, 133:*411–426, 1949.

47. Plate, W.P.: Dysgerminoma of the ovary in a patient with wirilism. *Acta Endocrinol, 14:*227–234, 1953.

48. Blocksma, R.: Bilateral dysgerminoma of the ovary with pseudohermaphroditism. *Am J Obstet Gynecol, 69:*874–878, 1955.

49. Santesson, L., and Marrubini, G.: Clinical and pathological survey of ovarian embryonal carcinomas, including so-called "mesonephromas" "Schiller), or "mesoblastomas" (Teilum), treated at the Radiumhemmet. *Acta Obstet Gynecol Scand, 36:*399–419, 1957.

50. Miller, O.J.: The sex chromosome anomalies. *Am J Obstet Gynecol, 90:*1078–1139, 1964.

51. Bieger, R.C., Passarge, E., and McAcams, A.J.: Testicular intratubular bodies. *J Clin Endocrinol, 25:*1340–1346, 1965.

52. Bradbury, J.T., and Bunge, R.G.: Gonadal dysgenesis: case report of a 6-year-old boy with a Fallopian Tube and an undifferentiated gonad. *J Clin Endocrinol, 18:*1006–1014, 1958.

53. Teter, J., and Boczkowski, K.: Testicular feminization with and without clitoral enlargement. *Am J Obstet Gynecol, 94:* 813–819, 1966.

54. Teter, J., and Boczkowski, K.: Les "Corps Intratubulaires" (Pseudo-Ovocytes) du Testicule Dysgenesique. *Rev Fr Endocrinol Clin, 8:*11–18, 1967.

55. Witschi, E., and Mengert, W.F.: Endocrine studies on human hermaphrodites and their bearing on interpretation of homosexuality. *J Clin Endocrinol, 2:*279–286, 1942.

56. Serment, H., and Piana, L.: *Tumeurs Endocrines Sexuelles de l'Ovarie.* Paris, Expansion Scientifique Francaise, 1964.

57. Warren, J.C., Erkman, B., Cheatum, S., and Holman, G.: Hilus-cell adenoma in a dysgenetic gonad with XX/XO mosaicism. *Lancet, 1:*141–143, 1964.

58. Hauser, G.A., Gloor, F., Stalder, G., Bodis, J., Keller, M., Goerre, J., and Gouw, W.L.: XX-chromosomal gonadal dysgenesis with granulosa-thecal cell tumor and feminization. *Schweiz Med Wochenschr, 90:*1486–1491, 1960.

59. Goldgerg, M.B., and Scully, A.L.: Gonadal malignancy in gonadal dysgenesis: papillary pseudomucinous cystadenocarcinoma in a patient with Turner's Syndrome. *J Clin Endocrinol, 27:*341–347, 1967.

60. Ober, W.B.: Embryonal carcinoma of testicular type arising in the gonad of a true hermaphrodite. *Jewish Memorial Hospital Bulletin, 7:*94–102, 1962.

61. Peyron, A., Patel, Poumeau-Delille, G., and Gozland: A Propos de Deux Cas d'Embryome du Testicule. *Bull Assoc Franc Cancer, 28:*646–657, 1939.

62. Pinkerton, J.H.: Gonadal dysgenesis complicated by virilizing embryonal carcinoma. *J Reprod Fertil, 9:*203–205, 1965.

63. Woodruff, H.D.: Neoplasms of dysgenetic gonads. *Am J Obstet Gynecol, 96:*822–823, 1966.

64. Taylor, H., Barter, R., and Jacobson, C.: Neoplasms of dysgenetic gonads. *Am J Gynecol, 96:*816–823, 1966.

65. Teter, J.: Rare gonadal tumors occurring in intersexes and their classification. *Int J Gynecol Obstet, 7:*183–198, 1969.

66. Teter, J., and Boczkowski, K.: Occurrence of tumors in dysgenetic gonads. *Cancer, 20:*1301–1310, 1967.

67. Van Campenhout, J., Lord, J., Vauclair, R., Lanthier, A., and Bcrard, M.: The phenotype and gonadal histology in XO/XY mosaic individuals: report of two personal

cases. *J Obstet Gynaecol Br Commonw,* 76:631–639, 1969.

68. Desjeux, J.F., Gagnon, J., Leboef, G., St-Rome, G., and Ducharme, J.R.: Huit Observations de Mosaique XO/XY Dont Une XO/XYq—Avec Gonadoblastome. *L'Union Med. du Canada, 98:*1667–1685, 1969.

69. Boczkowski, K., and Teter, J.: Clinical, histologic and cytogenetic observations in intersexuality. Report of 13 cases. *Obstet Gynecol, 27:*7–14, 1966.

70. Dominguez, C.J., and Greenblatt, R.B.: Dysgerminoma of the ovary in a patient with Turner's Syndrome. *Am J Obstet Gynecol, 83:*674–677, 1962.

71. Rochet, Y., Feroldi, J., Laurent, C., and Pollosson, E.: Une Observation Exceptionelle de Gonocytome Sur Syndrome de Turner. Caryotype XO. *Comptes Rendus de la Société Francaise de Gynécologie, 39:* 115–127, 1969.

72. Salet, J., de Gennes, L., de Grouchy, J., Musset, R., Pelissier, C., Yaneva, H., Sebacum, M., and Netter, A.: A Propos d'un Cas de Gonadoblastome 46,XX. *Ann Endocrinol* (Paris), *31:*927–938, 1970.

73. Lafferty, J.C., and Pandergrass, E.P.: Carcinoma of the testicle with metastasis of bone: report of two cases, one in a pseudohermaphrodite, *Am J Roentgen, 63:*95–101, 1950.

74. Halley, J.B.W.: Seminoma in a young male pseudohermaphrodite. *J Urol, 80:*856–859, 1963.

75. Morris, J.M.: The syndrome of testicular feminization in male pseudohermaphrodites. *Am J Obstet Gynecol, 65:*1192–1211, 1953.

76. Dewhurst, C.J.: The XY female. *Am J Obstet Gynecol, 109:*675–688, 1971.

77. Morris, J.M., and Mahesh, V.B.: Further observations on the syndrome "testicular feminization." *Am J Obstet Gynecol, 87:* 731–745, 1963.

78. Wachstein, M., and Scorza, A.: Male pseudohermaphroditism: a type showing female habitus, absence of uterus, and male gonads often associated with testicular tubular adenoma: report of case and

review of literature. *Am J Clin Pathol, 21:*10–23, 1951.

79. Boczkowski, K.: Genetical studies in testicular feminization syndrome. *J Med Genet, 5:*181–188, 1968.

80. Goldberg, M.B., and Maxwell, A.F.: Male pseudohermaphroditism proved by surgical exploration and microscopic examination: a case report with speculations concerning pathogenesis. *J Clin Endocrinol, 8:*367–379, 1948.

81. Hauser, B.A.: Testicular feminization. In Overzier, C. (Ed.): *Intersexuality,* London, Acad Pr, pp. 255–276, 1963.

82. Jones, H.W., and Scott, W.W.: *Hermaphroditism, Genital Anomalies and Related Endocrine Disorders.* Baltimore, Williams Wilkins, 1958.

83. Barr, M.L., Carr, D.H., Plunkett, E.R., Soltan, H.C., and Wiens, R.G.: Male pseudohermaphroditism and pure gonadal dysgenesis in sisters. *Am J Obstet Gynecol, 99:*1047–1055, 1967.

84. Cohen, M.M., and Shaw, M.W.: Two XY siblings with gonadal dysgenesis and a female phenotype. *New Engl J Med, 272:* 1083–1088, 1965.

85. Boczkowski, K., Teter, J., Tomaszewska, J., and Philip, J.: Gonadoblastoma (Gonocytoma III) in a boy with XO-XY mosaicism: case report with survey of lierature. *Acta Pathol Microbiol Scand, 71:* 46–51, 1967.

86. Borghi, A., Montali, E., Bigozzi, U., and Giusti, G.: XO/XY mosaicism in a phenotypic female with gonadoblastoma: attempt of classification of the clinical picture of the XO/XY mosaicism. *Helv Paediatr Acta, 20:*185–192, 1965.

87. Levin, B.: Roentgenologic aspects of gynecologic endocrinology. In Gold, Jay J. (Ed.): *Textbook of Gynecologic Endocrinology.* New York, Hoeber, pp. 265–324, 1968.

88. Teter, J.: Prognosis, malignancy, and curability of the germ-cell tumor occurring in dysgenetic gonads. *Am J Obstet Gynecol, 108:*894–900, 1970.

89. Teter, J.: Discrepancies concerning malignancy and prognosis of gonocytomas (go-

nadoblastomas) in dysgenetic gonads. *Obstet Gynecol, 36:*627–629, 1970.

90. Asadourian, L.A., and Taylor, H.B.: Dysgerminoma. an analysis of 105 cases. *Obstet Gynecol, 33:*370–379, 1969.

91. Pedowitz, P., Felmus, L.B., and Grayzel, D.M.: Dysgerminoma of the ovary. Prognosis and treatment. *Am J Obstet Gynecol, 70:*1284–1297, 1955.

92. Taylor, C.H., Jr., and Munnell, E.W.: Treatment of tumors of the ovary. In Pack, G.T. and Ariel, I.M. (Eds.): *Treatment of Cancer and Allied Diseases. Vol. 6 Tumors of The Female Genitalia.* New York, Harper and Row, p. 254, 1962.

93. Carpentier, P.J., Stolte, L.A.M., and Visschers, G.P.: Gonadal dysgenesis and testicular tumours. *Lancet, 1:*386–387, 1956.

94. Brogger, A., and Strand, D.: Contribution to the study of the so-called pure gonadal dysgenesis. *Acta Endocrinol,* (Kobenhavn) *48:*490–505, 1965.

95. Baron, J., Rucki, T., and Simm, S.: Familial gonadal malformations. *Gynaecologia,* (Basel), *153:*298–308, 1962.

96. Unpublished cases observed in Department of Clinical Endocrinology, Medical Academy in Warsaw, Poland.

97. Michalkiewicz, W., Simm, S., Przybora, L., Baron, J., and Warenik, S.: Gonadal dysgenesis in patients with normal body proportions in the light of clinical cytogenetic and histological investigations. *Endokrynol Pol, 17:*81–92, 1966.

98. Ferrier, P.E., Ferrier, S.A., Scharer, K.O., Genton, N., Hedinger, C., and Klein, D.: Disturbed gonadal differentiation in a child with XO/XY/XYY mosaicism: relationships with gonadoblastoma. *Helv Paediatr Acta, 22:*479–490, 1967.

99. Lewis, F.J.W., Mitchel, J.P., and Foss, G.L.: XY/XO mosaicism. *Lancet, 1:*221–222, 1963.

100. Miller, O.J., Breg, R., and Jailer, J.N.: *Human Chromosome Newsletter, 1:*6–7, 1960.

101. Goodlin, R.C.: Karyotypic analysis as an aid in sex determination. *Western J Surg, 70:*27–30, 1962.

102. Gagnon, J., and Cadotte, M.: Gonadoblastome et Aberrations Chromosomiques, *Congres International des Medecins de Langue Francaise.* Montreal, Canada, September 25–30, 1967, pp. 53–54.

103. Sadasivan, G., and Ebenezer, L.N.: Gonadoblastoma (Gonocytoma 3) with XO-XX-XY mosaicisim. *Indian J Med Res, 56:*310–313, 1968.

104. Schuster, J., and Motulsky, A.G.: Exceptional sex-chromatin pattern in male pseudohermaphroditism with XX/XY/XO mosaicism. *Lancet, 1:*1074–1075, 1962.

CHAPTER 11

CANCER IN ISRAEL: SOME ETHNIC CONSIDERATIONS

BARUCH MODAN

THE PRESENCE OF A heterogeneous population in Israel on the one hand, and the relatively small area of the country, with less than 30 general hospitals serving the total community on the other, provide a unique opportunity for studying inter-ethnic differences in the incidence of malignant disorders. This data may facilitate the assessment of the respective roles of genetic and environmental factors in carcinogenesis.

Population

The major ethnic groups in Israel are as follows:

European-born Jews

Primarily, Jews of European origin, the main subgroups of which originate from Poland, Russia and Rumania. To a much lesser extent, this group comprises persons coming from the U.S., Canada, Central and South America, South Africa, Rhodesia and Australia.

African-born Jews

Primarily, immigrants from Morocco, Algiers, Tunisia, Libya and to a much lesser extent, from Egypt.

Supported in part by Research Agreement No. 06-125-15 from the U.S. Public Health Service, and by a grant from the Israel Cancer Association.

Asian-born Jews

Immigrants coming from the Middle East, i.e. Syria, Iraq, Iran and Turkey, as well as Yemen.

Israeli-born Jews

Arabs

Born either in Israel, or in the surrounding countries.

The population distributions of these five groups differ significantly, with the majority of the European population being in the older age group, and the majority of the African and Asian in the younger age groups. In the Israeli born group, almost 80 percent of the population are younger than 20 years of age. Consequently, comparison of crude total rates for each of the populations would be inappropriate. Similarly, due to the small number of the Israelis in the older age group, and a lower rate of hospital referrals and under-reporting among Arabs, at least among adults, valid comparisons, at present, can only be made between the 3 foreign-born Jewish groups.

Incidence

Studies conducted by our group[1-13] and by other investigators[14] indicate that in most tumor categories, incidence is higher among the European born group, both males and females. This is particularly evident in cancer of the colon and rectum, breast, corpus uteri, ovary, brain tumors and malignant melanoma.

In contrast, cancer of the cervix, and of the nasopharynx present a higher incidence among the non-European population, while in thyroid neoplasms no inter-ethnic differences in incidence may be seen.

In addition, in some sites, the non-European population segment demonstrates a decrease rather than an increase in cancer rates in older age. The latter finding could be attributed either to an ignorance of the actual year of birth, leading to errors in the population denominator in the respective age categories, or to a lower frequency of histological confirmation.

Further analysis reveals a number of specific points of interest in some of the cancer sites:

Female Genital Organs

Cancer of the corpus uteri and of the ovary which are considerably more frequent in the European-born, present a parallel pattern with the one observed for breast cancer, and are in contrast with cervical cancer, which occurs most frequently among the North African-born. Consequently, while among the European-born the incidence of cancer of the corpus in older age is about three times higher than that of cancer of the cervix, the incidence of cervical cancer is twice as high as carcinoma of the corpus among the African-born. The Asian-born present an intermediate pattern with an equal incidence of both sites.

Comparison of incidence rates for cancer of the cervix by continent may be misleading. A more refined breakdown, by country of origin, *within* the North African group reveals a strikingly higher incidence among women originating from Morocco. Furthermore, when this sub-group is removed from

the total North African category, the incidence in the rest of North African countries becomes similar to that among women originating from the Middle East.

Gastrointestinal Neoplasms

The relative incidence of cancer of the alimentary tract varies among European versus Asian and versus African-born immigrants. The ratio is highest for cancer of the colon and rectum, (about 3:1), intermediate for gastric cancer, and close to unity for the esophagus, indicating different etiology for each site.

Of interest is also the fact that in the elderly, incidence of colorectal cancer is relatively higher in males among the European-born, while among the non-Europeans it is higher in females.

Lymphoma

The comparative incidence of malignant lymphoma reveals a varying pattern with age, being relatively higher in the non-Europeans below the age of 40, while in older age the incidence is higher in the European-born. This could be related to a differential occurrence of two distinct patterns of disease—nodal and extranodal.[15] Thus, extranodal lymphoma, where the original manifestation is organ-oriented, is more prevalent in younger age and in the non-European segment, while the nodal form, in which original symptomatology occurs in a lymph node, is more prevalent in older age and in the European-born group.

A most interesting sub-entity in this category is small intestinal lymphoma, which was originally observed, but never actually described, by Brandsteter. In contrast with Caucasian populations among whom the median age for the appearance of small intestinal lymphoma is 40 years and above, the Mediterranean entity affects primarily children and young adults. It is quite frequently associated with malabsorption which occasionally serves as the first symptom, and may precede the full blown lymphomatous course, by as much as 4 years.[16] In Israel, this syndrome has been noted almost exclusively in patients of African and Asian origin, as well as among Arabs. Similarly, a considerable proportion of the cases described in other countries, such as France, North Africa, and Mexico were diagnosed among Jews of Sephardic origin.[17,18] Seligman and Rambaud[18] have recently reported the presence of a light chain molecule in this disease category.

The possibility that this condition should be considered as analogous to that of Burkitt's lymphoma with different site predilection and mode of transmission has been raised,[15] but never proven.

Leukemia

The incidence of leukemia also varies according to age. While there are no differences among the ethnic groups between 20 and 49 years of age, the rate is higher in the African-born in the 10 to 19 age group, and in the European group in older age.

The higher incidence in the African-born teenagers has been apparent for the past 10 years.[19] The hypothesis that this may be related to the mass treatment of this cohort by scalp irradiation for tinea capitis in the early 1950's is currently under our investigation. On the other hand, the higher incidence in the elderly Europeans represents primarily a chronic lymphatic leukemia.

Gallbladder and Biliary Tract

Gallbladder cancer is relatively more frequent among European-born women, but not among the men, than among those born in Asia and Africa; the overall male/female ratio is extremely low—1:4.5. In contrast,

for biliary tract cancer there are no ethnic differences in the incidence with respect to sex; the sex ratio is 1:1.6 and the frequency of gallstones approximates the reported figures for the general population.

These findings suggest that the etiology of the two sites differs, and confirm that cholelithiasis should be considered as a precancerous condition in gallbladder neoplasms.

The notion of a causal relationship between gallbladder cancer and cholelithiasis is based on the following observations:[20] 1) presence of gallstones in the vast majority of patients with cancer of the gallbladder; 2) a similar male/female ratio in cancer of the gallbladder patients and in those with cholelithiasis; 3) similarly higher frequency (70–80%) of gallstones in both males and females with cancer of the gallbladder, despite the higher frequency of gallstones in females in the general population; 4) a higher incidence of cancer of the gallbladder among the European-born females in Israel than in Asian-and African-born, and lack of this pattern among males; again, in parallel with a similarly higher frequency of gallstones among European-born females and no difference among males; 5) the similarly high frequency among women of gallstones in cancer of the gallbladder of all ethnic groups, despite the marked difference in the incidence of both gallstones and cancer of the gallbladder, when estimated separately in each ethnic group; and 6) the long period of previous abdominal complaints in the vast majority of patients with cancer of the gallbladder.

Malignant Melanoma

The excessive incidence rate of this tumor site among European-born is the highest we have observed. The low risk among the non-European groups indicates the presence of a protective mechanism offered by a darkly pigmented skin and is compatible with the hypothesis that sunlight exposure plays a major role in the etiology of this disease.[21] This hypothesis is supported by the following facts: a) the higher incidence among females as compared to males is limited to tumors occurring on the upper and lower extremities, b) a higher incidence among the more veteran European-born; and c) an excess among the Israeli-born of European parentage, irrespective of sex or age group.

Childhood Malignancies

Differences in incidence rates among children may provide an opportunity to assess the effect of different parental origin, within a similar physical environment. It is of interest, therefore, that in marked contrast with the differences noted among the foreign born adults, a comparison of the combined incidence of childhood malignancies reveals only minimal interethnic differences. This might be attributed either to a different etiology of childhood malignancies or to a similarity in environmental conditions. However, further information on this subject is needed in order to evaluate this problem more comprehensively.

Elucidation of Hereditary Versus Environmental Factors

The patterns discussed above do not enable one to conclude a prior that the differences observed are either genetically or environmentally determined. The marked heterogeneity of the Jewish sub-groups has been contributed to by both cultural influences and cross-breeding with the surrounding communities in the East and Europe alike. Furthermore, due to the interrelationship between common biological ancestry

and familial cultural environment, even family studies cannot always distinguish these two factors.

On the other hand, the sudden recent mixture in modern Israel could enable one to measure changes in disease pattern in relation to changes in physical and cultural environment. This evaluation will be more complicated in the future if the rate of inter-ethnic marriage is high. At the present stage, however, the frequency of inter-ethnic marriage, although rising, could not yet affect the disease risk among the second generation Israelis and one, therefore, can and should, measure those disease entities where the latent period is short.

So far, a change in disease pattern according to the length of residence in Israel has been determined for gastric cancer, malignant melanoma and childhood leukemia. In each of these three sites a definite change in pattern emerges. Thus, the gastric cancer incidence among *recent* immigrants is higher than in more veteran ones, independent of age, sex and origin. In contrast, as mentioned above, incidence of melanoma is higher in the more *veteran* European-born, as compared to those who immigrated more recently.

Rates for childhood leukemia are highest in each of the foreign-born groups as compared to their counterpart, Israelis, with a striking gradient starting with the foreign-born children, decreasing through the Israeli-born of foreign parentage, to the native Israelis of native parentage.[22]

Limited as they are, these observations suffice to demonstrate that environmental changes lead to changes in cancer risk, in a manner similar to that observed in several other chronic diseases.[23]

The inter-ethnic comparisons in Israel reveal also a striking similarity to the findings of Dorn and Cutler's ten city study[24] in the U.S. This conclusion is based on the following

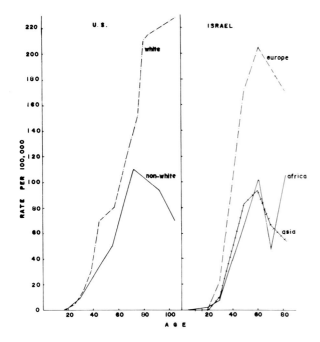

Figure 11–1. Comparison of mean annual incidence of Cancer of the Breast in Israel and in the U.S. by main ethnic groups.

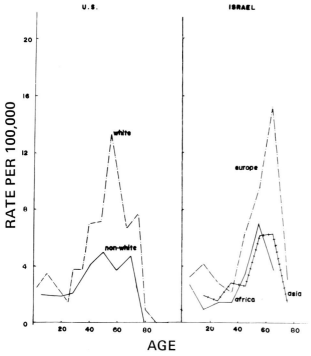

Figure 11–2. Comparison of mean annual incidence of Malignant Brain Tumors in Israel and in the U.S. by main ethnic groups.

observations: a) A relatively excessive rate in most tumor sites in the European-born Israeli and the U.S. Whites; b) A similar population pattern for cancers of the uterine corpus, ovary, and breast, in contrast with that of the uterine cervix; c) A change in the relative ethnic standing of the main cancerous lesions of the gastrointestinal tract; d) Equal rates for cancer of the thyroid; e) A decrease in cancer incidence in the oldest age category in the non-European segment in Israel and the blacks in the U.S., possibly due to incomplete data and error in diagnosis, as well as unreliable population statistics for these segments of the population; f) A lower sex ratio for cancer of the colon and the rectum among non-European-born Europeans and U.S. Blacks; g) Minimal inter-ethnic differences in childhood, for all tumor categories combined; h) Change in the relative incidence among migrants with length of residence in their new home country.

These similarities are illustrated in Figures 11–1 and 11–2 by a comparison of inter-ethnic differences for selected cancer sites in Israel and the U.S.

Now, if a common genetic background could be assumed for the parallel sub-groups in these two populations, our findings would have supported a genetic predisposition. However, the U.S. black population originated from Central Africa, while the non-European population in Israel immigrated from North Africa and the Middle East. Similarly, the Israeli European population originated primarily from Poland, Russia and Rumania, and, therefore, differs in many respects from the bulk of the American white population.

An alternative hypothesis would be a similarity in certain biochemical parameters such as, for instance, Glucose-Six-phosphate Dehydrogenase Deficiency.[25,26] Although this explanation cannot be ruled out completely at present, it does not seem likely in view of the almost identical pattern among the North

African and Asian-born immigrants in Israel, despite the marked difference in the frequency of the enzyme deficiency. Consequently, another common denominator for both communities should be looked for. One which seems to be most applicable is socio-economic gradient. This would also support Higginson's[27] concept that almost 90 percent of cancer could be attributed to environmental factors.

If differences in cancer incidence related to the socio-economic status are so prominent, then we are faced with three different types of malignant neoplasms: 1) sites associated with high socio-economic status, particularly, breast, corpus uteri, colon and rectum; 2) those more prevalent in the lower socio-economic groups, e.g. uterine cervix; and 3) sites that might be attributed to either endogenous factors, or alternately, to environmental ones that operate to a similar extent in all socio-economic levels.

The fact that more recent data from the U.S., based on the 1969 cancer survey conducted by Cutler, *et al.*,[28] demonstrate an increase of cancer incidence among the blacks, does not refute this hypothesis. On the contrary, it may suggest that with an up-grading of the socio-economic standards, differences in cancer incidence tend to disappear.

Needless to say, neither the relationships we observed, nor their interpretation are simple. The two non-European Israeli groups which represent by and large the same socio-economic level, differ in their rates for cancer of certain sites. For instance, esophageal cancer occurs less frequently in the North African group than in either the Asian or European-born,[29] and is particularly frequent among migrants originating from Yemen and Iran. Furthermore, preliminary results reveal that while there is essentially no difference in the incidence of laryngeal cancer[30] by continent of origin, when rates are computed on the basis of *country* of origin, a high risk area along the Mediterranean basin emerges, i.e. rates are significantly higher in immigrants originating from Bulgaria, Greece and Turkey.

These exceptions indicate that for some cancer sites the general and over-simplified social gradient hypothesis is not sufficient. It is possible, therefore, that in some sites a genetically determined characteristic, such as Glucose-Six-Phosphate Dehydrogenase deficiency or a similar biochemical or anthropometric component, yet to be described, may play a role in risk differences. A good, but by no means comprehensive

example is malignant melanoma, where the racial gradient both in Israel and in the U.S. can be easily attributed to a gradient in skin complexion and in the quantity of skin pigment, between the respective groups.

Finally, from the viewpoint of prevention, the expected general rise in living standards will probably abolish some of the differences in cancer incidence between distinct population groups. However, major efforts should be directed to impede the possible increase in incidence of those forms of cancer which are prevalent in communities with high socio-economic standards.

REFERENCES

1. Tulchinsky, D., and Modan, B.: Epidemiological aspects of cancer of the stomach in Israel. *Cancer, 20:*1311, 1967.

2. Shani, M., Modan, B., Steinitz, R., and Modan, M.: The incidence of breast cancer in Jewish females in Israel. *Harefuah, 71:* 337, 1966.

3. Mass, N., and Modan, B.: Cancer of the colon and rectum in Israel. *J Natl Cancer Inst, 42:*529, 1969.

4. Cohen, A., and Modan, B.: Some epidemiological aspects of brain tumors in Israel. *Cancer, 22:*1323, 1968.

5. Modan, B., Eisenstein, Z., and Virag, I.: Thyroid cancer in Israel. *Br J Cancer, 23:*488, 1969.

6. Modan, B., Virag, I., and Modan, M.: Survival in childhood malignancies. *J Natl Cancer Inst, 43:*349, 1969.

7. Virag, I., and Modan, B.: Some epidemiological aspects of childhood malignancies. *Cancer, 23:*137, 1969.

8. Modan, B., Sharon, Z., Shani, M., and Sheba, C.: Some epidemiological aspects of ccrvical and endometrial carcinoma. *Pathol Microbiol, 35:*192, 1970.

9. Modan, B., and Kallner, H.: Gastro-intestinal cancer in Israel. *Isr J Med Sci, 7:*1475, 1971.

10. Modan, B.: Role of ethnic in cancer development. *Isr J Med Sci. 10:*1112, 1974.

11. Modan, B., Hart, J., and Shani, M.: Epidemiological aspects of gallbladder and biliary tract neoplasms. *Am J Publ Health, 62:*36, 1972.

12. Movshovitz, M., and Modan, B.: Role of sun exposure in the etiology of malignant melanoma: Epidemiologic inference. *J Nat Cancer Inst, 51:*777, 1973.

13. Matalon, M., Modan, M., Paz, B., and Modan, B.: Malignant trophoblastic disorders. Some epidemiological aspects and relationship to hydatidiform mole. *Am J Obstet Gynecol, 112:*101, 1972.

14. Schenker, J.G., Polishuk, W.Z., and Steinitz, R.: An epidemiologic study of carcinoma of the ovary in Israel. *Isr J Med Sci, 4:*820, 1968.

15. Modan, B., Shani, M., Goldman, B., and Modan, M.: Nodal and extranodal malignant lymphoma in Israel. *Br J Haematol, 16:*53, 1969.

16. Shani, M., Modan, B., Goldman, B., Brandsteter, S., and Ramot, B.: Primary gastrointestinal lymphoma. *Isr J Med Sci, 5:*1173, 1969.

17. Jinich, H., Rojas, E., Webb, J.A., and Kelsey, J.R.: Lymphoma presenting as malabsorption. *Gastroenterology, 54:*421, 1968.

18. Seligmann, M., and Rambaud, J.D.: IgA abnormalities in abdominal lymphoma (â-chain disease) *Isr J Med Sci, 5:*151, 1969.

19. Davies, A.M., Modan, B., Djaldetti, M., and de Vries, A.: Epidemiological observations on leukemia in Israel. *Arch Intern Med, 108:*86, 1961.

20. Hart, J., Modan, B., and Shani, M.: Cholelithiasis in the etiology of gallbladder neoplasms. *Lancet, 1:*1151, 1971.

21. Lee, J.A.H., and Merril, J.M.: Sunlight and the aetiology of malignant melanoma: a synthesis. *Med J Aust, 2:*846, 1970.

22. Royston, I., and Modan, B.: Comparative mortality of childhood leukemia and lymphoma among the immigrants and native born in Israel. *Cancer, 22:*385, 1968.

23. Medalie, J.H., Levene, C., Papier, C., Goldbourt, U., Dreyfuss, F., Oron, D., Neufeld, H.N., and Riss, E.: *New Engl J Med, 285:* 1348, 1971.

24. Dorn, H.F., and Cutler, S.J.: *Morbidity from cancer in the United States.* Public Health Monograph No. 56, U.S. Dept. HEW, Washington, D.C. 1959.

25. Sheba, C., Szeinberg, A., Ramot, B., and Adam, A.: Epidemiologic surveys of deleterious genes in different population groups in Israel. *Am J Public Health, 52:*1101, 1962.

26. Deaconsfield, P., Rainsbury, R., and Kalton, G.: Glucose-6-phosphate dehydrogenase deficiency and the incidence of cancer. *Oncologia, 19:*11, 1965.

27. Higginson, J.: Distribution of different patterns of cancer. *Isr J Med Sci, 4:*457, 1968.

28. Cutler, S.: Personal communication.

29. Shani, M., and Modan, B.: Esophageal cancer in Israel, a clinico-epidemiological study, (in preparation).

30. Shiloh, S., and Modan, B.: Epidemiological aspects of cancer of the larynx in Israel, (in preparation.)

CHAPTER 12

ENDOCRINE TUMOR GENETICS

——————— CHARLES E. JACKSON AND LESTER WEISS ———————

Introduction

LYNCH AND KRUSH[1] have emphasized that one of the major rewards of the study of cancer genetics is that it provides the physician with an extra clinical tool in the identification of patients at risk of developing cancer at specific anatomic sites. Some of the best support for this opinion comes from the study of heritable tumor endocrinopathies. Certain nonmalignant neoplasms (such as parathyroid adenomas) will be discussed since genetic investigation of these conditions may help provide a better understanding of the relationship between hyperplasia, adenoma, and carcinoma. The endocrine system is unique in that neoplasia of various glands may be associated with abnormal function manifest by either an excess or a deficiency of specific hormones.[2] The malfunction at times may be readily ascertained so that the neoplasms can be detected even in asymptomatic relatives of affected patients. The extremely practical value of human genetic studies in endocrinology is illustrated in the finding of hyperparathyroidism in early and curable stages by simple serum calcium determinations within families[3] and in the finding of medullary thyroid cancers by calcitonin determinations after calcium infusion.[4,5] Although most of the familial endocrine neoplastic conditions are inherited by an autosomal dominant mode (similar to most other hereditary tumors),[6] the specific mode of

Sponsored in part by U.S. Public Health Service Grant AM 14876.

inheritance will be discussed with each entity.

Although heritable malignancies occur in most endocrine glands, little information is available on the mechanism of origin of these neoplasms. Knudson,[7] in a statistical study of hereditary and nonhereditary retinoblastoma, developed the theory that this cancer is caused by two mutational events— in the dominantly inherited form one mutation is inherited via germinal cells and the second occurs in somatic cells whereas in the nonhereditary form both mutations occur in somatic cells. Knudson and Strong[8] have postulated that data on the familial incidence, age of onset, and multiplicity of neuroblastomas and adrenal pheochromocytomas are compatible with the same two mutational models for these tumors. The study of heritable tumor endocrinopathies may lead eventually to some understanding of the causation of such mutational events.

McKusick's catalog[9] of Mendelian inheritance in man will continue to provide an excellent reference source on clinical genetics (including the subject of endocrine tumors), in that it is updated periodically. Rimoin and Schimke's book[10] *Genetic Disorders of the Endocrine Glands* outlines in greater detail many of the clinical and endocrinological features of the conditions discussed in this chapter.

Endocrine Neoplasia Syndromes

Two distinct hereditary endocrine neoplasia syndromes involving several endocrine glands will be discussed separately instead of under the specific organs involved. These have been designated[11] multiple endocrine neoplasia type I (tumors of the pituitary gland, pancreatic islet cells and parathyroid glands) and multiple endocrine neoplasia type II (medullary carcinoma of the thyroid, pheochromocytoma, and parathyroid tumors). These are thought to be independent entities. The parathyroid adenomas are common to the two conditions but in the type II syndrome they are thought to occur secondary to the calcitonin production from the medullary thyroid carcinomas. A comparison of endocrine involvement in these two endocrine neoplasia syndromes is summarized in Table 12-I.

Wermer[12] in 1954 first reported the familial nature and the mode of inheritance of the multiple endocrine adenomatosis syndrome. In 1953, however, Underdahl, Woolner, and Black[13] had emphasized the occurrence of multiple adenomas of the pituitary, pancreatic islet cells and parathyroid glands in 8 patients. The clinical features of multiple endocrine adenomatosis (MEA) or endocrine neoplasia type I were summarized well by Ballard, Frame, and Hartsock[14] (Table 12-II). The increasing number of reports[15-23] of this condition show that it is not rare in clinical practice. Most cases of

hereditary hyperparathyroidism are thought to be a part of this larger multiple endocrine adenomatosis syndrome.[3] Since hyperparathyroidism occurs in about 1 in every 1000 patients seen in general diagnostic clinics[24] and 1 in every 6 to 8 patients with hyperparathyroidism has the hereditary variety,[3,24,25] multiple endocrine adenomatosis should occur in about every 6000 to 8000 patients. In a study[26] of the families of 100 consecutive patients with parathyroid adenomas at Henry Ford Hospital we encountered eleven patients who were found to have others in the family affected. Multiple endocrine tumors were present in members of 5 of these families (Fig. 12-1).

The pheochromocytoma-medullary thyroid carcinoma syndrome (endocrine neoplasia type II) was described by Steiner, Goodman, and Powers[11] as a separate entity. Since the earliest recognition of the association of the two conditions together in the same patient,[27] many families with this syndrome have been reported.[28-38]

Establishment of the presence of calcitonin in medullary thyroid cancer[39] and the refinement of the technique for radioimmunoassay for calcitonin[40] have led to procedures which enable the early detection of medullary thyroid cancer within families. Our experience at Henry Ford Hospital[5] is

TABLE 12-I
COMPARISON OF THE TWO ENDOCRINE NEOPLASIA SYNDROMES

	Type I	*Type II*
Synonyms	Multiple Endocrine Adenomatosis	Pheochromocytoma—medullary thyroid carcinoma
Inheritance	Autosomal Dominant	Autosomal Dominant
Involvement		
Pituitary	Common	——
Thyroid	Infrequent	Common
Parathyroid	Common	Infrequent
Adrenal cortex	Common	2° to ectopic ACTH
Adrenal Medulla	——	Common
Pancreatic Islets	Common	——
Peptic Ulcer	Common	——
Mucosal Neuromas	——	Common

Modified from D.C. Rimoin, and R.N. Schimke, *Genetic Disorders of the Endocrine Glands* (St. Louis, C.V. Mosby, 1971).

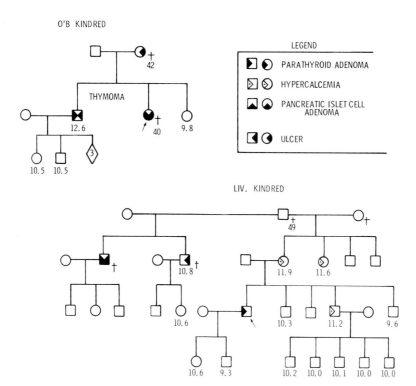

Figure 12–1. Two of the five families with multiple endocrine adenomatosis encountered in a genetic study of 100 consecutive patients with parathyroid adenomas (From C.E. Jackson *et al.*, The Importance of Heredity in Hyperparathyroidism," (1971).

typical of those institutions which have applied the calcitonin assay to the genetic detection of this neoplasm. Figure 12–2 illustrates the calcitonin response to calcium infusion in the 20 positive individuals in 3 families studied. The pedigree of the largest family, shown in Figure 12–3, illustrates the autosomal dominant mode of inheritance. The penetrance is high as measured by the calcitonin determinations. No pheochromocytomas have been found in 2 of these 3 families even though a total of 27 individuals are known to be affected in the two families. Both pheochromocytoma and medullary thyroid carcinoma were present in the third family.

In studies of 21 relatives of 10 apparently sporadic cases of medullary thyroid cancer, calcitonin determinations have been nega-tive—all of these were unilateral except the tenth case who had bilateral medullary thyroid cancers and pheochromocytomas. Her son had a negative calcitonin study but had positive catecholamines in the urine. At surgery he was found to have bilateral pheochromocytomas (Fig. 12–4). The bilaterality of tumors in inherited medullary thyroid carcinomas is similar to that observed in retinoblastoma,[7] with familial pheochromocytoma[11] and also with the tendency of multiple involvement in hereditary hyperparathyroidism.[3] This may be another example of the two mutational etiology (somatic and genetic) of hereditary neoplasms proposed by Knudson and Strong.[8]

The spectrum of involvement with this syndrome[10] consists of medullary thyroid carcinoma and pheochromocytoma each

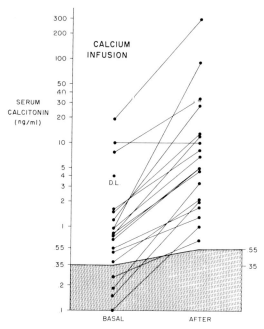

Figure 12–2. Maximum calcitonin responses to 4 hour infusion of calcium (15 mg/kg) in 20 positive individuals of 3 medullary thyroid carcinoma families. (From M.A. Block, *et al.,* "Medullary Thyroid Carcinoma Detected by Serum Calcitonin in Assay," *Archives of Surgery,* 104:579–586 (1972).

alone or combined together, medullary thyroid carcinoma combined with mucosal neuromas and neurofibromas,[32,35,41,42] and pheochromocytomas combined with neurofibromas[43] or with hemangioblastomas of retina or cerebellum.[44] Adrenal hyperplasia with Cushing's syndrome associated in this syndrome is thought to be secondary to ectopic adrenocorticotropic hormone production.[45]

It has been suggested[46,47] that substances produced by hyperplastic primordial cells of the pancreatic islets (nesidioblasts) stimulate changes in the other glands affected in the type I syndrome. Weichert[48] presented a theory explaining both multiple endocrine syndromes as a dysplasia of neural ectoderm. However, no completely satisfactory patho-

genetic mechanism has been proposed for these endocrine neoplastic syndromes.

Pituitary

Ballard, Frame, and Hartsock[14] noted anterior pituitary tumors in 65 percent of 85 patients with the MEA syndrome (Table 12-II). The earliest report of familial endocrine tumors[49] may be that of Goliath in the Bible (if we assume that his gigantism was related to acromegaly) where it states that he was born to a giant and his 3 brothers were also giants (Fig. 12–5). Table 12-III illustrates the pituitary involvement in Ballard, Frame, and Hartsock's MEA series.[14] Other families with only acromegaly[50] are reported but they may represent an incomplete expression of the MEA syndrome.

TABLE 12-II
FREQUENCY OF ADENOMATOUS OR
HYPERPLASTIC INVOLVEMENT OF THE
VARIOUS ENDOCRINE GLANDS IN
85 REPORTED MEA CASES

Pituitary	64.9%
Pancreas	81.2%
Parathyroid	88.2%
Adrenal	37.6%
Thyroid	18.8%

From H.S. Ballard, B. Frame, and R.J. Hartsock, "Familial Multiple Endocrine Adenoma-peptic Ulcer Complex," *Medicine, 43:*481–516 (1964).

TABLE 12-III
TYPE OF INVOLVEMENT IN THE MAJORITY
OF THE 55 CASES OF PITUITARY TUMORS
FROM 85 MEA CASES

Acromegaly, eosinophilic hyperplasia or adenoma	27.3%
Chromophobe adenoma	42.0%
Basophilic and eosinophilic adenomatous hyperplasia	3.6%
Eosinophilic and chromophobe adenoma	3.6%
Basophilic adenoma	3.6%
Enlarged sella	7.2%

From H.S. Ballard, B. Frame, and R.J. Hartsock, "Familial Multiple Endocrine Adenoma-peptic Ulcer Complex," *Medicine, 43:*481–516 (1964).

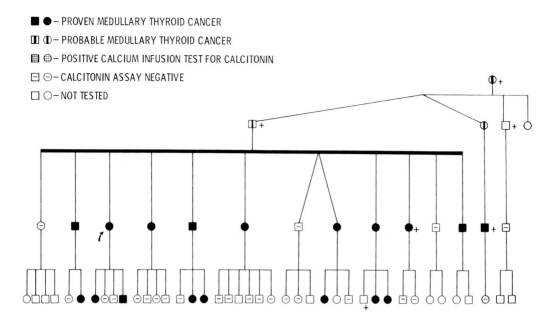

Figure 12–3. Pedigree of a kindred of medullary thyroid carcinoma (From M.A. Block *et al.,* "Medullary Thyroid Carcinoma Detected by Serum Calcitonin in Assay," *Archives of Surgery,* 104:579–586 (1972).

The Forbes-Albright syndrome of galactorrhea associated with amenorrhea has been reported in a mother and daughter[51] and as a part of the MEA syndrome.[52]

Posterior pituitary or neurohypophyseal tumors have not been reported in families. Pinealomas[53] have been reported in 3 of 7 siblings affected by secondary sexual precocity, hirsutism, pigmentation, and diabetes mellitus. As our knowledge of the endocrine function of the hypophysis increases, hereditary cellular changes there may eventually be found to be responsible for inherited tumors of other endocrine glands.

logical factors except for the medullary thyroid carcinoma — pheochromocytoma syndrome already described. Papillary carcinoma is the most common type of thyroid malignancy; but only a few families have been reported.[54–57] Although medullary carcinoma comprises but 5 to 10 percent of the cancers of the thyroid[58] many families with this condition have been described, some[59,60] of which did not have associated pheochromocytomas. However, we consider these most likely to be part of the same endocrine neoplasia syndrome with variable expression.

Thyroid

Although thyroid tumors are among the most common endocrine malignancies, very little evidence is available for genetic etio-

Parathyroid

The parathyroid glands are the most commonly involved endocrine organs in the MEA syndrome. Ballard, Frame, and Hartsock[14] found the parathyroid to be involved in 88 percent of their 85 cases (Table 12-II). How-

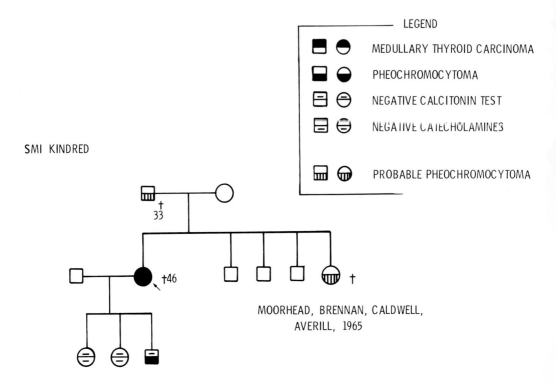

SMI KINDRED

MOORHEAD, BRENNAN, CALDWELL,
AVERILL, 1965

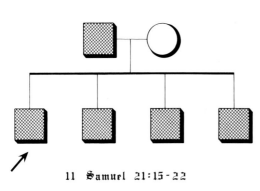

11 Samuel 21:15-22

Figure 12–5. Pedigree of Goliath. (From C.E. Jackson *et al.*, *Journal of The Indiana State Medical Association.* 55:1313–1316, 1960.

ever, the emphasis on hereditary hyperparathyroidism being a part of the MEA syndrome brings in many other families of affected cases which would make the frequency of parathyroid involvement much greater and other endocrine involvement relatively less. Multiple parathyroid involvement is more frequent (40% vs 15%) in hereditary hyperparathyroidism than in the sporadic disease.[3] Hyperplasia of the parathyroid glands is common in familial hyperparathyroidism[61] but adenomas and hyperplasia have been seen within different members of the same family.[3] Parathyroid carcinoma is rare[62] and so far no reports are known of this condition associated with hyperplasia or adenoma within one family. The occurrence of

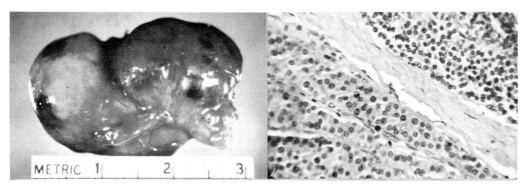

Figure 12–6. Gross and microscopic views of parathyroid adenoma removed from a woman later found to have pancreatic islet cell carcinoma at autopsy (From C.E. Jackson *et al., American Journal of Medicine,* 43:727–734, 1967. Adenomatous changes were noted in 2 different parathyroid cell types.

these conditions within one family would give us additional evidence for the suspected interrelationship of hyperplasia, adenoma, and carcinoma as is actually seen in pancreatic islet cell tumors.

Twenty-eight families of hereditary hyperparathyroidism were reviewed[63] in 1970 exclusive of those associated with the MEA syndrome. Since then other families have appeared in the literature.[64–66] The pedigrees of most reported families are compatible with an autosomal dominant mode of inheritance. Exceptions are the neonatal hyperparathyroidism in 2 brothers born to related but unaffected parents reported by Hillman, Scriver, and others[67] and other neonatal cases of parathyroid hyperplasia reviewed by Goldbloom, Gillis, and Prasad.[68]

Pancreas

The hormone secreting cells of the pancreas are the alpha cells secreting glucagon, the beta cells secreting insulin and the delta cells which secrete gastrin. Technological

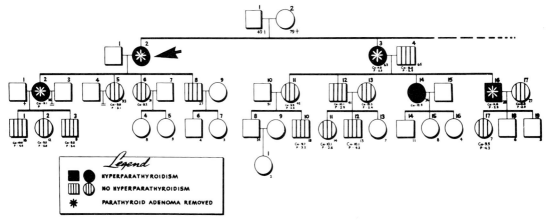

Figure 12–7. Pedigree of the family thought to represent simply hereditary hyperparathyroidism until the propositus (II-2, Figure 12–4) was shown to have pancreatic islet cell carcinoma and a pituitary adenoma (From C.E. Jackson, *et al., American Journal of Medicine,* 43:727–734, 1967.

advances have provided means of evaluating the various functions of the islet cells.[69] Adenomas or adenocarcinomas of these islet cells occur as a part of the multiple endocrine adenomatosis syndrome (Type I) described. The frequency of pancreatic islet cell carcinoma associated with adenomas or hyperplasia of pituitary and parathyroid glands attests to the close relationships of malignancy to these other conditions considered as benign neoplasms. Figure 12–6 shows the parathyroid tumor of a 58 year old woman who was thought to have only hereditary hyperparathyroidism until post mortem examination revealed a pituitary adenoma and metastasizing islet cell carcinoma. Others in her family[3] were found to have hyperparathyroidism (see pedigree Fig. 12–7). Were it not for the autopsy on the propositus, this family would have been thought to be representative of hereditary hyperparathyroidism rather than the endocrine neoplasia syndrome Type I.

Although islet cell tumors of the pancreas were described earlier in association with peptic ulceration, Zollinger and Ellison[70] in 1955 first postulated a humoral factor of pancreatic islet origin as the cause of the ulcers. The non-beta cell tumor is the primary lesion in this syndrome with more than 60 percent of the tumors being malignant according to Ptak and Kirshner.[71] The hormone gastrin has been found in high concentration in the pancreatic islet cell tumors[72] and high concentrations of gastrin have been found in serum of these patients by radioimmunoassay.[73] The assay procedure may provide as important a means of studying the families of patients with the Zollinger-Ellison (ZE) syndrome as the calcitonin assay has in families of medullary thyroid carcinoma patients.[4,5]

Many peptic ulcers were observed in the MEA family reported by Wermer.[12] It is not known what percentage of ulcers are secondary to islet cell tumors in patients with the MEA syndrome. Ptak and Kirshner[71] regard the ZE syndrome as the gastrin secreting pancreatic islet cell component of the MEA syndrome. Non-beta cell adenomas and carcinomas account for 60 percent of the islet cell tumors of the MEA syndrome with beta cell adenoma or carcinoma accounting for about 35 percent.[71] Patients with beta cell tumors present with symptoms of hypoglycemia associated with excessive insulin production. The ulcerogenic non-beta cell tumors are more frequently malignant than the beta cell tumors.[74]

Adrenal Cortex

Genetic disease of the adrenal cortex is not unusual. Congenital adrenal hypoplasia can be inherited as a sex linked recessive.[75] At least six different inborn errors of metabolism can result in adrenal hyperplasia.[10] However, malignancy involving the adrenal cortex in the absence of the multiple endocrine neoplasia Type I syndrome is quite rare. Aldosterone producing tumors of the adrenal cortex are considered to be a part of this MEA syndrome. In 1971 Mahloudju, Ronaghy, and Dutz[76] reported two siblings with virilizing adrenal carcinoma who were born to parents who were second cousins. There is at least one other report of adrenal carcinoma in siblings.[77] It appears that at least on rare occasions adrenal cortical carcinoma may be inherited as a simple Mendelian recessive trait.

Adrenal Medulla

Tumors of the adrenal medulla include pheochromocytoma, ganglioneuroma, and neuroblastoma. Although neuroblastomas are among the more common malignant neoplasms occurring during childhood, the prevalence does not approach the frequency of "neuroblastoma *in situ*" found by Beckwith and Martin[78] in autopsies of infants dying from other causes. They estimated that microscopic neuroblastoma occurs in approximately 1:2000 autopsies. Clinically manifest neuroblastomas occur in approximately 1:10,000 live born children. In view of the known tendency of neuroblastoma to undergo both spontaneous remission and maturation to ganglioneuroma,[79] it is reasonable to suppose that most of the neuroblastomas *in situ* undergo this type of change. If this is true, it is not surprising that familial neuroblastomas are not often found. Affected family members may not have manifest disease and, therefore, may not be discovered. Griffin and Bolande[80] reported two sisters with neuroblastomas diagnosed histologically. One died of pneumonia following the generally accepted therapy of surgery and deep x-ray therapy. At autopsy, areas of the tumor showed evidence of maturation to ganglioneuroma or ganglioneurofibroma. The parents refused therapy for the second child. The tumor in this child underwent transition and maturation to neurofibroma. A third sister had a small area of calcification in one adrenal gland. The findings in this family lend support to the hypothesis that the familial nature of neuroblastoma may be obscured by spontaneous maturation and/or regression. Chatten and Voorhess[81] reviewed the previously reported familial neuroblastomas in a report of a family in which neuroblastomas were found in three of four siblings. Of significance was the finding of an abnormally elevated output of dopamine and norepinephrine in the mother of these children. It is possible that at least some neuroblastomas are inherited as Mendelian dominant traits with variation in expression due to regression and/or maturation. Others may represent new dominant mutations. More recently, Hardy and Nesbit[82] reported a family in which two siblings had neuralcrest tumors. One had a right adrenal neuroblastoma, the other had a right adrenal ganglioneuroblastoma. A paternal cousin died of a neuroblastoma and three other paternal relatives died of tumors of the kidney or scalp in infancy or childhood. The authors suggest an autosomal dominant mode of inheritance with variation in expression due to maturation and regression.

Knudson and Strong,[8] after summarizing the current literature on familial incidence of neuroblastoma and adding two familial cases from 60 cases of neuroblastoma at M.D. Anderson Hospital, offer an alternate hypothesis regarding the genetics of this tumor. They suggest that these tumors are due to two mutational events. Two somatic mutations can result in nonfamilial neuroblastoma. In other families there is a gonadal mutation that is transmitted in a Mendelian fashion. In the genetically disposed individuals a single somatic mutation results in a neuroblastoma.

Pheochromocytomas of the adrenal medulla are discussed under the endocrine neoplasia syndromes. Although there are families in which pheochromocytomas are inherited as a Mendelian dominant condition without evidence of other endocrine tumors,[83,84] these families may represent endocrine neoplasia Type II families in which only the pheochromocytomas have been found thus far. Since pheochromocytoma may occur fairly frequently as a familial condition and since 7 percent are malignant,[85] relatives of affected individuals (especially those with bilateral involvement) should have urinary catecholamines assayed to detect these tumors in early stages.

Gonads

Individuals with abnormalities of sexual development have an unusually high incidence of gonadal neoplasms. Abnormal sexual development may be due to gross sex

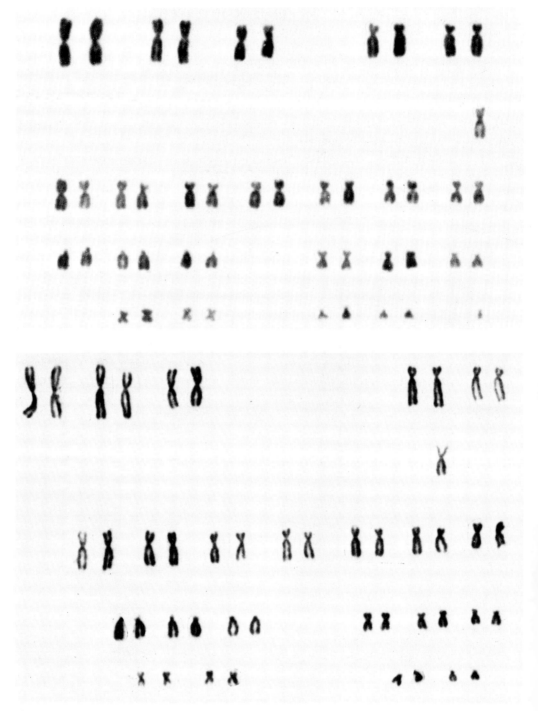

Figure 12–8. Giemsa stained karyotype from a mosaic individual with unilateral gonadal dysgenesis. (A) 46,XY cell line. (B) 45,X cell line.

chromosome abnormalities or to single gene defects. An understanding of the basic mechanisms of normal sexual development is essential to the proper interpretation and management of abnormalities that occur in the developmental process. Prompt and correct management in addition to being essential for optimal physical and psychological development includes prophylactic surgery in situations where the risk of neoplasm is high. The development of anatomic sex depends upon a series of inter-related sequential events. The sex chromosome constitution of the individual determines the development of the gonad which in turn determines the development of the internal ductal system and the external sexual phenotype.[86]

Errors at any stage of sexual development can result in a dysgenetic gonad that has a high risk of neoplastic change. The most common errors in sexual development are the result of errors of chromosomal sex. The sex chromosome abnormalities that have the highest frequency are apparently not related to the development of gonadal neoplasia. These are Turner's syndrome (45,X), Klinefelter's syndrome (47,XXY), and the XYY syndrome. Patients with Klinefelter's syndrome, however, do have a risk of breast neoplasia that is considerably higher than that of normal males.

Some individuals have some cells with one sex chromosome constitution, and other cells with a different sex chromosome constitution. This situation is known as mosaicism. When one cell line has a normal male karyotype (46,XY), and the other has only a single X chromosome, (45,X), abnormal gonadal development results (Fig. 12–8). Typically,

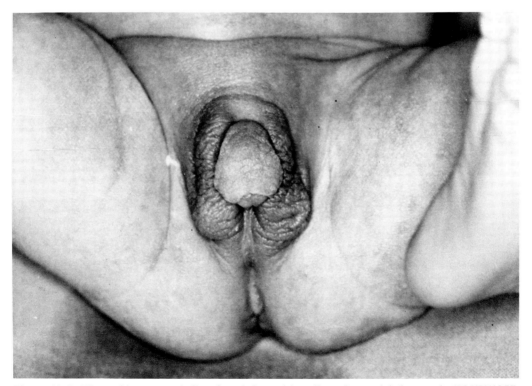

Figure 12–9. The ambiguous genitalia of an infant with unilateral gonadal dysgenesis (46,XY/45,X).

a fibrous streak replaces one gonad and a dysgenetic gonad is present on the opposite side. This dysgenetic gonad usually contains some testicular elements. In accord with the mechanism of sex determination, the ductal system on the side with the streak gonad is the female derivative of the Müllerian ducts. On the other side, the testicular remnant induces the development of the male Wolffian duct. The external genitalia are variable, depending on the degree of masculinization induced by the circulating androgen produced by the gonad. Some have phenotypes that are almost those of a normal female, while others have marked phallic enlargement and labial-scrotal fusion. The latter individuals may resemble cryptorchid males. Most 46,XY/45,X mosaics have ambiguous genitalia and can be identified in the neonatal period (Fig. 12–9). When a newborn has ambiguous genitalia, appropriate studies will define the situation so that a proper assignment of sex rearing can be made. In 1964 Robinson, Priest, and Bigler[87] described the development of gonadoblastoma in a patient with this syndrome. Since the initial report, the risk of tumor formation has been repeatedly documented. Prompt and accurate diagnosis of these patients not only results in the proper assignment of sex but permits the prophylactic removal of the abnormal gonad. At the usual age of puberty appropriate hormonal replacement therapy must be given to develop secondary sex characteristics.

True hermaphrodites have the same risk of gonadal neoplasm as do the patients described above. These individuals have both ovarian and testicular elements. The external genitalia are again variable but many have ambiguous genitalia. Several different karyotypes have been described. Most are mosaics. In some only one cell line has been found, usually 46,XX, but some have had 46,XY karyotypes. The reason for the abnormal gonadal development in the 46,XX and the 46,XY individuals is not clear. They may have an undiscovered mosaic cell line or a previously present mosaic cell line that has disappeared. The variable ductal system and external genitalia develop in accordance with the principles of normal sexual development and depend upon the presence or absence of the locally acting inducer substance and on the circulating androgen. When these individuals are identified, the abnormal gonad should be removed to prevent the development of gonadal tumors.

Another genetic cause of gonadal neoplasm is the testicular feminization syndrome. It is apparently an inborn error of metabolism that results in end organ unresponsiveness. Individuals with the testicular feminization syndrome are phenotypic females. They have labia minora and majora and a vagina. At puberty they usually develop normal female secondary sex characteristics. They function sexually as females. Some patients are diagnosed during childhood when they present with an inguinal hernia containing a gonad. At the time of herniorrhaphy the gonad is found to be a testis. On further exploration the patient is found to have a normal vagina, no uterus and a ductal system derived from the Wolffian

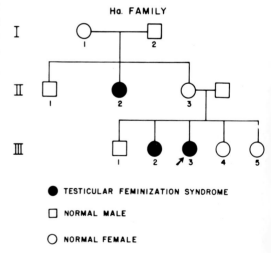

Figure 12–10. Pedigree of family with testicular feminization syndrome.

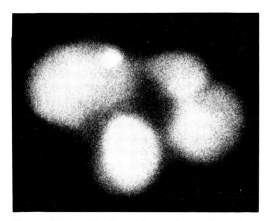

Figure 12–11. Nucleus of a polymorphonuclear cell of the propositus of family with testicular feminization (Figure 12–10). This has been stained with quinacrine mustard and viewed with fluorescence microscopy to demonstrate the brightly fluorescent F body (the distal portion of the Y chromosome).

ducts. Alternatively, girls with testicular feminization syndrome may present with a chief complaint of primary amenorrhea or infertility. The description of a family that follows is used as an example of how these families can be evaluated.

CASE HISTORY: L. H. is a 17 year old white female who was referred to the Henry Ford Hospital Genetic Counseling Clinic because she was found to have a chromatin negative buccal smear by her gynecologist whom she had consulted because of primary amenorrhea. Breast development had started and pubic and axillary hair appeared at 14 years of age. She had never menstruated. The family history revealed that she had three phenotypic sisters and one brother (Fig. 12–10). "Sister" II-2 had amenorrhea and "aunt" I-2 was infertile. Physical ex-

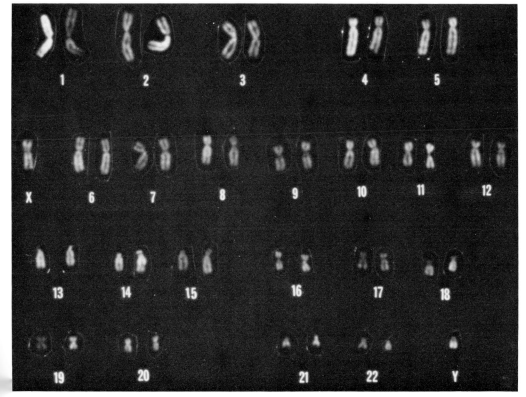

Figure 12–12. The normal male karyotype (46,XY) of the propositus of family with testicular feminization shown in Figure 12–10 (quinacrine mustard stain and fluorescence microscopy).

amination revealed a normal female except that no uterus was palpable on bimanual examination. Repeat buccal smear confirmed that the proband was chromatin negative. A peripheral blood smear was stained with quinacrine mustard and examined with fluorescence microscopy (Fig. 12–11). A brightly fluorescent spot was noted in the nucleus of the white cells. This F body indicates the presence of a Y chromosome and is the fluorescent heterchromatic distal portion of the Y chromosome. Chromosome analysis (Fig. 12–12) confirmed the normal male karyotype. The patient's "sister" (Fig. 12–10, II-2) had identical findings. The other siblings were normal. An exploratory laparotomy revealed no uterus and testes and Wolffian duct derivatives bilaterally. These were removed and the patient is being given estrogen maintenance therapy. By appropriate diagnosis and management not only the proband but her sister had the benefit of prophylactic orchidectomy to prevent the development of testicular neoplasm.

Whenever the diagnosis of testicular feminization is made, appropriate family studies should be undertaken. In the maternal families and among the siblings of these patients there is an excessive number of females in the ratio of three females to each male. Of the females, one in three have the testicular feminization syndrome. This syndrome is either inherited as a sex linked recessive or a sex limited dominant. In either case, the affected chromosomal males are infertile. There is a group of patients with 46,XY karyotypes and female phenotypes who differ from those with testicular feminization in that they have a uterus and fallopian tubes. These patients are also at risk of developing gonadal tumors. Therefore, these dysgenetic gonads should be prophylactically removed. Patients with dysgenetic gonads have been reported to have seminomas, teratomas, teratocarcinomas, embryonal carcinoma, and gonadoblastomas.

Even in the absence of dysgenetic gonads there is evidence for genetic determinants in the origin of ovarian tumors. Jackson[88] reported the occurrence of ovarian dysgerminoma in two and possibly three generations of a Jamaican family. Accardo and Condorelli[89] reported arrhenoblastoma in two sisters. Benign ovarian dermoid cysts have been reported in triplets,[90] and Lynch,[91] Liber,[92] and Lewis and Davidson[93] have reported familial instances of ovarian carcinoma.

The influence of genetic factors on the development of testicular tumors in other than dysgenetic gonads is not clear. Cryptorchid testes are usually thought to have a higher incidence of neoplasia than those that are normally descended.[94] Although polygenetic inheritance is usually thought to be important in the developmental defect known as cryptorchidism, it has been reported in as many as four consecutive generations.[95] In the absence of cryptorchidism, genetic factors in the development of testicular tumors are even more difficult to identify. Tiltman[96] reported his findings, and reviewed the literature related to the racial incidence of testicular tumors and found a higher incidence in the Caucasian than in the non-Caucasian population. Racial differences are at least compatible with the concept that genetic factors are involved. Testicular tumors have been found in brothers[97] and in identical twins.[98] The incidence of concordance in twins is low enough to indicate that the major factors in the development of testicular tumors in otherwise normal testes are non-genetic.

Non-Endocrine Hormone Secreting Tumors

The non-endocrine malignancies which secrete hormones or hormone-like substances causing the ectopic hormone syndromes (Table 12-IV) will not be discussed.[99,100]

TABLE 12-IV
SUMMARIZATION OF ECTOPIC HORMONE SYNDROMES

Hormone	Condition	Tumor
Adrenocorticotropin	Cushing Syndrome	Lung (oat cell; bronchial adenoma) thymus; pancreas; thyroid (medullary)
Parathormone	Hyperparathyroidism	Kidney; lung (squamous); pancreas; ovary; many squamous sites
Arginine-Vasopressin	Inappropriate Antidiuresis	Lung (oat cell)
Erythropoietin	Erythocytosis	Cerebellum (hemangioblastoma); liver; uterus
Gonadotropins	Gynecomastia (adults)	Lung (large cell)
	Precocious puberty	Liver (hepatoblastoma, hepatoma)
Thyrotropin	Hyperthyroidism	Trophoblast; lung
Insulin?	Hypoglycemia	Retroperitoneal mesoderm; liver
Serotonin	Carcinoid Syndrome*	Carcinoid tumors (intestine, ovary, bronchus) Lung (oat cell) Thyroid (medullary) Pancreas (adenocarcinoma and islet cell)

Modified from G.S. Omenn, "Ectopic Polypeptide Hormone Production By Tumors." *Annals of Internal Medicine, 72:*136–138 (1970).

* A.S. Patchefsky, *et al.,* "Hydroxyindole-producing Tumors of the Pancreas: Carcinoid-islet Cell Tumor and Oat Cell Carcinoma," *Annals of Internal Medicine, 77:*53–61 (1972).

Study of these syndromes may contribute to our knowledge of hormone secretion and even possibly lead to the discovery of new hormones. For example, the occurrence of a vitamin D resistant rickets-like syndrome with sclerosing hemangiomas (and its disappearance after excision of the tumors)[101] may eventually lead to the discovery of a hormonal substance responsible for this syndrome.

Summary and Conclusions

Relationships between genetics, endocrinology and cancer harbor a potential for elucidation of etiology, pathogenesis and hopefully, for improved control. Implications for these assumptions are found in recent studies. For example, in calcium stimulation studies of calcitonin levels in families of patients with the medullary thyroid carcinoma-pheochromocytoma syndrome, three patients with a previously undescribed condition of "C-cell hyperplasia" of the thyroid have been reported.[102,103] It was proposed that this "C-cell hyperplasia" may be the early change in patients destined to develop medullary thyroid carcinoma and therefore the premalignant stage of the neoplasm. The possibility was considered[102] that this condition may represent the genetic mutational event occurring prior to the second somatic mutation of the proposed two mutational theory of hereditary cancer.[8]

REFERENCES

1. Lynch, H.T., and Krush, A.J.: Cancer genetics. *South Med J, 64:*suppl. 1:26–40, 1971.

2. Schimke, R.N.: Familial tumor endocrinopathies. *Birth Defects: Original Article Series. 7:*55–65, 1971.

3. Jackson, C.E., and Boonstra, C.E.: The relationship of hereditary hyperparathyroidism to endocrine adenomatosis. *Am J Med, 43:*727–734, 1967.

4. Melvin, K.E.W., Miller, H.H., and Tashjian, A.H. Jr.,: Early diagnosis of medullary

carcinoma of the thyroid gland by means of calcitonin assay. *N Engl J Med, 285:* 1115–1120, 1971.

5. Block, M.A., Jackson, C.E., and Tashjian, A.H. Jr.,: Medullary thyroid carcinoma detected by serum calcitonin assay. *Arch Surg, 104:579–586,* 1972.

6. Lynch, H.T.: Genetic factors in carcinoma. *Med Clin North Am, 53:923–939,* 1969.

7. Knudson, A.G. Jr.: Mutation and cancer: Stastical study of retinoblastoma. *Proc Natl Acad Sci USA, 68:820–823,* 1971.

8. Knudson, A.G. Jr., and Strong, L.C.: Mutation and cancer: Neuroblastoma and pheochromocytoma. Personal communication.

9. McKusick, V.A.: *Mendelian Inheritance in Man. Catalogs of Autosomal Dominant, Autosomal Recessive and X-linked Phenotypes,* 3rd ed., Baltimore, Johns Hopkins, 1971.

10. Rimoin, D.C., and Schimke, R.N.: *Genetic Disorders of the Endocrine Glands.* St. Louis, Mosby, 1971.

11. Steiner, A.L., Goodman, A.D., and Powers, S.R.: Study of a kindred with pheochromocytoma, medullary thyroid carcinoma, hyperparathyroidism and Cushing's disease: Multiple endocrine neoplasia type 2. *Medicine, 47:371–409,* 1968.

12. Wermer, P.: Genetic aspects of adenomatosis of endocrine glands. *Am J Med, 16:363–371,* 1954.

13. Underdahl, L.O., Woolner, L.B., and Black, B.M.: Multiple endocrine adenomas: Report of 8 cases in which the parathyroids, pituitary and pancreatic islets were involved. *J Clin Endocrinol Metab, 13:20–47,* 1953.

14. Ballard, H.S., Frame, B., and Hartsock, R.J.: Familial multiple endocrine adenoma-peptic ulcer complex. *Medicine, 43:481–516,* 1964.

15. Moldawer, M.: Multiple endocrine tumors and Zollinger-Ellison syndrome in families: One or two syndromes? A report of two new families. *Metabolism, 11:153–166,* 1962.

16. Johnson, G.J., Summerskill, H.J., Anderson, V.E., and Keating, F.R. Jr.: Clinical and genetic investigation of a large kindred

with multiple endocrine adenomatosis. *N Engl J Med, 277:*1379–1385, 1967.

17. Stocks, A.E.: Problems of the syndrome of familial multiple endocrine adenomas. *Aust Ann Med, 16:*278–288, 1967.

18. Snyder, N., Scurry, M.T., and Deiss, W.P., Jr.: Five families with multiple endocrine adenomatosis. *Ann Intern Med, 76:*53–58, 1972.

19. Assan, R., Tchobroutsky, G., Rosselin, G., Kopf, A., Welti, J.J., and Dérot, M.: Les Polyandénomatoses: *Presse Med, 76:* 2259–2262, 1968.

20. Delaney, J.P., and Jacobson, M.E.: Multiple endocrine adenomatosis. *Minn Med, 51:* 1731–1734, 1968.

21. Karbach, H.B., and Galindo, D.L.: Familial endocrine adenomatosis. *Tex Med, 66:* 54–63, 1970.

22. Craven, D.E., Goodman, A.D., and Carter, J.H.: Familial multiple endocrine adenomatosis. *Arch Intern Med, 129:*567–569, 1972.

23. Maurer, W., Walser, A., and Gloor, F.: Hypophysenadenom, hyperparathyreoidismus und hyperthyreose. *Schweiz Med Wochenschr, 96:*536–542, 1966.

24. Boonstra, C.E., and Jackson, C.E.: Serum calcium survey for hyperparathyroidism: Results in 50,000 clinic patients. *Am J Clin Pathol, 55:*523–526, 1971.

25. Jackson, C.E., and Frame, B.: Relationship of hyperparathyroidism to multiple endocrine adenomatosis. *Birth Defects: Original Article Series, 7:*66–68, 1971.

26. Jackson, C.E., Frame, B., and Block, M.A.: The importance of heredity in hyperparathyroidism. *Proceedings of the IV International Congress of Human Genetics,* 1971, p. 94.

27. Sipple, J.H.: The association of pheochromocytoma with carcinoma of the thyroid gland. *Am J Med, 31:*163–166, 1961.

28. Cushman, P., Jr.: Familial endocrine tumors: Report of two unrelated kindred affected with pheochromocytomas, one also with multiple thyroid carcinomas. *Am J Med, 32:*352–360, 1962.

29. Manning, P.C., Jr., Molnar, G.D., Black, B.M., Priestley, J.T., and Woolner, L.B.:

Pheochromocytoma, hyperparathyroidism and thyroid carcinoma occurring coincidentally.: Report of a case. *N Engl J Med, 268*:68–72, 1963.

30. Nourok, D.S.: Familial pheochromocytoma and thyroid carcinoma. *Ann Intern Med, 60*:1028–1040, 1964.

31. Schimke, R.N., and Hartmann, W.H.: Familial amyloid-producing medullary thyroid carcinoma and pheochromocytoma: A distinct genetic entity. *Ann Intern Med, 63*:1027–1039, 1965.

32. Williams, E.D., and Pollock, D.J.: Multiple mucosal neuromata with endocrine tumours: A syndrome allied to von Recklinghausen's disease. *J Pathol Bact, 91*: 71–80, 1966.

33. Ljungberg, O., Cederquist, E., and von Studnitz, W.: Medullary thyroid carcinoma and phaeochromocytoma: A familial chromaffinomatosis. *Br Med J, 1*:279–281, 1967.

34. Huang, S., and McLeish, W.A.: Pheochromocytoma and medullary carcinoma of thyroid. *Cancer, 21*:302–311, 1968.

35. Schimke, R.N., Hartmann, W.H., Prout, T.E., and Rimoin, D.L.: Syndrome of bilateral pheochromocytoma, medullary thyroid carcinoma and multiple neuromas: A possible regulatory defect in the differentiation of chromaffin tissue. *N Engl J Med, 279*:1–7, 1968.

36. Sarosi, G., and Doe, R.P.: Familial occurrence of parathyroid adenomas, pheochromocytoma, and medullary carcinoma of the thyroid with amyloid stroma (Sipple's Syndrome). *Ann Intern Med, 68*: 1305–1309, 1968.

37. Slavotinek, A., de la Lande, I.S., and Head, R.: Medullary thyroid carcinomas with bilateral phaeochromocytomas. *Aust Ann Med, 17*:320–326, 1968.

38. Miller, H.H., Melvin, K.E.W., Gibson, J.M., and Tashjian, A.H., Jr.: Surgical approach to early familial medullary carcinoma of the thyroid gland. *Am J Surg, 123*:438–443, 1972.

39. Melvin, K.E.W., and Tashjian, A.H., Jr.: The syndrome of excessive thyrocalcitonin produced by medullary carcinoma of the thyroid. *Proc Natl Acad Sci USA, 59*: 1216–1222, 1968.

40. Tashjian, A.H., Jr., Howland, B.G., Melvin, K.E.W., and Hill, C.S., Jr.: Immunoassay of human calcitonin: Clinical measurement, relation to serum calcium and studies in patients with medullary carcinoma. *N Engl J Med, 283*:890–895, 1970.

41. Cunliffe, W.J., Hudgson, P., Fulthorpe, J.J., Black, M.M., Hall, R., Johnston, I.D.A., and Shurster, S.: A calcitonin-secreting medullary thyroid carcinoma associated with mucosal neuromas. Marfanoid features, myopathy and pigmentation. *Am J Med, 48*:120–126, 1970.

42. Williams, E.D., Brown, C.L., and Doniach, I.: Pathological and clinical findings in a series of 67 cases of medullary carcinoma of the thyroid. *J Clin Pathol, 19*:103–113, 1966.

43. Campbell, C.B., and Mortimer, R.H.: A functioning malignant phaeochromocytoma occurring in a patient with neurofibromatosis. *Aust Ann Med, 17*:331–333, 1968.

44. Nibbelink, D.W., Peters, B.H., and McCormick, W.F.: On the association of pheochromocytoma and cerebellar hemangioblastoma. *Neurology, 19*:455–460, 1969.

45. Melvin, K.E.W., Tashjian, A.H., Jr., Cassidy, C.E., and Givens, J.R.: Cushing's syndrome caused by ACTH-and calcitonin-secreting medullary carcinoma of the thyroid. *Metabolism, 19*:831–838, 1970.

46. Brown, R.E., and Still, W.J.S.: Nesidioblastosis and the Zollinger-Ellison syndrome. *Am J Dig Dis, 13*:656–663, 1968.

47. Vance, J.E., Stoll, R.W., Kitabchi, A.E., Buchanan, K.D., Hollander, D., and Williams, R.H.: Familial nesidioblastosis as the predominant manifestation of multiple endocrine adenomatosis. *Am J Med, 52*: 211–227, 1972.

48. Weichert, R.F., III: The neural ectodermal origin of the peptide-secreting endocrine glands. *Am J Med, 49*:232–241, 1970.

49. Jackson, C.E., Talbert, P.C., and Caylor, H.D.: Hereditary hyperparathyroidism. *J Indiana State Med Assoc, 53*:1313–1316, 1960.

50. Leva, J.: Ueber familiäre akromegalie. *Med Klin, 11:*1266–1268, 1915.

51. Linquette, M., Herlant, M., Laine, E., Fossati, P., and Dupont-Lecompte, J.: Adénome à prolactine chez une jeune fille dont la mère était porteuse d'un adénome hypophysaire avec aménorrhée galactorrhée. *Ann Endocrinol* (Paris), *28:*773–780, 1967.

52. Briggs, R., and Powell, J.R.: Chiari-Frommel syndrome as a part of the Zollinger-Ellison multiple endocrine adenomatosis complex. *Calif Med, 111:*92–96, 1969.

53. Rabson, S.M., and Mendenhall, E.N.: Familial hypertrophy of pineal body, hyperplasia of adrenal cortex and diabetes mellitus. *Am J Clin Pathol, 26:*283–290, 1956.

54. Robinson, D.W., and Orr, T.G.: Carcinoma of the thyroid and other diseases of the thyroid in identical twins. *Arch Surg, 70:*923–928, 1955.

55. Camiel, M.R., Mulé, J.E., Alexander, L.L., and Benninghoff, D.L.: Association of thyroid carcinoma with Gardner's syndrome in siblings. *N Engl J Med, 278:*1056–1058, 1968.

56. Smith, W.G.: Familial multiple polyposis: Research tool for investigating the etiology of carcinoma of the colon. *Dis Colon Rectum, 11:*17–31, 1968.

57. Block, M.A.: Familial medullary carcinoma of the thyroid. *GP, 39:*105–107, 1969.

58. Fletcher, J.R.: Medullary (solid) carcinoma of the thyroid gland: A review of 249 cases. *Arch Surg, 100:*257–262, 1970.

59. Friedell, G.H., Carey, R.J., and Rosen, H.: Familial thyroid cancer. *Cancer, 15:*241–245, 1962.

60. Block, M.A., Horn, R.C., Jr., Miller, J.M., Barrett, J.L., and Brush, B.E.: Familial medullary carcinoma of the thyroid. *Ann Surg, 166:*403–412, 1967.

61. Cutler, R.E., Reiss, E., and Ackerman, L.V.: Familial hyperparathyroidism. A kindred involving eleven cases, with a discussion of primary chief cell hyperplasia. *N Engl J Med, 270:*859–865, 1964.

62. Holmes, E.C., Morton, D.L., and Ketcham, A.S.: Parathyroid carcinoma: A collective review. *Ann Surg, 169:*631–640, 1969.

63. Jackson, C.E., and Mock, L.F.: Genetic modes of transmission in metabolic bone disease. *Clin Orthop, 68:*238–240, 1970.

64. Carey, M.C., and Fitzgerald, O.: Hyperparathyroidism associated with chronic pancreatitis in a family. *Gut, 9:*700–703, 1968.

65. Cholod, E.J., Haust, M.D., Hudson, A.J., and Lewis, F.N.: Myopathy in primary familial hyperparathyroidism. *Am J Med, 48:*700–707, 1970.

66. Goldsmith, R.E., Gall, E.A., Altemeier, W.A., Weinstein, A., and Zolme, E.: Hyperparathyroidism: Therapy and response, with a test for assessment of response. *Ann Intern Med, 75:*395–405, 1971.

67. Hillman, D.A., Scriver, C.R., Pedvis, S., and Shragovitch, I.: Neonatal familial primary hyperparathyroidism. *N Engl J Med, 270:*483–490, 1964.

68. Goldbloom, R.B., Gillis, D.A., and Prasad, M.: Hereditary parathyroidism hyperplasia: A surgical emergency of early infancy. *Pediatrics, 49:*514–523, 1972.

69. Arky, R.A., and Knopp, R.H.: Evaluation of islet-cell function in man. *N Engl J Med, 285:*1130–1131, 1971.

70. Zollinger, R.M., and Ellison, E.H.: Primary peptic ulcerations of the jejunum associated with islet cell tumors of the pancreas. *Ann Surg, 142:*709–728, 1955.

71. Ptak, T., and Kirsner, J.B.: The Zollinger-Ellison syndrome, polyendocrine adenomatosis and other endocrine associations with peptic ulcer. *Adv Intern Med, 16:*213–242, 1970.

72. Gregory, R.A., Tracy, H.J., French, J.M., and Sircus, W.: Extraction of a gastrin-like substance from a pancreatic tumour in a case of Zollinger-Ellison syndrome. *Lancet, 1:*1045–1048, 1960.

73. McGuigan, J.E., and Trudeau, W.L.: Immunochemical measurement of elevated levels of gastrin in the serum of patients with pancreatic tumors of the Zollinger-Ellison variety. *N Engl J Med, 298:*1308–1313, 1968.

74. Floquet, J., Laurent, J., Florentin, P., Rauber, G., Grignon, G., Floquet, A.: Les tumeurs du pancréas endocrine: Considérations morphologiques et histogénétiques. *Presse Med, 77:*87–90, 1967.

75. Weiss, L., and Mellinger, R.C.: Congenital adrenal hypoplasia: An X linked disease. *J Med Genet, 7:*27–32, 1970.

76. Mahloudji, M., Ronaghy, H., and Dutz, W.: Virilizing adrenal carcinoma in two sibs. *J Med Genet, 8:*160–163, 1971.

77. Fraumeni, J.F., Jr., and Miller, R.W.: Adrenalcortical neoplasms with hemihypertrophy, brain tumors and other disorders. *J Pediatr, 70:*129–138, 1967.

78. Beckwith, J.B., and Martin, R.F.: Observations on the hystopathology of neuroblastomas. *J Pediatr Surg, 3:*106–110, 1968.

79. Bolande, R.P.: *Cellular Aspects of Developmental Pathology.* Philadelphia, Lea and Febiger, 1967.

80. Griffin, M.E., and Bolande, R.P.: Familial neuroblastoma with regression and maturation to ganglioneurofibroma. *Pediatrics, 43:*377–382, 1969.

81. Chatten, J., and Voorhess, M.L.: Familial neuroblastoma. *N Engl J Med, 277:*1230–1236, 1967.

82. Hardy, P.C., and Nesbit, M.E., Jr.: Familial neuroblastoma: Report of a kindred with a high incidence of infantile tumors. *J Pediatr, 80:*74–77, 1972.

83. Carman, C.T., and Brashear, R.E.: Pheochromocytoma as an inherited abnormality: Report of the tenth affected kindred and review of the literature. *N Engl J Med, 263:*419–423, 1960.

84. Moorhead, E.L. II., Brennan, M.J., Caldwell, J.R., and Averill, W.C.: Pheochromocytoma: A familial tumor, a study of eleven families. *Henry Ford Hosp Med Bull, 13:*467–478, 1965.

85. Hermann, H., and Mornex, R.: *Human Tumours Secreting Catecholamines: Clinical and Physiopathological Study of the Pheochromocytomas.* New York, MacMillan, 1964.

86. Jost, A.: Embryonic sexual differentiation. In Jones, H.W., Jr., and Scott, W.W. (Eds.): *Hermaphroditism, Genital Anomalies, and Related Endocrine Disorders.* Baltimore, Williams & Wilkins, 1958.

87. Robinson, A., Priest, R.E., and Bigler, P.C.: Male pseudohermaphrodite with XY/XO

mosaicism and bilateral gonadoblastomas. *Lancet, 1:*111–112, 1964.

88. Jackson, S.M.: Ovarian dysgerminoma in three generations. *J Med Genet, 4:*112–113, 1967.

89. Accardo, M., and Condorelli, B.: Arrenoblastoma in due Sorelle. *Riv Patrol Clin Sper, 7:*171–188, 1966.

90. Feld, D., Labes, J., and Nathanson, M.: Bilateral ovarian dermoid cysts in triplets. *Obstet Gynecol, 27:*525–528, 1966.

91. Lynch, F.W.: A clinical review of 110 cases of ovarian carcinoma. *Am J Obstet Gynecol, 32:*753–777, 1936.

92. Liber, A.F.: Ovarian cancer in mother and five daughters. *Arch Pathol, 49:*280–290, 1950.

93. Lewis, A.C.W., and Davison, B.C.C.: Familial ovarian cancer. *Lancet, 2:*235–237, 1969.

94. Dixon, F.J., and Moore, R.A.: Tumors of the male sex organs. *Atlas of Tumor Pathology,* Washington, D.C., Armed Forces Institute of Pathology, 1952.

95. Perrett, L.J., and O'Rourke, D.A.: Hereditary cryptorchidism. *Med J Aust, 1:*1289–1290, 1969.

96. Tiltman, A.J.: The racial incidence of testicular tumours. *S Afr Med J, 43:*97–98, 1969.

97. Hutter, A.M., Jr., Lynch, J.J., and Shnider, B.I.: Malignant testicular tumors in brothers: A case report. *JAMA, 199:*1009–1010, 1967.

98. Villani, U.: Concordant tumors of the testicles in monozygotic twins. *Urol Int, 22:*353–365, 1967.

99. Omenn, G.S.: Ectopic polypeptide hormone production by tumors. *Ann Intern Med, 72:*136–138, 1970.

100. Patchefsky, A.S., Solit, R., Phillips, L.D., Craddock, M., Harrer, W.V., Cohn, H.E., and Kowlessar, O.D.: Hydroxyindole-producing tumors of the pancreas: Carcinoid-islet cell tumor and oat cell carcinoma. *Ann Intern Med, 77:*53–61, 1972.

101. Salassa, R.M., Jowsey, J., and Arnaud, C.D.: Hypophosphatemic osteomalacia associated with "nonendocrine" tumors. *N Engl J Med, 283:*65–70, 1970.

102. Jackson, C.E., Tashjian, A.H., and Block, M.A.: Detection of medullary thyroid cancer by calcitonin assay in families. *Ann Intern Med, 78:*845–852, 1973.

103. Wolfe, H.J., Melvin, K.E.W., Cervi-Skinner, S.J., AlSaadi, A.A., Juliar, J.F., Jackson, C.E., and Tashjian, A.H.: C-Cell hyperplasia preceding medullary thyroid carcinoma. *N Engl J Med, 289:*437–441, 1973.

CHAPTER 13

CANCER OF THE LUNG: HOST AND

ENVIRONMENTAL INTERACTION

GEORGE K. TOKUHATA

Host Factor and Environment

TO RECOGNIZE THE role of the host in the etiology of disease the nature and extent of genetic-environmental interaction must be understood. In all probability this concept of interaction applies to the majority of diseases, but is particularly true in chronic degenerative conditions and neoplastic processes. The genetic component which is inherited would differentiate the host resistance and susceptibility either by itself or more often in interaction with the environment to which he is exposed. The constitutional configuration encompassing both genotype and phenotype would determine how and to what extent the host responds to any or all of his environmental stimuli, physical, biological or psychosocial.

The way in which different hosts would react to the external environment can vary between two theoretical extremes. At one end, mutations or gene alterations may impart their effects universally; at the other end, the expression of the genotype may be subtle and influenced strongly by the environmental conditions. Many neoplastic processes are assumed to be at or closer to the latter extreme.

Because of the fact that man's environment is heterogenous and complex, and the majority of the genetically conditioned diseases are likely to involve multiple, rather than single, genes which are subject to modification by a variety of environmental influences, the generalized term "host factor" is often used to denote individual differences in disease susceptibility. In this sense the term "host factor" is interchangeable with that of "constitutional factor" which relates to both genotypic and phenotypic characteristics of the individual. Phenotypic characteristics are the results of genetic-environmental interaction. The interplay between genetic and environmental forces in most instances cannot be clearly delineated, however.

There is also something fundamental in the role of the host. Many diseases, including neoplasms, are sex or age dependent or both. Differences in physiology, particularly the endocrine function, and in social norms and activities between men and women as well as variations in the state of aging process can lead to differential biological processes and pathological manifestations under certain environmental conditions.

Many environmental variations are adaptive while some others may cause changes in the biology of the host in order to accommodate his survival. Those who fail to accommodate such changes may be selected out in the course of evolution. The genetic constitution of the host reacts differently to environmental agents depending upon the nature and intensity of their physiological insults. It is important to recognize that no genotype possesses the ability to withstand all environmental hazards; by the same token, not all aberrant genotypes are always impaired; some aberrant genotypes may benefit by living in certain special environments or by carefully avoiding certain environmental exposures.

The body's homeostasis is limited which

may give rise to the development of a disease including neoplasm. This limitation or threshold in the host defense mechanism, however, varies from one individual to another; thus, exposure to the same environmental risk does not necessarily result in the same impairment of health in all individuals. The operation of the host factor, more often than not, would increase or decrease the susceptibility of a given individual to a disease which can be shown to be induced primarily by an environmental factor or agent.

Carcinogenesis is a complex process which usually involves both host factors and specific environmental agents or conditions. Some agents by themselves cause irreversible alterations in cells which may lead to the malignant transformation or the production of cancer when other requirements, yet to be identified, are met, while others may primarily promote the carcinogenic process which was initiated by some other mechanism within a genetically susceptible host.[1] All forms of malignancy, if they originate in a genetic carrier, may be classified as "prezygotic."

In view of the great variety of carcinogens in our environment including many chemicals and physical properties, it is reasonable to assume that cancer may result from some change within the somatic cell. In this sense any mutagenic agent could be carcinogenic, provided the mutagenic action is extended over many mitotic cycles. Several investigators have suggested that the chemical carcinogen works by activating or by causing a mutation in a latent virus.[2-3]

While the importance of the host factor in cancer is well recognized, it is generally agreed that the time of onset of neoplastic disease is not very strictly determined genetically because of the heterogenous environmental exposure of different hosts. It is also generally held that the organ site at which a tumor is likely to develop is largely

under genetic control. It should also be recognized that certain environmental factors, as conventionally considered, may in fact have a significant genetic underlay, and that such factors, when combined with some other host factors, could produce a powerful synergistic interaction in the etiology of cancer.

Epidemiology of Lung Cancer

Statistical data from a large number of countries in different parts of the world have for some years been showing a notable and steady increase in age-adjusted mortality from cancer of the lung. In some countries, e.g. England and Wales, the increase appears to have started at least 40 years ago; in others, such as Japan and Chile, it has been noted only during the last decade or two.[4]

Although part of the increase in lung cancer must be ascribed to improved diagnosis in recent years, it is generally agreed that in many countries the greater part of the observed increase is real. It is clear that lung cancer now represents a major health hazard in many countries. A number of studies have been conducted in search of the etiology of lung cancer. For the purpose of our present discussion, only a limited number of such studies will be reviewed briefly.

Cigarette Smoking

The relationship between cigarette smoking and lung cancer has been the major focus of research attention during the past two decades. At least 29 major retrospective studies and seven large prospective studies have firmly established a statistical association between cigarette smoking and lung cancer in man. Despite the fact that statistical methods cannot establish proof of a causal relationship in an association, the Advisory Committee to the Surgeon General of the U.S. Public Health Service has concluded that cigarette smoking is a major causal factor in human lung cancer.[5]

However, a number of investigators, though accepting the existence of a statistical association, have questioned its significance in terms of causal hypothesis. Some of these doubts have been on the basis of a possible *genetic underlay* which might determine both smoking and lung cancer.[6] Others have supported some type of constitutional theory[7-10] or have claimed that the observed associations are *spurious* because of selection biases in the design of study.[11] Also, many experiments on inhalation of cigarette smoke in animals have failed to produce a single cancer similar to the most prevalent type of lung cancer in humans.[12]

The fact that a small but not insignificant proportion of lung cancer cases does occur among nonsmokers clearly indicates the presence of other etiological factors. The inability to account for the higher lung cancer incidence in the lower economic classes entirely by differences in smoking habits also suggests the existence of other causal variables. Several environmental factors have been implicated.

Occupational Hazards

Certain occupations have been identified as being hazardous with respect to the incidence of lung cancer. For example, evidence was found for an excess of lung cancer mortality among chromate workers and nickel processing workers in refineries.[13-14] Among uranium miners an excess risk has also been indicated.[15] In addition, significant excess of lung cancer deaths has been reported among coal gas workers[16] and asbestos workers[17] in England. In other studies in the U.S. asbestos insulation workers were found to have a seven to eight times greater risk of dying from bronchogenic carcinoma.[18-19]

The evidence for possible importance of arsenic as a factor in the causation of lung cancer has been evaluated by Hueper.[20] The major points of evidence cited include (a) the universality of arsenic in many ores and in the atmosphere in and near smelters, (b) the widespread use of arsenic as an insecticide and the consequent exposure of workers in insecticide manufacture, agricultural workers, and those handling or consuming crops with arsenic residues, and (c) reports of a relatively high incidence of lung cancer in people living around smelters processing arsenic containing ores.

Investigation of cancer incidence among Japanese industrial employees resulted in a significant finding that exposure to kerosene and other petroleum by-products may increase the risk of lung cancer.[21] In a prospective study of white males employed in beryllium extracting companies Mancuso[22] found a much greater rate of lung cancer particularly among those who had prior chemical diseases of the respiratory system.

Two important points should be brought to attention in evaluating the significance of these occupational hazards to lung cancer. First, the population exposed to industrial carcinogens is relatively small and these agents, therefore, cannot fully account for the increasing lung cancer risk in the general population. Second, smoking histories are not usually obtained in studies of industrial hazards; therefore, the role of smoking of itself or as a contributing factor in the presence of industrial carcinogens cannot be assessed properly.

Modernization and Air Pollution

In all countries where detailed studies of lung cancer have been undertaken, the incidence has been higher in urban than in rural areas. Having allowed for any possible influence of the difference in smoking habits, there still remain some urban/rural differences in lung cancer rate which cannot be fully explained. Several investigators have noted a gradient among nonsmokers, light cigarette smokers and pipe smokers by density of population, but no gradient among heavy smokers.[23] These data suggest that there is an important *urban* factor, yet to be identified, in the production of lung cancer. Differing standards of diagnosis, different occupational exposures, and the effect of air pollution have been put forward as contributing factors in relation to the *urban* factor.

Among chemicals known to be carcinogenic in animals, benzpyrene and other polycyclic hydrocarbons have been thought by many to be particularly important. These compounds come mainly from the incomplete combustion of coal and from the exhausts of internal combustion engines. Air pollution due to these and other industrial sources could be a factor of some importance in the etiology of lung cancer, but its importance is generally considered to be much less than that of cigarette smoking. Stocks[24] has estimated that approximately two thirds to three fourths of the lung cancer deaths in men would result from cigarette smoking and the remaining from air pollution and possibly other factors. His estimates have not been substantiated, however.

Less direct evidence has been presented in other studies that lung cancer death rate is higher among migrants from Great Britain to New Zealand, South Africa and Australia, respectively,[25–26] and that migration of rural people into urban areas subjects them to lung cancer risk greater than for lifetime urban residents.[27] Again, interpretation of these data in reference to urban living and air pollution is difficult; obviously many factors are involved.

Previous Respiratory Infections

Relatively few well designed studies have been reported in which the effect of prior respiratory disease, particularly infections, on the development of lung cancer was directly evaluated. In a retrospective study of the smoking lung cancer relationship, Doll and Hill[28] included inquiry into a history of previous respiratory infections. They found a significant excess of antecedent chronic bronchitis and pneumonia among lung cancer patients even when the smoking factor was taken into account.

However, Beebe,[29] in his study of World War veterans, found no evidence of an increased lung cancer risk with an antecedent history of influenza, pneumonia or chronic bronchitis, but he did find a significant association between mustard gas exposure and lung cancer. Smoking histories were taken into account in his study.

Recently a statistically significant association was reported between bullous disease of the lung and cancer of the lung in a chest disease of the lung and cancer of the lung in a chest disease screening program.[30] In contrast, the examination of the past illness histories of lung cancer patients for comparison with control subjects in another recent study did not support the hypothesis that prior illness patterns might be predictive.[31]

The observations on previous respiratory illnesses in relation to lung cancer are too few in number to draw any definitive conclusions at present. Ascertainment of accurate and complete data on such variables, particularly in a retrospective study, would be extremely difficult.

Experimental Observations

Lung cancer has been induced in animals by radioactive substances,[32] by chemical carcinogens,[33] and by air pollutants plus influenza virus.[34] These studies have demonstrated the occurrence of extensive atypical hyperplastic changes in the bronchial epithelium of experimental animals preceding the appearance of lung cancer. These cellular changes are generally similar to those seen in the bronchial epithelium of heavy cigarette smokers. The hyperplastic lesions in animals do not invariably develop into cancer, however. This appears to be the case also in man.[35]

The susceptibility of various tissues to chemically induced tumor formation is also influenced, to some degree, by the metabolism of the tissue, thus by aging process, and by hormonal factors as evidenced by higher tissue susceptibility in female mice. Female mice are more susceptible to pulmonary metastases from tumors originating in other organ sites than male mice. In contrast, primary lung tumors occur with greater frequency in male mice.[36]

There have also been several reports linking pulmonary tumor susceptibility to specific genes in inbred strains of mice.[37-38] These investigators have demonstrated that genetic factors exert a determining influence on the spontaneous development and induction of lung tumors (adenomas) in mice. The relative importance of genes for susceptibility to these lung tumors is indicated by an incidence ranging from a few tumors to over 90 percent, depending on the inbred strain examined.

Lung Cancer and Smoking in Families

Although the possible importance of genetic factors in lung cancer has long been speculated upon,[39-54] direct evidence of its role in a human population has not been reported. Data indicating the presence of significant familial aggregation of lung cancer, while allowing for the effects of cigarette smoking and other important environmental factors, would provide some suggestive evidence. Tokuhata conducted such a study in Baltimore in which both the history of lung cancer and of smoking habits were evaluated in detail over three generations, beginning with the probands and control index subjects and extending to their parents, siblings, and offspring. Data on the spouses of the index subjects were also ascertained for comparative purposes. Complete details of this study have been reported elsewhere.[55-59]

In the present report we shall discuss some of the data from this study in the light of host and environmental interaction, and present the results of statistical tests for a genetic hypothesis on smoking using new, unreported data from the same study. On the basis of the major findings of our study, together with the results of other studies, a new genetic hypothesis was formulated in the etiology of human lung cancer and smoking.

Familial Aggregation of Lung Cancer

To determine the presence of familial aggregation of lung cancer, the lung cancer mortality among relatives of a group of 270 lung cancer probands was compared with that of relatives of a comparable group of 270 individuals selected as index controls. In this comparison the effects of several host and environmental factors such as cigarette smoking, sex, age, and generation (category of relatives) were taken into account.

As shown in Table 13-I, the observed mortality of lung cancer was greater than expected in all categories of the proband relatives, including both males and females as well as both smokers and nonsmokers. The overall difference for all relatives being considered together was statistically significant, indicating that the proband relatives had a significantly increased risk of dying from lung cancer either in association with, or independently of, the history of cigarette smoking. As an indication of the possible influence of the environmental factor common to members of married couples, spouses of the probands and those of the index controls were compared with respect to lung cancer mortality. There were no significant differences in such mortality among the spouses; this was true for both wives and husbands of the index subjects.

Since the index controls were selected within the adjacent residential neighborhood and the majority of the relatives were also residing in the same geographic areas, the possible effects on lung cancer of such additional environmental factors as atmospheric pollution, socioeconomic status and ethnic background are assumed to be fairly homogeneous. From the totality of these observations it would appear that some inherent biological factor plays an important role in the etiology of lung cancer in man.

Another suggestive evidence in support of the implicated genetic hypothesis in human lung cancer was also presented by Tokuhata who conducted a similar study in New York State.[60] He compared lung cancer mortality rates between blood relatives of lung cancer patients admitted to the Roswell Park Memorial Institute and those

of comparable noncancer patients admitted to the same Institute. The history of smoking on these relatives was not obtained, however.

Familial Aggregation of Smoking Habits

Familial aggregation of smoking habits was analyzed differently because of the fact that data were not initially ascertained through smoking history. It has been well established that lung cancer patients are much more likely to be cigarette smokers than those who do not have such disease. Our analysis was focused on three separate, but related questions: (a) Are the relatives of the lung cancer probands also more likely to be smokers than the counterparts of the controls? (b) Is the smoking pattern in the families of the lung cancer group different from that of the control group? (c) Is there a clear association between the smoking habits of offspring and that of parents? To answer these questions we employed several different methods that have been developed in epidemiology and human genetics.

Lung Cancer Proband Families Compared with Control Families: The inter-familial aggregation of smokers was determined by comparing the actually observed number of

TABLE 13-I
NUMBER OF RELATIVES AND OBSERVED AND EXPECTED NUMBERS OF LUNG CANCER
DEATHS AMONG SMOKERS AND NONSMOKERS OF THE PROBAND RELATIVES

Proband Relatives	Nonsmokers			Smokers			Smokers and Nonsmokers		
	No. of Relatives	Obs. No. of Lung Ca.	Exp. No. of Lung Ca.	No. of Relatives	Obs. No. of Lung Ca.	Exp. No. of Lung Ca.	No. of Relatives	Obs. No. of Lung Ca.	Exp. No. of Lung Ca.
Mothers	259	5	2.0	7	0	0.0	266	5	2.0
Sisters	405	3	1.2	155	0	0.0	560	3	1.2
All Females	664	8	3.2	162	0	0.0	826	8	3.2
Fathers	190	3	0.0	70	2	1.1	260	5	1.1
Brothers	188	1	0.0	350	21	9.0	538	22	9.0
All Males	378	4	0.0	420	23	10.1	798	27	10.1
Total	1,042	12	3.2	582	23	10.1	1,624	35	13.3

smokers among the blood relatives of the lung cancer probands with the number of smokers that would be expected as calculated by applying the age-sex-generation specific proportion of smokers found in the control

TABLE 13-II
OBSERVED AND EXPECTED NUMBERS OF CIGARETTE SMOKERS AMONG PROBAND RELATIVES*

Category of Relatives	Number of Relatives	Number of Smokers	
		Observed	*Expected***
Fathers	261	70	58.4
Brothers	560	363	322.5
Sons	215	141	150.8
All Males	1,036	574	531.7
Mothers	268	7	5.4
Sisters	585	160	129.9
Daughters	199	116	91.1
All Females	1,052	283	226.4
Parents	529	77	63.8
Siblings	1,145	523	452.4
Offspring	414	257	241.9
All Relatives	2,088	857	758.1

*Those with unknown smoking status, unknown ages, or those under 20 years of age are excluded.
**Computed on the basis of the age-specific smoking proportion of the control relatives.

relatives. This method was used in order to take into account possible differences in the sex, age, and generation factors of the two family populations which may be related to the smoking habits.

As shown in Table 13-II, the observed number was significantly greater than expected in both sexes, i.e. both male and female relatives of the probands manifested a greater risk of being smokers than those of the controls. The data further showed that this excess frequency of smokers was actually accounted for by the siblings of the index subjects. A similar trend was also observed among parents and children; however, the difference was not statistically significant.

Index Subjects in Relation to Their Relatives: The intra-familial aggregation of smokers was determined by comparing the proportion of smokers among those relatives whose index subjects are also smokers with that among those relatives whose index subjects are nonsmokers. This comparison was made in each of the proband and control

TABLE 13-III
PERCENTAGE OF CIGARETTE SMOKERS AMONG RELATIVES ACCORDING TO CIGARETTE SMOKING STATUS AND PROBAND-CONTROL IDENTITY OF THE INDEX SUBJECTS

Category of Relatives	Proband Group		Control Group		Combined Group	
	Index Subjects, Smokers	*Index Subjects, Nonsmokers*	*Index Subjects, Smokers*	*Index Subjects, Nonsmokers*	*Index Subjects, Smokers*	*Index Subjects, Nonsmokers*
Father	27.9	15.0	30.4	12.0	28.9	12.5
Mother	2.8	0.0	3.1	0.0	2.9	0.0
Brother	65.0	62.9	66.9	46.7	65.7	49.0
Sister	27.6	20.7	27.4	14.1	27.5	15.0
Son	66.0	63.0	72.8	67.6	68.7	66.7
Daughter	58.3	58.3	47.1	42.3	53.7	45.3
All Males	55.7	51.2	58.3	43.1	56.7	44.4
All Females	26.8	27.4	24.7	17.5	26.0	19.1
All Parents	15.2	7.5	16.7	6.0	15.8	6.2
All Siblings	45.8	43.8	47.6	31.5	46.4	33.2
All Offspring	62.3	60.8	60.2	55.0	61.4	56.2
Total	41.1	40.0	41.8	30.7	41.3	32.2

Note: Percentage of smokers is computed against those for whom smoking information is available.

family populations as well as in the combined population.

The data in Table 13-III clearly indicate that, within the combined population, there is significant aggregation of smokers in families. Specifically, those parents and siblings whose index subjects are smokers are much more likely to be smokers than those whose index subjects are nonsmokers. Although more than twice as large a proportion of the male as the female relatives are actually smokers, the same mode of aggregation was revealed in both sexes.

The data also show a striking difference when the proband and control families were considered separately. As mentioned earlier, the overall frequency of smokers among the proband relatives was significantly greater than that among the control relatives. No such relationship was found among the spouses of the index subjects.

It should be noted that about 40 percent of the proband relatives reported a history of regular smoking regardless of the smoking status of the index subjects. This generally increased and *diffuse* frequency of smokers among the proband relatives suggests that there may be something inherent in the biological makeup common to all blood relatives of the probands which is related to the habit of smoking. Environmental influences in the induction of smoking habit, if it existed, cannot explain this observation at least within the lung cancer proband families.

It has been pointed out that the control relatives were much less likely to be smokers than the proband relatives as a whole. The data further show that approximately 40 percent of those control relatives whose index subjects were smokers, as compared with about 30 percent of those control

TABLE 13-IV
NUMBER AND PERCENTAGE OF CIGARETTE SMOKERS AMONG OFFSPRING ACCORDING
TO PARENTAL MATING TYPE ON SMOKING HABITS

Parental Mating Type	Number of Families	Male Offspring			Female Offspring			All Offspring		
		Total	Smokers	Percent Smokers	Total	Smokers	Percent Smokers	Total	Smokers	Percent Smokers
Both Smokers	7	16	15	93.8	14	11	78.6	30	26	86.7
One Smoker	171	509	380	74.7	412	119	28.9	921	499	54.2
Neither Smoker	85	274	196	71.5	171	42	24.6	445	238	53.5
Total (Proband Families)	263*	799	591	74.0	597	172	28.8	1,396	763	54.7
Both Smokers	5	14	13	92.9	11	6	54.5	25	19	76.0
One Smoker	152	413	258	62.5	268	73	27.2	681	331	48.6
Neither Smoker	110	333	184	55.3	213	28	13.1	546	212	38.8
Total (Control Families)	267**	760	455	59.9	492	107	21.7	1,252	562	44.9
Both Smokers	12	30	28	93.3	25	17	68.0	55	45	81.8
One Smoker	323	922	638	69.2	680	192	28.2	1,602	830	51.8
Neither Smoker	195	607	380	62.6	384	70	18.2	991	450	45.4
Total (Combined Families)	530	1,559	1,046	67.1	1,089	279	25.6	2,648	1,325	50.0

* Seven families are excluded.
** Three families are excluded.
Notes: (a) Offspring includes index subjects and their siblings 20 years of age or over.
(b) Occasional smokers are considered as nonsmokers.
(c) Siblings whose smoking information or parental smoking information is not available are excluded.

relatives whose index subjects were non-smokers, were actually smokers; a difference which is statistically significant. This *selective* intra-familial aggregation of smokers may be due to genetic factors, or common environmental factors, or more likely to be due to both.

Parents in Relation to Offspring: The pattern of smoking habit was analyzed in a more direct *parent-offspring* construct. Since a number of children of the index subjects under study were still younger than 20 years, this generation was not included. The data for this analysis, therefore, pertain to the older generations, i.e. parents and siblings of the index subjects. More specifically, siblings of the index subjects plus index subjects themselves constitute offspring.

As shown in Table 13-IV, the relative frequency of matings in which both parents are smokers was about the same in the proband and control groups. The like frequency in which one parent is a smoker was slightly greater in the proband group. In contrast, matings in which neither parent is a smoker was much more common in the control group. There was a high degree of statistical association between the parental smoking habits and the smoking habits of their offspring. Specifically, in both the proband and control families, offspring are much more likely to be smokers when parents are in fact smokers; this is particularly true when both parents are smokers. An additional analysis indicated that the average age of the parents did not differ appreciably according to their mating type with respect to smoking.

The difference between one parent smoker and neither parent smoker groups in the proportion of offspring who smoke was relatively small, and the actual proportions in these two groups were much smaller when compared with the proportion in the both parents smoker group. The relative frequency

of smokers among the male offspring according to the parental mating type was generally less variable than that among the female offspring. From the statistical association such as shown here, it is not possible to clearly differentiate the source of influence between genetic factors and familial environmental factors, however.

Testing a Genetic Hypothesis on Smoking

Although smoking habit is considered by many observers as being influenced by environmental factors, there is sufficient evidence to suggest that genetic factors may also play a significant role in the induction of such habits.[61-65] At present neither the acquired nor the inherited factor in smoking is completely understood.

It is conceivable that smokers and non-smokers are genotypically different, and that the underlying inherent factor, presumably common to all smokers, could be so expressed phenotypically as to be detectable by conventional methods of analysis used in population genetics. In testing a genetic hypothesis it is necessary to make an *a priori* assumption regarding the mode of inheritance of the trait under investigation. For the purpose of the present analysis we formulated a working hypothesis that the smoking habit is an expression of a simple, autosomal recessive trait. The data subjected to this analysis were also derived from the same familial study of lung cancer and smoking conducted by Tokuhata.

To test the recessive hypothesis stated above, the statistical data were arranged in the following order. First, we selected from the original index subjects those who were smokers; second, among such smokers we further selected those neither of whose parents was a smoker; and third, we then identified smokers in each sibship. This procedure was applied to each of the proband and control groups as well as to the combined group. Since each family was ascertained through one index subject who was a smoker, the criterion of "single ascertainment through affected individuals (smokers) whose parents are not affected (nonsmokers)" might be justified.

The number of sibships finally included, the number of smokers, the total number of individuals, the estimate of segregation ratio, and the significance test in each of the two and combined groups of families are given in Table 13-V.

An estimate of the segregation ratio was computed according to the Weinberg-Fisher method[66] in which correction was made for an inflated selection bias. Specifically, families with no smokers were not observed, which would result in a considerable inflation in the proportion of homozygous recessives. The estimate of proportion was 0.264 in the proband families, 0.219 in the control families, and 0.244 in the combined families. All of these estimates, particularly the combined average, correspond very closely to the theoretically expected value of 0.250; these observations are consistent with the recessive hypothesis being tested.

Because of the fact that the index control subjects were those who did not have lung cancer and were selected without any prior knowledge of their smoking habits, we assumed that the relative frequency of smokers in these families may not deviate significantly from that for all families in the general population. To this extent, we might be justified in employing the assumption of "complete ascertainment through affected individuals (smokers) whose parents are not affected (nonsmokers)." Under this assumption another test for the same recessive hypothesis was made.

The data pertaining to the control families were rearranged in such a way that the observed and expected numbers of smokers could be compared according to the size of family. The expected number was computed by the Lenz-Hogben method.[67] As shown in Table 13-VI, the overall observed number of smokers was only slightly larger than would be expected, but the difference was well within the limit of random variation. Again, the result of this analysis is consistent with the recessive hypothesis being tested.

In evaluating the results of these tests for a genetic hypothesis, several points should

TABLE 13-V
ESTIMATE OF SEGREGATION RATIO FOR SMOKING (BASED ON AUTOSOMAL, RECESSIVE HYPOTHESIS): SINGLE ASCERTAINMENT THROUGH SMOKERS WHOSE BOTH PARENTS ARE NONSMOKERS

	(N)	(R)	(T)	(P)	(σ^2)	(σ)	95% Confidence Limits:	
Family Group	No. of Sibships	No. of Smokers	Total No. of Individuals	Estimated Proportion of Smokers*	Variance of Proportion	Standard Error	Upper	Limit
Controls	58	100	250	0.219	0.000890	0.029	0.277	0.161
Probands	74	139	320	0.264	0.000790	0.028	0.320	0.208
Combined	132	239	570	0.244	0.000421	0.021	0.286	0.202

*Proportion of smokers was estimated according to the following Weinberg-Fisher method: (R.A. Fisher, "Effect of Methods of Ascertainment upon Estimation of Frequencies," *Ann Eugen*, London, 6:13–25, 1934)

$$P = \frac{R - N}{T - N}$$ R = No. of smokers. T = Total No. of individuals. N = Number of sibships considered.

Variance (σ^2) was computed according to the following method:

$$\sigma^2 = \frac{PQ}{T - N} \quad \text{where} \quad Q = 1 - P$$

TABLE 13-VI
OBSERVED AND EXPECTED NUMBERS OF SMOKERS ACCORDING TO SIZE OF SIBSHIP
(BASED ON AUTOSOMAL, RECESSIVE HYPOTHESIS): COMPLETE ASCERTAINMENT
THROUGH SMOKERS WHOSE BOTH PARENTS ARE NONSMOKERS

Size of Sibship (S)	No. of Sibships (N_s)	Total No. of Individuals ($S \times N_s$)	Observed Smokers	Expected Smokers (R)*	Variance ($\sigma_R{}^2$)
2	7	14	9	8.000	0.8572
3	8	24	8	10.378	2.1038
4	10	40	13	14.628	4.2005
5	7	35	11	11.472	3.5125
6	8	48	19	14.598	6.2076
7	5	35	15	10.098	4.8512
8	1	8	3	2.223	1.1724
9	1	9	5	2.433	1.3802
Total	47	213	83	73.830	24.2854

Notes: (a) Data from control families.
(b) Sibships of size one were excluded.
*Computed according to the Lenz-Hogben formula (J.B.S. Haldane, "Method for Investigating Recessive Characters in Man," *J Genet, 25*:251–255, 1932)

$$R = \sum \frac{sp}{1 - q^s} N_s \qquad \sigma_R{}^2 = \sum N_s \left[\frac{spq}{1 - q^s} - \frac{s^2 p^2 q^2}{(1 - q^s)^2} \right]$$

$$P = \tfrac{1}{4} \qquad q = 1 - p = \tfrac{3}{4}$$

95% confidence limits on the expected number:

Upper limit = 73.83 + 9.64 = 83.47
Lower limit = 73.83 − 9.64 = 64.19

be kept in mind. First, there is no completely satisfactory single technique currently available with which to test genetic hypotheses on the smoking habit. The primary methodological difficulty is that of inability to delineate the nature and extent of environmental influences.

Second, although we have tested a simple, autosomal, recessive hypothesis, and the data we used appear to fit the theoretical model, other genetic hypotheses can also be formulated. Lilienfeld[68] has also cautioned that nongenetic characteristics can fit a simple recessive mode of inheritance, particularly when data are derived from a relatively small sample.

Third, if smokers and nonsmokers are genotypically different, it is conceivable that the genotype associated with the smoking habit may be pleiotropic having multiple phenotypic expressions. In other words, smoking in such a person may represent only one of several socially related habits, e.g. alcoholism, drug dependence, and certain behavioral characteristics such as neuroticism.[69-70]

Fourth, entertaining a genetic hypothesis in smoking one recognizes that there is a problem of sex difference. This is important particularly because of apparent dimorphism with respect to both smoking and lung cancer. It should be noted, however, that both men and women are equally liable to lung cancer if they are nonsmokers, but men are more liable than women if they are smokers. No simple explanation is available for the difference among smokers. It may be that men smoke more than do women. It is also possible that such a difference may be due to certain physiological (e.g. hormone) or biochemical makeup of men and women. In testing the recessive hypothesis on smoking we were unable to separate the data by sex mainly due to limited sample size.

Fifth, in the absence of needed information to determine the validity of many assumptions usually required in testing genetic hypotheses, such as "random mating," "equal probability of ascertainment," "equal environmental influence," etc., the results of our genetic analyses of smoking remain inconclusive. However, our data should provide a preliminary basis for further epidemiologic-genetic studies of human populations, hopefully of larger sizes.

Interaction between Smoking and and Family History of Lung Cancer

Our study has indicated that the importance of inherent biological predisposition to lung cancer is nearly equal to that of cigarette smoking which has been known to be the most significant single factor. Therefore, a separate, and more detailed analysis was made in order to identify the relative liability of each of these two significant factors under different circumstances, and also to evaluate how the risk of lung cancer mortality can change according to the presence or absence of these two factors in the same individual.

Specifically, we first compared the difference in lung cancer mortality between the proband and control relatives among smokers and nonsmokers separately. We then compared the difference in lung cancer mortality between smokers and nonsmokers within the proband and control groups separately. The former analysis made it possible to estimate the effect of the familial host factor upon cancer of the lung in the absence of cigarette smoking, whereas the latter made it possible to estimate the influence of cigarette smoking on the same disease in the absence of the familial host factor. The results of these analyses are summarized in Table 13-VII.

When the influence of cigarette smoking was held constant, the relative lung cancer mortality among the proband relatives was 4.0 times greater than that among the control relatives. Likewise, in the absence of familial host factor, the relative lung cancer mortality among cigarette smokers was 5.3 times greater than that among nonsmokers. These results suggest that the relative importance of cigarette smoking in the pathogenesis of cancer of the lung is slightly greater than that of the host susceptibility to lung cancer. In terms of the actual risk of lung cancer mortality the influence of smoking is approximately 32 percent greater.

When only cigarette smokers were considered, the lung cancer mortality was 2.6 times greater in the proband group than in the control group, whereas among nonsmokers it was four times greater in the proband than in the control group. This suggests that the familial host factor was more evident or discriminative in the absence of the influence of cigarette smoking.

Within the proband group, those relatives who smoked, as compared with those who did not, had 3.4 times a greater lung cancer mortality, whereas within the control group those relatives who smoked had a 5.3 times greater mortality. In other words, the relative

TABLE 13-VII

PERCENTAGE OF LUNG CANCER DEATHS AMONG RELATIVES ACCORDING TO CIGARETTE SMOKING AND PROBAND-CONTROL STATUS, AND RELATIVE RISK OF LUNG CANCER MORTALITY IN TERMS OF PROBAND/CONTROL RATIO AND SMOKER/NONSMOKER RATIO

| Family Group | Relatives | | | Ratio (Smokers/Nonsmokers) |
	Smokers	Nonsmokers	Total	
Probands	3.82%	1.11%	2.08%	3.4 (fold)
Controls	1.47%	0.28%	0.65%	5.3 (fold)
Total	2.78%	0.70%		4.0 (fold)
Ratio (Probands/Controls)	2.6 (fold)	4.0 (fold)	3.2 (fold)	

TABLE 13-VIII
LUNG CANCER MORTALITY RATIO AND RELATIVE LIABILITY AMONG RELATIVES
ACCORDING TO CIGARETTE SMOKING AND FAMILIAL HISTORY OF LUNG CANCER

Family Group	Individual Characteristics		Population at Risk	Lung Cancer Deaths	Mortality Ratio per 1,000	Relative Liability
	Cigarette Smoking	*Familial History*				
Probands (A)	Yes	Yes	602	23	38.2	13.64
Controls (B)	Yes	No	475	7	14.7	5.25
Probands (C)	No	Yes	1,080	12	11.1	3.96
Controls (D)	No	No	1,055	3	2.8	1.00

lung cancer mortality in association with cigarette smoking was almost twice in the control what it was in the proband relatives. Several possible explanations may follow: (a) The control relatives, presumably lacking the host susceptibility to lung cancer, were more *sensitive* to the carcinogenic effect of cigarette smoking, or these relatives had a more clear effect of cigarette smoking without being clouded by the familial host factor. (b) The proband relatives, being influenced by the familial factor responsible for the common host susceptibility to lung cancer, did not produce as much difference in the lung cancer mortality due to cigarette smoking.

Another way of presenting the relative influence of, and mutual relationship or interaction between these two factors is to determine the lung cancer mortality in the following four groups of relatives: (A) those proband relatives who smoked; (B) those control relatives who smoked; (C) those proband relatives who did not smoke; and (D) those control relatives who did not smoke.

These four groups of relatives were compared in terms of relative liability as expressed in the ratio of percent lung cancer deaths with the use of group D, the lowest risk group, as a common base. As shown in Table 13-VIII, group A had a 13.6 times greater relative liability and the relative liability decreased to 5.3 times in group B and 4.0 times in group C. The direction of differences in the lung cancer mortality was quite consistent in each sex as well as in each parent and sibling category.

The distribution of these relative liability ratios among the four groups of relatives seems to form an exponential-like curve, rather than a linear one, which suggests that the combined risk of cigarette smoking and the familial host factor are multiplicative or synergistic, rather than additive.

Measure of Interaction between Study Factors

One of the most difficult, and often neglected, methodological problems in analyzing multiple factors of possible etiologic importance is the method of evaluating interaction of two or more such factors with respect to the disease under investigation. Few specific statistical techniques for this purpose have been discussed in this context. In the following we have illustrated one such technique in which two such factors were related to each other. A more detailed discussion of multiple causality in chronic disease, together with some suggested statistical methods of analysis has been presented elsewhere.[71]

For the purpose of our discussion, let us consider cancer of the lung as the disease under investigation. Let us also choose two specific factors, cigarette smoking and urban living, both of which have been found to be associated with cancer of the lung. In addition, we assume that both cases (lung cancer patients) and controls (persons without lung cancer) are representative groups in a general population.

As illustrated in Figure 13–1, each of the selected groups of cases and controls can be distributed in a 2 × 2 contingency table. Specifically, in the case group a person who smokes is denoted as "A" as compared with a person who does not smoke being denoted as "a"; likewise, a person who lives in the urban area is marked as "B" as compared

with a person who does not live in the urban area being marked as "b." Thus, "AB" persons represent those lung cancer patients who smoke cigarettes and live in the urban area; "Ab" persons represent those patients who smoke, but do not live in the urban area; "aB" persons represent those patients who do not smoke, but live in the urban area; and "ab" persons represent those patients who neither smoke nor live in the urban area.

In the control group a similar 2 × 2 contingency table would be established. In this group a person who smokes is labeled as "A′" in contrast to "a′", a nonsmoker; "B′" a person who lives in the urban area in contrast to "b′," a nonurban resident. According to these markings, "A′B′" persons would represent those control subjects who smoke cigarettes and live in the urban area; "A′b′" those control subjects who smoke, but do not live in the urban area; "a′B′" those control subjects who do not smoke, but live in the urban area; and "a′b′" those control subjects who neither smoke nor live in the urban area.

The question before us is *whether or not there is an "interaction" between cigarette smoking (A factor) and urban living (B factor) with respect to lung cancer.*

If combination of "A" and "B" factors produces a "booster" or "synergistic" effect in the pathogenesis of lung cancer, "A" and "B" should be more closely related within the case group than within the control group. Therefore, the degree of association between "A" and "B" in the case group would be greater than that between "A′" and "B′" in the control group.

The degree of this association within the case group can be measured as (AB)(ab)/(aB)(Ab). Likewise, the degree of same association within the control group can be measured as (A′B′)(a′b′)/(a′B′)(A′b′).

Thus, an estimated measure of "interaction" between cigarette smoking and urban

Cases (with disease)

		(present)	(absent)
		A	B
(present)	B	AB	aB
(absent)	b	Ab	ab

Controls (without disease)

		(present)	(absent)
		A′	a′
(present)	B′	A′B′	a′B′
(absent)	b′	A′b′	a′b′

AB (or A′B′) – Those with both A and B characteristics.
Ab (or A′B′) – Those with only A characteristic.
aB (or a′B′) – Those with only B characteristics
ab (or a′b′) – Those with neither characteristics

Figure 13–1

living in relation to lung cancer can be expressed as follows:

$$\frac{(AB)(ab)}{(aB)(Ab)} \bigg/ \frac{(A'B')(a'b')}{(a'B')(A'b')} = \frac{(AB)(ab)(a'B')(A'b')}{(aB)(Ab)(A'B')(a'b')}$$

To test significance of this "interaction," an adjusted Chi square value (d.f. = 1) may be computed according to the following formula:

$$\frac{(|AB - A'B'| - \frac{1}{2})^2}{A'B'} + \frac{(|Ab - A'b'| - \frac{1}{2})^2}{A'b'}$$

$$+ \frac{(|aB - a'B'| - \frac{1}{2})^2}{a'B'} + \frac{(|ab - a'b'| - \frac{1}{2})^2}{a'b'}$$

where:

$$AB + Ab + aB + ab = A'B' + A'b' + a'B' + a'b'$$

How the familial history of lung cancer (probable genetic host factor) and cigarette smoking "interact" with each other in the pathogenesis of lung cancer can also be evaluated by the same procedure described above. In this evaluation, the following four groups of individuals would be identified in a 2×2 contingency table for each of the case and control groups; "those with a suspected genetic factor who also smoke cigarettes"; "those with a suspected genetic factor who do not smoke"; "those without a suspected genetic factor who smoke cigarettes"; and "those without a suspected genetic factor who do not smoke."

One conceptual complication might emerge in dealing with the smoking factor. That is, those who reject genetic hypotheses of smoking habits would consider this factor as merely "environmental" in nature. However, those who are inclined to support genetic hypotheses may be willing to treat this as either a "genetic" or at least "constitutional host" factor. We consider smoking a "constitutional host" factor in which probably both genetic and environmental influences exist in the induction of the habit, and which also serves as a carcinogenic agent.

Genetic Hypotheses on Lung Cancer and Smoking

In the light of known association between lung cancer and smoking, apparent biological predisposition to lung cancer, and suggestive evidence implicating the role of a constitutional host factor in smoking, several possible genetic hypotheses may be formulated. Undoubtedly, other factors are of etiological importance in cancer of the lung; however, for the purpose of our present

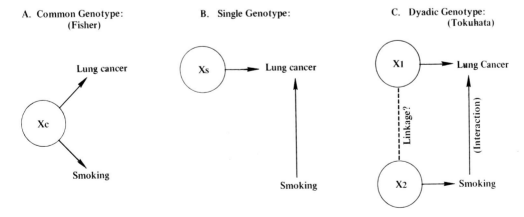

Figure 13–2

discussion such other factors are not considered. Theoretical models of three genetic hypotheses are illustrated in Figure 13–2.

Common Genotype Hypothesis

According to Fisher's "common genotype" hypothesis, smoking and lung cancer may coexist in the same individual without direct causal relationship between them because both smoking habits and lung cancer are phenotypic expressions of a "common genotype." According to his theory, selection of smokers would automatically provide a population in which pulmonary cancer would appear on the basis of genetic susceptibility. Fisher's conclusions were based on the preliminary results of a study of smoking habits among adult twin pairs where the degree of concordance was much higher for the monozygous twins than for the dizygous twins.

Fisher's theory has been challenged by some investigators on the ground that the twin data on which his argument was based were biased, and that the history of cancer in twins whose smoking habits are known has not been documented sufficiently. More data on smoking habits and medical histories are needed regarding other siblings, offspring, and parents. Our data on the familial study of lung cancer and smoking, as discussed earlier, are not consistent with the "common genotype" hypothesis.

Single Genotype Hypothesis

Investigators who accept a genetic hypothesis in lung cancer, but do not agree with Fisher's theory nor with any biological basis for the induction of smoking habits may choose to entertain another alternative, "single genotype" hypothesis. In this theoretical construct a person may inherit certain biological predisposition to lung cancer, and if he is exposed to the influence of a strong environmental agent, such as cigarette smoke, would increase his probability of developing the disease. Actually, this type of hypothesis, in a very broad sense, may be applicable to almost any disease entity. While "single genotype" hypothesis may be acceptable to many investigators, its specificity would be sacrificed when one particular disease, e.g. cancer of the lung, is considered. Furthermore, this type of simple hypothesis cannot adequately explain some of the major findings of our study of lung cancer and smoking in families.

Dyadic Genotype Hypothesis

Based on the results of his familial study of lung cancer and smoking, Tokuhata has formulated a still different hypothesis, "dyadic genotype." The theoretical reasoning behind his hypothesis was derived mainly from his several significant, and specific findings that (a) lung cancer aggregates in families independently of smoking, (b) smoking aggregates in families irrespective of lung cancer, (c) the degree of association between lung cancer and the familial host factor (history of lung cancer in family) is nearly as strong as that between lung cancer and smoking, and (d) the risk of developing lung cancer is the same for both men and women who do not smoke cigarettes.

Tokuhata maintains, further, that there is a strong synergistic interaction, or multiplicative rather than additive effect, between cigarette smoking and the constitutional host susceptibility to lung cancer. The specific mechanism of such interaction (possible genetic linkage or primarily postzygotic phenomenon) is unknown, however. This view on the host-environmental interaction is supported by his findings that those who smoke cigarettes and also have the familial host factor are exposed to a 14-fold greater risk than those who do not have either of the two characteristics, and that the risk decreases for those who smoke without the familial host factor (5-fold) and those who have the familial host factor but do not smoke (4-fold).

These familial statistical data have been employed by Burch[72] to estimate the approximate size of the lung cancer carrier sub-population in the U.S.

Within the theoretical framework of the proposed "dyadic genotype" hypothesis, the following four different phenotypes, as observed in our population, may be explained: (a) "cigarette smokers who develop lung cancer (X_1X_2 genotype)," (b) "cigarette smokers who do not develop lung cancer (X_2 genotype)," (c) "nonsmokers who develop lung cancer (X_1 genotype)," and (d) "nonsmokers who do not develop lung cancer (genotypes without X_1 or X_2)."

From these phenotypic variations the following questions can also be answered: (a) Who is resistant to lung cancer even with the influence of smoking, or why do many smokers not develop lung cancer? (b) Who is liable to lung cancer even without the influence of smoking, or why do some nonsmokers develop lung cancer?

Conclusions

The available data to support the implicated role of a genetic factor in lung cancer and in smoking are still incomplete. In a larger study of the familial aggregation of lung cancer and smoking it would be possible and desirable to analyze separately adenocarcinoma and other types of bronchogenic carcinoma. This would be particularly important because adenocarcinoma is not usually associated with smoking. Future studies of lung cancer and smoking should also consider evaluation of cytogenetic and biochemical characteristics of the implicated genotype.

Although single genes may be involved in a few exceptional neoplastic and preneoplastic states such as retinoblastoma and precancerous colonic polyposis, genes for susceptibility to human cancer are generally assumed to be multiple. Whether multiple genes for susceptibility may also be operating in the case of human lung cancer has not been established. The linkage (in a genetic sense) between multiple genes related to the habit of smoking and cancer of the lung is a theoretical possibility at present. Also, the mode of inheritance or transmission has not been established.

Our present knowledge is still limited regarding the biology of smoking habits. Studies of the characteristics of smokers have been numerous and varied; e.g. physique or somatotype, height and weight and their ratios, musculinity, anthropometric measures, physiological variables, physical activities, and personality types. However, genetics of these characteristics themselves has not been adequately evaluated or determined. Future studies of smoking habits should also consider other related behavioral characteristics such as drinking and drug dependence which may have a common constitutional basis. Furthermore, such studies should be related to the pathogenesis of cancer of the lung within the conteet of a family population.

While the basic biological makeup of an individual may not be conducive to the development of a smoking habit, he may, as often assumed, acquire the habit under a favorable social environment and *vice versa*. However, no study has yet demonstrated the way in which such an apparent environmental influence may reinforce or interfere with the suggested biological susceptibility.

Since cancer of the lung occurs in both men and women who do not smoke, susceptibility genes acting alone or in combination with some exogenous or additional endogenous factors can be effective without exposure to tobacco smoke. The development of lung cancer, therefore, is not invariably linked to hypothetical genes responsible for the habit of smoking. However, as our data have suggested, cigarette smoking may add an extrinsic determinant which can increase the incidence of lung cancer beyond that which would otherwise prevail in the same population. The rising tendency in recent decades of the incidence of lung cancer may be partially due to changing diagnostic practice, but more importantly due probably to changing environment with which the host genotype interacts rather than due to changing genic pool or genome itself. Recent studies of aryl hydrocarbon hydroxylase in lung cancer patients may help elucidate this problem.[73]

REFERENCES

1. Berenblum, I.: A speculative view: The probable nature of promoting action and its significance in the understanding of the mechanism of carcinogenesis. *Cancer Res, 14:*471, 1954.
2. Stanley, W.M.: Biochemistry and biophysics of viruses. *In* Doerr, R., and Hallauer, C. (Eds.): Handbuch der Virusforschung. Springer, Vienna, 1938.
3. Duran-Reynols, F.: Studies on the combined effects of fowl pox virus and methylcholanthrene in chickens. *Ann NY Acad Sci, 54* (6):977, 1952.
4. Epidemiology of Cancer of the Lung. *WHO Techn Rep Ser,* 192, 1960.
5. Smoking and Health: Report of the Advisory Committee to the Surgeon General of the Public Health Service. *Pub Hlth Serv Pub* No. 1103.
6. Fisher, R.A.: Lung cancer and cigarettes? *Nature, 182:*108, 1958.
7. Cohen, J., and Heimann, R.K.: Heavy smokers with low mortality. *Ind Med Surg, 31:*115, 1962.
8. Eastcott, D.F.: The epidemiology of lung cancer in New Zealand. *Lancet, 1:*37, 1956.
9. Haag, H.B., and Hamner, H.R.: Smoking habits and mortality among workers in cigarette factories. *Ind Med Surg, 26:*559, 1957.
10. Rigdon, R.H.: Consideration of the relationship of smoking to lung cancer: With a review of the literature. *South Med J, 50 :* 524, 1957.
11. Berkson, J.: Smoking and lung cancer; some observation on two recent reports. *J Am Stat A, 53:*28, 1958.
12. Little, C.C.: Report of the Scientific Director, Tobacco Industry Research Committee, N.Y., 1957.
13. Seltser, R.: Special report to the Surgeon General's Advisory Committee on Smoking and Health.
14. Taylor, F.H.: The relationship of mortality and duration of employment as reflected by a cohort of chromate workers. *AJPH, 56:* 218, 1966.
15. Wagoner, J.K., Archer, V.E., Carroll, B.E., Holaday, D.A., and Lawrence, P.A.: Cancer mortality patterns among United States uranium miners and millers, 1950 through 1962. *J Natl Cancer Inst* (in press).
16. Doll, R.: The causes of death among gas workers with special reference to cancer of the lung. *Br J Indust Med, 9:*180, 1952.
17. Doll, R.: Mortality from lung cancer in asbestos workers. *Br J Indust Med, 12:*81, 1955.
18. Selikoff, I.J., Hammond, E.C., and Churg, J.: Asbestos exposure, smoking, and neoplasia. *JAMA, 204:*106, 1968.
19. Dunn, J.E., and Weir, J.M.: Cancer experience of several occupational groups followed prospectively. *AJPH, 55:*1367, 1965.
20. Hueper, W.C.: A quest into the environmental causes of cancer of the lung. *Pub Health Monogr.* No. 36, 1955.
21. Tsuchiya, K.: The relation of occupation to cancer, especially cancer of the lung. *Cancer, 18:*136, 1965.
22. Mancuso, T.F.: Relation of duration of em-

ployment and prior respiratory illness to respiratory cancer among beryllium workers. *Environ Res, 3:*251, 1970.

23. Stocks, P., and Campbell, J.M.: Lung cancer death rates among nonsmokers and pipe and cigarette smokers: An evaluation in relation to air pollution by benzpyrene and other substances. *Br Med J, 2:*923, 1955.

24. Stocks, P., and Campbell, J.M. ibid.

25. Dean, G.: Lung cancer in Australia. *Med J Aust, 1:*1003, 1962.

26. Eastcott, D.F.: The comparative mortality experience from cancer of certain sites between indigenous non-Maori population, and immigrants from Great Britain. Report of the British Empire Cancer Campaign (N.Z.), Branch Cancer Registration Scheme, Department of Health, Wellington, N.Z., 1955.

27. Haenszel, W., Loveland, D.B., and Sirkin, M.G.: Lung cancer mortality as related to residence and smoking histories. I. White males. *J Natl Cancer Inst, 28:*947, 1962.

28. Doll, R., and Hill, A.B.: A study of the etiology of carcinoma of the lung. *Br Med J, 2:*1271, 1952.

29. Beebe, G.W.: Lung cancer in World War I veterans: Possible relation to mustard-gas injury and 1918 influenza epidemic. *J Natl Cancer Inst, 25:*1231, 1960.

30. Stoloff, I.L., Karnofsky, P., and Magilner, L.: The risk of lung cancer in males with bullous disease of the lung. *Arch Environ Health, 22:*163, 1971.

31. Stavraky, K.M.: A study of precursor illness in lung cancer patients. *J. Chronic Dis, 23:*691, 1971.

32. Kuschner, M., Laskin, S., Nelson, N., and Altschuler, B.: Radiation induced bronchogenic carcinoma in rats. *Am J Pathol, 34:*554, 1958.

33. Summary of meeting on pathogenesis of lung cancer—Toronto. Special communication to the Surgeon General's Advisory Committee on Smoking and Health.

34. Kotin, P., and Wiseley, D.V.: Production of lung cancer in mice by inhalation exposure to influenza virus and aerosols of hydrocarbons. *Progr Exp Tumor Res, 3:*186, 1963.

35. Auerback, O., Stout, A.P., Hammond, E.C., and Garfinkel, L.: Bronchial epithelium in former smokers. *New Engl J Med, 267:*119, 1962.

36. Markello, R.: Maternal age selection and chemically induced tumors in mice. *Ann NY Acad Sci, 71:*897, 1958.

37. Burdette, W.J.: Induced pulmonary tumors. *J Thorac Surg, 24:*427, 1952.

38. Heston, W.E.: Effects of genes located on chromosomes III, V, VII, IX, and XIV on the occurrence of pulmonary tumors in the mouse. *Proc Intern Genetics Symposia,* Cytologia Suppl. *219:*224, 1937.

39. Joint Report of the Study Group on Smoking and Health: Smoking and Health. *Science, 125:*1129, 1957.

40. Parnell, R.W.: Smoking and cancer. *Lancet, 1:*963, 1951.

41. Heath, C.W.: Differences between smokers and nonsmokers. *AMA Arch Intern Med, 101:*377, 1958.

42. Lilienfeld, A.M.: Emotional and other selected characteristics of cigarette smokers and nonsmokers as related to epidemiological studies of lung cancer and other diseases. *J Natl Cancer Inst, 22:*259, 1959.

43. LeShan, L.: Psychological states as factors in the development of malignant disease: A critical review. *J Natl Cancer Inst, 22:*1, 1959.

44. Rigdon, R.H., and Kirchoff, H.: Cancer of the lung from 1900 to 1930. *Surg Gynecol Obstet, 107:*105, 1958.

45. Platt, R.: Life (biological, not biographical). *Lancet, 1:*61, 1956.

46. Lacassagne, A.: Present-day aspects of research on the etiology of pulmonary tumors; Osler oration. *Can Med Assoc J, 75:*894, 1956.

47. Gsell, O.: Kinishe studien zur etiologie des brnchialkalzinoma. *Deutsch Med Wochonschr, 81:*496, English summary, 553, 1956.

48. Motulsky, A.G.: Drug reactions, enzymes, and biochemical genetics. *JAMA, 165:*835, 1957.

49. Berkson, J.: The statistical study of association between smoking and lung cancer. *Proc Mayo Clinic, 30:*319, 1955.

50. Fisher, R.A.: Cancer and smoking. *Nature* (London), *182:*596, 1958.

51. Friberg, L.: Smoking habits of monozygotic and dizygotic twins. *Br Med J, 1:*1090, 1959.
52. Norton, H.W.: Letter. *American Scientist, 47:* 141, 1959.
53. Goodhart, C.B.: Cancer-proneness and lung cancer. *Practitioner* (London), *182:*578, 1959
54. Shettles, L.B.: Biological sex differences with special reference to disease, resistance, and longevity. *J Obstet Gynecol Br Commonw, 65:*288, 1958.
55. Tokuhata, G.K., and Lilienfeld, A.M.: Familial aggregation of lung cancer in humans. *J Natl Cancer Inst, 30:*289, 1963.
56. Tokuhata, G.K.: Smoking habits in lung-cancer proband families and comparable control families. *J Natl Cancer Inst, 31:*1153, 1963.
57. Tokuhata, G.K.: Familial factors in human lung cancer and smoking. *AJPH, 54:*24, 1964.
58. Tokuhata, G.K.: Familial factors in lung cancer and smoking. *In* Genetics and the Epidemiology of Chronic Diseases. Proceed. of Symposium on Contributions of Genetics to Epidemiologic Studies of Chronic Diseases. *Public Health Serv Pub* No. 1163, U.S. Dept. HEW, 1965.
59. Abelin, T. and Tokuhata, G.K.: Maternal age at birth and susceptibility to lung cancer. *Lancet,* Nov. 27, 1121, 1965.
60. Tokuhata, G.K., and Lilienfeld, A.M.: Familial aggregation of lung cancer among

hospital patients. *Public Health Rep, 78:* 277, 1963.
61. Fisher, R.A.: op cit.
62. Friberg, L.: op cit.
63. Seltzer, C.C.: Why people smoke. *Appl Ther, 4:*1023, 1962.
64. Heath, C.W.: op cit.
65. Parnell, R.W.: op cit.
66. Fisher, R.A.: Effect of methods of ascertainment upon estimation of frequencies. *Ann Eugen* (London), *6:*13, 1934.
67. Haldane, J.B.S.: Method for investigating recessive characters in man. *J Genet, 25:*251, 1932.
68. Lilienfeld, A.M.: A methodological problem in testing a recessive genetic hypothesis in human disease. *AJPH, 49:*199, 1959.
69. Lilienfeld, A.M.: op cit.
70. Kissen, D.M.: The significance of personality in lung cancer in man. *Ann NY Acad Sci, 125:*820, 1966.
71. Tokuhata, G.K.: Epidemiology of Chronic Diseases: With Emphasis on Multiple-Factor Approach. Monog., Division of Research and Biostatistics, Pennsylvania State Department of Health, Harrisburg, Pa., 1970.
72. Burch, P.R.J.: Genetic carrier frequency for lung cancer. *Nature, 202:*711, 1964.
73. Kellermann, G., Shaw, C.R., Kellermann, M.L.: Aryl Hydrocarbon Hydroxylase Inducibility and Bronchogenic Carcinoma. *New Eng J Med, 289:*934–937, 1973.

CHAPTER 14

HEREDITARY FACTORS IN LEUKEMIA
AND LYMPHOMA

CLARK W. HEATH, JR.

THE POSSIBLITY THAT hereditary factors contribute to the etiology of human leukemia and lymphoma has received scientific attention from the time when these diseases were first recognized. Evidence bearing on the subject has come from many sources and involves many different kinds of data. To review these data is a complex task and not one which at present can be expected to yield definitive etiologic answers. Considerable information does exist, however, to indicate that hereditary factors are important in this group of diseases, and from such information tentative hypotheses can perhaps be drawn.

Before embarking on a review of the subject, three points, each of which unfortunately increases the complexity of an already complex field, deserve emphasis. First, the terms "leukemia" and "lymphoma," as commonly used, encompass a spectrum of disease which includes several quite separate entities. While distinctions between disorders are not always clearcut (for instance, the entities of CLL* and LS merge in adults as do ALL and LS in children), clinical, therapeutic, and epidemiologic features allow one

*The following abbreviations are used throughout this chapter:

> AL = Acute leukemia
> AGL = Acute granulocytic leukemia
> ALL = Acute lymphocytic leukemia
> CGL = Chronic granulocytic leukemia
> CLL = Chronic lymphocytic leukemia
> HD = Hodgkin's disease
> LS = Lymphosarcoma
> RCS = Reticulum cell sarcoma
> MM = Multiple myeloma

readily to recognize basic differences and to distinguish among different disease groups. By these means, the leukemias can be sorted into at least 3 separate varieties (CGL, CLL, and the acute leukemias) and the lymphomas into at least as many (HD, LS, RCS, and, included for the purposes of the present review, MM). In view of these differences it is important that the etiology of different forms of leukemia or lymphoma be considered separately.

The second point is that the etiology of any form of leukemia or lymphoma, as with most cancers, involves almost certainly the interaction of multiple factors, both environmental and genetic. The question of heredity in leukemia and lymphoma, therefore, should not be viewed as an all or none affair, but as a matter of degree: to what extent do genetic factors contribute to leukemia/lymphoma etiology, not is one individual case or one type of leukemia/lymphoma genetically determined while another results exclusively from irradiation, chemical exposure, or viral infection. In all likelihood all such modes of causation operate in all cases, the degree of involvement of any one mode depending to some extent on the type of leukemia or lymphoma concerned.

The third point concerns the term "genetic," a word widely used to denote not just inheritance but any aspect of gene structure and function. In the realm of leukemia and lymphoma this has encompassed such non-inherited genetic problems related to leukemogenesis as x-ray-induced chromosomal aberrations and Down's syndrome. While

233

such situations do not, strictly speaking, come under the heading of hereditary factors, they will be included in this review because of their genetic nature in a broad sense.

Part of the evidence that heritable factors play a role in human leukemia and lymphoma comes from the fact that they clearly do so in other species. Data in animals, of course, are far more complete than in man because of our ability in other species to conduct rigorous experiments with inbred lines and because short generation times facilitate genetic observations. Mice are the animals most thoroughly studied, and in that species the role of genetic factors in leukemogenesis is now quite clear.[1] No simple mode of single-gene recessive-dominant Mendelian inheritance seems involved. Instead, genetic influences take the form of a multifactorial polygenic complex in which numerous genetic traits interact with various environmental factors to produce the end result of leukemia/lymphoma. It seems logical to assume that similar broad etiologic patterns govern human disease, as they also may in bovine disease.[2] It is hard to envision how so complex a causal pattern can be true for one species but not for another, however great the species gap. The fact that evidence of genetic factors is not as readily apparent in man as in mice can easily be attributed to man's outbred state, since observations in mice depend fundamentally on the existence of inbred strains for their clarity.

By necessity, evidence from studies in man himself is virtually all indirect. This leads inevitably to difficulty in judging the relative roles of genetic and environmental factors, since persons who share genetic bonds within a family or racial group usually share a common environment as well. Be this as it may, and acknowledging that this kind of reservation needs always to be kept in mind, one can arrange the evidence from human studies into the following three categories: (1) studies of case distributions in different races, (2) studies of case distributions within family groupings, including incidence among sibs and in twin sets, and (3) studies of case associations with known genetic disorders, genetic markers, or genetic traits.

Racial Distributions

Data from studies of racial distribution suggest genetic factors in the etiology of at least two forms of leukemia/lymphoma. The most striking evidence concerns CLL, which is only rarely encountered in Far Eastern races. Published reports suggest that this type of leukemia is uncommon in Japanese in Japan,[3,4] Chinese in Singapore,[5] Indians in India[6,7] and Maoris in New Zealand.[8] Among these various groups CLL accounts for less than 5 percent of all leukemia while among other races in western countries this percentage approaches 30 percent. The incidence among Japanese has been most thoroughly studied, and the idea that rareness of CLL in this group may reflect genetic rather than cultural factors is supported by a study of Japanese immigrants to the U.S. among whom the deficiency in CLL seems to persist despite their new surroundings.[9]

The other disorder showing an unusual racial pattern is MM in which incidence among blacks in the United States exceeds that among whites by about a two-fold margin.[10,11] Since selective underdiagnosis of cases among blacks makes this a minimal estimate of racial difference, and since other forms of leukemia and lymphoma are less common among blacks than whites, especially at older ages,[12] it seems quite possible that this particular racial pattern reflects a true genetic predisposition of MM.

Numerous other racial differences have been described for various forms of leukemia and lymphoma,[13] and particularly for leukemia of every sort in Jewish people,[14,15] but none are as striking as the two examples cited above. While any or all may well reflect elements of genetic variation in susceptibility to leukemia/lymphoma, confounding factors such as differences in case ascertainment as well as differences in environmental settings make interpretations hazardous. Worth particular mention, however, may be age patterns observed in different racial groups for childhood ALL.[16] While incidence rises to a sharp peak at age 4 to 5 in whites in Britain and the United States, no such peak in incidence is seen in native Japanese or in U.S. blacks. Whether this phenomenon reflects genetic, environmental, or merely diagnostic differences is uncertain since data for recent years have suggested that age peaks similar to that seen in whites may now be developing in the other two racial groups.[17]

Familial Distributions

Incidence in Relatives

The most direct approach to the question of hereditary factors in human leukemia and lymphoma is to measure the frequency of such disease in relatives of patients. Unfortunately the results of such studies have proved hard to interpret. The first comprehensive investigation, beyond a smaller series of cases described in 1937,[18] was reported in 1947 by Videbaek from Denmark.[19] Among 209 patients with leukemia, 17 were found to have at least one leukemic relative (8.1 percent) compared with only one (0.5 percent) among 200 controls. Although this difference seemed at first clear-cut, it was soon pointed out[20,21] that on the basis of mortality statistics leukemia was grossly under-reported in the control group, a reflection, one would suppose, of greater awareness of leukemia in families that have had recent experience with the disease than in families that have not. In any case, when data for first degree relatives

were examined separately, the difference between cases and controls became smaller.

Since that time, numerous studies of familial incidence have been conducted,[22-34] most concerned only with leukemias, but at least three[28,29,32] with lymphomas as well. Although in some studies familial incidence has appeared moderately increased,[18,22,28, 29,31-34] no striking increases have been found, and in no study can environmental influences be ruled out as an explanation for findings.

Next to the leukemias, HD has received the closest attention. In the large case series assembled by Razis, et al.,[29] the frequency of HD in relatives of patients with HD was estimated to be about 3 times higher than in the general population. MacMahon, however, in reviewing published accounts of familial HD[35] found that, on the whole, cases within families tended more often to have similar dates of diagnosis than similar ages at diagnosis. Such an observation suggests that environmental factors play a stronger role in familial aggregation than does heredity, a possibility which may especially be true for HD.

With regard to the leukemias, several studies,[18,26,29,34] together with various reports concerning individual families,[36-40] have suggested that the tendency for familial occurrence, and hence the likelihood of having genetic origin, may be stronger for cases of CLL than for cases of other sorts. Gunz in particular has stressed this possibility.[34] In his survey of leukemia in New Zealand, seven of 54 patients with CLL were found to have sibs with chronic leukemia (4 CLL, 3 CGL).This contrasts with an expected incidence among family members of less than one case, calculated from New Zealand mortality statistics and corrected for age and year of death.

Childhood leukemia has been the particular subject of attention in several studies, some of which have suggested that the incidence of leukemia may be about 4 times increased among sibs of leukemic children. The earliest study to focus exclusively on childhood leukemia found no indications of increased leukemia incidence among sibs or other relatives of 249 patients.[30] In a subsequent case-control study, however, involving 459 patients, Miller found a significant excess of cases among sibs (six cases compared with one expected),[41] an observation which was independently corroborated in a larger British case-control series where 1,798 leukemia patients had nine sibs with leukemia compared with an expectation of 1.5.[42,43] The question, however, of leukemia risk to sibs of leukemia patients is not yet clearly settled since efforts to confirm the findings of these two studies by matching for sibs among childhood cancer deaths in the United States have thus far yielded negative results, except for the special situation of twins.[44,45]

Many of the studies cited above have examined the occurrence of cancer and of other hematologic diseases (notable pernicious anemia) in addition to leukemia/lymphoma in relatives of patients with leukemia and lymphoma. Again, while some have suggested that various of these other sorts of disease are more frequent in such families,[19,22,32] the data present problems in interpretation and in any case do not suggest clear-cut patterns. In neither of the two childhood leukemia case-control series[41,43] was an excess of cancer other than leukemia found among sibs, and the same to date has been true of death certificate studies in the United States.[44,45] The possibility, however, that undetected relationships may exist between leukemia and cancer of other sorts within families should not be ruled out too quickly, witness the observation in the latter study[45] of four children with leukemia/lymphoma, each of whom had a sib recorded as having died of cancer of the colon, a distinctly unusual site for malignancy in childhood.

Multiple Case Families

The medical literature contains numerous accounts of individual families in which more than one case of the various forms of leukemia and lymphoma have occurred. Most attention has been given to the leukemias, but reports concerning familial lymphoma[29] as well as MM[46] are plentiful. Occasional families have also been described containing multiple cases of myeloproliferative or reticuloendothelial disease, often resembling leukemia and lymphoma.[47,48]

While most reports of familial leukemia or lymphoma involve pairs of cases in individual families, occasional families have been described in which as many as 6 cases have occurred (Table 14-I). No attempt will be made here to review reports of families containing fewer than four cases. A fairly complete compilation, however, of all multiple-case families has been made by Zuelzer and Cox[49] in an analysis of cell-type frequency and concordance in relation to familial leukemia. They conclude that, on the whole, cell types within families tend to be concordant, a fact which may be taken to indicate the operation of genetic factors, but which may also reflect the fact that concordant situations are more likely to be recorded in the medical literature than are discordant ones. Among the three varieties of concordance examined (AL-AL, CGL-CGL, CLL-CLL), CLL concordance seemed unusually frequent (39 percent of 102 families) and CGL unusually rare (8 percent) when compared with expected frequencies of leukemic cell types in the general population. About half of all concordant multiple leukemia case families involved AL. These comparisons, although crude and imprecise, suggest that hereditary factors may be a greater force in CLL than in AL, but that in CGL they play at best a minor role.

In the absence of any striking tendency for leukemia/lymphoma to recur in families, it is

TABLE 14-I
LIST OF FAMILIES REPORTED IN THE MEDICAL LITERATURE IN WHICH 4 OR
MORE CASES OF LEUKEMIA OR LYMPHOMA HAVE OCCURRED

Author	Year of Report	Number of Cases in Family	Diagnosis	Description
Decastello[36]	1939	4	4 CLL	2 generations. 3 of 5 adult sibs and the son of one.
Videbaek[50]	1947	4	2 CLL, 1 CGL 1 eosinophilic leukemia	3 generations. 2 adult sibs (CLL, CGL), a grandson of one (eos. L), and a nephew (CLL).
Anderson[51]	1951	5	5 ALL	1 generation. 5 of 8 childhood sibs.
Johnson, Peters[52]	1957	4	3 AL, 1 LS	1 generation. 4 of 12 adult sibs. Parents first cousins.
Steinberg[30]	1960	4	3 AL, 1 LS	1 generation. 4 of 7 childhood sibs. Parents second cousins.
Gordon[53]	1963	4	4 AL	2 generations. 2 sibs age 2 and 29 and 2 adult maternal aunts.
Heath, Moloney[54]	1965	5	5 AGL	3 generations. 3 adult sibs, the daughter of one and that daughter's son age 7.
Gunz, et al.[55]	1966	4	4 ALL	1 generation. 4 of 8 childhood sibs including both members of a dizygous twin set.
Kajii, et al.[56]	1968	4	3 RCS, 1 LS	1 generation. 4 of 8 adult sibs.
McPhedran, et al.[39]	1969	6	6 CLL	1 generation. 2 sets of first cousin adult sibships containing 3 cases each, one among 5 sibs, the other among 10.
McPhedran, et al.[39]	1969	4	4 AL	3 generations. 4 adult cases: a woman, her daughter, and 2 cousins.
Ferguson, Lynn[57]	1970	4	4 AL	4 generations. 3 adults and a 14-year-old girl in direct line of descent.
Snyder, et al.[58]	1970	6	6 AGL	3 generations. 3 of 6 childhood sibs, one adult maternal great uncle, his adult sister, and her adult son.
Potolsky, et al.[59]	1971	6	2 CLL, 2 RCS, 2 LS	1 generation. 6 of 10 adult sibs.

hard to assess the significance of two or even three cases in individual family groups. Since the diseases themselves are rare, however, the fact that as many as four, five, and six cases have occurred in certain families is by itself strong evidence that familial factors do influence etiology: the likelihood that such impressive case aggregates might result from chance is vanishingly small.

To date 14 such families have been recorded in the medical literature, nine containing four cases, two containing five, and three containing six (Table 14-I).[30,36,39, 50-59] All but two[56,59] involve primarily cases of leukemia, and in all but one[50] there is clear similarity, if not concordance, of cell type or tumor histology within families. As indicated before, such diagnostic concordance supports the concept that genetic factors do play an etiologic role in these disorders.

No particular diagnosis seems dominant in this series of families. Cases of AL are most often involved (nine families), and in only two families are cases exclusively CLL.[36,39] With the exception of one case in the family described by Videbaek,[50] CGL is not represented at all in the series. Again, this would seem to indicate that familial factors have little role in the etiology of this particular form of leukemia.

In two families there was evidence of consanguinity,[30,52] a fact which raises the question of precisely how genetic factors in human leukemia/lymphoma may be inherited. Consanguinity is a rare phenomenon in most human populations, and its presence, therefore, in these two families and in others like them[40] cannot be easily dismissed as unrelated to leukemia occurrence. However, since inbreeding is only rarely encountered as a background for cases of leukemia/lymphoma, it seems unreasonable to think that such occasional consanguinity reflects a general state of simple single-gene recessive inheritance. It does seem consistent, though, with what we know regarding genetic factors in experimental leukemia, where severe inbreeding of selective lines can greatly accentuate the appearance of leukemia in mice by increasing the pool of genes which contribute to leukemia/lymphoma proneness.

The relevance of such a concept to human leukemogenesis has recently been emphasized by a study conducted in Japan[60] where consanguinity in the general population is not unusual. In a series of 18 families in which two or more sibs had leukemia, evidence of consanguinity was significantly more frequent (nine families, 50 percent) than in multiple case families in which patients were less closely related (one of 18 families, 6 percent) or in families containing only one case (nine of 200 families, 4.5 percent).

Twin Studies

Analysis of case occurrence among twins can be a powerful tool for assessing potential genetic etiology in any disease. However, although considerable attention has been given to leukemia in twins over the past decade, interpretation of findings is still far from clear. In 1964 MacMahon and Levy, in an analysis of 77 leukemic twins drawn from several extensive registries of childhood leukemia, demonstrated that leukemia concordance

was greatly increased for monozygous twins in childhood.[61] This observation confirmed the conjecture of earlier authors[62] and supported the impression one gets on scanning the 25 or so instances of concordant twin leukemia which have been adequately documented to date in the medical literature.[49] The MacMahon-Levy series of cases contained five concordant pairs, each like sexed, at least two clearly monozygotic, data indicative of a concordance rate in identical twins under age 15 of about 20 percent. These findings, including this estimate of concordance, were later confirmed in a series of leukemic twins assembled for California-born children[63] as well as in an ongoing national registry of childhood leukemia deaths.[44,45] They were not supported, however, in British data[64] were no concordant twin cases were found in a case sample quite large enough to produce several, given the level of concordance found in American studies. The reasons for this discrepancy are not yet clear.

If one assumes, however, that the degree of concordance described by MacMahon and Levy is in fact true for monozygous twins under age 15, it does not necessarily follow that this reflects genetic influence. In fact, as pointed out by Zuelzer and Cox in an exhaustive review of the topic,[49] the observation of twin concordance in childhood leukemia may be more easily reconciled with a concept of environmental leukemogenesis affecting the fetus (or fetuses) late in gestation. In support of this idea is the close resemblance of twin leukemia to neonatal leukemia and the fact that, although concordant twin leukemia has been reported in adults,[38,65] it is an extremely rare event beyond childhood. Among children the distribution of cases by age and sex more closely parallels neonatal leukemia than childhood leukemia as a whole in that the sex ratio seems reversed (female cases exceed male) and the age peak occurs under age 1 rather than at age 4 to 5.[49]

One possible explanation for these facts, an alternative to the genetic hypothesis, involves the theory that, since monozygous twins are probably all hematopoietic chimeras by virtue of shared placental circulation, leukemia in one twin may easily transplant itself to the other.[66,67] The end result, concordant twin leukemia, would thus be prominent only in monozygous twins, would be mostly confined to very young children, and would show close similarities in cell type and time of leukemia occurrence within twin sets. (The latter features have been characteristic of virtually all instances of concordant twin leukemia reported to date.[44,45,49,61,62]) Needed to support this theory will be evidence from cytogenetic or other cellular studies which might identify the leukemic process in both members of an affected twin pair as arising from a single cell line. Thus far, work of this sort (cytogenetics) has been attempted in two twin sets, but in neither have results been conclusive.[68,69]

Genetic Case Associations

A further approach to the study of genetic factors in leukemia/lymphoma, beyond assessing racial and familial incidence directly, has been to look for associations with known genetic disease or with possible genetic markers. While most such investigations, as pointed out previously, do not on the whole deal with strictly hereditary situations, they are pertinent to the broader question of genetic contributions to leukemia/lymphoma etiology. We shall deal with this area in three parts: (1) chromosomal disorders, (2) immune disorders, and (3) genetic markers.

Chromosomal Disorders

In several disease situations the occurrence of leukemia can be linked to chromosomal abnormalities of one sort or another. The most prominent of these involves the association of leukemia with Down's syndrome (mongolism), a disorder involving mitotic nondisjunction of chromosome G-21. Reports of leukemia occurring in patients with Down's syndrome have appeared in the medical literature since 1930,[70] but recognition of the association did not become widely established until the mid 1950's.[71-74] It now is evident from various surveys[75-79] that cases of leukemia occur about 20 times more often in patients with Down's syndrome than in the general population and that this risk in all likelihood extends to all age groups.[76] Estimates of risk in children, however, may often be exaggerated because of the occasional occurrence at very young ages of reversible disorders of granulopoiesis, which are probably related to heightened susceptibility to infection in Down's syndrome but which may often be mistaken for true leukemia.[49,80-84] It is perhaps these cases which account for the fact that the age peak for childhood leukemia in Down's syndrome occurs somewhat earlier than in childhood leukemia generally.[40,79]

The mechanism of leukemogenesis in Down's syndrome is unclear. Since leukemia is a disorder of cellular proliferation and is often itself associated with chromosomal derangements, it seems not unreasonable to link it to Down's syndrome on a chromosomal level. However, cytogenetic abnormalities reported in leukemia associated with Down's syndrome show no patterns different from leukemia generally, and there seems no particular reason to relate leukemogenesis as a whole to disorders of chromosome 21. In addition, leukemia in Down's syndrome shows the same general distribution of cell type as is seen in the population at large.[85] It is worth noting, however, that while risk of leukemia is increased in Down's syndrome, risk of lymphoma is not,[79] at least in so far as one can separate these two tumor groups.

In addition to its association with G-21 trisomy, leukemia has been reported in occasional patients with other forms of chromosomal nondisjunction:[17,86] Klinefelter's syndrome and other forms of sex chromosome nondisjunction,[87-94] D 13-15 trisomy,[95,96] as well as D/G translocation Down's syndrome.[97] While such reports are not so numerous that one can generalize regarding predisposition to leukemia in nondisjunction states (most are considerably rarer than G-trisomy Down's syndrome itself), some support for such a concept does come from the occasional finding of families in which leukemia or lymphoma and various forms of nondisjunction (G-trisomy, Klinefelter's syndrome) have been found to coexist in separate family members.[98-104] In addition, some evidence suggests that the frequency of Down's syndrome may be slightly increased (no more than 5-fold) among sibs of leukemic children.[41] The latter findings, however, have not been borne out elsewhere.[43]

The concept that leukemogenesis may be related to underlying chromosomal abnormalities is also supported by data concerning various population groups which exhibit increased levels of chromosomal breakage.[105-108] Some of these involve inherited tendencies for chromosome fragility while in others breakage is environmentally acquired. In the first category are the disorders of Bloom's syndrome and Fanconi's anemia, both determined by recessive inheritance, and both associated with increased risk of leukemia in affected individuals.[109-113] In the latter category are the well-known situations where risk of developing leukemia is distinctly increased following exposure to varying doses of ionizing irradiation[3,114-117] as well perhaps as following exposure to benzene and its derivatives.[118]

A final piece of evidence regarding the relation of cytogenetic abnormalities to leukemogenesis concerns the Philadelphia (Ph[1])

chromosome which is present in all cells of myeloid descent in virtually every clinically typical case of CGL.[119,120] While it appears to be an acquired rather than an inherited defect, the Ph[1] chromosome does seem intimately involved with the pathogenesis of CGL.[49] This is particularly apparent in the terminal phases of CGL when it is common for acute leukemia to appear.[121] Since AL in this setting seems generally to develop in Ph[1]-positive cells, often with aneuploid evolution resulting in cell lines containing multiple Ph[1] chromosomes,[122] one can conclude that here again is a situation where an underlying chromosomal disorder (the Ph[1] chromosome) leads directly to increased risk of leukemia (albeit a special case of leukemogenesis in a preexisting leukemic state).

Immune Disorders

Evidence of hereditary influences in the origins of leukemia and lymphoma are also reflected in the association of both sorts of disease with inherited disorders of immune function.[17] These include Bruton-type X-linked agammaglobulinemia[123] and hereditary ataxia-telangiectasia[124,125] but are paralleled by observations of lymphoma and lymphocytic leukemia in immune deficiency disorders of other sorts (reviewed by Fraumeni,[17] and by Gatti and Good.[126] From this constellation of disease associations one gets the distinct impression that tumors of lymphoid or reticuloendothelial origin are closely related etiologically to functional disorders of such tissues,[17,106,108] but that leukemias of the granulocytic and myeloid sorts do not share in the association with immune disorders. Such a pattern seems reasonable etiologically, and it provides further grounds for considering different forms of leukemia and lymphoma separately.

Additional evidence concerning genetic relationships between lymphoid malignancy and immune function has come from observations in relatives of such patients. Evidence has been presented of immunologic abnormalities in asymptomatic relatives of patients with Waldenstrom's macroglobulinemia,[127] in the mothers and sibs of children with ALL,[128] and in the healthy members of two sibships in which multiple cases of CLL and other lymphoreticular malignancies have occurred.[40,59] Conceivably in such families an inherited propensity for immune dysfunction predisposes to the development of lymphoid tumors. Such a hypothesis, however, is speculative at present, since it is entirely possible that immunologic defects in such settings are more a matter of environment than of heredity.

Genetic Markers

The search for genetic markers in leukemia and lymphoma has followed several different directions but as yet has not uncovered clear-cut patterns. Standard blood group distributions appear to be unremarkable.[129,130] However, a possible relationship of CLL to haptoglobin patterns (deficiency in type 1/1 and excess in type 2/1) has been described,[131] although not yet confirmed by other workers. Studies of histocompatibility genetic types have also been done, partly on the grounds that in mice a strong relationship exists between the H2 histocompatibility system and susceptibility to certain forms of viral leukemia.[132,133] Observations in human populations, however, are still in a preliminary stage, and much further work needs yet to be done. In acute leukemia, while one study suggested an association with the haplotype HL-A2/HL-A12 and an absence of HL-A1 antigen,[134] several others have found no departures from normal.[135-138] In HD, however, two separate studies have suggested that the frequency of HL-A5 antigen is distinctly increased.[139,140]

Cytogenetic studies have been extensively used to search for marker chromosomes that might indicate genetic origins for leukemia, lymphoma, and other cancers. No such markers have been found. The Ph[1] chromosome has proved to be an acquired feature of CGL, as shown by its absence in marrow cells of persons whose identical twins have developed Ph[1]-positive CGL.[141-146] The so-called Christchurch chromosome (Ch[1]), reported in 1962 as a possible genetic marker in some cases of CLL,[147-149] has subsequently come to be considered as probably a normal morphologic variant of the G 21–22 chromosome group.[1501-152] Among other forms of leukemia and lymphoma no consistent evidence of chromosome markers has appeared, cytogenetic abnormalities when present varying from patient to patient and being restricted to malignant cell lines.[153-156]

A final potential genetic marker concerns variations in susceptibility of cells to viral transformation. With recent interest focusing on the role of viruses in oncogenesis, studies have been made concerning the *in vitro* susceptibility of human cells to known tumor virus. These have led to a technique employing SV-40 virus and human fibroblasts which when applied to patients with Down's syndrome and with Fanconi's anemia has demonstrated greatly increased susceptibility to transformation.[157,158] Since similar susceptibility was also found in the parents of patients with Fanconi's anemia,[157] it has been suggested that this measure of transformation sensitivity may serve as a genetic marker for identifying persons or family groups at particular risk of developing malignancy.[159] To date the procedure has yet to be widely applied. That it may prove useful in genetic studies of leukemia, however, is suggested by the finding of increased SV-40 transformation in three individuals (one patient and two first degree relatives) belonging to a family in which multiple cases of AL have occurred.[58]

Summary

There is evidence from many sources that hereditary and genetic factors contribute to the multifactorial etiology of human leukemia and lymphoma: studies of incidence in different races, observations concerning the occurrence of leukemia and lymphoma in relatives of patients and in certain multiple case families, and the association of various forms of leukemia and lymphoma with assorted chromosomal and immunologic disorders, many of which themselves have hereditary and genetic origins. The hereditary component of leukemia/lymphoma etiology is in all likelihood polygenic, its influence varying from one specific disease type to another. Although in no type has it been possible clearly to distinguish hereditary influences from environmental ones, hereditary factors seem to play less of a role in CGL and HD and more of a role in CLL. Distinct racial patterns exist in CLL (and possibly also in MM); CLL also appears to have a greater tendency for cases to cluster in families than do other varieties of leukemia. Studies of leukemia incidence in twins, theoretically a useful way to distinguish between genetic and environmental causes, have produced striking evidence of disease concordance in monozygous childhood twins which, however, may be less a matter of genetic origin and more one of antenatal leukemia spread by way of shared placental circulation.

Chromosomal studies, which have contributed greatly to our understanding of mechanisms of leukemogenesis and the cellular nature of leukemia/lymphoma, have revealed no evidence of inherited cytogenetic defects which might be construed as genetic markers. However, genetic indicators of other sorts seem likely to be important: variations in immune capacity relative to leukemogenesis, variations in histocompatibility genotypes, and patterns of cellular response to viruses and other agents capable of triggering malignant disease. At the present time, genetic studies focused on areas such as these offer particular promise for improving our understanding of how hereditary and genetic factors contribute to leukemia/lymphoma etiology.

REFERENCES

1. Heston, W.E.: Genetic factors in the etiology of cancer. *Cancer Res. 25:*1320–1326, 1965.

2. Croshaw, J.E., Jr., Abt, D.A., Marshak, R.R., Hare, W.C.D., Switzer, J., Ipsen, J., and Dutcher, R.M.: Pedigree studies in bovine lymphosarcoma. *Ann NY Acad Sci, 108:* 1193–1202, 1963.

3. Brill, A.B., Tomonaga, M., and Heyssel, R.M.: Leukemia in man following exposure to ionizing radiation. A summary of the findings in Hiroshima and Nagasaki, and a comparison with other human experience. *Ann Intern Med, 56:*590–609, 1962.

4. Finch, S.C., Hoshino, T., Hoga, T., Ichimaru, M., and Ingram, R.H., Jr.: Chronic lymphocytic leukemia in Hiroshima and Nagasaki, Japan. *Blood, 33:*79–86, 1969.

5. Wells, R., and Lau, K.S.: Incidence of leukaemia in Singapore and rarity of chronic lymphocytic leukaemia in Chinese. *Br Med J, 1:*759–763, 1960.

6. Firkin, B., and Moore, C.V.: Clinical manifestations of leukemia. *Am J Med, 28:* 746–776, 1960.

7. Reddy, G., and Bhargava, K.: Leukaemia. *J Assoc Phys India, 8:*171–176, 1960.

8. Gunz, F.W.: Incidence of some aetiological factors in human leukaemia. *Br Med J, 1:* 326–327, 1961.

9. Haenszel, W., and Kurihara, M.: Studies of Japanese migrants. I. Mortality from cancer and other diseases among Japanese in the United States. *J Natl Cancer Inst, 40:* 43–68, 1968.

10. MacMahon, B., and Clark, D.W.: The inci-

dence of multiple myeloma. *J Chronic Dis,* *4*:508–515, 1956.

11. McPhedran, P., Heath, C.W., Jr., and Garcia, J.: Multiple myeloma in metropolitan Atlanta, Georgia: racial and seasonal variations. *Blood, 39*:866–873, 1972.

12. McPhedran, P., Heath, C.W., Jr., and Garcia, J.: Racial variations in leukemia incidence among the elderly. *J Natl Cancer Inst, 45:* 25–28, 1970.

13. Dameshek, W., and Gunz, F.W.: Leukemia. New York, Grune & Stratton, 1964, pp. 30–33.

14. MacMahon, B., and Koller, E.K.: Ethnic differences in the incidence of leukemia. *Blood, 12*:1–10, 1957.

15. Graham, S., Gibson, R., Lilienfeld, A., Shuman, L., and Levin, M.: Religion and ethnicity in leukemia. *Am J Public Health, 60*:266–274, 1970.

16. Court Brown, W.M., and Doll, R.: Leukaemia in childhood and young adult life. *Br Med J, 1*:981–988, 1961.

17. Fraumeni, J.F., Jr., and Miller, R.W.: Epidemiology of human leukemia: recent observations. *J Natl Cancer Inst, 38*:593–605, 1967.

18. Ardashnikov, S.N.: Genetics of leukaemia in man. *J Hyg, 37*:286–302, 1937.

19. Videbaek, A.: Heredity in human leukemia and its relation to cancer. (Opera ex domo biologiae hereditariae humanae universitatis Hafnensis) Vol 13, Copenhagen, Munksgaard, 1947.

20. Busk, T.: Some observations on heredity in breast cancer and leukemia. *Ann Eugenics, 14*:213–229, 1948.

21. Gorer, F.A., and Videbaek, A.: Heredity in human leukemia and its relation to cancer (a review). *Ann Eugenics, 14*:346–348, 1949.

22. Gross, L., and Matte, M.L.: Occurrence of tumors and leukemia in members of families suffering from leukemia. *NY State J Med, 48*:1283–1284, 1948.

23. Amiotti, P.L.: Sulla incidenza dei tumori nei familiari di bambini leucemici. *Minerva Pediatr, 5*:449–450, 1953.

24. Kaliampetsos, G.: Kommen Blutkrankheiten und Karzinome unter den Verwandten von Leukämie-kranken gehäuft vor? *Dtsch*

Med Wochenschr, 79:1783–1785, 1954.

25. Guasch, J.: Hérédité des leucémies. *Sang, 25:* 384–421, 1954.

26. Morganti, G., and Cresseri, A.: Nouvelles recherches génétiques sur les leucémies. *Sangre, 25*:421–453, 1954.

27. Revol, L., Millet, C., and Thivollet: A propos l'étiologie de la leucose aiguë; étude de 193 cas. *Sang, 25*:825–840, 1954.

28. Devore, J.W., and Doan, C.A.: Studies in Hodgkin's syndrome. XII. Hereditary and epidemiologic aspects. *Ann Intern Med, 47*:300–316, 1957.

29. Razis, D.V., Diamond, H.D., and Craver, L.F.: Familial Hodgkin's disease: its significance and implications. *Ann Intern Med, 51*:933–971, 1959.

30. Steinberg, A.G.: The genetics of acute leukemia in children. *Cancer, 13*:985–999, 1960.

31. Gunz, F.W.: Genetic factors in the genesis of leukemia. *Proc XI Cong Int Soc Hemat, 183–193,* 1966.

32. Rigby, P.G., Rosenlof, R.C., Pratt, P.T., and Lemon, H.M.: Leukemia and Lymphoma. *JAMA, 197*:25–30, 1966.

33. Rigby, P.G., Pratt, P.T., Rosenlof, R.C., and Lemon, H.M.: Genetic relationships in familial leukemia and lymphoma. *Arch Intern Med, 121*:67–70, 1967.

34. Gunz, F.W., and Veale, A.M.O.: Leukemia in close relatives—accident or predisposition? *J Natl Cancer Inst, 42*:517–524, 1969.

35. MacMahon, B.: Epidemiology of Hodgkin's disease. *Cancer Res, 26*:1189–1200, 1966.

36. Decastello, A.: Beitrag zur Kenntnis der familiären Leukämie. *Med Klin, 35*:1255–1257, 1939.

37. Reilly, E.B., Rapaport, S.I., Karr, N.W., Mills, H., and Carpenter, G.E.: Familial chronic lymphatic leukemia. *Arch Intern Med, 90*:87–89, 1952.

38. Gunz, F., and Dameshek, W.: Chronic lymphocytic leukemia in a family, including twin brothers and a son. *JAMA, 164:* 1323–1325, 1957.

39. McPhedran, P., Heath, C.W., Jr., and Lee, J.: Patterns of familial leukemia. Ten cases of leukemia in two interrelated families. *Cancer, 24*:403–407, 1969.

40. Fraumeni, J.F., Jr., Vogel, C.L., and DeVita, V.T.: Familial chronic lymphocytic leukemia. *Ann Intern Med, 71:*279–284, 1969.

41. Miller, R.W.: Down's syndrome (mongolism), other congenital malformations, and cancers among the sibs of leukemic children. *New Engl J Med, 268.*393–401, 1963.

42. Stewart, A., Webb, J., and Hewitt, D.: A survey of childhood malignancies. *Br Med J, 1:*1495–1508, 1958.

43. Barber, R., and Spiers, P.: Oxford survey of childhood cancers: progress report II. *Monthly Bull Min Health, 23:*46–52, 1964.

44. Miller, R.W.: Death from childhood cancer in sibs. *New Engl J Med, 279:*122–126, 1968.

45. Miller, R.W.: Deaths from childhood leukemia and solid tumors among twins and other sibs in the United States 1960–67. *J Natl Cancer Inst, 46:*203–209, 1971.

46. Alexander, L.L., and Benninghoff, D.L.: Familial multiple myeloma. *J Natl Med Assoc, 57:*471–475, 1965.

47. Randall, D.L., Reiquam, C.W., Githens, J.H., and Robinson, A.: Familial myeloproliferative disease: a new syndrome closely simulating myelogenous leukemia in childhood. *Am J Dis Child, 110:*479–500, 1965.

48. Miller, D.R.: Familial reticuloendotheliosis: concurrence of disease in five siblings. *Pediatrics, 38:*986–995, 1966.

49. Zuelzer, W.W., and Cox, D.E.: Genetic aspects of leukemia. *Semin Hematol, 6:* 4–25, 1969.

50. Videbaek, A.: Familial leukemia. A preliminary report. *Acta Med Scand, 127:* 26–52, 1947.

51. Anderson, R.C.: Familial leukemia. A report of leukemia in five siblings with a brief review of the genetic aspects of this disease. *Am J Dis Child, 81:*313–322, 1951.

52. Johnson, M.J.E., and Peters, C.H.: Lymphomas in four siblings. *JAMA, 163:*20–25, 1957.

53. Gordon, R.D.: Hereditary factors in human leukaemia: report of four cases of leukaemia in a family. *Australasian Ann Med, 12:*202–207, 1963.

54. Heath, C.W., Jr., and Moloney, W.C.: Familial leukemia. Five cases of acute leukemia in three generations. *New Engl J Med, 272:*882–887, 1965.

55. Gunz, F.W., Fitzgerald, P.H., Crossen, P.E., Mackenzie, I.S., Powles, C.P., and Jensen, G.R.: Multiple cases of leukemia in a sibship. *Blood, 27:*482–489, 1966.

56. Kajii, T., Neu, R.L., and Gardner, L.I.: Chromosome abnormalities in lymph node cells from patient with familial lymphoma. *Cancer, 22:*218–224, 1968.

57. Ferguson, S.W., and Lynn, T.N.: Familial leukemia: a report of 4 cases of acute leukemia in 4 consecutive generations. *South Med J, 63:*1337–1340, 1970.

58. Snyder, A.L., Li, F.P., Henderson, E.S., and Todaro, G.J.: Possible inherited leukaemogenic factors in familial acute myelogenous leukaemia. *Lancet, 1:*586–589, 1970.

59. Potolsky, A.I., Heath, C.W., Jr., Buckley, C.E. III, and Rowlands, D.T., Jr.: Lymphoreticular malignancies and immunologic abnormalities in a sibship. *Am J Med, 50:*42–48, 1971.

60. Kurita, S., and Kamei, Y.: Genetics of familial leukemia. *Jap J Hum Genet, 14:* 163–179, 1969.

61. MacMahon, B., and Levy, M.A.: Prenatal origin of childhood leukemia. Evidence from twins. *New Engl J Med, 270:*1082–1085, 1964.

62. Pearson, H.A., Grello, F.W., and Cone, T.E., Jr.: Leukemia in identical twins. *New Engl J Med, 268:*1151–1156, 1963.

63. Jackson, E.W., Norris, F.D., and Klauber, M.R.: Childhood leukemia in California-born twins. *Cancer, 23:*913–919, 1969.

64. Hewitt, D., Lashof, J.C., and Stewart, A.M.: Childhood cancer in twins, *Cancer, 19:* 157–161, 1966.

65. Tokuhata, G.K., Neely, C.L., and Williams, D.L.: Chronic myelocytic leukemia in identical twins and a sibling. *Blood, 31:* 216–225, 1968.

66. Wolman, I.J.: Parallel responses to chemotherapy in identical twin infants with concordant leukemia. *J Pediatr, 60:*91–95, 1962.

67. Clarkson, B.D., and Boyse, E.A.: Possible explanation of the high concordance for

acute leukaemia in monozygotic twins (letter to editor). *Lancet, 1:*699–701, 1971.

68. Whang-Peng, J., Freireich, E.J., Oppenheim, J.J., Frei, E., and Tjio, J.H.: Cytogenetic studies in 45 patients with acute lymphocytic leukemia. *J Natl Cancer Inst, 42:* 881–897, 1969.

69. Hilton, H.B., Lewis, I.C., and Trowell, H.R.: C-group trisomy in identical twins with acute leukemia. *Blood, 35:*222–226, 1970.

70. Brewster, H.F., and Cannon, H.E.: Acute lymphatic leukemia: report of a case in eleventh month mongolian idiot. *New Orleans Med Surg J, 82:*872–873, 1930.

71. Bernard, J., Mathé, G., and Delorme, J-Cl.: Les leucoses des trés jeunes enfants. *Arch Franc Pediat, 12:*470–502, 1954.

72. Merritt, D.H., and Harris, J.S.: Mongolism and acute leukemia. *Arch Dis Child, 92:* 41–44, 1956.

73. Krivit, W., and Good, R.A.: The simultaneous occurrence of leukemia and mongolism. *J Dis Child, 91:*218–222, 1956.

74. Krivit, W., and Good, R.A.: Simultaneous occurrence of mongolism and leukemia. Report of a nationwide survey. *J Dis Child, 94:*289–293, 1957.

75. Lashof, J.C., and Stewart, A.: Oxford survey of childhood cancers. Progress report III: leukaemia and Down's syndrome. *Monthly Bull Minist Health* (London), *24:*136–143, 1965.

76. Wald, N., Borges, W.H., Li, C.C., Turner, J.H., and Harnois, M.C.: Leukemia associated with mongolism (letter to editor). *Lancet, 1:*1228, 1961.

77. Holland, W.W., Doll, R., and Carter, C.O.: The mortality from leukaemia and other cancers among patients with Down's syndrome (mongols) and among their parents. *Br J Cancer, 16:*178–186, 1962.

78. Jackson, E.W., Turner, J.H., Klauber, M.R., and Norris, F.D.: Down's syndrome: variation of leukaemia occurrence in institutionalized populations. *J Chronic Dis, 21:*247–253, 1968.

79. Miller, R.W.: Neoplasia and Down's syndrome. *Ann NY Acad Sci, 171:*637–644, 1970.

80. Ross, J.D.: Moloney, W.C., and Desforges, J.F.: Ineffective regulation of granulopoiesis masquerading as congenital leukemia in a mongoloid child. *J Pediatr, 63:* 1–10, 1963.

81. Engel, R.R., Hammond, D., Eitzman, D.V., Pearson, H., and Krivit, W.: Transient congenital leukemia in 7 infants with mongolism. *J Pediatr, 65:*303–305, 1964.

82. Germain, D., Monnet, P., Roux, J.-F., Salle, B., Rosenberg, D., Berger, Cl., and David, M.: Les leucoblastoses transitoires de la trisomie 21. *Ann Pédiat 43:*504–510, 1967.

83. Wegelius, R., Väänänen, I., and Koskela, S.-L.: Down's syndrome and transient leukemia-like disease in a newborn. *Acta Paediat* (Uppsala), *56:*301–306, 1967.

84. Drescher, J., Halsband, H., Brunck, H.-J., and Tolksdorf, M.: Abnormal hämatopoese mit hepatosplenomegalie bei neugeborenen mit Down-syndrom. *Z Kinderheilk, 104:* 135–169, 1968.

85. Fraumeni, J.F., Jr., Manning, M.D., and Mitus, J.: Acute childhood leukemia: epidemiologic study by cell type of 1,263 cases at the Children's Cancer Research Foundation in Boston, 1947–65. *J Natl Cancer Inst, 46:*461–470, 1971.

86. Fraumeni, J.F., Jr.: Clinical epidemiology of leukemia. *Semin Hematol, 6:*26–36, 1969.

87. Augustine, J.R., and Jaworski, Z.F.: Unusual testicular histology in "true" Klinefelter's syndrome. *Arch Pathol, 66:*159–164, 1958.

88. Mamunes, P., Lapidus, P.H., Abbott, J.A., and Roath, S.: Acute leukaemia and Klinefelter's syndrome (letter to editor). *Lancet, 2:*26–27, 1961.

89. Tough, I.M., Court Brown, W.M., Baikie, A.G., Buckton, K.E., Harnden, D.G., Jacobs, P.A., King, M.J., and McBride, J.A.: Cytogenetic studies in chronic myeloid leukaemia and acute leukaemia associated with mongolism. *Lancet, 1:*411–417, 1961.

90. Bousser, J., and Tanzer, J.: Syndrome de Klinefelter et leucemie aiguë, a propos d'un cas. *Nouv Rev Franc Hemat, 3:*194–197, 1963.

91. MacSween, R.N.M.: Reticulum cell sarcoma

and rheumatoid arthritis in a patient with XY/XXY/XXXY Klinefelter's syndrome and normal intelligence. *Lancet, 1:*460–461, 1965.

92. Borges, W.H., Nicklas, J.W., and Hamm, C,W.: Prezygotic determinants in acute leukemia. *J Pediatr, 70.*180–184, 1967

93. Lewis, F.J.W., Poulding, R.H., and Eastham, R.D.: Acute leukaemia in a XO/XXX mosaic (letter to editor). *Lancet, 2:*306, 1963.

94. Wertelecki, W., and Shapiro, J.R.: 45,XO Turner's syndrome and leukaemia (letter to editor). *Lancet, 1:*789, 1970.

95. Shade, H., Schoeller, L., and Schultz, K.W.: D-trisomie (Pätau-Syndrom) mit kongenitaler myeloischer leukämie. *Med Welt, 50:*2690–2692, 1962.

96. Zuelzer, W.W., Thompson, R.I., and Mastrangelo, R.: Evidence for a genetic factor related to leukemogenesis and congenital anomalies: chromosomal aberrations in pedigree of an infant with partial D trisomy and leukemia. *J Pediatr, 72:*367–376, 1968.

97. German, J.L., III, DeMayo, A.P., and Bearn, A.G.: Inheritance of an abnormal chromosome in Down's syndrome (mongolism) with leukemia. *Am J Hum Genet, 14:*31–43, 1962.

98. Buckston, K.E., Harnden, D.G., Baikie, A.G., and Woods, G.E.: Mongolism and leukaemia in the same sibship (letter to editor). *Lancet, 1:*171–172, 1961.

99. Thompson, M.W., Bell, R.E., and Little, A.S.: Familial 21-trisomic mongolism coexistent with leukemia. *Can Med Assoc J, 88:* 893–894, 1963.

100. Verresen, H., vanden Berghe, H., and Creemers, J.: Mosaic trisomy in phenotypically normal mother of mongol. *Lancet, 1:* 526–527, 1964.

101. Conen, P.E., Erkman, B., and Laski, B.: Chromosome studies on a radiographer and her family: report of one case of leukemia and two cases of Down's syndrome. *Arch Intern Med, 117:*125–132, 1966.

102. Ebbin, A.J., Heath, C.W., Jr., Moldow, R.E., and Lee, J.: Down's syndrome and leukemia in a family. *J Pediatr, 73:*917–919, 1968.

103. Baikie, A.G., Buckton, K.E., Court Brown, W.M., and Harnden, D.G.: Two cases of leukaemia and case of sex chromosome abnormality in same sibship. *Lancet, 2:* 1003–1004, 1961.

104. Miller, O.J., Breg, W.R., Schmickel, R.D., and Tretter, W.: A family with an XXXXY male, a leukaemic male, and two 21 trisomic mongoloid females. *Lancet, 2:*78–79, 1961.

105. Miller, R.W.: Radiation, chromosomes and viruses in the etiology of leukemia. Evidence from epidemiologic research. *New Engl J Med, 271:*30–36, 1964.

106. Miller, R.W.: Relation between cancer and congenital defects in man. *New Engl J Med, 275:*87–93, 1966.

107. Miller, R.W.: Persons with exceptionally high risk of leukemia. *Cancer Res, 27:*2420–2423, 1967.

108. Miller, R.W.: Relation between cancer and congenital defects: an epidemiologic evaluation. *J Natl Cancer Inst, 40:*1079–1085, 1968.

109. Garriga, S., and Crosby, W.H.: The incidence of leukemia in families of patients with hypoplasia of the marrow. *Blood, 14:* 1008–1014, 1959.

110. Bloom, G.E., Warner, S., Gerald, P.S., and Diamond, L.K.: Chromosome abnormalities in constitutional aplastic anemia. *New Engl J Med, 274:*8–14, 1966.

111. Gmyrek, D., Witkowski, R., Syllm-Rapaport, I., and Jacobasch, G.: Chromosomal aberrations and abnormalities of red-cell metabolism in a case of Fanconi's anemia before and after development of leukaemia. *German Med Monthly, 13:*105–111, 1968.

112. Prigozhina, E.L., Stavrovskaya, A.A., Zakharov, A.F., Lelikova, G.P., and Streljukhina, N.V.: Congenital anomalies of the karyotype in human acute leukemia. *Vop Onkol, 14:*58–64, 1968.

113. Sawitsky, A., Bloom, D., and German, J.: Chromosomal breakage and acute leukemia in congenital telangiectatic erythema and stunted growth. *Ann Intern Med, 65:*487–495, 1966.

114. Biszozero, J.O., Jr., Johnson, K., and Ciocco, A.: Radiation-related leukemia in Hiro-

shima and Nagasaki, 1946–1964. I. Distribution, incidence, and appearance time. *New Engl J Med, 274:*1095–1101, 1966.

115. Court Brown, W.M., and Doll, R.: Mortality from cancer and other causes after radiotherapy for ankylosing apondylitis. *Br Med J, 2:*1327–1332, 1965.

116. MacMahon, B.: Prenatal x-ray exposure and childhood cancer. *J Natl Cancer Inst, 28:* 1173–1191, 1962.

117. Modan, B., and Lilienfeld, A.M.: Polycythemia vera and leukemia—the role of radiation treatment. A study of 1,222 patients. *Medicine, 44:*305–344, 1965.

118. Vigliani, E.C., and Saita, G.: Benzene and leukemia. *New Engl J Med, 271:*872–876, 1964.

119. Nowell, P.C., and Hungerford, D.A.: Chromosome studies in human leukemia. II. Chronic granulocytic leukemia. *J Natl Cancer Inst, 27:*1013–1035, 1961.

120. Tough, I.M., Jacobs, P.A., Court Brown, W.M., Baikie, A.G., and Williamson, E.R.D.: Cytogenetic studies on bonemarrow in chronic myeloid leukaemia. *Lancet, 1:*844–846, 1963.

121. Heath, C.W., Jr.: Formal discussion: epidemiology of acute leukemia and Burkitt's tumor. *Cancer Res, 27:*2439–2440, 1967.

122. Hammouda, F., Quaglino, D., and Hayhoe, F.G.J.: Blastic crisis in chronic granulocytic leukaemia. Cytochemical, cytogenetic, and autoradiographic studies in four cases. *Br Med J, 1:*1275–1281, 1964.

123. Page, A.R., Hansen, A.E., and Good, R.A.: Occurrence of leukemia and lymphoma in patients with agammaglobulinemia. *Blood, 21:*197–206, 1963.

124. Peterson, R.D.A., Kelly, W.D., and Good, R.A.: Ataxia-telangiectasia: its association with defective thymus, immunological-deficiency disease and malignancy. *Lancet, 1:*1189–1193, 1964.

125. Hecht, F., Koler, R.D., Rigas, D.A., Dalinke, G.S., Case, M.P., Tisdale, V., and Miller, R.W.: Leukaemia and lymphocytes in ataxia-telangiectasia (letter to editor). *Lancet, 2:*1193, 1966.

126. Gatti, R.A., and Good, R.A.: Occurrence of malignancy in immunodeficiency diseases.

A literature review. *Cancer, 28:*89–98, 1971.

127. Seligman, M., Danon, F., Mihaesco, C., and Fudenberg, H.H.: Immunoglobulin abnormalities in families of patients with Waldenström's macroglobulinemia. *Am J Med, 43:*66–83, 1967.

128. Sutton, R.N.P., Bishun, N.P., and Soothill, J.F.: Immunological and chromosomal studies in first-degree relatives of children with acute lymphoblastic leukaemia. *Br J Haematol, 17:*113–119, 1969.

129. Best, W.R., Limarzi, L.R., and Poucher, H.G.: Distribution of blood types in the leukemias (abstract). *J Lab Clin Med, 34:* 1587, 1949.

130. Kay, H.E.M., and Shorter, R.G.: Blood groups in leukaemia and the reticuloses. *Vox Sang, 1:*255–258, 1956.

131. Veale, A.M.O., and Gunz, F.W.: Haptoglobins and leukaemia. *Proc Univ Otago Med Sch, 45:*36–38, 1967.

132. Lilly, F., Boyse, E.A., and Old, L.J.: Genetic basis of susceptibility to viral leukaemogenesis. *Lancet, 2:*1207–1209, 1964.

133. Ellman, L., Green, I., and Martin, W.J.: Histocompatibility genes, immune responsiveness, and leukaemia. *Lancet, 1:*1104–1106, 1970.

134. Walford, R.L., Finkelstein, S., Neerhout, R., Konrad, P., and Shanbrom, E.: Acute childhood leukaemia in relation to the HL-A human transplantation genes. *Nature, 225:*461–462, 1970.

135. Kourilsky, F.M., Dausset, J., Feingold, J., Dupuy, J.M., and Bernard, J.: Etude de la repartition des antigenes leucocytaires chez des malades attients de leucémie aigue en remission. In *Advances in Transplantation.* Copenhagen, 1968, pp. 515–522.

136. Thorsby, E., Bratlie, A., and Lie, S.O.: HL-A genotypes of children with acute leukaemia. A family study. *Scand J Haematol, 6:* 409–415, 1969.

137. Lawler, S.D., Klouda, P.T., Hardisty, R.M., and Till, M.M.: Histocompatibility and acute lymphoblastic leukemia (letter to editor). *Lancet, 1:*699, 1971.

138. Batchelor, J.R., Edwards, J.H., and Stuart, J.: Histocompatibility and acute lympho-blastic leukemia (letter to editor). *Lancet, 1*:699, 1971.

139. Zervas, J.D., Delamore, I.W., and Israëls, McG.: Leucocyte phenotypes in Hodg-kin's disease. *Lancet, 2*:634–635, 1970.

140. Forbes, J.F., and Morris, P.J.: Leucocyte antigens in Hodgkin's disease. *Lancet, 2*: 849–851, 1970.

141. Goh, K., and Swisher, S.N.: Identical twins and chronic myelocytic leukemia. Chro-mosomal studies of a patient with chronic myelocytic leukemia and his normal iden-tical twin. *Arch Intern Med, 115*:475–478, 1965.

142. Goh, K., Swisher, S.N., and Herman, E.C., Jr.: Chronic myelocytic leukemia and identical twins. Additional evidence of the Philadelphia chromosome as postzygotic abnormality. *Arch Intern Med, 120*:214–219, 1967.

143. Dougan, L., Scott, I.D., and Woodliff, H.J.: A pair of twins one of whom has chronic granulocytic leukaemia. *J Med Genet, 3*: 217–219, 1966.

144. Woodliff, H.J., Dougan, L., and Duesti, P.: Cytogenetic studies in twins, one with chronic granulocytic leukaemia. *Nature, 211*:533, 1966.

145. Jacobs, E.M., Luce, J.K., and Cailleau, R.: Chromosome abnormalities in human can-cer. Report of a patient with chronic myelocytic leukemia and his nonleukemic monozygotic twin. *Cancer, 19*:869–876, 1966.

146. Kosenow, W., and Pfeiffer, R.A.: Chronisch-myeloische Leukämie bei eineiigen Zwil-lingen. *Dtsch Med Wochenschr, 94*:1170–1176, 1969.

147. Gunz, F.W., Fitzgerald, P.H., and Adams, A.: An abnormal chromosome in chronic lymphocytic leukaemia. *Br Med J, 2*: 1097–1099, 1962.

148. Fitzgerald, P.H., and Hamer, J.W.: Third case of chronic lymphocytic leukaemia in a carrier of the inherited Ch^1 chromosome. *Br Med J, 3*:752–754, 1969.

149. Fitzgerald, P.H.: Abnormal length of the small acrocentric chromosomes in chronic lymphocytic leukemia. *Cancer Res, 25*: 1904–1909, 1965.

150. Court Brown, W.M.: Chromosomal abnor-mality and chronic lymphatic leukaemia (letter to editor). *Lancet, 1*:986, 1964.

151. Fitzgerald, P.H., Crossen, P.E., Adams, A.C., Sharman, C.V., and Gunz, F.W.: Chro-mosome studies in familial leukemia. *J Med Genet, 3*:96–100, 1966.

152. Juberg, R.C., and Jones, B.: The Christchurch chromosome (G_p-). Mongolism, erytho-leukemia and an inherited G_p- chromo-some (Christchurch). *New Engl J Med, 282*:292–297, 1970.

153. Sandberg, A.A., Ishihara, T., Kikuchi, Y., and Crosswhite, L.H.: Chromosomal dif-ferences among the acute leukemias. *Ann NY Acad Sci, 113*:663–716, 1964.

154. Reisman, L.E., Mitarii, M., and Zuelzer, W.W.: Chromosome studies in leukemia: evidence for the origin of leukemic stem lines from aneuploid mutants. *New Engl J Med, 270*:591–597, 1964.

155. Reisman, L.E., Zuelzer, W.W., and Thomp-son, R.I.: Further observations on the role of aneuploidy in acute leukemia. *Cancer Res, 24*:1448–1455, 1964.

156. Fitzgerald, P.H., Adams, A., and Gunz, F.W.: Chromosome studies in adult acute leu-kemia. *J Natl Cancer Inst, 32*:395–417, 1964.

157. Todaro, G. J., Green, H., and Swift, M.R.: Susceptibility of human diploid fibroblast strains to transformation by SV40 virus. *Science, 153*:1252–1254, 1966.

158. Todaro, G.J., and Martin, G.M.: Increased susceptibility of Down's syndrome fibro-blasts to transformation by SV40. *Proc Soc Exp Biol Med, 124*:1232–1236, 1967.

159. Miller, R.W., and Todaro, G.J.: Viral trans-formation of cells from persons at high risk of cancer. *Lancet, 1*:81–82, 1969.

CHAPTER 15

WISKOTT-ALDRICH SYNDROME

NORMAN C. NEVIN

THE WISKOTT-ALDRICH syndrome, a severe disease of infancy and childhood, is characterized by eczema, thrombocytopenia and recurrent infections. Although first described in 1937 by Wiskott,[1] it was not until seventeen years later that Aldrich, *et al.*[2] adumbrated the clinical features in detail and suggested a sex-linked recessive mode of inheritance. Affected males have a profound immunologic disturbance;[3-6] low isohemagglutinin titers, low serum IgM levels, lymphocytopenia, and depletion of tissue lymphocytes. Although patients seldom survive beyond the age of ten years, dying of overwhelming viral or bacterial infection or from hemmorrhage during infancy, some have survived to die of malignant disease later in childhood. Lymphoreticular malignancy has been reported in more than 10 percent of cases.[7,8]

Clinical Features

The presenting clinical aspects are those derived from the triad of eczema, thrombocytopenia and increased susceptibility to infections.

Eczema with onset in the first year of life, is a constant feature, involving face, upper arms (Fig. 15–1) and legs with sparing of the abdomen and back; a distribution similar to that of infantile atopic eczema. It is the most benign aspect of the syndrome. The severity is variable and often an eczematous area is the site of infection and hemorrhage[9] (Fig. 15–2).

Thrombocytopenia usually presents in the first few weeks of life. The hemorrhagic tendency, however, is extremely variable. Some patients have frequent severe epistaxes, hematuria or rectal bleeding, whereas others have only petechial eruptions (Fig. 15–3), bleeding gums, or melena. Occasionally, bleeding from a circumcision wound,[10] or subperiosteal hemorrhage[11] may herald the onset of the disease.

Increased susceptibility to infection, the third characteristic abnormality of the triad, is also apparent within the first year of life. Patients are susceptible to a wide variety of infectious agents including gram-negative and gram-positive bacteria, fungi, viruses and *pneumocystis carinii.*[5] The infections involve essentially every organ and all body surfaces. Superficial pyogenic infections are common and include furunculosis, impetigo and conjunctivitis. Purulent otitis media due to beta hemolytic streptococcus, pseudomonas or proteus is often a chronic condition. Other frequent infections are pneumonia and cellulitis of eczematoid areas. Other clinical features are variable and include hepatosplenomegaly[4,12] and lymphodenopathy.[13] Some patients have unexplained transient arthritis involving several large joints.[5]

Pathogenesis

The basic defect in the Wiskott-Aldrich syndrome must account for the abnormalities in two seemingly unrelated organ systems: lymphocytes and platelets.

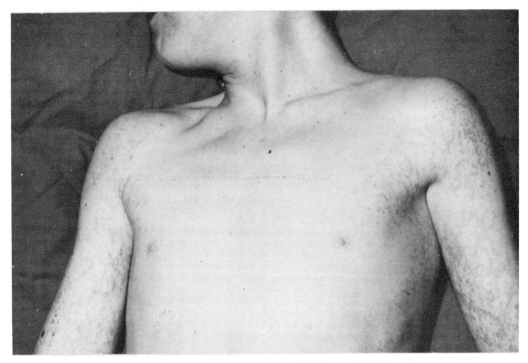

Figure 15–1. Eczema involving upper arms in Wiskott-Aldrich syndrome.

Immunologic Disorder

Patients have an immunologic disturbance but the degree of the deficit may be variable. Both humoral and cellular immune responses are affected.[6]

Isohemagglutinin titers are usually very low or absent but some may be within the lower limit of the normal range.[4,10] Frequently, serum IgM levels are low and serum IgA levels may be raised.[14,15] In some patients the serum IgE level is also elevated.[15]

Early in the course of the disease cell-mediated immunity is intact but with time, affected individuals become anergic to delayed hypersensitivity skin tests and *in vitro* lymphocyte responses to phytohemagglutinin and antigens. Depletion of thymus-dependent small lymphocytes in peripheral lymphoid tissues and circulation and the development of a cell-mediated immune deficiency are relatively late occurrences.[5]

There is a general failure to respond with antibody synthesis to polysaccaride of lipopolysaccharide antigens.[5] This primary inability to produce antibodies to polysaccharide antigens could explain the low serum IgM levels, small lymphocyte depletion, functional deficiency of the thymus-dependent lymphoid system, excessive proliferation of the reticuloendothelial cells, the extraordinary susceptibility to all types of infectious agents and even the high frequency of lymphoreticular malignancies which occur in the Wiskott-Aldrich syndrome.[7,8]

Thrombocytopenia

The exact cause of the thrombocytopenia is not clear; megakaryocytes may or may not be present in bone marrow aspirates[10,16] and donor platelets have a normal survival time,[17,18] indicating an intracorpuscular defect rather than increased destruction. A recent investigation[19] demonstrated a failure of platelet aggregation in response to adrenaline and an abnormality in platelet metabolic response to stimulation with polystyrene particles and adrenaline. The authors suggested that a single basic defect in energy metabolism causing a failure in "regulators of oxidative phosphorylation probably residing in the cell granules," might account for an intrinsic platelet defect and a defect in macrophage processing antigen.

Pathological Features

Apart from hemorrhage involving gastrointestinal tract, skin, adrenal glands and brain, and infection such as pneumonia, purulent otitis media and meningitis, significant autopsy findings are related to the lymphoreticular system. The thymus may be small[4,5] with histologic evidence of atrophy.

Although lymphadenopathy often may be an impressive feature, histological studies indicate that the lymph node enlargement is due primarily to reticulum cell hyperplasia.[4] However, it may be that the degree of reticulum cell hyperplasia is related to the age of the patient and to the number of infectious diseases which the patient has experienced.

Histologically, there is a characteristic depletion of lymphocytes in the follicles of the lymph nodes and the Malpighian corpuscles of the spleen and infiltration of the visceral organs and brain by reticulum cells, plasma cells and histiocytes.[4,10,16,20]

Inheritance

The Wiskott-Aldrich syndrome is inherited in a sex-linked recessive manner (Fig. 15–4). Aldrich, et al.[2] described a family which included 40 males, 16 of whom died in infancy

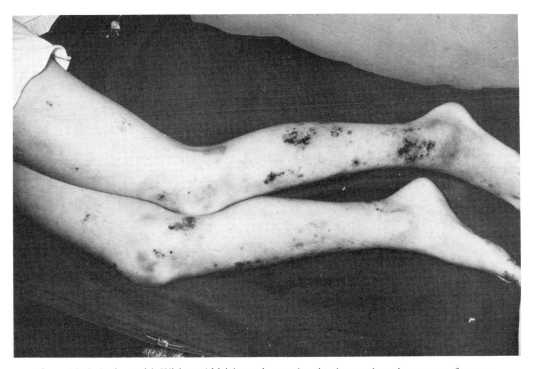

Figure 15–2. Patient with Wiskott-Aldrich syndrome showing hemorrhage into areas of eczema.

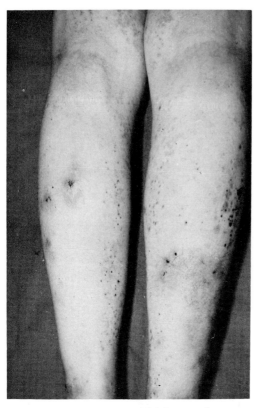

Figure 15–3. Typical petechial haemorrhages on dorsum of legs in patient with the Wiskott-Aldrich syndrome.

and 10 of whom had eczema, otitis, and bloody diarrhoea. Several recent reviews of reported cases[4,10-12,16,20,21] have indicated that the syndrome may be considerably broader in clinical manifestation than was originally thought and that both sex-linked and sporadic varieties may exist. Incomplete expression of the genetic defect may occur, as illustrated by instances of eczema alone or of abnormal bleeding without unusual susceptibility to infection in male relatives of severely affected patients. The condition has been described in male twins.[22] Affected individuals usually died in the first few years of life, but recently some long-term survivals have been reported. Mandl, *et al.*[23] described a 24-year-old male with a sporadic variety of the syndrome.

Several techniques to detect carriers (heterozygotes) for the gene for the Wiskott-Aldrich syndrome have been proposed. Wolff[4] suggested that "low IgM . . . may prove a valuable genetic marker to facilitate the identification of carriers." He studied three mothers (2 definite and 1 probable carrier) of patients of the Wiskott-Aldrich syndrome; the serum IgM level, in one was low, in another equivocal, and in the third,

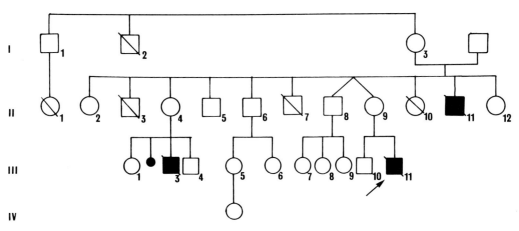

Figure 15–4. Pedigree of family with Wiskott-Aldrich syndrome.

normal. In addition, the serum IgM level in three female sibs (possible carriers) was also variable. In eight female relatives (2 definite carriers, 1 probable carrier, and 5 possible carriers) from three families of patients with the Wiskott-Aldrich syndrome, we found normal serum IgM levels.[24] Stiehm and McIntosh[21] also found normal serum immunoglobulin levels in carriers.

Van den Bosch and Drukker[25] proposed that low platelet counts may be useful in identifying carriers. Again, in the eight carriers we have investigated, platelet counts were within the normal range.[24]

A more definitive method of carrier identification was recently suggested by the finding of Kuramoto, *et al.*[9] that a failure of platelet aggregation in response to adrenaline and an abnormality in platelet metabolic response to stimulation by polystyrene particles and adrenaline not only in 3 boys with the Wiskott-Aldrich syndrome, but also in their mother. In collateral studies, they also observed a deficient aggregation of platelets with adenosine diphosphate (ADP) and collagen. We also noted an abnormal response of platelet aggregation to adrenaline in two definite carriers and in two of the five possible carriers.[24] Although the abnormal response of platelet aggregation to adrenaline is not consistent, it may have some value in genetic counseling.

Treatment

Several forms of therapy have been attempted. Splenectomy may have a temporary effect on the platelet count. Splenectomy, however, is contra-indicated in patients with the Wiskott-Aldrich syndrome even in the presence of severe thrombocytopenia, as almost all patients died with serious infectious sequelae following the operation.[26] Bone marrow transplantation has been successfully employed in some cases. A 2-year-old boy with the Wiskott-Aldrich syndrome has been treated by bone-marrow transplantation.[27] An initial attempt to transplantation without extensive preparation of the recipient failed. Subsequently, the recipient was prepared with a 4-day course of cyclophosphamide followed by bone-marrow transplantation from a sister identical for major transplantation antigens. Twenty-two months after transplantation the patient had no evidence of graft-versus-host disease.[28] However, long-term sequelae in bone-marrow transplantation recipients has not yet been adequately evaluated. An interesting approach was that of Levin, *et al.*[29] who attempted immunologic reconstitution of patients with the Wiskott-Aldrich syndrome with transfer factor (a dialysate of peripheral blood leucocytes). In 3 out of 5 patients, there was a marked improvement in the clinical condition, although platelet counts were not dramatically altered. In the other 2 patients there was no improvement. Stiehm and McIntosh[21] treated two patients with prolonged trials of periodic plasma infusions accompanied by γ-globulin injections but without any remarkable effects on platelets or resistance to infection.

Predisposition to Malignancy

Malignancy, particularly of the lymphoreticular system, is increased in the Wiskott-Aldrich syndrome. Although accurate estimates of the incidence of malignancy among such patients are not available, approximately one in ten of these children die of malignancy.[7,8]

In 1961, Coleman, *et al.*[20] first emphasized this association of malignant disease with the Wiskott-Aldrich syndrome. Their patient who died age 20 months, had a malignant reticuloendotheliosis involving the brain, meninges, lungs, oesophagus, larynx, spleen, and lymph nodes. Since then, thirteen further patients with the Wiskott-Aldrich syndrome have died with associated malignant lesions (Table 15-I). The majority of malignancies have been of lymphoreticular origin.[16,20, 30-36] The mean age at death of 11 patients in whom the age of death is recorded, is 7 years 6 months.

In a family reported by Ten Bensel, *et al.*[30] in which four brothers in sibship of seven had the Wiskott-Aldrich syndrome, two brothers died from neoplastic disease; one aged 3 years with myelogenous leukaemia and the other, aged 6 years 6 months with an anaplastic reticulum cell sarcoma. Oppenheimer, *et al.*[37] described a patient with the Wiskott-Aldrich syndrome who also died with leukemia. Their patient manifested the type of response seen in acute leukemia two months prior to death

and at autopsy the bone marrow was completely replaced with undifferentiated cells. Two patients with the Wiskott-Aldrich syndrome developed a nonlymphoid tumor.[38,39] The oncogenetic mechanism in the Wiskott-Aldrich syndrome is unknown. It has been suggested that the recurrent infection with hyperplasia of the reticulum cell may play an aetiological role in this form of malignancy.[31] However, the raised incidence of malignancy in the course of the disease may be due primarily to the immunologic disturbance. Almost every form of primary immunologic disturbance is associated with a distinctive malignancy. The frequency of malignancy in immuno-deficiencies has been estimated as approximately 10,000 times greater than the general age-matched population.[8]

TABLE 15-I
MALIGNANCY IN PATIENTS WITH THE WISKOTT-ALDRICH SYNDROME

Author	Year	Age at Death	Type of Cancer
Coleman, *et al.*	1961	1 year 8 months	Malignant reticuloendotheliosis
Kildeberg	1961	2 years 6 months	Malignant reticuloendotheliosis
CPC	1962	20 years	Reticulum cell sarcoma
Amiet	1963	7 years 10 months	Astrocytoma
Pearson, *et al.*	1966	8 years 9 months	Disseminated lymphoma
	1966	8 years	Malignant lymphoma
Ten Bensel, *et al.*	1966	6 years 6 months	Malignant reticuloendotheliosis
	1966	3 years	Myelogenous leukaemia
Chaptal, *et al.*	1966	9 years	Thymosarcoma
Rádl, *et al.*	1967	13 years 6 months	Lymphosarcoma
Huber	1968	*	Malignant reticulosis
Brand & Marinkovich	1969	3 years 1 month	Malignant reticuloendotheliosis
Oppenheim, *et al.*	1970	*	Acute leukaemia
Rupprecht & Huff	1971	*	Multiple leiomyosarcoma

* = Not recorded.

REFERENCES

1. Wiskott, A.: Familiärer, angoborener Morbus Werlhofli? *Mschr f Kinderheilk, 68:*212–216, 1937.
2. Aldrich, R.A., Steinberg, A.G., and Campbell, D.C.: Pedigree demonstrating a sex-linked recessive condition characterized by draining ears, eczematoid dermatitis and bloody diarrhoea. *Pediatrics, 13:*133–139, 1954.
3. Peterson, R.D., Cooper, M.D., and Good, R.A.: The pathogenesis of immunologic

deficiency diseases. *Am J Med, 38:*579–604, 1965.
4. Wolff, J.A.: Wiskott-Aldrich syndrome: Clinical, immunologic and pathologic observations. *J Pediatr, 70:*221–232, 1967.
5. Cooper, M.D., Chase, H.P., Lowman, J.T., Krivit, W., and Good, R.A.: Immunologic defects in patients with Wiskott-Aldrich syndrome. In *Immunologic Deficiency Diseases in Man.* Birth Defects

Original Articles Series, Vol. IV, No. 1., 378–387, 1968.

6. Blaese, R.M., Strober, W., Brown, R.S., and Waldmann, T.A.: The Wiskott-Aldrich Syndrome. A Disorder with a possible Defect in Antigen processing or recognition. *Lancet, i:*1056–1061, 1968.

7. Good, R.A.: In Smith, Richard T., and Landy, Maurice, (Eds.): *Immune Surveillance.* New York and London, Acad Pr, 1970, pp. 439–451.

8. Gatti, R.A., and Good, R.A.: Occurrence of malignancy in immunodeficiency diseases. A Literature Review. *Cancer, 28:*89–98, 1971.

9. Strivastava, R.N.: Wiskott-Aldrich Syndrome. *Arch Dis Child, 42:*604–607, 1967.

10. Krivit, W., and Good, R.A.: Aldrich's syndrome (thrombocytopaenia, eczema and infection in infants): Studies of the Defence Mechanisms. *Am J Dis Child, 97:*137–153, 1959.

11. Rivera, A.M., and Biehusen, F.C.: Aldrich's syndrome. Report of a case with subperiosteal haemorrhage. *J Pediatr, 57:*86–88, 1960.

12. Cassimos, C., Anastasea-Vlahou, C., Kattamis, C., and Kanavakis, E.: Aldrich's syndrome (thrombocytopenia, eczema and recurrent infections). Report of a case. *Am J Dis Child, 100:*904–917, 1960.

13. Root, A.W., and Speicher, C.E.: The triad of thrombocytopenia, eczema and recurrent infections (Wiskott-Aldrich syndrome) associated with milk antibodies, giant cell pneumonia and cytomegalic inclusion disease. *Pediatrics, 31:*444–454, 1963.

14. West, C.D., Hong, R., and Holland, N.H.: Immunoglobulin levels from the newborn period to adulthood and in immunoglobulin deficiency states. *J Clin Invest, 41:* 2054–2064, 1962.

15. Berglund, G., Finnström, O., Johansson, S.G.O., and Möller, K.L.: Wiskott-Aldrich syndrome—a study of 6 cases with determination of the immunoglobulins A, D, G, M, and ND. *Acta Paediatr Scand, 57:* 89–97, 1968.

16. Kildeberg, P.: The Aldrich syndrome. Report of a case and discussion of pathogenesis. *Pediatrics, 27:*362–369, 1961.

17. Pearson, H.A., Shulman, N.R., Oski, F.A., and Eitzman, D.V.: Platelet Studies in the Wiskott-Aldrich syndrome. *J Pediatr, 67:* 955, 1965.

18. Krivit, W., Yunis, E., and White, J.G.: Platelet survival studies in Aldrich syndrome. *Pediatrics, 37:*339–341, 1966.

19. Kuramoto, A., Steiner, M., and Baldini, M.G.: Lack of platelet response to stimulation in the Wiskott-Aldrich syndrome. *New Engl J Med, 282:*475–479, 1970.

20. Coleman, A., Leikin, S., and Guin, G.H.: Aldrich's Syndrome. *Clin Proc Child Hosp (Wash), 17:*22–27, 1961.

21. Stiehm, E.R., and McIntosh, R.M.: Wiskott-Aldrich syndrome: review and report of a large family. *Clinical Exp Immunol, 2:* 179–189, 1967.

22. Cummins, L., Searer, W., Levenson, S., and Geppert, L.: Aldrich syndrome in twins. *Am J Dis Child, 98:*579–580, 1959.

23. Mandl, M.A.J., Watson, J.I., and Rose, B.: The Wiskott-Aldrich syndrome. Immuno-pathologic Mechanisms and a Long-term survival. *Ann Intern Med, 68:*1050–1059, 1968.

24. Nevin, N.C., Bridges, J.M., Mayne, E.E., Moore, W.M.A., and Otridge, B.W. The Wiskott-Aldrich syndrome: The detection of carriers. (Unpublished).

25. Van Den Bosch, J., and Drukker, J.: Het syndroom van Aldrich; een klinisch en genetisch onderzoek van enige Nederlandse families. *Maandschr Kindergeneesk, 32:* 359–373, 1964.

26. Weiden, P.L., and Blaese, R.M.: Hereditary thrombocytopenia: Relation to Wiskott-Aldrich syndrome with special reference to splenectomy. Report of a family and review of the literature. *J Pediatr, 80:*226–234, 1972.

27. Bach, F.H., Albertini, R.J., Joo, P., Anderson, J.L., and Bortin, M.M.: Bone-marrow transplantation in a patient with the Wiskott-Aldrich Syndrome. *Lancet, ii:*1364–1366, 1968.

28. Bach, F.H. quoted Levin, *et al,* 1970.

29. Levin, A.S., Spitler, L.E., Stites, D.P., and Fudenburg, H.H.: Wiskott-Aldrich Syndrome, A Genetically Determined Cellular Immunologic Deficiency: Clinical and

Laboratory Responses to Therapy with Transfer Factor. *Proceedings of the National Academy of Sciences, 67:*821–828, 1970.

30. Ten Bensel, R.W., Stadlan, E.M., and Krivit, W.: The development of malignancy in the course of the Aldrich syndrome. *J Pediatr, 68:*761–767, 1966.

31. Brand, M.M., and Marinkovich, V.A.: Primary malignant reticulosis of the brain in Wiskott-Aldrich syndrome. Report of a case. *Arch Dis Child, 44:*536–542, 1969.

32. Pearson, H.A., Shulman, N.R., Oski, F.A., and Eitzman, D.V.: Platelet survival in the Wiskott-Aldrich Syndrome. *J Pediatr, 68:* 754–760, 1966.

33. Rádl, J., Masopust, J., Houstek, J., and Hrodek, O.: Paraproteinaemia and Unusual Dys-γ-globulinaemia in a Case of Wiskott-Aldrich Syndrome. An Immunochemical Study. *Arch Dis Child, 42:*608–614, 1967.

34. Huber, J.: Experience with various immunologic deficiencies in Holland. In Good, R.A., and Bergsma, D. (Eds.): *Immunologic Deficiency Diseases in Man.* Birth Defects Original Article Series, Vol. 4, New York, 1968, 53–66.

35. Chaptal, J., Royer, R., Jean, R., Alagille, D., Bonnet, H., LaGarde, E., Robinet, M., and Rieu, D.: Syndrome de Wiskott-Aldrich avec survie prolongée (9 ans). Evolution mortelle par thymosarcome. *Arch Franç de Pédiatrie, 23:*907–920, 1966.

36. Clinicopathological Conference. Rademacher's disease. Diminished Immunity of an Unusual form complicated by lymphadenopathy. *Am J Med, 32:*80–95, 1962.

37. Oppenheim, J.J., Blaese, R.M., and Waldmann, T.A.: Defective lymphocyte transformation and delayed hypersensitivity in Wiskott-Aldrich syndrome. *J Immunol, 104:* 835–844, 1970.

38. Amiet, Von A.: Aldrich-syndrom: Beobachtung zweier Fälle. *Ann Paediatr, 201:*315–335, 1963.

39. Rupprecht, L., and Huff, D.: quoted Gatti, R.A., and Good, R.A., 1971.

CHAPTER 16

THE GENETICS OF RETINOBLASTOMA

HAROLD F. FALLS

RETINOBLASTOMA IS A HIGHLY malignant intraocular tumor of early childhood and is hereditary in certain circumstances (Fig. 16–1).

Incidence

The literature suggests a frequency of occurrence which varies between 1 in 17,000 births to 1 in 34,000. Although not totally substantiated, it is postulated that there is an increasing incidence of the disease: 1 in 34,000 (1931) births to 1 in 14,000 (1961).[1,2] Perhaps this is a consequence of the lessening mortality rate subsequent to earlier diagnosis and more efficient therapy.

Sex

The literature indicates a minimal preponderance of male sex involvement. Most authorities do not agree.

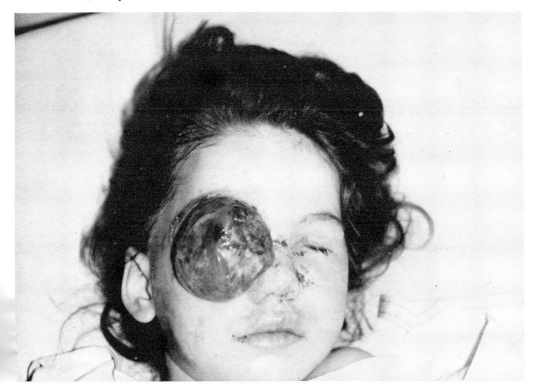

Figure 16–1. Ocular and Orbital Extension of Retinoblastoma.

Age of Manifestation

Retinoblastoma may be observed at birth. Some authors insist that the tumor is congenital. In the vast majority of cases (70%) the diagnosis is made before two years of age. It is most exceptional for the tumor to become manifest after seven years of age. Cases, however, have been reported as late as the fifties and even sixties.

Race

It is hinted but not adequately documented that retinoblastoma is rarer in the black race.

Mutation Rate

The mutation rate per generation has been reported as varying from 1.76×10^{-7}, 2.3×10^{-5} to 2.9×10^{-5}.

Heredity

All authorities agree that the tumor is hereditary,[4] transmission being autosomal dominant but with reduced penetrance 20 to 80 percent. Approximately 8 percent of all cases of retinoblastoma are hereditary.

A recently evolved hypothesis suggests that retinoblastoma is caused by at least two mutational events.[5] In the hereditary form of the tumor one mutation is transmitted via the germinal cells and a second mutational event occurs in the somatic retinal cells. It is suggested that in the nonhereditary variety of retinoblastoma both mutations occur in the somatic cells. Based upon observations of 48 new cases of retinoblastoma and the experience of the literature, Knudson postulates further that the second mutation produces an average of three retinoblastoma per individual in those who inherit the first mutation (germinal).

In employing Poisson's distribution statistics he[5] states that this number (three) can best explain the occasional individual who gets no tumor, those who develop bilateral tumors as well as those who have multiple tumors in only one eye.

Most recently reported,[6] and perhaps the causation of the above-mentioned second mutation, is the demonstration of RNA-directed DNA-polymerase activity in retinoblastoma. The researchers used various templates to demonstrate the above activity and found this enzyme in retinoblastoma to be similar to the RNA-directed polymerase activity found in oncogenic RNA viruses.

Unilateral and Bilateral Manifestation

Most cases of retinoblastoma are unilateral—65 to 80 percent; 20 to 35 percent[6] are bilateral. It is assumed that each tumor is in fact a *de novo* mutation. In general the diagnosis of the tumor is made earlier in life in the bilateral than the unilateral cases. There is agreement that the vast majority of bilateral cases are hereditary and that only 8 to 25 percent of unilateral cases exhibit genetic transmission. Of interest in this regard are the findings of Ellsworth[7] which intimate that in his involved families affected children occurred in 67 to 80 percent of the cases when the parent exhibited bilateral involvement. In contrast only 42 to 50 percent of the cases showed affected children when the affected parent was a unilateral case.

Cytogenics

Certain occurrences may be etiologically related to a partial deletion in D chromosome.[8]

Twins

At least ten examples of monozygotic twin involvement are known and discordance is reported in only one pair.

Diagnosis

By ophthalmoscopy, in eyes of normal size, normal anterior chamber and in early cases, the ophthalmologist observes a solitary or multi-focic, slightly elevated whitish-pink, smooth, rarely nodular lesion (Fig. 16–2). When the tumor exhibits superficial pearly white or deep chalky calcium deposits the finding is pathognomonic (Fig. 16–3).

To the laity the most common sign is a white pupil—"cat's eye reflex" (Fig. 16–4). The next most prevalent manifestation is strabismus. Less common findings in order of their frequency are glaucoma, uveitis, poor vision, orbital cellulitis, nystagmus, hyphema and hypopyon.

Increasing in frequency is the diagnosis of retinoblastoma by alert pediatricians and generalists upon routine examination of their patients. It goes without saying, moreover, that all newborns in retinoblastoma families should be subjected to meticulous

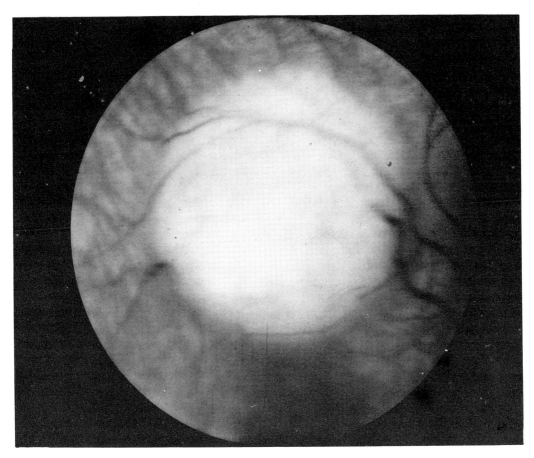

Figure 16–2. Solitary Retinoblastoma.

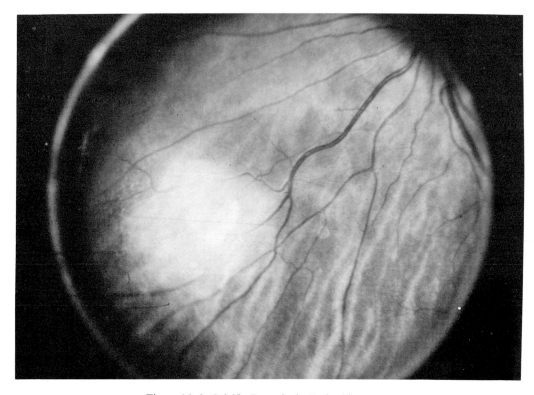

Figure 16–3. Calcific Deposits in Retinoblastoma.

ophthalmoscopic examination under anesthesia at birth and at three month intervals up to the age of at least two years.

Differential Diagnosis

Any disease of the eye which presents with a "white pupil" should be suspect of retinoblastoma. The following are among many entities:

Pseudoglioma—Norrie's Disease

This entity presents congenital or early phthisis of the eyes, an associated hearing defect, mental retardation, cataract (very rarely seen in retinoblastoma), and a sex-linked recessive mode of inheritance.

Larval Granulomatosis (*Toxocara Canis and Catis*)

The spectrum of a localized solitary retinal granuloma, or a violent endophthalmitis may be the consequence of ocular toxocara infestation. Eosinophilia may or may not be diagnostically helpful. A history of intimate contact with an infested puppy or kitten should be suggestive.

Retrolental Fibroplasia

A history of prematurity, low birth weight, exposure to high oxygen levels, or maternal hypoxia is most suggestive. With the ophthalmoscope bilateral retinal gliosis, retinal folds and aberrant vessel distribution may be observed. The anterior chambers may be shallow and the eyes smaller than normal.

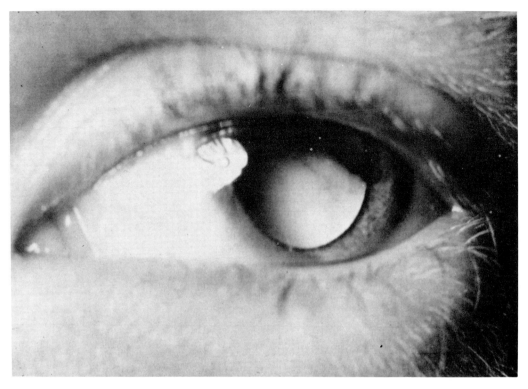

Figure 16–4. "Cat's-eye Reflex" from Retinoblastoma.

Persistent Hyperplastic Primary Vitreous

The affected eye of full term infants is usually smaller than normal and exhibits a dense gray retrolental membrane which may invade the lens. The anterior chamber is usually shallow. Elongated ciliary processes—cicatricial contracture—are almost pathognomonic.

Coats' Disease

When the eye is extensively involved this entity is most difficult to differentiate from retinoblastoma. The presence in a male of unilateral aneurysmal vasculature in association with widespread glittery exudation, the absence of calcium flecks and optic atrophy is suggestive of Coats' disease.

Angiomatosis Retinae

In a dominant family history the appearance of a large aneurysmal peripheral lesion in the retina with associated feeder sausage-shaped and beaded retinal vessels and widespread exudate suggests von Hippel Lindau's entity. When associated with widespread retinal detachment, the diagnosis is usually dependent on the pathological study of the enucleated eye.

Other Entities

Among other diseases in the differential diagnoses of retinoblastoma, one must include metastatic disease (viral meningococcosis), birth trauma, hemorrhage, congenital retinal detachment, incontinentia pigmenti, trisomy D and so on.

Genetic Counseling

It is axiomatic, of course, to insist that no genetic prognostication be undertaken until the physician has performed a most meticulous ophthalmoscopic examination of the patient, the parents (to rule out spontaneous regression) and when feasible the immediate relatives. In addition a very thorough pedigree is requisite.

Based upon personal experience and that of the literature, the following statements, with license to flexibility, can be made.

1. Assuming normal parents subsequent involvement of siblings of a sporadic case occurs in 1 to 6 percent of cases.
2. Assuming normal parents and the occurrence of more than one affected offspring subsequent involvement of siblings can be anticipated in 50 percent of the cases. This expectancy is conditioned by a 40 to 80 percent penetrance of the gene.
3. Assuming a unilateral affected parent and an affected offspring subsequent siblings can be anticipated to be affected in 50 percent of the cases. This expectancy is modified by a 40 to 50 percent penetrance.
4. Assuming a bilateral affected parent and affected offspring subsequent siblings can be expected to be affected in 50 percent of the cases. This expectancy is conditioned by a 67 to 89 percent penetrance of the gene.
5. Normal individuals (clinically) who have affected parents or siblings may be carriers and should be so informed (1.5–10% to 25% of cases).

REFERENCES

1. Hemmes, G.D.: Morbiditet en prognose van retinoblastoma (glioma retinae). *Nederl tijdschr genecsk, 11:*211, 1958.

2. Francois, J.: Recent data on the heredity of retinoblastoma. In Boniuk, M., (Ed.): *Ocular and Adnexal Tumors.* St. Louis, Mosby, 1964, p. 123.

3. Falls, H.F., and Neel, J.V.: Genetics of Retinoblastoma. *Arch Ophthalmol, 46:*367, 1951.

4. Falls, H.F.: The Inheritance of Retinoblastoma. *JAMA, 133:*171, 1947.

5. Knudson, A.G., Jr.: Mutation and Cancer: Statistical study of retinoblastoma. *Proc Natl Acad Sci,* U.S.A., *68:*4, 820–823, 1971.

6. Albert, D.M., and Reid, T.W.: RNA-directed DNA-polymerase activity in retinoblastoma. (In press.)

7. Ellsworth, R.M.: The practical management of Retinoblastoma. *Trans Am Ophthalmol Soc, 67:*462, 1969.

8. Jensen, R.D., and Miller, R.W.: Retinoblastoma: Epidemiologic Characteristics. *New Engl J Med, 285:*307–311, 1971.

CHAPTER 17

OCCURRENCES OF CENTRAL NERVOUS SYSTEM TUMORS, WITH SPECIAL REFERENCE TO RELATIVE GENETIC FACTORS

GABRIEL M. MULCAHY AND WILLIAM L. HARLAN

Introduction

THE AIM OF THIS presentation is to review the significance of the genetic factor in relation to what is known concerning the etiology and pathogenesis of central nervous system tumors, both in humans and experimentally. Factors of known or possible importance in the development of these tumors will be reviewed, irrespective of their genetic import or lack thereof, and the relevance to such factors of genetics and genetic influences will be considered where applicable. The aim is not merely to review genetic factors in the etiology of brain tumors, but to attempt to review and appraise the importance of genetic factors in relation to our total understanding, such as it is, of the etiology and pathogenesis of CNS tumors.

Our review will deal chiefly with malignant tumors of the central nervous system, but will include also benign intracranial and intraspinal tumors, such as meningioma; and also neuroblastoma, which on occasion may occur in the brain,[1-3] but which is generally found as an extracranial tumor developing in relation to adrenal medulla or other elements of the sympathetic nervous system. On the other hand, pituitary tumors and chemodectomas will not be considered in this chapter, although the former may be necessarily mentioned in certain contexts.

Since our review is of a literature of many countries employing diagnostic terms of various systems of nomenclature, we have in general adopted the practice of retaining the diagnostic terms employed by authors of original reports. To do otherwise, in an attempt to adhere to any particular system of pathologic classification in a uniform manner, would often require conversion of the diagnostic terms employed in authors' reports to the categories of the chosen classification, and it seems inappropriate to attempt such changes simply on the basis of the necessarily limited pathologic data commonly furnished with journal articles.

Fortunately, the problem of differing schemata of pathologic classification is not a barrier to exploration and review of this subject, since the several major older and more recent classifications of nervous system neoplasms,[4-12] despite their many points of difference, share substantial agreement on the nature of broad categories of tumors, and even on the identity of specific tumor types, such as astrocytoma, oligodendroglioma, medulloblastoma, and meningioma. Thus, adherents of any classification will have an understanding of the meaning of such terms as these, and of more general terms, such as glioma, which will be included in the discussion to follow.

This is not to deny that use of a single pathologic classification for CNS neoplasms would be highly desirable, and would have the potential of better definition of the epidemiology of tumor occurrences, and also their experimental induction.

Comparative and Experimental Evidence Relating to the Etiology and Pathogenesis of CNS Tumors

Evidence concerning natural occurrence and experimental induction of CNS tumors in animals may be summarized under several headings: species variation, chemical induction, viral induction, immunologic susceptibility, radiation, and interactions of various of these factors.

Species, Breed, and Strain Variation

The incidence of spontaneous brain tumors appears to vary among species, and even among breeds or strains of a single species. It may be fairly inferred that genetic differences in constitution probably contribute greatly to this variation in tumor susceptibility.

Many reports of surveys of tumor incidence in animals, while providing much valuable data, give only limited information concerning the incidence of neural tumors,[13-24] at least in some instances due to lack of provision in the surveys for routine and complete pathologic examination of the central nervous system.

Nevertheless, much information is available. Fraser found thirty-two astrocytomas, believed to be spontaneously occurring, on examination of the brains of approximately 10,000 mice which had been used in various experiments dealing with scrapie.[25] Interestingly, although this population included several different strains of mice, 29 of the 32 astrocytomas were found in VM strain mice, which accounted for only 4,000 of the total population. Two of the other three mice with astrocytomas were VM crosses. Anticipating our section on the relationship between brain tumors and congenital defects, it is pertinent to note that certain developmental anomalies, including cleft palate and cranial meningocele, were observed by

Fraser more frequently in VM strain mice than in the other strains examined.

Employing animals which had been used in previous toxicologic research, Bots, *et al.* found three brain tumors considered of spontaneous origin in 1100 albino Wistar rats,[26] and Schardein, *et al.* found six neural tumors, three central and three peripheral, in 5086 Sprague-Dawley-derived albino rats of various age groups, but including many very young rats.[27] Thompson and Hunt found four tumors thought to be spontaneously occurring in the brains of 177 albino Sprague-Dawley rats which had been used previously in experiments involving consumption of either irradiated or nonirradiated diets, and most of which had been allowed to live out their life-spans.[28] Neoplasms found were an ependymoma, a papilloma of choroid plexus, a meningioma, and a pinealoma.[29]

A relatively recent tabulation of reports of spontaneously occurring tumors in the guinea pig omits any mention of glial tumors of the central nervous system, although tumors of other organs appear to occur in this animal with some frequency after three years of age.[30]

Much of the information available on brain tumors in animals has emphasized occurrences in dogs. Luginbühl has reported brachycephalic dogs, particularly boxers, as accounting for a very high percentage of CNS tumors of various species submitted for pathologic diagnosis.[31,32] Of 163 dogs with CNS tumors, 57, which appears to be a disproportionate number, were brachycephalics. Of even greater interest, a later series showed that of 42 oligodendrogliomas encountered in dogs, 80 percent were in brachycephalics.[33]

Similar findings have been recorded by others. Hayes and Schiefer reported on 23 brain tumors of carnivores, 19 of which were in dogs and 4 in cats.[34] Fifteen of the 19 dogs, including 10 boxers, were from brachycephalic breeds. The composition of the population of animals-at-risk from which the animals with brain tumors were drawn was not stated. All four tumors from cats were meningiomas, a finding in accord with that of Luginbühl that 8 of 155 cat brains had one or more meningiomas on careful postmortem examination.[35]

In a report on neoplasia of various systems in the boxer, Howard and Nielsen found many more tumors in this breed than in their control animals.[36] Neoplasms found in increased number in the boxer included particularly mesenchymal tumors of the skin; but also neoplasms of the cardiovascular, hemolymphatic, alimentary, endocrine, and nervous systems, and seminoma. Because of the high incidence of tumors of the reticuloendothelial system, the authors speculated on the possibility that the boxer may have an immunologic deficiency.

Case reports of interest include that of Taylor, *et al.* dealing with a 14-year-old Boston terrier, one of the brachycephalic breeds, with a thalamic oligodendroglioma.[37]

While Misdorp, in a review of congenital tumors in animals, notes the lack of reports of congenital retinoblastoma and neuroblastoma in lower animals,[38] as compared to the finding of these tumors as congenital lesions in man, there have been reports of neuroblastoma of presumed adrenal medullary origin in a 15-year-old Irish setter and a two-year-old boxer;[39] and of retinoblastoma in a 9-year-old Welsh corgi.[40]

The literature also contains reports on multiple neurofibromatosis in a cow and her male calf;[41] on bovine acoustic neurinoma;[42] on ependymoma in deer;[43] and on astrocytoma associated with gliosis of domestic fowl.[44]

On examination of the central nervous system of 12,000 very young monkeys, most of which had been used for neurovirulence tests of live polio vaccine, Jungherr found only eight lesions which may be diagnosed with high probability as tumors: lumbar meningiomatosis in one animal, lipoma of the choroid plexus in another, and a peculiar lesion, endotheliomatosis of the lumbar cord, in six others.[45] It is quite possible, of course, that examination of older monkeys would show more numerous tumors with a different spectrum of histopathologic types.

Thus, although much of the evidence comes from data and observations not rigidly controlled, it would appear that there are striking differences in incidence of CNS tumors among various species, and within a single species according to breed or strain. These differences may be best explicable on the basis of genetic differences among the species, breeds, and strains concerned.

Chemical Induction

There is a long history to chemical induction of brain tumors.[46,47] For well over 30 years, investigators have been able to induce brain tumors in mice and rats by means of intracerebral implantation of chemicals such as methylcholanthrene.[48-53] Seligman and Shear, and also Zimmerman and Arnold, further demonstrated that tumors of various histopathologic types, including astrocytoma, oligodendroglioma, and spongioblastoma polare, could be induced in mice by means of implantation of the same chemical substance, methylcholanthrene.[48,51] Very early in these investigations, Zimmerman and Arnold found that different strains of mice differed in their responses to implanted pellets of methylcholanthrene.[54] Intracranial tumors were readily produced in C3H mice (25 of 42 animals), but less commonly in dba mice (2 of 19). Furthermore, in parallel experiments, no tumors were produced in rats, rabbits, guinea pigs, and dogs.[55] Species and strain, therefore, were shown to be factors of possible importance in determining susceptibility to the neoplasm-inducing effect of intracerebrally implanted carcinogen.

Many resorptive carcinogens have been used also for induction of intracranial tumors, especially in recent years. These agents, which need not be inoculated intracerebrally to accomplish tumor induction, but may be administered intravenously or orally, include 2-acetylaminofluorene,[56,57] N,N'-2, 7-fluorenylenebisacetamide,[58] lead subacetate,[59] and other compounds, particularly the nitrosoureas.[60-62]

Abundant new opportunities for experimental investigation of CNS tumors have been provided by the availability of carcinogens of the resorptive type. Thus far, nitrosourea compounds have been used for this purpose chiefly in experiments on rats, and have been responsible for induction of brain tumors of many different histopathologic patterns in this species. In the case of ethylnitrosourea, it has been demonstrated that fetal and newborn rats are particularly susceptible to the effects of the carcinogen, as compared with older animals.

There is evidence that brain tumors are induced by nitrosoureas in other species as well as the rat,[60] e.g., in the dog,[63] but more complete information on species susceptibility remains to be elucidated. Already, however, it is known that fetal rats of various inbred strains differ in their susceptibility to transplacental induction of CNS tumors by ethylnitrosourea.[64]

Viral Induction

There is substantial information, dating from the early work of Vázquez-López, that many viruses may be used to induce brain tumors in experimental animals.[65,66] Species in which neuroepithelial or intracranial mesodermal tumors of diverse histopathology can be virally induced include mouse, rat, hamster, guinea pig, dog, cat, rabbit, mastomys, calf, chicken, duck, and turkey.[67,68] Viruses capable of inducing tumors in one or more of these species include adenovirus type 12, various strains of Rous sarcoma virus (RSV), simian vacuolating virus (SV40), simian adenovirus 20 (SV20), simian adenovirus 7, polyoma virus, bovine papilloma virus, chicken embryo-lethal orphan (CELO) virus (an avian virus), and the Harvey murine leukemia-sarcoma virus.[68-72]

Since the susceptibility of many species to viral induction of CNS tumors has been well documented, it would seem a mistake to ascribe great importance to the genetic constitution as predisposing to tumor induction by viruses. For example, as tabulated by Rabotti, strains of Rous sarcoma virus can induce CNS tumors in ten different species of very different genomes.[68]

On the other hand, although Yaba virus-induced tumor has been transplanted successfully to monkey brain,[73] various breeds of monkeys have resisted direct CNS tumor induction by virus inoculation,[68,74] and this resistance may well be due to limited genetic susceptibility.

There is also a limited amount of evidence for species variation in regard to dose of oncogenic virus required for induction of intracranial neoplasms.[74] It may be that under conditions of experimental induction of CNS tumors so far employed, viral dose often has been so great as to overwhelm host attempts at resistance, and to obscure genetic differences in susceptibility to tumor induction. In this connection, it is of particular interest that, generally speaking, CNS tumors can be induced by viruses in various species only in very young animals, up to 24 to 48 hours old.[68] Outside this very short period of susceptibility, tumors can be induced only with great difficulty.

It will be of interest to learn if means will be found to more readily accomplish tumor induction by viruses in older animals, thereby providing an additional basis for comparing genetic similarities and differences among species, and perhaps permitting detection of more heterogeneity of response to viral challenge than has been demonstrated up to now. Such heterogeneity, if found, could be explicable on a genetic basis.

Radiation

There have been isolated reports of induction of brain tumors in animals by ionizing radiation,[67] including glioblastoma multiforme in monkeys[75] and malignant glioma in the rabbit,[76] but there has been no evidence linking susceptibility to such induction to genetic factors.

Immunologic Susceptibility

Among factors implicated in the development of brain tumors, alteration in immune status of the host has been given considerable attention.

Learning that immunologic response is of consequence in the pathogenesis of and resistance to neoplasia has been one of the more important achievements of the broad field of modern immunobiology. It has been demonstrated that immunity to specific tumors can be induced, and that host immunologic response, therefore, may play some part in inhibiting tumor growth.[77-79]

The concept of immunosurveillance, which has been developed by several workers, and which may be considered both a derivative, and a stimulus to discovery of the new immunologic knowledge, postulates a mechanism whereby the immune system is continuously involved in the destruction of cells of malignant potential arising *de novo* due to the effects of oncogenic stimuli of whatever type.[80-83]

More recently, Prehn has summarized evidence that a limited immunologic reaction in the face of tumor challenge may stimulate rather than inhibit tumor growth, i.e., that minimal immune reactivity, less than that sometimes adequate to inhibit neoplastic growth, may actually promote and accelerate tumor growth.[84-86]

Although immunologic mechanisms regulating tumor growth are as yet poorly understood, they have been found to have specific pertinence to occurrences of human brain tumors. Evidence for this statement, including information on occurrences of brain tumors in genetic disorders of immune deficiency, and in transplant recipients receiving immunosuppressive therapy, is presented below in subsequent sections of this chapter.

At this point, however, it should be noted that, as shown in experimental work, the brain has some degree of immunologic competence, although presumably less than that of other tissues.[87] Thus the brain is not completely "privileged" in an immunologic sense, i.e., it is not totally and indiscriminately receptive of all tissues of foreign antigenicity. Scheinberg, *et al.* have shown that after transplantation of glioma to isologous mouse brain, and then radiation cure of the lesion, some degree of induced immunity could be demonstrated on subsequent transplant challenge.[87] In other experiments, also using an isologous system in mice, these investigators induced immunity to intracerebral implants of glioma by prior intradermal injection of glioma emulsion, but not with emulsion of normal brain.[88,89]

Age has been shown to be a factor affecting the success of attempts at heterotransplantation of tumors. Janisch was able to successfully transplant human brain tumors to the brains of very young albino rats (less than 48 hours old), but had virtually no success with older animals.[90]

Administration of antilymphocyte serum to recipient animals can also affect the success of attempts at tumor transplantation. Ridley has demonstrated that transplants of two hamster tumors, polyoma virus-induced spindle cell sarcoma, and estrogen-induced kidney tumor, will grow well in the brains of ALS treated 150 gram rats, while normal untreated rats reject the transplants.[91] Nevertheless, Ridley was unable to successfully transplant human glioma to the brains of ALS treated rats.

The basis of immunocompetence of the brain, however limited in function or widely applicable it may prove to be, remains to be further worked out. The recent finding of tumor-specific soluble and membrane-bound antigens in a rat astrocytoma cell line[92] provides information which may be highly relevant to one path of exploration towards resolution of this question.

The potential importance of genetic factors in determining immunologic susceptibility or resistance to CNS tumor growth, both in experimental animals and in humans, requires delineation, but well-known relationships involving determination by genes of protein and antigenic structure presuppose a genetic influence on immunologic function.

Aspects of immunologic susceptibility bearing more specifically on human CNS tumors will be given further consideration below.

Interactions of Etiologic Factors

It need not be postulated that individual etiologic factors act singly in inducing brain tumors, for the possibilities are obvious that neoplasms may result through pathogenetic pathways involving incremental or interacting effects of two or more etiologic factors, such as oncogenic viruses and chemicals. In fact, the scope of the present contribution is to attempt to view such genetic factors as may pertain to CNS neoplasms in the perspective of possible relationships between genetic influences and other factors thought to be operative.

Several possible examples of interacting factors contributing to brain tumor induction and growth may be cited. Ikuta and Zimmerman have reported virus-like particles in reactive glial cells of the precancerous lesions induced by implantation of pellets of methylcholanthrene, benzpyrene, and dibenzanthracene into mouse brain.[93,94]

Rubin, *et al.* have found virus-like particles in murine ependymoblastoma induced with methylcholanthrene.[95] The latter workers noted that these particles, while not proven to be oncogenic, occurred selectively in tumor cells.

In experiments with 1000 mice, divided by age into five groups, Perese found that age was a factor in determining the rate of glioma induction in response to implantation of methylcholanthrene pellets in brain.[96] Bridges, also producing gliomata in mice by intracerebral implantation of methylcholanthrene, reported that mice deficient in thiamine died of their gliomata sooner than those mice given adequate dietary thiamine.[97] He stated the opinion, however, that the worsened prognosis was probably due to greater susceptibility to hemorrhage within the tumor in the thiamine deficient animal, rather than to a greater susceptibility to carcinogenesis resulting from thiamine deficiency.

Specific consideration of the central nervous system aside, involvement of multiple etiologic and modifying factors in neoplastic development has long been postulated and/or observed.[98 – 101] Chang and Hildemann, for example, in genetic experiments with two strains of mice, one susceptible and one relatively resistant to polyoma virus, found evidence leading these investigators to the conclusion that susceptibility to polyoma virus tumorigenesis may be due to a single autosomal gene with incomplete penetrance.[102]

In this context, multiple interacting factors would seem to deserve consideration as possibly operative in the development of brain tumors.

Genetic Factors Relating to the Epidemiology and Clinical Correlations of Human CNS Tumors

In this section we will review the epidemiology and certain clinical correlations of human CNS tumors, including points of genetic as well as nongenetic interest.

Epidemiology of CNS Tumors

The importance of the brain tumor problem is reflected in Kurland's report that 1 percent of deaths in the resident population of Rochester, Minnesota, is due to primary intracranial neoplasms.[103] Van der Drift and Magnus found that, in six age groups surveyed, neoplasms are by far the most common of space-occupying intracranial lesions.[104] For the age group under fifteen, CNS cancer is second only to leukemia in cancer mortality tables.[105] Contrary to a once common opinion, epidemiological studies, dating from the 1950's, and including both clinical and post-mortem ascertainment, give some indication that brain tumor incidence increases with advancing age.[103,106] Percy, *et al.*, also reporting on the experience with the resident population of Rochester, Minnesota, and compiling information on CNS neoplasms occurring during the years 1935 through 1968, found the age-specific incidence of primary brain tumors to increase steadily with age, although not at a uniform rate of increase;[107] and Guomundsson, in a study of the population of Iceland, found that age-specific incidence rates for primary brain tumors ranged from 3.4 per 100,000 for the age group birth-to-nineteen years, to 28.5 per 100,000 for the age group 80 plus.[108] Data from the Israeli Central Tumor Registry, however, while indicating increasing rates of age-specific CNS tumor incidence through the seventh decade, also indicated a decline in incidence beyond age 70, perhaps, in the latter instance, due to a lack of available information concerning the pathologic status of the central nervous system in individuals from this age group.[109,110]

In a series of 497 primary intracranial tumors documented during the course of 17,000 autopsies, Cooney and Solitare found those age 60 or older accounting for approximately 35 percent of the total number of tumors, including 27 percent of glioblastomas, 43 percent of cranial nerve tumors, 37 percent of meningiomas related to cause of death, and 82 percent of meningiomas occurring as incidental findings.[111]

There are several reservations required in evaluating available epidemiologic information concerning brain tumor incidence and prevalence. In some studies the information has come from death certificates, with the known limitations on accuracy implicit therein, including hasty preparation, lack of pathologic verification, either at autopsy or with surgical specimens, and remoteness of the investigator from his primary source material. Hospital statistics, another source of information, suffer from the obvious selectivity of hospital admissions, and the lack of well defined total population bases from which hospital populations are drawn.

Berg has pointed to the lack of provision for means of establishing precise histopathologic diagnosis in most cancer epidemiology studies, and he has called, in fact, for studies taking due account of the pathologic nature, including specific histologic subtypes, of cancers under epidemiologic investigation.[112]

Autopsy studies, on the other hand, while providing firm pathologic documentation, have drawbacks of their own. They are frequently performed on a highly selective basis, both in respect to total deaths within an individual hospital (a low autopsy rate), and, even more, in respect to total deaths occurring in the population residing in the geographic area in which an individual hospital is located. There can be no assurance that the results of autopsy examinations performed selectively will provide mortality data representative of that of the total population of any given area. The inherent inability of the autopsy examination to provide full morbidity information, as opposed to mortality data, for a given individual and for a given population, further limits the epidemiologic value of investigations limited solely to post-mortem examinations.

Another consideration relating to autopsies, as Huntington, *et al.* have pointed out, is that post-mortem examinations are frequently not performed on medical examiners' cases.[113] These workers demonstrated that careful examination of the central nervous system in medico-legal cases uncovers an important group of fatal primary brain tumors undiagnosed during life, and expressed the opinion that the results of their study could be duplicated in other jurisdictions were appropriate efforts to be made.

Despite the admirable manner in which the many obstacles to the gathering of reliable information have been hurdled or circumvented by individual investigators, it is still true that we are lacking much of the information concerning brain tumor occurrences and associations which could be obtained in a broad-scale prospective study attempting complete epidemiologic, clinical, and pathologic ascertainment of a large population in a defined geographic area. To our knowledge, such a study has not yet been performed.

Nevertheless, much valuable data has been obtained, both from autopsy studies, and from broader population surveys. The post-mortem examination has provided especially interesting information in respect to particular aspects of brain tumor incidence. Peers, for example, in a review of autopsy material, found no significant year-to-year variation in CNS tumor incidence during the period 1896 through 1934.[114] Andersson, reviewing post-mortem examinations on psychiatric patients, found approximately 2 percent with primary intracranial neoplasms, the majority of which had not been diagnosed antemortem.[115]

In an autopsy series concerned with geriatric patients, Harenko found a 3.1 percent incidence of primary brain tumors, chiefly meningiomas,[116] while Wood, *et al.* found

that of 100 patients with asymptomatic meningiomas encountered at autopsy, 16 percent had multiple lesions.[117] In a pediatric autopsy series, Regelson, *et al.* found tumors of neural origin, including brain tumors, neuroblastomas, and retinoblastomas, to account for 21 percent of all cancers.[118]

Likewise, large population surveys have produced a great deal of informative data. Goldberg and Kurland, in a study of mortality statistics of 26 countries, found a geographically uniform pattern of age-adjusted death rates for nervous system tumors, with values falling in the narrow range of 3.8 to 5.6 per 100,000 per year in most countries.[119] Only Chile, Japan, and Mexico, on the one hand, and Israel, on the other, with lower and higher rates, respectively, seemed to be exceptions, and the values for these countries were considered as perhaps at least partially explicable on the basis of differences in patterns of medical practice and also in the processes of collecting and handling data.

As would be expected, studies dealing with incidence rates of CNS tumors, rather than death rates, have tended to produce somewhat higher figures than those mortality rates quoted above.[120–122]

Especially interesting are the results of the above-mentioned Rochester, Minnesota, study of CNS tumors reported by Percy, *et al.*[107] The work of these investigators was supported by the high quality of the medical records maintained by the Mayo Clinic and its affiliated institutions, and, very importantly, by the relatively high autopsy rate of 45 to 60 percent that has been achieved for all deaths occurring among residents of Rochester. Of the 153 primary CNS neoplasms encountered by these workers in their period of study (1935–1968), 95 percent were histologically confirmed, and of a total of 174 primary intracranial tumors, including the CNS tumors plus 21 pituitary tumors,

36 percent were first diagnosed at autopsy, more than half of these autopsy-discovered tumors being meningiomas. Incidence rates for the population of Rochester were calculated as 12.5 per 100,000 per year for primary brain tumors (not including pituitary tumors), and 1.3 per 100,000 for primary spinal cord tumors. Other findings of this careful survey included a higher incidence of meningioma in females than in males, but in contrast to the findings of some other reports, no significant differences in incidence according to sex were found for other brain and spinal cord tumors. Five-year survival rate was 22 percent for gliomas and 59 percent for meningiomas. There was no consistent change in the pattern of tumor incidence over the period of the years surveyed, although a lower tumor incidence rate was noted in the first decade of the study period, as compared to subsequent years.

In this connection, it is worthy of note that United States statistics, based on death certificates, suggest a trend of increasing incidence of CNS tumors since 1950.[123] This trend would seem in need of corroboration and, if not artifactitious, in need of explanation.

An average annual incidence of 12.8 nervous system tumors per 100,000 population was derived from the data of the Israeli national tumor registry mentioned above, with this figure including the incidence of neurofibroma, neuroblastoma, and pituitary tumors, as well as brain and spinal cord tumors.[109,110] There was pathologic verification of only 69 percent of recorded neoplasms, however, and only three-fourths were brain tumors. Spinal cord was involved in 7 percent of cases, and peripheral nerves in 12 percent.

A survey of occurrences of cerebral tumor over a three-year period in Gothenburg, Sweden, indicated an incidence of 11.4 per 100,000 per year for primary neoplasms.[124]

In his careful studies on the population of Iceland, Guomundsson found a rate of 7.8 per 100,000 per year for primary brain tumors (but including a small number of pituitary tumors), with 95 percent confidence limits ranging from 6.6 to 9.3 per 100,000; and 1.1 per 100,000 for spinal cord tumors.[108] In almost all instances, he was able to obtain histopathologic verification of cerebral tumors occurring in his population under study.

Guomundsson's conclusion from his own and other studies, a conclusion we believe to be very close to the truth, is that the annual incidence of primary CNS tumors is of the order of 10 per 100,000, with 90 percent of these tumors occurring in the brain.

Additional evidence for uniformity of distribution of brain tumor in various geographic areas has been provided by Kurtzke, who on examining mortality rates in subdivisions of the United States and Denmark, found the rate within each subdivision similar to that of the particular country as a whole.[125] This pattern, he thought, was more consistent with endogenous or multifactorial causation of brain tumors than with causation by a single exogenous agent, since, if the latter were to be postulated, its uniform geographic distribution would have to be postulated also.

Despite the similarities of distribution in various geographic areas, however, and of considerable interest from the genetic viewpoint, there appear to be differences in brain tumor incidence, and in the distribution of histopathologic types of brain tumor, among various racial and ethnic groups.

In the Israeli tumor registry material, for example, Leibowitz, *et al.* found an incidence of brain tumor of 11.5 per 100,000 per year among immigrants from Europe, compared to an age-adjusted figure of 6.0 per 100,000 among immigrants from Africa.[109,110] In another report from Israel, Cohen and Modan found a lower incidence of brain tumors in the Arabic as compared to the

Jewish population; and a higher incidence of malignant brain tumor in European and Israeli-born residents than in Asian and African-born.[120] In data from New York City, Newill found brain tumor recorded as the cause of death among Jews with a frequency 1.8 times that of the non-Jewish population.[126] Seidman, studying age-adjusted death rates in New York City, found CNS cancer less common in Negroes than in whites, and more common in Jewish females than in the total group of non-Puerto Rican white females.[127]

United States national statistics, in similar fashion, have indicated a lower than expected mortality rate due to nervous system tumors in nonwhite populations, as compared to whites,[123] and a racial difference in incidence of CNS tumors has been suggested also by other sources.[128-130]

On the other hand, recent reports from Nairobi and Dakar indicate the presence of a substantial CNS tumor problem among Africans.[131,132]

Other interesting manifestations of CNS tumor occurrences which have been reported in surgical and/or autopsy series include a greater relative frequency of ependymoma in certain Asiatic countries, such as Thailand[133] and India,[134] and a greater relative frequency of pinealoma in Japan,[135] as compared to Western series. Another facet of the subject, however, is that the death rate due to cancer of the nervous system has been found to be lower among Japanese living in Japan than in Japanese living in the United States.[136]

Newill found no essential difference in death rates due to brain tumor in native-born and foreign-born white residents of New York City,[126] but Choi, et al. found support for the possibility that the foreign-born population of Minnesota may have a higher mortality due to brain tumor than does the native-born.[137]

Obviously, many different hypotheses may

be put forward in an attempt to explain these various findings.

Innis has used epidemiologic data to support the importance of the genetic factor in development of neoplasia. He has pointed out that, while in a country such as the Netherlands brain and nervous system tumors are more common in children than is leukemia, at the same time, in widely scattered geographic areas, including Australia, England and Wales, Canada, and New Zealand, children of populations of substantially British heredity have a greater incidence of leukemia than nervous system tumors, and with about the same ratio between the two forms of cancer in each of these countries.[138] Innis' thesis is that genetic constitution predetermines occurrences of childhood cancer, regardless of widely differing environmental exposures, even such as those encountered on different continents.

In addition to the information summarized above concerning world-wide incidence of central nervous system tumors, and variations in incidence among various racial and ethnic groups, there are many other interesting facets of central nervous system tumor occurrences. These will be described below.

Congenital Central Nervous System Tumors

The occurrence of congenital central nervous system tumors, defined as those CNS tumors found to be present at birth or becoming symptomatic within three months thereafter; and including astrocytoma, oligodendroglioma, ependymoma, medulloblastoma, spongioblastoma, teratoma, and meningioma, has been documented in many individual reports, and summarized in several reviews.[139-158] In some instances the congenital neoplasm has occurred together with a malformation of one or another type, as, for example, in the case of the infant with ependymoma and cardiovascular and urinary system anomalies reported by Krohn and Hjelt;[153] and others to be mentioned below.

Lombardi and Passerini reported that of 347 spinal cord tumors in a surgical series, nineteen, or 5 percent, including lipomas, dermoids, epidermoids, and a teratoma, could be considered as of congenital origin.[159]

Many instances of congenital neuroblastoma have been reported,[160-167] including a disseminated lesion associated with antenatal death.[168] Beckwith and Perrin, in fact, have developed the concept of *in situ* neuroblastoma as a microscopic finding in the adrenals of one of 100 to 300 infants under three months of age coming to autopsy, and thus occurring with a frequency more than 40 times the rate of occurrence of clinically manifesting neuroblastoma.[169] In 69 percent of their cases the *in situ* lesions were associated with severe anomalies, chiefly of the cardiovascular system. Guin, *et al.* reported on adrenal neuroblastoma in eleven infants, all less than three months of age, with six of the lesions being of *in situ* type.[170] None of the eleven tumors produced symptoms or metastasized. In eight of the eleven infants, severe congenital malformations were associated, but the authors doubted the validity of this association between congenital anomalies and neuroblastoma.

Thus, the risk of developing central nervous system tumors, and neuroblastoma, is present even before birth.

Association of Central Nervous System Tumors with Other Tumors, Both Intracranial and Extracranial, Thought Usually to be of Sporadic Occurrence

When brain tumors occur, they may do so in association with other tumors, either neural or nonneural. Known associations between brain tumors and hereditary syndromes with neoplastic involvement of nervous and other tissues will be summarized below in another section of this chapter, but mention will be made here of reports of associations of CNS tumors with both neural and nonneural tumors not known to be of hereditary origin.

Multiple primary cancers involving various organs are encountered with some frequency,[118,171-173] but the explanation for this finding has been the subject of controversy.

On the basis of long-term follow-up of patients of the Ellis Fischel Hospital, Spratt and Hoag concluded that persons living to great age may expect a high risk of multiple cancers, simply on a statistical basis, but that prior cancer of several different sites investigated, of which the central nervous system was not one, does not affect the subsequent risk for development of new neoplasms.[174] On the other hand, Kuehn, *et al.* suggested a more specific type of association involving primaries of breast, colon, and genitalia in multiple occurrences,[175] and Warren and Gates felt that chance alone did not explain the frequency of occurrences of multiple malignant tumors.[173]

In specific regard to the nervous system, there are numerous reports of primary neural tumors that are either multicentric or associated with other primary neural tumors of different pathologic type.[176-179] While, as intimated above, multiple primary CNS tumors may occur as manifestations of a hereditary syndrome, e.g., neurofibromatosis,[180] there are numerous examples of such occurrences in the absence of neurofibromatosis or other recognized hereditary disease. For example, Batzdorf and Malamud found five of 209 gliomas to be multicentric;[181] and there are reports of multiple meningiomas and meningiomatosis occurring even in the absence of neurofibromatosis.[182,183] Likewise, multiple ganglioneuromata of the central nervous system have been reported in the absence of neuro-fibromatosis.[184]

In a review of the literature concerning multiple primary brain tumors, Madonick, *et al.* reported the most frequent combination of diverse types to be glioblastoma multiforme and meningioma.[185] Other combinations reported have included glioblastoma multiforme and cystic piloid astrocytoma;[186] oligodendroglioma and meningioma;[187] glioblastoma multiforme and fibrosarcoma;[188] and meningioma and malignant glioma.[189]

CNS tumors have also been reported in association with many types of extracranial as well as intracranial nonneural tumors. Regelson, *et al.*, in the study referred to above involving an autopsy series of 150 children with cancer, found that three of the 150 had the combination of brain tumor with other primary malignant tumor.[118] A five-year-old boy had both acute lymphoblastic leukemia and cerebellar neuroastrocytoma. A 13-year-old girl, whose father and paternal grandfather also developed neoplasms at about the same time, had both adenocarcinoma of colon and cerebral neuroastrocytoma; and another girl had both cerebral glioblastoma multiforme and hepatocarcinoma. Only in the second of these three cases was there a suggestion of any of the familial tumor syndromes to be discussed below. This study also included other interesting associations: a patient with retinoblastoma subsequently developing widespread Hodgkin's disease; adrenal neuroblastoma and rhabdomyoma of the heart, the latter of particular interest because of its known relationship to tuberous sclerosis;[190] and bilateral retinoblastoma treated by surgery and radiation, with later onset of maxillary fibrosarcoma. The possibility of induction by virus attracted the interest of Regelson and his co-workers as a possible explanation for the double primaries with CNS malignant component.

Sorenson reported astrocytoma and meningioma of brain with carcinoma of rectum;[191] and Dodge, *et al.* reported bilateral granulosa cell tumor of ovary and later an intraspinal neurofibroma in a 14-year-old girl whose father and brother were said to have died of "brain tumor."[192] A female with breast cancer, and years subsequently, thymoma, two astrocytomas, and low serum values for gamma globulin fractions, has been reported;[193] as has a patient with meningioma, craniopharyngioma, and ovarian cystadenoma;[194] another with cerebral astrocytoma and pituitary adenoma;[195] and as have patients with other combinations of intracranial and extracranial tumors.[196-198]

Mere coincidence may be the explanation for some of these reports of multiple tumor occurrences, and in other instances it is possible that the individual tumors involved in the multiple occurrences are associated in an etiological sense. There is the possibility, for example, that some of these instances of multiple occurrences may represent incompletely manifesting forms of one or another of the familial cancer syndromes; or could actually be assigned to one of these syndromes were additional clinical and pathologic information available concerning illnesses of family members. Such possibilities, however, must at present remain speculation.

Diabetes and Brain Tumors

The literature records disagreement concerning the risk for cancer among diabetics,[199-201] although there is good evidence that death due to carcinoma of the pancreas is more common in diabetics than in the general population.[202]

In regard to the nervous system, Aronson and Aronson have reported on a large autopsy series showing a paucity of gliomas and metastatic cancers in the brains of diabetics, although the frequencies of intracranial meningioma and acoustic neurinoma were the same in both diabetics and nondiabetics.[203] As mentioned in a previous section, however, when considering the results of such an autopsy series, one must keep in mind the factor of selectivity operative in performance of autopsies, since this factor may affect over-all statistical results.

ABO Blood Groups and CNS Tumors

Data are conflicting on the question of whether brain tumors are associated with any particular ABO group. There are reports that group A is excessively represented in patients with intracranial neoplasms;[204] of decreased frequency of groups O and B in patients with astrocytoma;[205] and of increased frequency of group B with meningioma.[206] Pearce and Yates, in studying ABO group distribution among patients with various tumors of the central nervous system, found only one clear difference between their study and control groups, namely, a reduction in frequency of group O with astrocytoma (not including glioblastoma), and this particularly in cases diagnosed since 1945 in individuals under 20 years of age.[207] Strang, *et al.* found male but not female patients with cerebral astrocytoma to have an excessive frequency of blood group A.[208] On the other hand, there have been several studies indicating a normal ABO group distribution in patients with various types of CNS tumors, including astrocytoma.[209-212]

Occurrence of CNS Tumors in Relation to Immunologic Status of the Host

The question of the immunobiology of brain tumors has been introduced above in the section on experimental tumors, and will be referred to briefly below in a later section in respect to specific immunodeficient diseases of genetic origin, ataxia-telangiectasia

and the Wiskott-Aldrich syndrome. Still other information relating to our knowledge of immunologic aspects of human brain and nervous system tumors will be briefly presented at this point, including discussion of the following: 1) development of neoplasms in transplant recipients; 2) morphologic and humoral evidence of immunity; and 3) spontaneous regression of neural tumors, specifically neuroblastoma.

Neoplasms Associated with Allotransplantation: One of the results of introduction of widespread renal homografting in recent years is that a number of kidney recipients are developing neoplasms, including many of the lymphoma group.[213-215] Pierce, *et al.*, for example, while not reporting cerebral involvement, found that of 151 kidney recipients, three developed reticulum cell sarcoma, an incidence calculable as more than 100 times greater than expected.[216]

Starzl, *et al.* have reported both on the experience of their own group in Denver, and on information submitted to an unofficial registry maintained in that city, and receiving data from transplantation centers throughout the world.[217]

They divided their own patients into two groups. In Group I were 195 patients receiving renal transplants and followed for at least three years, with the exception of 41 patients dying within four months after surgery. Of the remaining 154 patients truly at risk, fifteen (9.7%) developed neoplasms. Azothioprine and prednisone had been used in treatment of all of these 154 patients, while the later members of this group (I) had been treated also with horse antilymphocyte globulin. Splenectomy had been employed for more than 90 percent of these patients and thymectomy had been done on 45 patients, either before or after transplantation. For the most part, the fifteen tumors, including twelve carcinomas and three lymphomas, were easily treated, but two lesions, both reticulum cell sarcoma, were fatal. All three lymphomas involved the brain, two exclusively so.

In Group II were 111 more recent recipients, followed for periods varying from six months to three years. No neoplasms had occurred in this group at the time of the report of Starzl and his co-workers. These patients had received the triple drug regimen of azothioprine, prednisone, and ALG, and, as in Group I, splenectomy had been performed in more than 90 percent. There was no good explanation for the absence of tumors in Group II patients.

The data of the unofficial registry, listing cases from throughout the world, included 42 tumors developing in 41 kidney and one cardiac recipients. Twenty-one of the forty-two were mesenchymal tumors, most commonly reticulum cell sarcoma. Eight of the 42 had been splenectomized but none had had thymectomy. All 42 patients had received azothioprine and prednisone, and ten had received ALG in addition.

Schneck and Penn have reported that in the combined experience of the Colorado group and the world registry there were 22 lymphomas, eleven of which involved the brain.[218] Most tumors affecting brain were reticulum cell sarcomas. In eight patients, the brain was the sole organ involved by malignant lymphoma.

Dismissing the possibility of actual transplantation of tumor from donor to recipient as generally unsupported by evidence, Schneck and Penn summarized four remaining explanations that could relate to the origin of tumors in transplant recipients: 1) continuous antigenic stimulation of host reticuloendothelial system by foreign antigens of the donor tissue; 2) chromosome breakage due to the action of immunosuppressive drugs; 3) loss of a usually protective surveillance mechanism due to the action of immunosuppressive drugs on host reticuloendothelial system; and 4) proliferation in the host of oncogenic virus.

Clearly, one may postulate that two or more of these possibilities may contribute together to the genesis and development of particular neoplasms.

Pierce, *et al.* have expressed the opinion that the fact that lymphomas seem to develop with azothioprine therapy only in the presence of transplanted tissue, at least so far as recorded experience goes, tends to favor a combination of explanations 1 and 3; while a disproportionate number of lymphomas, as compared to other tumor types developing in transplant recipients, militates against the conclusion that possibility 3 is solely determining.[216] These workers also point to a high incidence of lymphoma in graft-versus-host disease in certain mouse strains as supporting the concept that lymphoma development in allotransplantation is dependent upon stimulation of host reticuloendothelial tissue by donor transplanted antigen.

Possibility four has received support from the experimental work of Hirsch, *et al.*, who showed activation of leukemia virus in mice receiving both skin homografts and anti-lymphocyte serum, but not either alone.[219]

Potentiation of viral carcinogenesis by immunosuppression has been demonstrated in mice.[220] Of special genetic interest, as indicated by Allison, is that the relative resistance of C57BL mice to polyoma virus tumors can be overcome by means of immunosuppression, and may be due, therefore, to early development of cellular immunity in this particular strain, presumably on a hereditary basis.[220]

Penn, *et al.*, in speculating on a possible virus etiology of the tumors found in transplant recipients, have pointed out that herpes infections have been common in transplant recipients, and also that two human strains of herpes virus, the Epstein-Barr virus and herpes hominis II, have been associated, at least, with malignant disease, the former virus with Burkitt's lymphoma, and the latter with cervical carcinoma.[221] Of related interest is Spencer's finding of an apparent increased incidence of three viral diseases, common warts, cytomegalovirus disease, and shingles, in renal transplant recipients.[222] The significance of these observations in respect to transplant recipients developing brain tumors remains to be established.

More information concerning the incidence of neoplasia following the transplantation of kidneys from identical twins would help to throw light upon the relative weight to be assigned to each of the four etiologic-pathogenetic possibilities listed by Schneck and Penn.

The history of thymectomy of some of the transplant recipients developing tumors would not seem to be of great importance as an etiological factor, chiefly because many other tumor-affected transplant recipients had not received this treatment. In addition, although there is evidence in mice that aged neonatally thymectomized animals have increased susceptibility to lymphoreticular tumors,[223] it would appear that thymectomy in human adults does not lead to increased tumor incidence.[224]

Very interesting, of course, is the question of why the brain should seem to be so peculiarly vulnerable to lymphoid malignancy in transplantation patients receiving immunotherapy. One explanation advanced is that the brain is a relatively favorable site for implantation of foreign cells, or growth of tumor cells, because its relative lack of lymphoid tissue provides for lessened host immunologic resistance. This explanation involves the concept of brain as an "immunologically privileged site,"[218,225,226] which is supported in part by evidence for a lack of lymphatics in the brain.[227]

Not all recorded cases of malignant lymphoma of brain in patients receiving immunosuppressive therapy have been associated with transplantation. Lipsmeyer reported the case of a 27-year-old female with systemic

lupus erythematosus, and undergoing immunosuppression therapy, who developed a lesion described as cerebral reticulum cell sarcoma; but Lipsmeyer also commented on the possibility that the development of tumor in this patient could have been related to the autoimmune nature of systemic lupus, as well as to the immunosuppressive therapy received.[228]

Kinlen has pointed out the need to accumulate information on tumor incidence in patients who are not transplant recipients, but who are receiving immunosuppressive therapy for conditions such as the nephrotic syndrome, rheumatoid arthritis, and Crohn's disease.[229]

While the appearance of lymphoid tumors in individuals undergoing immunosuppression may suggest that the immunologic resistance of brain is relatively easily overcome, at least in comparison with other body sites; by the same token, the fact that such neoplasms occur only infrequently in the general population could be interpreted as an indication that some degree of immunocompetence of brain is normally present. Indeed, the experimental work already referred to indicates that the brain is not completely privileged in an immunologic sense.

Morphologic, Chemical, and Humoral Factors: From the preceding discussion, it may be concluded that the brain offers some degree of resistance to tumor growth, but that this resistance is only limited. On the clinical level, and in rather striking contrast to the rarity of extracranial metastases from human brain tumors,[230,231] is Earle's finding that, in an autopsy series of adult males, 11 percent of extracranial malignancies, excluding basal cell and squamous cell carcinomas of skin, metastasized to the brain.[232] This high incidence of metastasis to brain could be interpreted, perhaps, as consistent with the concept of immunological privilege of this organ.

Concerning primary human brain tumors, there is a limited amount of information available in respect to tumor antigens and antibodies. An immunologically specific material in both neural neoplasms and normal neural tissue has been reported;[233] and Catalano, et al., in examining CNS tumors for common antigens characteristic of virus-induced tumors, found an antigen present in cell cultures from human meningiomas, detectable by reaction with antibody found in sera of patients with meningioma.[234] Cross-reactivity of this antibody with gliomatous tissue was also found.

Trouillas has reported a "carcino-fetal" glial antigen present in glioblastomas and also in fetal brain,[235,236] perhaps analogous to the fetal proteins reported with hepatoma,[237] and with gastrointestinal malignancy.[238,239] The relationship between protein S 100, unique to the nervous system, and various types of experimental and human tumors, has been the subject of much recent interest.[240-245] Mahaley, however, while noting the occurrence of antigen common to glioblastoma, normal brain, and nonneural tissues, states that there is as yet no *in vitro* confirmation of glioma-specific antigen or antibody.[246,247]

Wilkins has found a serum fraction which, when obtained from patients with CNS malignancy, stimulates an experimental model system of liver regeneration, but when obtained from patients with benign CNS neoplasms, inhibits the same system.[248] In addition, there has been a report suggesting that in sera and buffy coats of patients with glioma of the brain, there are factors capable of inhibiting *in vitro* growth of the autogenous tumors.[249]

The morphologic aspects of immunity to glioma are also of interest. Considering the possibility that lymphocytic infiltration of gliomas may be an indicator of host resistance, Ridley and Cavanagh found that of 93 patients dying with glioma at London Hospital, the tumors of 30 percent showed significant, and 28 percent slight, lymphocytic infiltration, while the remaining 42 percent showed none.[250] The possibility that the lymphocytes, when present, were necrosis-associated could not be excluded.

In the neuroblastoma series of Lauder and Aherne, most tumors had at least some degree of lymphocytic infiltration, and there was a positive correlation between associated lymphocytic infiltration and survival time of the patient.[251]

Neoplastic Regression: For cancer generally, many reports of spontaneous regression have been tabulated.[252] In regard to the nervous system, most of the instances of spontaneous tumor regression or maturation have concerned either neuroblastoma[253-257] or retinoblastoma,[258-261] although a rare report concerning astrocytoma is also on record.[262] For example, Gross, et al. have reported what they consider two undoubted spontaneous cures of neuroblastoma, with respective periods of follow-up of twenty and twenty-five years.[253]

Certain cautions must be kept in mind when evaluating reports of tumor regression. In an excellent commentary, although one not directed specifically to neural lesions, Kidd reminds us that in many reported cases of spontaneous tumor regression there are defects in the case histories, including an especially important one, lack of histopathologic verification.[263]

A particularly interesting body of knowledge has been developing during the last several years, in large part due to the work of the Hellströms, concerning immunologic mechanisms relating to neuroblastoma and possibly to its spontaneous regression.[264-268] It may be that these mechanisms will prove to be determined, at least in part, by genetic factors. Specifically, it has been shown that lymphocytes from patients with neuroblastoma inhibit growth of neuro-blastoma cells *in vitro*, both neuroblastoma cells of autogenous origin and those of other patients, but not fibroblast cultures from the same tumor donors.

These findings have been interpreted as consistent with the concept that neuro-blastoma neoplasms from different individuals have common tumor-specific antigen. The *in vitro* inhibitory capacity of lympho-cytes from an individual patient does not correlate well with his ability to resist neo-plastic growth, however, since lymphocytes of neuroblastoma patients with progressive disease, and of those neuroblastoma patients free of symptoms, are capable of similar levels of *in vitro* inhibitory activity. The ex-planation for this paradoxical finding may lie in the phenomenon of immunological en-hancement, i.e., serum blocking antibodies may be present *in vivo* in the clinically aggres-sive cases, and be united with tumor cells in such a way as to protect them from attack by immune lymphocytes.

In respect to this question, it is notable, and perhaps indicative of the importance of the subject, that sera of patients with pro-gressively growing neuroblastoma, but not sera of asymptomatic, successfully treated neuroblastoma patients, are capable of block-ing the inhibitory effect of immune lym-phocytes on growth of neuroblastoma cells *in vitro*.

The ability of lymphocytes to inhibit the growth of plated neuroblastoma cells has been found also in family members of pa-tients with neuroblastoma. Twelve of six-teen mothers of patients with neuroblastoma have exhibited this inhibitory capacity, as has a number of healthy siblings. These find-ings have been viewed as possibly consistent with a viral etiology of neuroblastoma, in-volving formation of common tumor-specific antigen characteristic of virus-induced neo-plasms.

The abilities to form humoral antibody and to respond with cellular immunity would seem to be central to the biology of the Hellströms' investigations. Both of these abilities could be genetically conditioned. Certainly, if neuroblastoma results from viral infection, it is still to be explained why the virus attacks only certain individuals; or if the infection is more widespread, as seems more likely, why the infection results in neo-plasia only in selected individuals, not in all. The Hellströms' *in vitro* system for study of protective and enhancement mechanisms in neuroblastoma and other tumors would seem to provide opportunities for search for specifically genetic components influencing tumor growth.

In what amounts to an extension of the work cited above, Levy, *et al.* have found that lymphocytes from patients with brain tumors may be cytotoxic to autogenous tu-mor cells *in vitro*, with some indication of cross-reactivity between glioblastomas oc-curring in different individuals, and between glioblastoma and melanoma.[269]

Radiation

There have been several reports linking exposure to radiation to development of human primary intracranial and intraspinal tumors, particularly meningiomas and tu-mors of mesenchymal origin such as fibro-sarcoma.[270-278] Only a few cases of glioma following therapeutic radiation have been recorded.[75] Of particular interest, children with a history of *in utero* exposure to radia-tion have been found to have a 40 percent increase in cancer mortality,[279-281] includ-ing CNS cancer mortality.[279]

In the Ann Arbor series of thymus-irradi-ated children there appeared to be an increase in number of subsequently developing ma-lignant tumors, including two tumors of the brain, but the observed increase was not of statistical significance.[282]

In any case, we are not aware of any firm evidence indicating a genetic susceptibility to radiation-induced CNS tumors in man.

Virus Causation of CNS Tumors in Man

Viruses have not yet been shown to be causative agents of human brain tumors, but particles resembling the oncogenic C-type viruses have been described in association with a few brain tumors, and papova-like viruses of possibly oncogenic potential have been found in the brains of patients with subacute sclerosing panencephalitis (SSPE) and progressive multifocal leuko-encephalopathy (PML).[66] Quite recently, JC virus, a new human papovavirus, has been isolated from the brain of a patient with PML and found to induce gliomas in hamsters following intracerebral inoculation.[283]

Particles resembling papovavirus, and closely similar to particles seen in a case of PML, have been found also on electron microscopic examination of a human choroid plexus papilloma.[284]

The finding of an antigen common to mammalian RNA oncogenic viruses in human glial tumors, as described by Trouillas, was considered as strongly supporting a virus etiology for the tumors concerned.[285] This antigen was also found in fetal brain and intestine and was thought to be related to what Trouillas has called the carcino-fetal glial antigen.

Again, we are not aware of any firm evidence concerning occurrence in humans on a genetic basis of altered susceptibility to viral induction of CNS neoplasms.

Trauma as a Factor in CNS Tumors

No clear link between trauma and brain tumors has been established, except in the instances of a number of cases of meningioma

in which a causal relationship may be inferred because of well documented specifics of time and site of injury.[286-293] No genetic factor has been identified in the development of these CNS tumors of traumatic origin.

Chemical Causation of CNS Tumors in Humans

There is almost no evidence dealing directly with the subject of chemical induction of CNS tumors in humans, although some of the experimental evidence cited above may prove to have pertinence. Interestingly enough, in this regard, while certain nitro-sourea compounds have been used to induce brain tumors in animals, other nitrosoureas have been used to treat brain tumors in the mouse and in man.[294-297]

Also of interest is an isolated report from Ohio of some years ago. Mancuso found that among a group of workers in the rubber industry, 8.2 percent of deaths due to cancer involved a CNS tumor, as compared to a figure of 3.1 percent for male residents of Ohio.[298] This report, although very interesting, would seem to require extensive follow-up and corroboration.

More recently, exposure to chemical carcinogens in contaminated water supplies has been suggested, but not proved, as an explanation for a detected clustering of brain tumors in six counties of eastern Kentucky.[299] Alternative explanations for the clustering, including a genetic explanation, have not been ruled out.

Miscellaneous Epidemiologic Factors

This section concerns some of the remaining epidemiologic considerations relating to CNS tumors in man, but will not include associated congenital malformations and specifically genetic factors to be presented in some detail in subsequent sections.

Associations have been suggested between CNS tumors and a maternal history of previous abortion;[212] and between CNS and retinal neoplasms and infection by Toxoplasma gondii.[300-302] An isolated report associates CNS neoplasm and congenital lues.[303] There appears to be a negative association between brain tumor and history of use of alcohol.[212] Differences in sex-ratios for various CNS tumor types have been noted,[137] as mentioned above in referring to somewhat contrary findings.

Instances have been found also of CNS tumor occurring together with myasthenia gravis, and with multiple sclerosis, disorders in which autoimmune factors have been implicated. Evidence for a genetic component is present in these disorders but seems to be quite limited.[304]

Papatestas, *et al.* have reported that 94 extra-thymic malignant neoplasms, including five CNS tumors, occurred in 1243 patients with myasthenia gravis.[305] The incidence of neoplasms in these patients increased after the onset of myasthenia, but prior to this onset, was actually lower than expected. For those myasthenia patients treated with thymectomy, the incidence of malignant tumors decreased to expected levels.

There is evidence suggesting the possibility of a relationship between the pathogenesis of multiple sclerosis, with its characteristic demyelinating lesions, and slow infection with the measles virus, or one of several other viruses.[306-308] Of considerable interest are the gliomatous tumors, including astrocytoma, oligodendroglioma, and glioblastoma, which have been reported in association with this disease.[309-312] Mathews and Moossy, who reported a case manifesting Charcot-Marie-Tooth disease, a hereditary disorder, as well as glioma and multiple sclerosis, thought that the tumor associations have been fortuitous, both in their own case and in others in the literature.[309] On the other hand, Brihaye, *et al.*, in reporting on a 62-year-old male with both multiple sclerosis and cerebral glioma, noted a close topographical relationship between the neoplastic and demyelinating lesions.[312]

CNS Tumors and Congenital Malformations

In the section below dealing specifically with the occurrence of CNS tumors in association with genetic disorders, we will list a number of genetic conditions which may be considered rightly as congenital malformations also, e.g. neurofibromatosis, tuberous sclerosis, and ataxia-telangiectasia.

Before proceeding to a discussion of CNS tumors occurring with these specific disorders, however, we believe it worthwhile to briefly review some of the information bearing on the relationship between CNS tumors and a wide spectrum of congenital malformations involving many organ systems and occurring usually on a sporadic basis.

The malformations found in association with CNS tumors may vary from microscopic findings to the most obvious type of gross deformity.

As an example of the former, abnormal cell collections in the posterior medullary velum have been described as the possible origin of cerebellar medulloblastoma.[313]

The association of CNS tumors with more obvious types of gross malformations in general parallels the documented associations between certain malignant tumors of other systems and congenital anomalies.[314-318]

In the specific context of the relationship between congenital defects and neural tumors or tumors closely related to the neuraxis, a number of interesting associations in individual cases has been reported. These include congenital medulloblastoma with gastrointestinal and genitourinary system anomalies;[319] congenital ependymoma with multisystem anomalies;[320] neuroblastoma *in situ* with congenital heart disease;[321] neuroblastoma with syndactyly and rib anomalies;[322] congenital teratoma within a myelomeningocele;[323] congenital teratoma, occurring in relation to spina bifida, and undergoing malignant change in adult life;[324] gliomatous neoplasm, in an infant with bilateral nasal proboscis, hamartoma of brain, arhinencephaly, and agenesis of the corpus callosum;[325] astrocytoma with arteriovenous malformation of overlying meninges;[326] glioblastoma multiforme with an adjacent arteriovenous angiomatous malformation;[327] ependymoma of the cauda equina with vascular malformation of the spinal cord;[328] glioblastoma with pulmonary arteriovenous fistula;[329] retinoblastoma with mental defect and hydrocephalus;[330] and retinoblastoma with dermatoglyphic anomalies.[331]

Of course, occurrences such as these in individual patients, or small numbers of patients, need not imply associations based on more than coincidence. For example, Miller, *et al.* were unable to confirm a significant relationship between neuroblastoma and congenital anomalies, although they found many individuals with both in their extensive survey.[332]

There has been a suggestion that cental nervous system tumors may be increased in Down's syndrome,[314] a disorder of abnormal chromosomal constitution. A pineal teratoma has been found in a patient with Klinefelter's syndrome, another disorder of abnormal chromosomal complement;[333] and cerebral astrocytoma and certain stigmata similar to those of Turner's syndrome have been reported in an individual possessing, just as three sisters and her father, an abnormal small metacentric chromosome.[334]

Many lipomas and other fatty lesions of the cauda equina have occurred in association with hydrocephalus and myelomeningocele.[335]

Gliomatous tumors have developed often with syringomyelia, a disorder for which there is some evidence of a genetic basis. This subject will be referred to below in the section on genetic diseases.

Fraumeni and Miller have reported on a very interesting series of 62 patients with adrenocortical neoplasms, 46 carcinomas and 16 adenomas. None represented the familial syndrome of multiple endocrine adenomatosis. Two of these patients also had astrocytoma; one had cerebral melanocytosis; and a number had various types of malformations, including GU anomalies, cutaneous pigmentations, and congenital hemi-hypertrophy.[336] Among the 62 patients were two children with developmental brain lesions and two with siblings with organic brain disease. In one family, the mother was said to have died of "cystic brain tumor."

Such provocative findings reinforce the need for acquisition of further information concerning the not yet well defined relationship between oncogenesis and teratogenesis.

CNS Tumors Associated with Genetic and Allied Disorders, and CNS Tumors Occurring on a Familial Basis

In the preceding pages we have reviewed much of over-all etiologic-pathogenetic import in regard to CNS tumors, with consideration of genetic factors where applicable. It remains to review occurrences of CNS tumors in a number of disorders of clearly and specifically genetic origin, including also parenthetic information on CNS tumor occurrences in allied disorders, in some respects similar to the genetic disorders, but less clearly of genetic origin, or known not to be of genetic origin; and to review reports of familial occurrences of brain tumors, occurrences of CNS tumors in syndromes of familial cancer involving multiple organ sites, and the results of surveys of relatives of patients with CNS tumors.

CNS Tumors Occurring with Neurocutaneous Disorders

The phacomatoses include disorders grouped together on the basis of having anomalies of the skin, eyes, and central nervous system, although associated anomalies may often affect other organs and systems as well; and of characteristically manifesting both tumorous malformations and true neoplasms.[337] Over the years, since neurofibromatosis and tuberous sclerosis, and later von Hippel-Lindau disease, were designated as phacomatoses by Van der Hoeve;[338] and Yakovlev and Guthrie included neurofibromatosis, tuberous sclerosis, and encephalotrigeminal angiomatosis in the category of congenital ectodermoses or neurocutaneous syndromes;[339] the list of these disorders has grown, to number presently in the dozens according to some accounts, and there have been multiple attempts at definition and classification.[337,340-344]

Until the inclusion of the multiple basal cell nevus syndrome as the "fifth phacomatosis" some years ago,[345] there were four more or less classical members of the group: neurofibromatosis, tuberous sclerosis, von Hippel-Lindau disease, and Sturge-Weber disease. Four of the five are disorders well established as of hereditary type, while the exception, Sturge-Weber disease, sometimes occurs on a familial basis.[337] Our discussion of CNS tumors associated with phacomatoses will include mention of all five of these disorders, plus others of related interest.

It should be noted that, because individual patients have seemed to exhibit signs characteristic of two or more of the neurocutaneous disorders,[346-350] there has been consideration of the question of whether there is a close relationship among those genes responsible for the clinical presentations of these disorders. In most cases, however, each of the phacomatoses is easily recognizable as a specific singular entity.

A point of interest is Willis' expressed opinion that neurofibromatosis, tuberous sclerosis, leptomeningeal melanosis, and like disorders, which he considers essentially hamartomatous in nature, will be shown ultimately to be inborn errors of metabolism caused by specific biochemical defects.[351]

Von Recklinghausen's Disease (Neurofibromatosis): Von Recklinghausen's disease is an example of an autosomal dominant condition[352] with multisystem involvement, its manifestations being not at all limited to the classic findings of multiple neurofibromas and café-au-lait spots of the skin. Associations with numerous types of congenital anomalies have been reported, as well as associations with tumors of the central nervous system, including true neoplasms of gliomatous type. In fact, in neurofibromatosis we have an illustrative example of an undeniably hereditary disorder which is at once responsible for malformation of the morphological structures of many organ systems in a manner that may be designated hamartomatous, and responsible also for the origin of benign and malignant neoplasms of the central nervous system. In the complexities and intricacies of their pattern in this disorder, the intertwining threads of genetics, congenital anomalies, and true neoplasia may reach a fullness of expression, however limited may be our capacity to read the message expressed.

Congenital anomalies which have been found in association with neurofibromatosis and are also related to the nervous system include syringomyelia,[353] hydromyelia,[354] meningocele,[355-358] mental defect,[359] abnormal response to muscle relaxants,[360] and others.[361-364] Anomalies of blood vessels, bone, and other tissues at sites remote from the neuraxis have likewise been found.[352,365-370]

Neoplasms which have been found in association with neurofibromatosis include sarcomas developing in neurofibromas;[371-373] neuroblastomas;[374,375] spinal ganglioneuromata;[376] pheochromocytomas;[344,377] various types of nonneural tumors;[373,377-379] and central nervous system tumors.[363,380-401] Among the CNS tumors which have occurred with neurofibromatosis are acoustic neurinoma, meningioma, spongioblastoma, ependymoma, astrocytoma, and glioblastoma. In some instances the CNS tumors have been multiple and of diverse type;[382] meningiomas have occurred both multiply and in the form of meningiomatosis;[387] and adrenal pheochromocytomas have been found in association with the CNS tumors occurring in this neurocutaneous disorder.[402-406] Tumors of the eye and optic nerve, particularly optic nerve gliomas, also occur in neurofibromatosis.[407-411]

The significance of the many reports of congenital anomalies and neoplasms in von Recklinghausen's disease is naturally open to various interpretations. Roberts, for example, thought the cerebral tumor he reported to be fortuitous in occurrence.[403] It would seem, however, that the numerous occurrences of tumor in a syndrome comprising multiple ectodermal, vascular, and skeletal defects suggest a common element in the etiology and pathogenesis of the defects and neoplasms found. Perhaps bearing on this point is the finding of Fialkow, *et al.*, on examination of neurofibromas from female patients affected by von Recklinghausen's disease and also heterozygous for the X-linked A and B genes for glucose-6-phosphate dehydrogenase, that these neurofibromas are of multiple cell origin.[412]

The report of Dörstelmann, *et al.*, concerning a family with three members of two generations showing concurrence for neurofibromatosis and another autosomal dominant trait, Huntington's chorea,[413] illus-

trates still another facet of the potential for von Recklinghausen's disease to interrelate with other disorders.

Bilateral Acoustic Neurinoma: Bilateral acoustic neurinomas have occurred on a hereditary basis in the presence of few signs suggestive of peripheral neurofibromatosis.[414-416] The relationship of this presentation to von Recklinghausen's disease is a nosological problem.

It is important to recognize, however, that bilateral acoustic neurinomas may be responsible for bilateral deafness, and may be transmitted as an autosomal dominant trait, even in the apparent absence of other manifestations of von Recklinghausen's disease. Other types of brain tumor, in some instances, occur together with the bilateral acoustic neurinomas.

Tuberous Sclerosis: Tuberous sclerosis, or Bourneville's disease, an autosomal dominant disorder in which there are characteristic CNS and skin lesions, and in which renal tumors, rhabdomyoma of the heart, and lesions of the eye and other organs occur,[417-421] is another example of a phacomatosis in which brain tumors may be found.[422-432]

While the multiple intraventricular nodules showing glial proliferation which are characteristic of CNS involvement in tuberous sclerosis would seem not to be tumors in the true sense, Kapp, *et al.* found seven of forty-eight cases of tuberous sclerosis to have brain tumors which caused elevations of intracranial pressure and which could be considered true neoplasms.[432] These tumors were present generally near the foramina of Monro, and although presenting considerable difficulty in pathologic diagnosis, were thought to be best classified as astrocytomas. The designation subependymal giant-celled astrocytoma is favored by Russell and Rubinstein for the gliomatous true neoplasms typically found in tuberous sclerosis.[8]

Von Hippel-Lindau Disease: Von Hippel-Lindau disease is another autosomal dominant disorder, but in this case the occurrence of an intracranial neoplasm is an integral part of the syndrome, and the neoplasm itself, usually cerebellar hemangioblastoma, together with retinal angiomatosis, pancreatic cyst, and benign and malignant renal lesions, accounts for the essential definition of the syndrome.[433-438] Not every affected individual, of course, manifests each finding. It is to be noted, however, that unlike the situation in tuberous sclerosis and, in some instances, neurofibromatosis, the intracranial neoplasm of von Hippel-Lindau disease is not in the glioma group, but is a neoplasm of vascular tissue.

Of special genetic interest, there are reports that chromosomal analyses of venous blood from von Hippel-Lindau patients show aberrations of number and structure, including particularly chromatid breaks.[439,440]

Although cerebellar hemangioblastoma is a characteristic finding in von Hippel-Lindau disease, there is not total coincidence of the neoplasm and the hereditary disorder. In the experience of Silver and Hennigar, only nine of forty patients with cerebellar hemangioblastoma had proven von Hippel-Lindau disease.[441]

Various reports enlarge the spectrum of pathologic changes in von Hippel-Lindau disease to include the following: posterior medullary hemangioblastoma;[442] spinal hemangioblastoma;[443,444] cerebral hemangioblastoma;[445] occurrence of hemangioblastoma of medulla, cerebellum, and lumbar spinal nerve root in the same patient;[446] and probable associations with pheochromocytoma.[447-449] The association of von Hippel-Lindau disease with syringomyelia has also been noted.[450]

There have been several reports of families with all affected members having cerebellar hemangioblastoma, but showing no evidence of retinal angiomatosis and few, if any, other signs of the von Hippel-Lindau syndrome.[451-454] Whether these cases represent a special form of the classical syndrome, or a distinct entity, or whether members of these families may in the future yet show retinal and other lesions, remains to be clarified. In particular, further pathologic studies on members of such families are essential.

Sturge-Weber Disease: Sturge-Weber disease, which includes the manifestations of nevus flammeus in the distribution of the trigeminal nerve, and ipsilateral meningeal angiomatosis with calcification of the underlying brain,[455] usually occurs on a sporadic basis, although familial cases have been recorded.[337,456]

There has been a report of choroid plexus papilloma in association with bilateral Sturge-Weber disease,[457] but glial tumors are not a feature of Sturge-Weber disease, or of a number of other disorders, both hereditary and nonhereditary, which involve various vascular lesions of the central nervous system.[458-467]

Multiple Basal Cell Nevus Syndrome: The multiple basal cell nevus syndrome, a disorder transmitted in an autosomal dominant pattern, and designated as the "fifth phacomatosis," comprises multiple skin neoplasms, often interpreted as basal cell carcinomas or trichoepitheliomas, ocular and skeletal anomalies,[468] and endocrine disturbances.[469,470] Medulloblastoma and other brain tumors have been found in several cases,[471-474] and there has been a report of an associated malignant melanoma of the iris.[475] Chromosomal anomalies, including chromatid breaks and gaps, and quadriradial figures, have been described as increased in number in leukocyte cultures from patients with this disorder.[476,477] In individual patients, the CNS tumor may be the first manifestation of the syndrome.[315]

Neurocutaneous Melanosis: The syndrome of giant pigmented hairy nevus of skin with melanosis of the brain and meninges, also referred to as neurocutaneous melanosis, and grouped with the phacomatoses, has been associated with development of primary leptomeningeal malignant melanoma and melanomatosis.[337,478,479] There has been no firm evidence for a hereditary factor in cases falling within this category of disorder,[480-489] although there has been some suggestion of a genetic influence on certain related anomalies of skin and meningeal pigmentation.[337]

Of the total number of cases of intracranial malignant melanoma, however, only a very small minority occurs on the basis of neurocutaneous melanosis. For example, Beresford found only one primary CNS tumor among 37 melanomas affecting the central nervous system.[490] Furthermore, primary melanomas of the central nervous system may occur in the absence of the skin lesions required for the diagnosis of neurocutaneous melanosis.[491-497]

Multiple Circumscribed Lipomatosis: Multiple circumscribed lipomatosis, manifested by the appearance in young adults of widely distributed subcutaneous tumors composed of adipose elements,[337,498] is probably transmitted as an autosomal dominant trait,[304] and has been classified with the phacomatoses by Koch[337] and by Van Bogaert.[340] The condition has been found in association with several neurological disorders, including neurofibromatosis.[499]

Of special interest is the finding of glioblastoma in two of the 42 patients in the series of Krabbe and Bartels.[498] Neither of these two patients seemed to have recognizable stigmata of von Recklinghausen's disease.

Encephalocraniocutaneous Lipomatosis: In a recent case report concerning a five-year-old mentally retarded boy, findings were reported as including unilateral lipomatosis of the scalp together with homolateral intracranial lipomas, leptomeningeal lipoangio-

matosis, and cerebral malformations and calcifications.[499] Lipomatosis of skull, eyelid, and heart was also described.

There was no positive hereditary history in this case, which was evaluated in terms of various case reports of patients with CNS lipomas among their findings, and which was proposed as representing a new neurocutaneous syndrome.

Nevus Unius Lateralis: An astrocytoma with accompanying diencephalic syndrome has been reported in a three-year-old boy with nevus unius lateralis, a condition which is notable for the unilateral location and unusual configuration of its verrucous and hyperpigmented skin lesions, but which has not been grouped with the neurocutaneous syndromes due to its customary lack of neurological involvement.[500] This reported association with astrocytoma may well be fortuitous, and, in any event, nevus unius lateralis is not known to be a disorder of genetic origin.

CNS Tumors Occurring with Immunodeficiency Disorders and Lymphomatoid Granulomatosis

We have summarized in earlier sections both experimental and clinical information relating to immunologic susceptibility to CNS tumors.

At this point it is pertinent to list two specific immune deficiency disorders of hereditary origin, ataxia-telangiectasia and the Wiskott-Aldrich syndrome, in which brain tumors have occurred,[501,502] and to mention briefly lymphomatoid granulomatosis, as recently described by Liebow, *et al.*, and its possible relationship to the immunologic deficiency disorders.[503]

Ataxia-Telangiectasia (Louis-Bar Syndrome): Medulloblastoma of cerebellum[504] and glioma of frontal lobe[505] have been reported with this disorder, which is generally considered inherited in an autosomal recessive pattern; is a type of spinocerebellar atrophy;[506] shows chromosomal breaks in cultured leukocytes;[507] and is further characterized by conjunctival and cutaneous telangiectasia, recurrent sinopulmonary infections, reduced levels of serum IgA and IgE, hypoplasia of thymic and lymphoid tissues, deficient cellular immunity, and a marked tendency towards development of malignant neoplasms, including leukemia, malignant lymphoma, and other solid tumors.[508] In their study of eighteen ataxia-telangiectasia patients, however, McFarlin, *et al.* did not find any case of brain tumor.[508]

Koch has listed ataxia-telangiectasia among the phacomatoses, thereby confirming the extensive overlapping of diagnostic categories that must be faced when attempting to classify such a disorder. Ataxia-telangiectasia is at once a congenital anomaly, a hereditary disorder, a phacomatosis (neurocutaneous disease), a disorder of impaired immunity, and a disorder with structural chromosomal aberrations.

Wiskott-Aldrich Syndrome: The Wiskott-Aldrich syndrome, the cardinal features of which are recurrent bacterial infections, eczema, and thrombocytopenia, has an X-linked recessive inheritance pattern, and, like ataxia-telangiectasia, includes abnormalities of both humoral and cellular immunity.[509] Affected individuals have developed malignant tumors, especially tumors of lymphoreticular type, and the brain is among the organs in which neoplasms have appeared.[501] There has been a report of primary malignant reticulosis of brain,[510] and an interesting family has been described in whigh malignant tumors of the reticuloendothelial system occurred in multiple organs, including the brain, in two of four boys with the syndrome.[511]

Lymphomatoid Granulomatosis: Lymphomatoid granulomatosis is a multisystem lymphoproliferative disease particularly affecting lung, but also other organs.[503] As delineated by Liebow, *et al.* the disorder may be a new entity but seems to be related to Wegener's granulomatosis. While lymphomatoid granulomatosis has not been shown to be hereditary or to be an immunodeficiency disorder, involvement of the central nervous system by lymphoproliferative lesions with neoplastic characteristics has occurred in this condition. Liebow and his co-workers have called attention to this point of similarity between lymphomatoid granulomatosis and the immunodeficiency disorders, especially the Wiskott-Aldrich syndrome.

Histopathologic Types of Tumors Occurring in Immunodeficient States: A point of some interest regarding the immunodeficient states is whether occurrences of tumor involve solely elements of the reticuloendothelial system, or also involve nonreticuloendothelial tissues. The answer to this question bears on the validity of the hypothesis that the immunosurveillance mechanism normally exerts effective control over continuously operative tendencies of cells of various tissues and organs towards neoplastic growth.[512,513] If this hypothesis is correct, then, in the face of immunologic deficiency, diverse tumor types originating in multiple organ systems should appear. On the other hand, if only reticuloendothelial tumors, such as lymphomas, appear when immunologic function is inadequate, these tumors could be postulated as occurring as a result of attempts at compensatory proliferation of the immunodeficient reticuloendothelial cells, with subsequent hyperplasia and neoplasia.

Insofar as the central nervous system is concerned, more information is required on the ratio of occurrences of reticuloendothelial to nonreticuloendothelial tumors in immunodeficiency states.

In respect to this question, there is considerable agreement that the microglial cells of the brain are among representatives of the reticuloendothelial system in the central nervous system.[514,515] The terms microglioma and reticulum cell sarcoma of brain are often used interchangeably.

Association of CNS Tumors with Other Hereditary and Familial Syndromes

Hereditary and Allied Disorders
1. Retinoblastoma
2. Familial Pheochromocytoma
3. Turcot Syndrome
4. Gaucher's Disease
5. Von Gierke's Disease
6. Paget's Disease of Bone
7. Werner's Syndrome
8. Alzheimer's Disease
9. Rubinstein-Taybi Syndrome
10. Blue Rubber-Bleb Nevus Syndrome & Maffucci's Syndrome
11. Multiple Hereditary Exostoses of Bone
12. Syringomyelia

In addition to those phacomatoses and immunodeficiency disorders mentioned above, CNS tumors have been associated with still other hereditary and familial disorders, including both those transmitted according to one of the simple Mendelian patterns, and those, such as certain syndromes of familial cancer, for which genetic mechanisms, insofar as they operate, have yet to be fully worked out.

Retinoblastoma, the hereditary transmission of which may occur, and if so, on an autosomal dominant basis, has been associated with nonneural tumors and with brain tumors.[516–518]

Both ependymoma of the spinal cord and adrenal pheochromocytoma have occurred in a 13-year-old female member of a family with the autosomal dominant condition of familial pheochromocytoma.[519] This patient had no specific stigmata of any of the neurocutaneous syndromes.

Multiple polyposis of the colon, also usually considered as an autosomal dominant trait, which occurs as a solitary finding and also as a component of certain other syndromes, has been found in an association with CNS tumors, including glioblastoma multiforme, now referred to as the polyposis-glioma syndrome or Turcot syndrome.[520–522] The pattern of inheritance of the Turcot syndrome is yet to be clarified.

There is an isolated report of astrocytoma occurring in Gaucher's disease.[523] The latter is generally transmitted in an autosomal recessive pattern, although dominant inheritance has been suggested for one subcategory.[304]

Hueper has linked the macromolecular structure of glycogen to a stated, but not detailed occurrence of gliomas of the brain in von Gierke's disease,[524,525] an autosomal recessive glycogen storage disorder.

Acoustic neurinoma,[526] meningioma,[527] and glioblastoma multiforme[528] have been found in association with Paget's disease of bone, which may have an X-linked mode of inheritance.[304]

Werner's syndrome, an autosomal recessive disorder, exhibits markedly diverse clinical and laboratory manifestations, including growth retardation, premature graying and loss of hair, cataracts, atrophy and hyperkeratosis of skin, mild diabetes, osteoporosis, joint deformities, soft tissue calcification, severe vascular disease, lessened viability of skin fibroblasts in culture, and, in males, testicular atrophy.[529–533] The first signs of the disorder appear as early as the second decade of life. On the basis of the various findings, the disease has been considered by many as one of premature aging, but critical analysis has brought this concept into serious question.[533,534] Of particular importance in the present context is the occurrence of neoplasms, both benign and malignant, in this disorder. Epstein, *et al.*, in a review of the literature and their own cases, found 13 of 125 patients to have developed tumors.[533] Three of these tumors were meningiomas, and the others included malignancies of various sites.

Alzheimer's disease, or presenile dementia, which probably occurs on a multifactorial basis, but which, on occasion, has manifested a dominant pattern of inheritance,[304] has been associated in one report with cerebral glioblastoma.[535]

Two CNS tumors have been found to date in the Rubinstein-Taybi syndrome, in which there have been suggestive indications, but no proof, that a genetic factor is operative.[536,537] This syndrome has also been referred to as the broad thumb-hallux syndrome, and includes in its manifestations a characteristic facies; mental, motor, and social retardation; and short stature.

Likewise, there has been a report of cerebellar medulloblastoma in the blue rubber-bleb nevus syndrome, a condition characterized by the presence of hemangiomatous lesions, perhaps hamartomas, of the skin and gastrointestinal tract, and for which there is some evidence for an autosomal dominant inheritance pattern.[538]

Maffucci's syndrome, which includes the finding of dyschondroplasia or enchondromatosis (as seen in Ollier's disease) together with cutaneous and subcutaneous angiomatous lesions, and which is a disorder for which there is very little evidence supporting the importance of a genetic etiological factor, has also occurred in association with CNS tumors, either proven or probable.[539,540]

It is of considerable interest, therefore, that one patient has been reported to combine the essential features of the blue rubber-bleb nevus and Maffucci syndromes.[541] This patient, however, did not show any sign of a CNS tumor. More information is needed concerning occurrences of CNS tumors in the blue rubber-bleb nevus and Maffucci syndromes, and concerning the relationship between these two disorders.

Another skeletal disorder, multiple hereditary exostoses of bone, which appears to be a dominant condition, but affects more males than females, has been associated with cerebellar astrocytoma in a recent case report.[542]

The relationship between syringomyelia and CNS tumors could have been discussed above in the section on congenital anomalies, but is referred to here because there is at least some evidence to support the possibility of genetic transmittance of this condition.[543]

Of the 38 patients with syringomyelia reported by Ferry, *et al.*, 75 percent also had intramedullary neoplasms.[544] Kosary, *et al.* reported a patient with both supratentorial meningioma and clinically diagnosed syringomyelia, and expressed the belief that the former led to the development of the latter.[545] From the literature and from his institution's files, Poser was able to gather 234 autopsy cases with both syringomyelia and neoplasia of the central nervous system.[543] In 32 of these 234 cases (13.7%), either von Recklinghausen's disease or von Hippel-Lindau disease was also present. The tumors tabulated included astrocytoma, ependymoma, and glioblastoma; and particularly, but not exclusively, involved the spinal cord. Poser also reported on a literature review of 245 autopsied cases of syringomyelia, finding 16.4 percent to have intramedullary tumor as well. He expressed the opinion that both syringomyelia and its associated neoplasms may be due to a single process involving faulty differentiation, perhaps related in some way to the pathogenesis of the phacomatoses.

Syndromes of Familial Cancer: Brain tumors occur also in certain syndromes of familial cancer, which have been the subject of much interest in recent years, and which have been delineated by means of study of unusual incidences within kindreds of multiple types of cancer, many of which are usually considered as sporadic in occurrence. Onset of cancer at an early age is another frequent finding in these syndromes.

Spongioblastoma multiforme was found in a complex of familial cancer including occurrences of osteogenic sarcoma and carcinoma of colon and adrenal gland;[546] and occurrences of glioma have been noted in a somewhat similar familial syndrome of osteogenic and other sarcomas, various carcinomas, and leukemia.[547]

Likewise, occurrences of brain tumor have been noted in the reports of Li and Fraumeni concerning familial aggregations of soft tissue sarcomas, breast cancer, and other tumors,[548,549] and in a more recent report by Lynch, *et al.* concerning similar families.[550]

It is of interest, as commented on by Li and Fraumeni,[549] and by Miller,[551] that families have been found in which rhabdomyosarcoma occurred in one child, and there were occurrences in two first degree relatives of brain tumor and adrenocortical carcinoma, respectively. Brain tumor and adrenocortical neoplasm, as mentioned above, in a previous section, have occurred also as double primaries in single individuals.

Additional reports of affected families are required in order to ascertain whether available reports of familial cancer syndromes with brain tumor occurrences represent somewhat varied manifestations of a single syndrome, or whether there are two or more such syndromes with distinctive attributes. Figure 17–1 and Table 17-I summarize the findings in a kindred currently under study by Dr. Lynch and his colleagues.

It should be noted that brain tumors seem not to be a prominent or common feature of certain other syndromes of familial cancer which have been reported.[552–554]

In respect to occurrences of tumors, including CNS tumors, within kindreds in the familial cancer syndromes referred to in this context, there is a need for evaluation of the

TABLE 17-I
TABLE INDICATING TUMOR REGISTRY IN A CANCER PRONE FAMILY
(Aggregation of Cancer of the Breast, Leukemia, Sarcoma, and Brain Tumors)

I.   1 Carcinoma, prostate

II.   1 Leiomyosarcoma, bladder
      2 Adenocarcinoma, colon
      3 "Tumor started in breast and metastasized to the pelvic organs"
      4 Carcinoma, breast
      5 Sarcoma, thigh
      6 Glioblastoma multiforme involving right cerebrum
      7 Squamous cell carcinoma, vocal cord (left)

III. 1 Squamous cell carcinoma, right vocal cord
      3 Osteogenic sarcoma, left distal femur
      4 Infratentorial glioma
      5 Adrenal cortical carcinoma
     11 Osteogenic sarcoma, right femur
     13 Carcinoma, breast
     18 Probable malignant neoplasm of right adrenal with intracranial metastasis
     24 Acute lymphatic leukemia
     25 Acute granulocytic leukemia
     28 Acute aleukemic lymphocytic leukemia
     29 Glioblastoma multiforme, right parietal lobe
     30 Carcinoma, left breast

IV.   8 Glioblastoma multiforme
      9 Osteogenic sarcoma, right fibula
     10 Glioblastoma multiforme
     13 Primary malignant brain tumor

findings in terms of the possible importance of environmental as well as genetic factors. One hypothesis to be excluded is that within the kindreds studied, neoplasia develops in individuals of a particular genetic susceptibility as a result of exposure to exogenous agents, such as oncogenic viruses.

Information relating to one possible pathogenetic mechanism in family cancer syndromes has been presented by Bottomley, *et al.*, who performed cytogenetic studies on peripheral blood of 27 of 405 members of a particular family, 37 of whom had developed some type of malignant neoplasia.[555] Tumors found in this family included carcinoma of breast, sarcoma, leukemia, and by history, brain tumor; and represented, therefore, a spectrum of pathologic tumor types similar to that described by Li and Fraumeni. Results of the chromosomal studies were

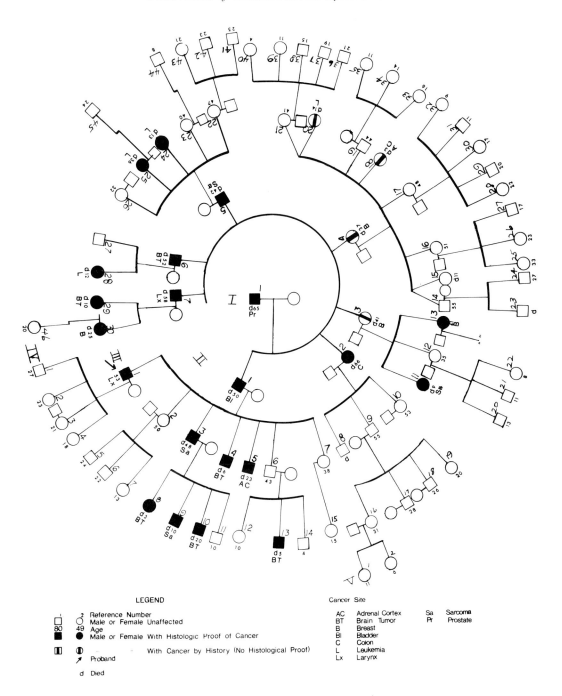

Figure 17–1. Pedigree of family with multiple cancers, including brain tumors. Family is currently under study by H.T. Lynch.

generally normal, although some individuals seemed to have increased numbers of aneuploid cells. Application of the chromosomal banding techniques may make future studies of this type more informative.

Reports offering a degree of support for concordance for cancer in marriage partners are of interest in respect to the problem of evaluating the importance of genetic as compared to environmental factors responsible for increased cancer incidence in particular kindreds.[556,557]

Susceptibility to Neoplasia of Individuals Heterozygous for Recessive Disorders — Fanconi's Anemia: Swift has reported the occurrence of a brain tumor and other malignancies in near relatives of patients with Fanconi's anemia, an autosomal recessive trait characterized by hypoplastic anemia, stunted growth, congenital anomalies, and chromosomal aberrations.[558] While leukemia and solid tumors often occur in patients with Fanconi's anemia,[559] who are homozygous for the gene responsible for this disorder, it is of exceeding interest that evidence is now coming forth to indicate an increased susceptibility to neoplasia even among individuals heterozygous for the defective gene. There is also evidence for increased susceptibility to neoplasia among individuals heterozygous for another precancerous autosomal recessive trait, ataxia-telangiectasia.[560]

The importance of these findings, as Swift has pointed out, is that because individuals heterozygous for these defective genes are much more numerous than homozygotes, heterozygotes may account for a significant portion of the total burden of neoplasia in the population. In New York State, for example, despite the rarity of Fanconi's anemia, it can be calculated that the prevalence of the gene in the population is one in three hundred individuals; and that heterozygotes for Fanconi's may represent 1 percent of all deaths from cancer and leukemia.

If heterozygotes for other rare precancerous autosomal recessive traits, such as Bloom's syndrome, ataxia-telangiectasia, and the Chediak-Higashi syndrome, share a similarly increased susceptibility to neoplasia, then the cumulative prevalence of genes for these disorders may account for a small but significant portion of the total problem of occurrences of cancer.[558]

The concept has also been advanced that double heterozygosity for the genes of two precancerous autosomal recessive traits may contribute to unexpectedly high incidences of neoplasia.[561]

Familial Occurrences of CNS Tumors

Reports of Individual Families: The subject of heredity and neoplasia has a vast literature;[562-568] and even apart from consideration of those genetic disorders discussed above, there are many reports of familial incidence of CNS tumors.[106,337,456,569-575]

In Table 17-II are tabulated instances of familial CNS tumors and neuroblastomas reported in the literature since the appearance of two prior tabulations,[572,575] somewhat less inclusive as to tumor types, of a decade and slightly more ago. Similar cases reported in the older literature may be referred to with the assistance of the references provided.

Although the number of reports of familial incidence of nervous system tumors is fairly large, familial incidence cannot be considered as synonymous with genetic etiology. Even if it could be proved, as is obviously not possible simply on the basis of case reports, that familial incidence represents something more than simple coincidence, this would still not mean that the familial occurrences were of hereditary nature, since the possibility of familial exposure to environmental agents responsible for induction of neoplasia would yet exist. Nevertheless, genetic origin is one possible ex-

TABLE 17-II

REPORTS OF FAMILIAL CNS TUMORS AND
NEUROBLASTOMAS SINCE REPORTS OF
KJELLIN *ET AL.* (1960)[575] AND METZEL (1963)[572]

Findings	Authors*
Glioblastoma multiforme in 3 sisters	Koch and Middendorf (1960)
Malignant glioma in identical twins	Fairburn and Urich (1971)
Glioblastoma in 2 brothers; in a second family, astrocytoma in two first cousins	Kaufman and Brisman (1972)
Glioblastoma and oligodendroglioma in brother and sister, respectively	Symonds (1960)
Glioblastoma and gliomatous tumor in brother and sister, respectively	Grosz and Plaschkes (1960)
Malignant astrocytoma in 3 siblings	Armstrong and Hanson (1969)
Oligodendroglioma in the frontal lobes of 2 brothers	Parkinson and Hall (1962)
Cerebellar medulloblastoma in 2 of 3 newborn hydrocephalic sisters	Belamaric and Chau (1969)
Cerebellar medulloblastoma in 2 brothers	Bickerstaff, et al. (1967)
Meningioma in mother and daughter	Joynt and Perret (1961)
Meningioma in mother and daughter	Joynt and Perret (1965)
Meningioma in brother and sister	Gaist and Piazza (1959)
Meningioma in 2 brothers and a female second cousin	Sahar (1965)
Intra-osseous meningioma in mother and daughter	Wagman, et al. (1960)
Meningioma in 2 brothers	Grunert, et al. (1970)
Optic glioma in 2 sisters; in a second family, spinal ependymoma in mother and astrocytoma of vermis in her son	Bromowicz, et al. (1971)
Papilloma of choroid plexus in brother and sister	Komminoth, et al. (1965)
Meningioma and hemangioblastoma in sister and brother, respectively	Chateau, et al. (1971)
Solitary spinal cord neurofibromas in a mother and two sons, with no other signs of von Recklinghausen's disease	Myers, et al. (1960)
Cervical cord tumors ("subependymoma") in two hemophiliac brothers, with syringomyelia also present in one (true neoplasms?)	Blaauw and Schenk (1971)
Congenital intraspinal extradural cysts in 3 siblings of a family also manifesting Milroy's disease and distichiasis (cysts apparently not neoplastic)	Bergland (1968)
Daughter dying at age 5 days with spina bifida and spinal cord sarcoma; her father having surgery for spinal cord neurinoma at age 50; and his brother for meningioma at age 43. No consanguinity in the family and no	Guomundsson (1970)

TABLE 17-II (CONTINUED)

Findings	Authors*
other signs of von Recklinghausen's disease	
Cavernous angiomata of brain in father and daughter (probably hamartomas)	Clark (1970)
Neuroblastoma or ganglioneuroblastoma in two siblings and a paternal cousin (possibly other types of infantile tumors in the family, but not verified)	Hardy and Nesbit (1972)
Neuroblastoma in two sisters, one of them trisomic for chromosome 13	Feingold, et al. (1971)
Neuroblastoma in 4 of 5 siblings, children of father with mild pectus excavatum and 3 café-au-lait spots, and mother with elevated catecholamine excretion. Congenital anomalies associated in 2 of 4 affected siblings	Chatten and Voorhess (1967)
Neuroblastoma in two siblings, and elevated urinary VMA in father	Wong, et al. (1971)
Neuroblastoma in two sisters. In one, histopathology suggestive of relationship to neurofibromatosis	Griffin and Bolande (1969)
Neuroblastoma in two related individuals, each from a family with a high incidence of cancer at multiple sites	Ullrich (1970)

* Reference numbers are 576–603, and 108 (Guomundsson).

planation for the observed clustering of CNS tumors within families. It may be postulated that a genetic factor is primarily responsible for the familial clustering of CNS tumors, or that there is a hereditary susceptibility to such tumors that operates in concert with environmental factors so as to result in the clustering phenomenon.

Histopathologic tumor types occurring with familial incidence, as listed in the older and more recent literature, have included glioblastoma, astrocytoma, oligodendroglioma, meningioma, and medulloblastoma. Koch has stated that familial gliomas and glioblastomas occur characteristically deep in the brain rather than in the cortical area.[337]

Specificity of histopathologic tumor type and of site of occurrence of tumor within the brain have been noted in a number of instances and been interpreted as militating against the possibility of mere coincidence being the sole explanation of familial occurrences. In the family reported by Parkinson and Hall, for example, not only did two siblings each have a frontal lobe tumor, but in each instance the tumor was an oligodendroglioma.[582]

Twin Studies: Identical twins, both concordant and discordant for CNS tumor, have been reported in the older literature, but instances of concordance for tumors of the same histopathologic type have been relatively few in number.[337,456,604]

More recent contributions have provided additional insight. In a review of childhood cancer deaths in unselected twins and singletons born in California during the period 1940 to 1964, Norris and Jackson found 54 instances of cancer other than leukemia among 145,708 individual twins born.[605] Of these 54 cases, 21 had brain tumors, two spinal cord tumors, one retinoblastoma, and five neuroblastomas. As compared to singletons, there was an over-all deficit of deaths due to cancer among twins, but cancer of the nervous system did not contribute to the deficit. In no case was there a record of a twin with CNS tumor or neuroblastoma having a co-twin dying of the same lesion. In two instances, however, co-twins of index twins with brain tumor died with pathologically unverified signs of central nervous system disease. Harvald and Hauge, in reporting on a series of twin pairs, both monozygotic and dizygotic, in which one twin had a CNS neoplasm, found no evidence of concordance for CNS tumors.[606] In a study of childhood leukemia and other cancers based on review of death certificates of children in the United States dying of cancer in the years 1960 to 1967, Miller found no instance of twins concordant for CNS neoplasms, although there was a pair of male twins dying of neuroblastoma, and a pair of female twins, one of whom died with glioblastoma multi-

forme, and the other of leukemia following osteosarcoma.[551,607]

Information available at the present time, therefore, does not offer support for the etiologic significance of the finding of concordance for CNS tumors in twins.

Surveys of Relatives of Patients with CNS Tumors: The information presented above on hereditary and familial occurrences of brain tumors does not provide us with data concerning the statistical importance of familial cases in relation to the total burden of brain tumor incidence. It would appear that such data would be best compiled from a large-scale prospective study of brain tumor patients and their families, with full documentation of clinical, genetic, and pathologic findings in subject and control groups from a defined population base. Although so complete a study has never been carried out, there have been conducted several surveys of relatives of patients with brain tumor.

In the studies of Harvald and Hauge, no significant hereditary factor was detected in the etiology of glioblastoma, astrocytoma, medulloblastoma, acoustic neurinoma, and meningioma;[608,609] and the same workers found no excess of deaths due to tumors of various extracranial sites in relatives of patients with glioblastoma, astrocytoma, and meningioma.[610] They found 15 cases of intracranial tumor among 6,757 relatives of 641 patients with CNS tumors, as compared to an expected number of 19.

Van der Wiel, on the other hand, reporting on an extensive experience in his very interesting monograph, found a greater number of brain tumors than expected statistically in relatives of probands with glioma of the brain.[456] Histopathologic types of the tumors of 100 probands included glioblastoma multiforme (38), cerebral astrocytoma (26), astroblastoma (6), medulloblastoma (7), spongioblastoma (6), cerebellar astrocytoma (6), ependymoma (5), oligodendroglioma (1), and glioma otherwise unclassified (5). Among 5,262 relatives of the 100 probands, there were seven who had died with verified glioma, one with meningioma, and five others with probable but unverified glioma. In the significantly smaller control group (2,228 individuals), there were no deaths due to glioma. Van der Wiel was able to calculate the mortality of probands' relatives due to glioma as four times that of the Netherlands as a whole.

Van der Wiel's monograph also explores the relationship between glioma of brain and status dysraphicus, which is described as a constitutional anomaly, manifesting many major and minor somatic stigmata, and associated with a predisposition to syringomyelia and certain other diseases. He found many probands with glioma to show stigmata of status dysraphicus, and found what he considered lethal forms of dysraphism, including spina bifida aperta, meningocele, and anencephaly, and milder forms also, more frequently in relatives of glioma patients than in the control population. It is of parenthetic interest that bulldogs, one of the brachycephalic breeds described above as peculiarly susceptible to brain tumors, are considered dysraphic animals. Café-au-lait spots were found in many probands with brain tumor (23%), and were more common in probands' relatives than in the control group. Furthermore, café-au-lait spots and status dysraphicus seemed to be positively associated in probands' relatives, but not in controls. In agreement with the findings of Hauge and Harvald, probands' relatives and controls showed no significant difference in mortality due to carcinoma of extracranial organs.

Van der Wiel felt that the café-au-lait lesions he observed may be related to a specific gene also influencing the development of gliomas, and concluded that gliomas may be manifestations of a pathologic process resembling those of the phacomatoses. In fact, Miller has suggested that the in-

creased incidence of familial brain tumors found in Van der Wiel's study may be due to the prevalence in the latter's study group of subclinical forms of hereditary conditions known to be associated with brain tumors, such as tuberous sclerosis and von Recklinghausen's disease.[315]

De Weerdt and Schut, in a questionnaire study not employing the case-control method, found no demonstrable familial correlation between occurrences of brain tumor and spina bifida.[611] These workers also expressed doubt that status dysraphicus, as described and studied by Van der Wiel, should be considered a single genetic entity.

In a study based on interviews with family members, Choi, *et al.* found twelve brain tumors among 2,104 relatives of 126 patients with verified CNS tumors, as compared to a finding of only three brain tumors among 2,404 relatives of 126 matched controls.[212] For the brain tumors occurring in relatives, however, pathologic verification was not obtained.

Metzel found that three of 393 gliomas investigated seemed to be occurring on a familial basis;[612] while Koch found evidence for familial occurrence in six of 350 cases of CNS tumor.[604] Pathological verification had been obtained, however, for only two-thirds of Koch's 350 cases, and for only four of the six familial occurrences.

In the families of 30 patients with brain tumor investigated by Pass, there was one instance of familial occurrence of brain tumor, and von Recklinghausen's disease was present in three other families.[613]

Findings of considerable interest have come also from the previously mentioned studies of Miller on deaths from childhood leukemia and other forms of cancer.[551,607] In his nationwide survey of death certificates for the years 1960 to 1967, and despite his negative findings for concordance of CNS tumors in twins, he found that among sibs other than twins, sib pairs with brain tumor

were found nine times more often than expected. There was also a significant and
quantitatively similar excess of families in
which one sibling had brain tumor, and
another a sarcoma of either muscle or bone.
Miller suggested that these striking occurrences in sibs could be on the basis of familial affliction with one of the phacomatoses,
such as von Recklinghausen's disease or
tuberous sclerosis, perhaps in subclinical
form; or could be developing as manifestations of one of the syndromes of familial
cancer.

It would appear, therefore, that family
studies conducted to date have not been
fully consistent in respect to data bearing on
the importance of familial incidence and genetic etiology of CNS tumors. At the same
time, illuminating and intriguing suggestions
concerning possible bases of familial occurrences have been proposed.

Cytogenetic Aspects of
CNS Tumor Occurrences

While the focus of this review is on genetic
factors contributing to the development of
CNS tumors, and relates directly, therefore,
to the constitution of germinal cells, it is also
appropriate to review briefly the cytogenetics
of CNS tumor cells. Indeed, malignant tumors generally may be considered genetic
diseases, since, as is well known, the alteration in tumor cells that is responsible for
neoplastic growth is passed from one generation of tumor cells to the next, i.e., the alteration is hereditable.

There is an abundant literature dealing
with cytogenetic findings in neoplasia, and
with the importance of these findings in neoplastic development and progression.[614-620]
Almost universally, human and experimental
malignant solid tumors have had abnormal
chromosomal complements, although there
are occasional reports, such as that of Nowell
and Morris dealing with "minimal deviation"

hepatomas, of malignancy with normal karyotype.[621] Possible interpretations which have
been considered for the chromosomal abnormalities of number and/or structure found
in malignant neoplasms include the following: 1) the chromosomal changes are primary
events resulting in malignancy; 2) the chromosomal changes are secondary effects of the
neoplastic process; 3) the chromosomal
changes and the malignancy are dual effects
of a primary causative factor; and 4) the
chromosomal changes, while not primary,
lead to the establishment of clones of malignant cells with a selective advantage for
neoplastic progression. The merits of these
interpretations remain controversial, but interpretation four has received considerable
support in the literature.

There is much information available concerning the chromosomes of both benign and
malignant central nervous system tumors.[622]
For the most part, malignant neural tumors
have demonstrated abnormalities of number
and/or structure,[623,624] although isolated
gliomas of low grade malignancy have been
found to have normal diploid chromosomal
complements;[625] and tissue culture techniques involving substantial periods of incu-
bation, as opposed to direct techniques of
analysis, have often yielded normal karyotypes,[626] presumably due to preferential
growth in culture of nonneoplastic host
cells.

Analyses of specific pathologic types of
CNS tumor have produced results worthy of
note. Several studies have described tissue
from meningiomas as having structural or
numerical anomalies of the G group. Loss of
a G group chromosome, shown recently to
be number 22, has been found frequently,[627-630] while a smaller number of
meningiomas has shown a Philadelphia-like
chromosome belonging to the G group.[631]
Numerical changes involving chromosomes
of groups other than G have been noted also,
as have marker chromosomes.[629,632-634]

In gliomatous tumors, including glioblastoma multiforme, highly variable abnormalities of number, and, in some instances, structure, have been described.[635–637] Notable has been a lack of uniformity of findings from case to case, even in tumors of the same histopathologic type. It is of interest that double minute chromosomes have been noted in several reports. For example, Mark and Granberg found double minutes in all or most cells of three of forty malignant gliomas, while five other tumors had double minutes in sporadic cells.[638] Kucheria has described a subependymal glioma with double minutes;[639] and Lubs, *et al.* have reported double minutes in cells of a tumor diagnosed as medulloblastoma, and in cells of peripheral blood and bone marrow from the affected individual.[640]

Double minutes have been reported also in isolated cases of neuroblastoma,[641,642] another tumor in which chromosomal changes have been quite variable.[643–648]

Despite these findings, however, double minutes are not found solely in neural neoplasms.[642] Such chromatin bodies have been found in sarcomatous mouse tumors induced by Rous sarcoma virus,[649] in Rous rat sarcoma,[650] in ascitic fluid from a case of human ovarian carcinoma complicated by infectious hepatitis,[651] and in human embryonic rhabdomyosarcoma.[652] Cox, *et al.* have found double minutes in direct preparations of cells from neuroblastoma, medulloblastoma, and rhabdomyosarcoma.[653]

In some, but not all, reports of occurrences of double minutes, there has been a history of previous radiation therapy.

Of related interest, abnormalities of number and structure have been found also in tissue taken from retinoblastomas,[654,655] tumors occurring in an organ with a highly specialized neural function.

Triploid and near triploid metaphase figures, and other chromosomal aberrations, are commonly found in human brain tumors of metastatic type.[656]

It may be anticipated that, in the near future, studies using the newly developed banding techniques will add greatly to our knowledge of the chromosomes of CNS tumors.

Finally, it may be noted that a form of chromosomal instability, characterized not by changes in chromosomal number but by a tendency to formation of spontaneous breaks, has been found in a number of precancerous genetic disorders, including ataxia-telangiectasia.[507] As noted above, brain tumors are among the neoplasms which have been associated with ataxia-telangiectasia. In this instance also, more than one interpretation is possible in regard to the relationship between the observed chromosomal changes, which are found in lymphocytes of peripheral blood, and the precancerous nature of the disorder.

Discussion

We have attempted to bring together information bearing on the relationship between genetic influences and occurrences of central nervous system tumors. It must be stated, however, that to the central question underlying our review, the degree to which genetic factors are important in respect to the total burden of central nervous system tumors occurring in the population, there is no precise answer presently available.

Still, it is clear that at least some CNS tumors occur as manifestations of specific hereditary syndromes, such as certain of the phacomatoses and immunodeficiency disorders. In addition, the multiplicity of interfacets between genetics and CNS tumors, both in animals and humans, is quite striking. In animals, both spontaneous occurrence and experimental induction appear to be influenced by the particular genetic constitution of the animal. In humans, epidemiologic information suggests the existence of differences in incidence among ethnic groups which could possibly be related to differences in genetic susceptibility; and associations of CNS tumors with numerous disorders, either definitely or possibly of genetic origin, have been reported. As we have tried to indicate above, these associations are well established in some instances, and in others merely isolated findings requiring additional corroboration.

Furthermore, there have been many reports of multiple occurrences of CNS tumors within individual families, in the absence of any known predisposing hereditary disorder. Whether such familial occurrences are of genetic origin is difficult or impossible to determine on the basis of only case reports.

At the same time, it need not be expected that genetic influences favoring the development of brain tumors will necessarily result in all cases in multiple tumor occurrences within individual families. It is in some cases known, and in other cases possible, that single occurrences of CNS tumor in families, such as may be found in families with von Recklinghausen's disease, other hereditary conditions listed above, and perhaps still others yet to be described, are occurring on a genetic basis.

Extended surveys of relatives of patients with CNS tumors have produced mixed results, but the weight of the evidence appears to support an increased, but not well quantified risk of developing CNS tumor for close relatives of affected individuals. How much of this increased risk for relatives may be due to familial occurrences of hereditary disorders known to predispose to CNS tumors, such as certain of the neurocutaneous syndromes, remains to be elucidated. Paradoxically, the few available twin studies do not support the importance of hereditary influences in occurrences of brain tumor.

Of course, it should be pointed out that certain occurrences of CNS tumors, e.g., meningiomas resulting from trauma, seem to be independent of any specific genetic influence.

It is of interest that our review of CNS tumors necessarily details many interfacets among congenital anomalies, neurocutaneous disorders, immunodeficiency diseases, other hereditary diseases, disorders of chromosomal instability, syndromes of familial cancer, and multiple tumor occurrences in a single individual. In particular, many conditions which may be classified as congenital anomalies, some of which have either dominant or recessive inheritance patterns, and some of which can be further subgrouped into hamartomatoses, or disorders of immune deficiency, and/or disorders of inborn chromosomal instability, exhibit a very interesting association with brain tumors. In some instances, there seems to be only a gradual, continuous change in findings between congenital anomaly and neoplasia. For example, in tuberous sclerosis the glial lesions present a spectrum of findings from the anomalous to the neoplastic, with no sharp demarcation between the two in individual cases.

A better understanding of the complex relationships among these various categories of disorder should yield a better understanding of the genetics of CNS tumors.

It would seem that a large-scale prospective study of CNS tumor patients and their relatives, preferably within the framework of a defined population base, could make a major contribution to information available concerning the significance of genetic factors relative to the total burden of CNS tumors in the population. Such a study should be solidly based in clinical medicine, epidemiology, pathology, and genetics. Included in the study should be examination of individuals for the presence of neurocutaneous disorders, even when appearing as formes frustes; a search for heterozygosity for the recessive precancerous traits, e.g., by viral transformation studies; accurate recording of data regarding consanguinity; pathologic verification of neoplasms, both intracranial and extracranial, and careful post-mortem study of deaths, in part in order to detect syndromes of familial cancer; and an attempt at detection of virus in families with multiple tumor occurrences. Of course, a well chosen control group is essential for any such study.

At the very least, a study of this type should give statistical data regarding familial occurrences of CNS tumors. Hopefully, clinical, genetic, and laboratory investigations would assist in achieving a second objective, that of determining the etiologic factors contributing to those familial occurrences encountered.

The prospects of success for such a study would be enhanced were additional means available for identifying formes frustes of the neurocutaneous disorders, and heterozygosity for the precancerous recessive traits. As we have discussed above, there is preliminary evidence that the individual heterozygous for certain of these precancerous recessive traits may be at risk for an increased incidence of neoplasia.

It is possible that basic investigations into various aspects of tumor etiology and pathogenesis, both those mentioned above, and others,[657-660] will help to provide direction as to specific biochemical, morphologic, immunologic, or other characteristics which could be searched for in family studies.

Although we cannot answer the central question as to the importance of the contribution of genetic factors to the total CNS tumor problem, it does seem to be true that in some cases of CNS tumor the genetic factor is the chief etiologic influence, while in certain other cases it is quite likely that the genetic factor is of importance.

Perhaps the following hypothesis may be put forward: CNS tumor will develop primarily on a genetic basis; or in the genetically susceptible individual, due to the effect of one or more adverse host or environmental factors. This hypothesis is not inconsistent with any data of which we are aware, and is supported by much of the information in this review.

Summary

There are numerous relationships between genetic factors and central nervous system tumors, both in humans and experimental animals.

In humans, central nervous system tumors occur in a number of hereditary disorders, such as von Recklinghausen's disease and tuberous sclerosis.

In addition, there are many reports of familial occurrences of CNS tumors, and several (but not all) family surveys have indicated that certain families have an increased incidence of CNS tumors. The extent of genetic influences in these familial occurrences requires further definition.

CNS tumors often occur in the apparent absence of any specific genetic influence, although general genetic susceptibility must be assumed.

At this time we are not able to quantify the importance of genetic influences in relation to the total problem of CNS tumor occurrences in the population. More information is needed.

It is suggested that a large-scale prospective study of brain tumor patients, their relatives, and suitable controls should be undertaken.

Acknowledgments

For assistance in review of the foreign literature, thanks are extended to H.A. Windhager, M.D., Department of Pathology, Jersey City Medical Center; J.C. Lee, M.D., Ph.D., formerly with the same department; W.A. Orlowski, D.D.S., Ph.D.,

Department of Oral Biology, College of Medicine and Dentistry of New Jersey, New Jersey Dental School; Miss Louise Niedbala; Miss Josephine Mulcahy; and Mrs. Vesna Mulcahy.

We also thank Mrs. Peggy Pridgen and Mrs. Doreen Puccio, both of Jersey City Medical Center, Mrs. Pridgen for typing the manuscript and Mrs. Puccio for clerical assistance.

REFERENCES

1. Durity, F.A., Dolman, C.L., and Moyes, P.D.: Ganglioneuroblastoma of the cerebellum. Case report. *J Neurosurg, 28:* 270–273, 1968.

2. Liss, L.: Neuroblastoma (malignant gangliocytoma) of the parietal lobe. *J Neurosurg, 17:*529–536, 1960.

3. Miller, A.A., and Ramsden, F.: A cerebral neuroblastoma with unusual fibrous tissue reaction. *J Neuropathol Exp Neurol, 25:* 328–340, 1966.

4. Cushing, H.: *Intracranial Tumours.* Thomas, Springfield, 1932.

5. Kernohan, J.W., and Sayre, G.P.: Tumors of the central nervous system. In *Atlas of Tumor Pathology.* Section X-Fascicles 35 and 37. Washington, Armed Forces Institute of Pathology, 1952.

6. Zülch, K.J., and Woolf, A.L. (Eds.): Classification of brain tumours. *Acta Neurochir* (Wien), Suppl. 10, pp. 1–217, 1965.

7. Zülch, K.J.: *Brain Tumors. Their Biology and Pathology.* 2nd Am Ed. New York, Springer, 1965.

8. Russell, D.S., and Rubinstein, L.J.: *Pathology of Tumours of the Nervous System,* 3rd Ed. Baltimore, Williams & Wilkins, 1971.

9. Rubinstein, L.J.: Tumors of the central nervous system. In *Atlas of Tumor Pathology,* Second series, Fascicle 6. Washington, Armed Forces Institute of Pathology, 1972.

10. Kernohan, J.W., Woltman, H.W., and Adson, A.W.: Intramedullary tumors of the spinal cord. A review of fifty-one cases, with an attempt at histologic classification. *Arch Neurol Psychiatry, 25:*679–701, 1931.

11. Harkin, J.C., and Reed, R.J.: Tumors of the peripheral nervous system. In *Atlas of Tumor Pathology,* Second series, Fascicle

3. Washington, Armed Forces Institute of Pathology, 1969.

12. Abell, M.R., Hart, W.R., and Olson, J.R.: Tumors of the peripheral nervous system. *Hum Pathol, 1:*503–551, 1970.

13. Madison, R.M., Rabstein, L.S., and Bryan, W.R.: Mortality rate and spontaneous lesions found in 2,928 untreated BALB/cCr mice. *J Natl Cancer Inst, 40:*683–685, 1968.

14. Hoag, W.G.: Spontaneous cancer in mice. *Ann NY Acad Sci, 108:*805–831, 1963.

15. Bailey, P.C., Leach, W.B., and Hartley, M.W.: Characteristics of a new inbred strain of mice (PBA) with a high tumor incidence: preliminary report. *J Natl Cancer Inst, 45:*59–73, 1970.

16. Smith, C.S., and Pilgrim, H.I.: Spontaneous neoplasms in germfree BALB/cPi mice. *Proc Soc Exp Biol Med, 138:*542–544, 1971.

17. Dorn, C.R., Taylor, D.O.N., Chaulk, L.E., and Hibbard, H.H.: The prevalence of spontaneous neoplasms in a defined canine population. *Am J Public Health, 56:* 254–264, 1966.

18. Dorn, C.R., Taylor, D.O.N., Frye, F.L., and Hibbard, H.H.: Survey of animal neoplasms in Alameda and Contra Costa Counties, California. I. Methodology and description of cases. *J Natl Cancer Inst, 40:*295–305, 1968.

19. Dorn, C.R., Taylor, D.O.N., Schneider, R., Hibbard, H.H., and Klauber, M.R.: Survey of animal neoplasms in Alameda and Contra Costa Counties, California. II. Cancer morbidity in dogs and cats from Alameda County. *J Natl Cancer Inst, 40:* 307–318, 1968.

20. Dorn, C.R.: Comparative oncology: dogs,

cats, and man. *Perspect Biol Med, 15:* 507–519, 1972.

21. Zaldivar, R.: Incidence of spontaneous neoplasms in beagles. *J Am Vet Med Assoc, 151:*1319–1321, 1967.

22. Priester, W.A., and Mantel, N.: Occurrence of tumors in domestic animals. Data from 12 United States and Canadian colleges of veterinary medicine. *J Natl Cancer Inst, 47:*1333–1344, 1971.

23. Moulton, J.E.: Occurrence and types of tumors in large domestic animals. *Ann NY Acad Sci, 108:*620–632, 1963.

24. Kent, S.P.: Spontaneous and induced malignant neoplasms in monkeys. *Ann NY Acad Sci, 85:*819–827, 1960.

25. Fraser, H.: Astrocytomas in an inbred mouse strain. *J Pathol, 103:*266–270, 1971.

26. Bots, G.Th.A.M., Kroes, R., and Feron, V.J.: Spontaneous tumors of the brain in rats. A report of 3 cases. *Pathol Vet, 5:*290–296, 1968.

27. Schardein, J.L., Fitzgerald, J.E., and Kaump, D.H.: Spontaneous tumors in Holtzman-source rats of various ages. *Pathol Vet, 5:* 238–252, 1968.

28. Thompson, S.W., and Hunt, R.D.: Spontaneous tumors in the Sprague-Dawley rat: incidence rates of some types of neoplasms as determined by serial section versus single section technics. *Ann NY Acad Sci, 108:*832–845, 1963.

29. Thompson, S.W., Huseby, R.A., Fox, M.A., Davis, C.L., and Hunt, R.D.: Spontaneous tumors in the Sprague-Dawley rat. *J Natl Cancer Inst, 27:*1037–1057, 1961.

30. Blumenthal, H.T., and Rogers, J.B.: Spontaneous and induced tumors in the guinea pig, with special reference to the factor of age. *Prog Exp Tumor Res, 9:*261–285, 1967.

31. Luginbühl, H.: A comparative study of neoplasms of the central nervous system in animals. In Zülch, K.J., and Woolf, A.L., (Eds.): *Classification of brain tumours.* Acta Neurochir (Wien), Suppl. 10, pp. 30–42, 1965.

32. Luginbühl, H.: Oligodendrogliomas in animals. In Zülch, K.J., and Woolf, A.L., (Eds.): *Classification of Brain Tumours.*

Acta Neurochir (Wien), Suppl. 10, pp. 173–180, 1965.

33. Luginbühl, H.: Comparative aspects of tumors of the nervous system. *Ann NY Acad Sci, 108:*702–721, 1963.

34. Hayes, K.C., and Schiefer, B.: Primary tumors in the CNS of carnivores. *Pathol Vet, 6:* 94–116, 1969.

35. Luginbühl, H.: Studies on meningiomas in cats. *Am J Vet Res, 22:*1030–1040, 1961.

36. Howard, E.B., and Nielsen, S.W.: Neoplasia of the boxer dog. *Am J Vet Res, 26:*1121–1131, 1965.

37. Taylor, R.F., Bucci, T.J., and Garvin, C.H.: Oligodendroglioma in a dog. *J Small Anim Pract, 13:*41–46, 1972.

38. Misdorp, W.: Tumors in newborn animals. *Pathol Vet, 2:*328–343, 1965.

39. Simon, J., and Albert, L.T.: Two cases of neuroblastomas in dogs. *J Am Vet Med Assoc, 136:*210–214, 1960.

40. Grice, H.C., and Hutchison, J.A.: Retinoblastoma in a dog. A clinico-pathologic report. *J Am Vet Med Assoc, 136:*444–447, 1960.

41. Simon, J., and Brewer, R.L.: Multiple neurofibromatosis in a cow and calf. *J Am Vet Med Assoc, 142:*1102–1104, 1963.

42. Sullivan, D.J., and Anderson, W.A.: Tumors of the bovine acoustic nerve—a report of two cases. *Am J Vet Res, 19:*848–852, 1958.

43. Kradel, D.C., and Dunne, H.W.: Brain tumors (ependymomas) in deer. *J Am Vet Med Assoc, 147:*1096–1098, 1965.

44. Wight, P.A.L., and Duff, R.H.: The histopathology of epizootic gliosis and astrocytomata of the domestic fowl. *J Comp Pathol, 74:*373–380, 1964.

45. Jungherr, E.: Tumors and tumor-like conditions in monkeys. *Ann NY Acad Sci, 108:*777–792, 1963.

46. Kirsch, W.M., and Schulz, D.: The chemical induction of brain tumors with carcinogenic hydrocarbons and miscellaneous agents. In Kirsch, W.M., Grossi-Paoletti, E., and Paoletti, P., (Eds.): *The Experimental Biology of Brain Tumors.* Thomas, Springfield, 1972, pp. 181–193.

47. Zülch, K.J.: The newest development of ex-

perimental induced tumors of the central nervous system. *J Génét Hum, 17:*511–529, 1969.

48. Seligman, A.M., and Shear, M.J.: Studies in carcinogenesis. VIII. Experimental production of brain tumors in mice with methylcholanthrene. *Am J Cancer, 37:* 364–395, 1939.

49. Alexander, L.: A note on the differential diagnosis of experimentally produced brain tumors and their relation to brain tumors in man. *Am J Cancer, 37:*395–399, 1939.

50. Weil, A.: Experimental production of tumors in the brains of white rats. *Arch Pathol, 26:*777–790, 1938.

51. Zimmerman, H.M., and Arnold, H.: Experimental brain tumors. I. Tumors produced with methylcholanthrene. *Cancer Res, 1:* 919–938, 1941.

52. Perese, D.M., and Moore, G.E.: Methods of induction and histogenesis of experimental brain tumors. *J Neurosurg, 17:*677–698, 1960.

53. Wahal, K.M., and Ansari, I.H.: Experimental brain tumours in albino mice. *Indian J Med Res, 56:*826–834, 1968.

54. Zimmerman, H.M., and Arnold, H.: Experimental brain tumors. IV. The incidence in different strains of mice. *Cancer Res, 4:* 98–101, 1944.

55. Zimmerman, H.M., and Arnold, H.: Chemical carcinogens and animal species as factors in experimental brain tumors. *J Neuropathol, 2:*416–417, 1943.

56. Vazquez Lopez, E.: Glioma in a rat fed with 2-acetyl-amino-fluorene. *Nature* (Lond), *156:*296–297, 1945.

57. Hoch-Ligeti, C., and Russell, D.S.: Primary tumours of the brain and meninges in rats fed 2-acetylaminofluorene. *Acta Un Int Contra Cancr, 7:*126–129, 1950.

58. Snell, K.C., Stewart, H.L., Morris, H.P., Wagner, B.P., and Ray, F.E.: Intracranial neurilemmoma and medulloblastoma induced in rats by the dietary administration of N, N′-2, 7-fluorenylenebisacetamide. *Natl Cancer Inst* Monogr. No. 5: 85–103, 1961.

59. Oyasu, R., Battifora, H.A., Clasen, R.A., McDonald, J.H., and Hass, G.M.: Induction of cerebral gliomas in rats with dietary lead subacetate and 2-acetylaminofluorene. *Cancer Res, 30:*1248–1261, 1970.

60. Druckrey, H., Ivankovic, S., Preussmann, R., Zülch, K.J., and Mennel, H.D.: Selective induction of malignant tumors of the nervous system by resorptive carcinogens In Kirsch, W.M., Grossi-Paoletti, E., and Paoletti, P., (Eds.): *The Experimental Biology of Brain Tumors.* Thomas, Springfield, 1972, pp. 85–147.

61. Koestner, A., Swenberg, J.A., and Wechsler, W.: Experimental tumors of the nervous system induced by resorptive N-nitrosourea compounds. *Progr Exp Tumor Res, 17:*9–30, 1972.

62. Grossi-Paoletti, E., Paoletti, P., Pezzotta, S., Schiffer, D., and Fabiani, A.: Tumors of the nervous system induced by ethylnitrosourea administered either intracerebrally or subcutaneously to newborn rats. *J Neurosurg, 37:*580–590, 1972.

63. Warzok, R., Schneider, J., Schreiber, D., and Jänisch, W.: Experimental brain tumours in dogs. *Experientia, 26:*303–304, 1970.

64. Druckrey, H., Landschütz, Ch., and Ivankovic, S.: Transplacentare Erzeugung maligner Tumoren des Nervensystems. *Z. Krebsforsch, 73:*371–386, 1970.

65. Vázquez-López, E.: On the growth of Rous sarcoma inoculated into the brain. *Am J Cancer, 26:*29–55, 1936.

66. Yohn, D.S.: Oncogenic viruses: expectations and applications in neuropathology. *Prog Exp Tumor Res, 17:*74–92, 1972.

67. Grove, A.S., Jr., Di Chiro, G., and Rabotti, G.F.: Experimental brain tumors, with a report of those induced in dogs by Rous sarcoma virus. *J Neurosurg, 26:*465–477, 1967.

68. Rabotti, G.F.: Experimental intracranial tumors of viral etiology. In Kirsch, W.M., Grossi-Paoletti, E., and Paoletti, P., (Eds.): *The Experimental Biology of Brain Tumors.* Thomas, Springfield, 1972, pp. 148–180.

69. Mancini, L.O., Yates, V.J., Jasty, V., and Anderson, J.: Ependymomas induced in hamsters inoculated with an avian adenovirus (CELO). *Nature* (Lond), *222:*190–191, 1969.

70. Ogawa, K., Hamaya, K., Fujii, Y., Matsuura, K., and Endo, T.: Tumor induction by adenovirus type 12 and its target cells in the central nervous system. *Gann, 60:* 383–392, 1969.

71. Merkow, L., Slifkin, M., Pardo, M., and Rapoza, N.P.: Studies on the pathogenesis of simian adenovirus-induced tumors. III. The histopathology and ultrastructure of intracranial neoplasms induced by SV20. *J Natl Cancer Inst, 41:*1051–1070, 1968.

72. Duffy, P.E.: Virus induced cerebral sarcoma. *J Neuropathol Exp Neurol, 29:*370–391, 1970.

73. Ausman, J.I., and Owens, G.: The production of a virus-induced tumor in the central nervous system of monkeys. *J Neurosurg, 21:*660–666, 1964.

74. Rabotti, G.F., and Haguenau, Fr.: Correlative biological and ultrastructural studies on Rous sarcoma virus in various hosts. *Bibl Haematol, 31:*31–33, 1968.

75. Haymaker, W., Rubinstein, L.J., and Miquel, J.: Brain tumors in irradiated monkeys. *Acta Neuropathol* (Berl), *20:*267–277, 1972.

76. Jentzer, A.: Premiers résultats d'application expérimentale de cobalt 60 dans le lobe frontal du lapin. *Confin Neurol, 19:*264–269, 1959.

77. Foley, E.J.: Antigenic properties of methylcholanthrene-induced tumors in mice of the strain of origin. *Cancer Res, 13:*835–837, 1953.

78. Prehn, R.T., and Main, J.M.: Immunity to methylcholanthrene-induced sarcomas. *J Natl Cancer Inst, 18:*769–778, 1957.

79. Klein, E., and Klein, G.: Tumour-associated antigens. Potential application in research, tumour therapy and tumour prevention. *Triangle, 11:*15–22, 1972.

80. Burnet, F.M.: Immunological surveillance in neoplasia. *Transplant Rev, 7:*3–25, 1971.

81. Burnet, F.M.: The concept of immunological surveillance. *Prog Exp Tumor Res, 13:*1–27, 1970.

82. Prehn, R.T.: Immunosurveillance, regeneration and oncogenesis. *Prog Exp Tumor Res, 14:*1–24, 1971.

83. Keast, D.: Immunosurveillance and cancer. *Lancet, 2:*710–712, 1970.

84. Prehn, R.T.: The immune reaction as a stimulator of tumor growth. *Science, 176:* 170–171, 1972.

85. Prehn, R.T., and Lappé, M.A.: An immunostimulation theory of tumor development. *Transplant Rev, 7:*26–54, 1971.

86. Prehn, R.T.: Perspectives on oncogenesis: does immunity stimulate or inhibit neoplasia? *J Reticuloendothel Soc, 10:*1–16, 1971.

87. Scheinberg, L.C., Levy, A., and Edelman, F.: Is the brain an "immunologically privileged site"? 2. Studies in induced host resistance to transplantable mouse glioma following irradiation of prior implants. *Arch Neurol, 13:*283–286, 1965.

88. Scheinberg, L.C., Suzuki, K., Davidoff, L.M., and Beilin, R.L.: Immunization against intracerebral transplantation of a glioma in mice. *Nature, 193:*1194–1195, 1962.

89. Scheinberg, L.C., Suzuki, K., Edelman, F., and Davidoff, L.M.: Studies in immunization against a transplantable cerebral mouse glioma. *J Neurosurg, 20:*312–316, 1963.

90. Janisch, W.: Heterotransplantation of human brain tumours with untreated albino rats of different age-groups. *Acta Un Int Contra Cancr, 20:* 1590–1591, 1964.

91. Ridley, A.: Antilymphocytic serum and tumour transplantation in the brain. *Acta Neuropathol* (Berl.), *19:*307–317, 1971.

92. Lim, R., and Kluskens, L.: Immunological specificity of astrocytoma antigens. *Cancer Res, 32:*1667–1670, 1972.

93. Ikuta, F., and Zimmerman, H.M.: The viral particles in the reactive cells of the brain induced by chemical carcinogens. *Int J Neurol, 5:*10–28, 1965.

94. Ikuta, F., and Zimmerman, H.M.: Virus particles in reactive cells induced by intracerebral implantation of dibenzanthracene. *J Neuropathol Exp Neurol, 24:*225–243, 1965.

95. Rubin, R., Ames, R.P., Sutton, C.H., and Zimmerman, H.M.: Virus-like particles in murine ependymoblastoma. *J Neuropathol Exp Neurol, 28:*371–387, 1969.

96. Perese, D.M.: Age and sex factors in experi-

mental brain tumors. *Surg Forum, 15:* 429–431, 1964.

97. Bridges, J.M.: The influence of dietary depletion of thiamine, riboflavin and niacin on the induction of gliomata in mice. *Br J Exp Pathol, 41:*169–175, 1960.

98. Foulds, L.: Multiple etiologic factors in neoplastic development. *Cancer Res, 25:*1339–1347, 1965.

99. Malmgren, R.A., Rabson, A.S., and Carney, P.G.: Immunity and viral carcinogenesis. Effect of thymectomy on polyoma virus carcinogenesis in mice. *J Natl Cancer Inst, 33:*101–104, 1964.

100. Diderholm, H., Estola, T., and Wesslén, T.: Effect of thymectomy on tumour production by polyoma virus in rabbits. *Acta Pathol Microbiol Scand, 66:*396–400, 1966.

101. Sigel, M.M., Scotti, T.M., Schulz, V.B., Dorsey, M., Jr., and Lefkowitz, S.S.: Age effects on the host and tissue response to Rous sarcoma virus (RSV). *Archiv Gesamte Virusforsch, 14:*422–430, 1964.

102. Chang, S., and Hildemann, W.H.: Inheritance of susceptibility to polyoma virus in mice. *J Natl Cancer Inst, 33:*303–313, 1964.

103. Kurland, L.T.: The frequency of intracranial and intraspinal neoplasms in the resident population of Rochester, Minnesota. *J Neurosurg, 15:*627–641, 1958.

104. Drift, J.H.A. van der, and Magnus, O.: Space occupying lesions in older patients. *Psychiatr Neurol Neurochir,64:*192–201, 1961.

105. Miller, R.W.: Fifty-two forms of childhood cancer: United States mortality experience, 1960–1966. *J Pediatr, 75:*685–689, 1969.

106. Kurland, L.T., Myrianthopoulos, N.C., and Lessell, S.: Epidemiologic and genetic considerations of intracranial neoplasms. In Fields, W.S. and Sharkey, P.C., (Eds.): *The Biology and Treatment of Intracranial Tumors.* Springfield, Thomas, 1962, pp. 5–47.

107. Percy, A.K., Elveback, L.R., Okazaki, H., and Kurland, L.T.: Neoplasms of the central nervous system. Epidemiologic considerations. *Neurology* (Minneap.), *22:* 40–48, 1972.

108. Guðmundsson, K.R.: A survey of tumours of the central nervous system in Iceland during the 10-year period 1954–1963. *Acta Neurol Scand, 46:*538–552, 1970.

109. Leibowitz, U., Yablonski, M., and Alter, M.: Epidemiology of tumors of the nervous system in Israel. *Isr J Med Sci, 7:*1491–1499, 1971.

110. Leibowitz, U., Yablonski, M., and Alter, M.: Tumors of the nervous system. Incidence and population selectivity. *J Chronic Dis, 23:*707–721, 1971.

111. Cooney, L.M., Jr., and Solitare, G.B.: Primary intracranial tumors in the elderly. *Geriatrics,* 27, No. 1, pp. 94–104, 1972.

112. Berg, J.W.: Some intercountry and intergroup differences in histological types of cancer. *J Chronic Dis, 23:*325–334, 1970.

113. Huntington, R.W., Jr., Cummings, K.L., Moe, T.I., O'Connell, H.V., and Wybel, R.: Discovery of fatal primary intracranial neoplasms at medicolegal autopsies. *Cancer, 18:*117–127, 1965.

114. Peers, J.H.: The occurrence of tumors of the central nervous system in routine autopsies. *Am J Pathol, 12:*911–932, 1936.

115. Andersson, P.G.: Intracranial tumors in a psychiatric autopsy material. *Acta Psychiatr Scand, 46:*213–224, 1970.

116. Harenko, A.: Aivokasvaimet geriatrisilla potilailla. *Duodecim,86:*765–771, 1970.

117. Wood, M.W., White, R.J., and Kernohan, J.W.: One hundred intracranial meningiomas found incidentally at necropsy. *J Neuropathol Exp Neurol, 16:*337–340, 1957.

118. Regelson, W., Bross, I.D.J., Hananian, J., and Nigogosyan, G.: Incidence of second primary tumors in children with cancer and leukemia. A seven-year survey of 150 consecutive autopsied cases. *Cancer, 18:* 58–72, 1965.

119. Goldberg, I.D., and Kurland, L.T.: Mortality in 33 countries from diseases of the nervous system. *World Neurol, 3:*444–465, 1962.

120. Cohen, A., and Modan, B.: Some epidemiologic aspects of neoplastic diseases in Israeli immigrant population. III. Brain tumors. *Cancer, 22:*1323–1328, 1968.

121. Ringertz, N. (Ed.): Cancer incidence in

Finland, Iceland, Norway and Sweden. A comparative study. *Acta Pathol Microbiol Scand* (A), Suppl. 224, 1971.

122. Brewis, M., Poskanzer, D.C., Rolland, C., and Miller, H.: Neurological disease in an English city. *Acta Neurol Scand,* Suppl. 24, Vol. 42, 1966.

123. Burbank, F.: Patterns in cancer mortality in the United States: 1950–1967. *Natl Cancer Inst,* Monogr. 33, 1971, pp. 406–414.

124. González Feria, L.: Sobre la frecuencia de los tumores cerebrales. *Rev Clin Esp, 94:* 226–228, 1964.

125. Kurtzke, J.F.: Geographic pathology of brain tumors. 1. Distribution of deaths from primary tumors. *Acta Neurol Scand, 45:* 540–555, 1969.

126. Newill, V.A.: Distribution of cancer mortality among ethnic subgroups of the white population of New York City, 1953–58. *J Natl Cancer Inst, 26:*405–417, 1961.

127. Seidman, H.: Cancer death rates by site and sex for religious and socioeconomic groups in New York City. *Environ Res, 3:*234–250, 1970.

128. Newbill, H.P., and Anderson, G.C.: Racial and sexual incidence of primary intracranial tumors. Statistical study of one hundred and thirty-three cases verified by autopsy. *Arch Neurol Psychiatry, 51:*564–567, 1944.

129. Oettlé, A.G.: Cancer in Africa, especially in regions south of the Sahara. *J Natl Cancer Inst, 33:*383–439, 1964.

130. Froman, C., and Lipschitz, R.: Demography of tumors of the central nervous system among the Bantu (African) population of the Transvaal, South Africa. *J Neurosurg, 32:*660–664, 1970.

131. Ruberti, R.F., and Poppi, M.: Tumours of the central nervous system in the African. *East Afr Med J, 48:*576–584, 1971.

132. Collomb, II., Girard, P.-L., Dumas, M., Lemercier, G., and Courson, B.: Gliomes de l'encéphale chez le noir Africain. *Bull Soc Med Afr Noire Lang Fr, 15:*221–230, 1970.

133. Shuangshoti, S., Tangchai, P., and Netsky, M.G.: Neoplasms of the nervous system in Thailand. *Cancer, 23:*493–496, 1969.

134. Dastur, D.K., and Lalitha, V.S.: Pathological analysis of intracranial space-occupying lesions in 1000 cases including children. Part 2. Incidence, types and unusual cases of glioma. *J Neurol Sci, 8:*143–170, 1968.

135. Araki, C., and Matsumoto, S.: Statistical reevaluation of pinealoma and related tumors in Japan. *J Neurosurg, 30:*146–149, 1969.

136. Smith, R.L.: Recorded and expected mortality among the Japanese of the United States and Hawaii, with special reference to cancer. *J Natl Cancer Inst, 17:*459–473, 1956.

137. Choi, N.W., Schuman, L.M., and Gullen, W.H.: Epidemiology of primary central nervous system neoplasms. I. Mortality from primary central nervous system neoplasms in Minnesota. *Am J Epidemiol, 91:* 238–259, 1970.

138. Innis, M.D.: Possible genetic basis of childhood neoplasia. *Med J Aust, 2:*1187–1189, 1970.

139. Barsky, P.: Congenital astrocytoma: definitive diagnosis at 30 days of age, with survival. *Can Med Assoc J, 98:*216–217, 1968.

140. Sandbank, U.: Congenital astrocytoma. *J Pathol Bacteriol, 84:*226–228, 1962.

141. Cooperman, E., Marshall, K.G., and Daria Haust, M.: Congenital astrocytoma. *Can Med Assoc J, 97:*1405–1407, 1967.

142. Masson, A., Heldt, N., Cronmuller, G., and Schneegans, E.: Astrocytome congénital du tronc cérébral. *Ann Pediatr* (Paris), *18:*789–795, 1971.

143. Lin, S., Lee, K.F., and O'Hara, A.E.: Congenital astrocytomas: the roentgenographic manifestations. *Am J Roentgenol Radium Ther Nucl Med, 115:*78–85, 1972.

144. DeSaussure, R.L., Miller, J.H., and Strickland, C.E.: Brain tumors in the newborn. *South Med J, 53:*918–921, 1960.

145. Chandor, S.B., and Osteraas, G.R.: Congenital glioma in a stillborn infant. *Milit Med, 134:*257–260, 1969.

146. Luse, S.A., and Teitelbaum, S.: Congenital glioma of brain stem. *Arch Neurol, 18:* 196–201, 1968.

147. Abbott, M., and Namiki, H.: Congenital

ependymoma. Case report. *J Neurosurg,* 28:162–165, 1968.

148. Fuste, F.G., Snyder, D.E., and Price, A.: Congenital spongioblastoma of the pons. *Am J Clin Pathol, 47*:790–796, 1967.

149. Greenhouse, A.H., and Neubuerger, K.T.: Intracranial teratomata of the newborn. *Arch Neurol, 3*:718–724, 1960.

150. Duckett, S., and Wilson, R.R.: Fetal spongioblastoma. *J Neuropathol Exp Neurol, 23*: 560–564, 1964.

151. Fine, R.D.: Medulloblastoma with onset in the newborn. *Aust NZ J Surg, 32*:167–169, 1962.

152. Svoboda, D.J.: Oligodendroglioma in a six-week old infant. *J Neuropathol Exp Neurol, 18*:569–574, 1959.

153. Krohn, K., and Hjelt, L.: A case of congenital ependymoma with malformations. The possibility of a common causative agent. *Ann Paediatr Fenn, 12*:73–75, 1966.

154. Mendiratta, S.S., Rosenblum, J.A., and Strobos, R.J.: Congenital meningioma. *Neurology* (Minneap), *17*:914–918, 1967.

155. Nagahara, S., Shirasawa, K., and Furuta, N.: Congenital brain tumor: report of an autopsy case of ependymoblastoma in six-months old infant. *Brain Nerve* (Tokyo), *13*:115–121, 1961. (Jap)

156. Wells, H.G.: Occurrence and significance of congenital malignant neoplasms. *Arch Pathol, 30*:535–601, 1940.

157. Raskind, R., and Beigel, F.: Brain tumors in early infancy—probably congenital in origin. *J Pediatr, 65*:727–732, 1964.

158. Solitare, G.B., and Krigman, M.R.: Congenital intracranial neoplasm. A case report and review of the literature. *J Neuropathol Exp Neurol, 23*:280–292, 1964.

159. Lombardi, G., and Passerini, A.: Congenital tumours of the spinal cord. *Acta Radiol* (Diagn) (Stockh), *5*:1047–1050, 1966.

160. Evans, A.R.: Congenital neuroblastoma. *J Clin Pathol, 18*:54–62 ,1965.

161. Schneider, K.M., Becker, J.M., and Krasna, I.H.: Neonatal neuroblastoma. *Pediatrics, 36*:359–366, 1965.

162. Becker, J.M., Schneider, K.M., and Krasna, I.H.: Neonatal neuroblastoma. *Progr. Clin Cancer, 4*:382–386, 1970.

163. Haber, S.L., and Bennington, J.L.: Maturation of congenital extra-adrenal neuroblastoma. *Arch Pathol, 76*:121–125, 1963.

164. Mackenzie, D.C., Ham, J.M., and Hyslop, R.S.: Congenital neuroblastoma. *Aust NZ J Surg, 34*:173–177, 1965.

165. Shuangshoti, S., and Ekaraphanich, S.: Congenital neuroblastoma and hyperplasia of islets of Langerhans in an infant. *Clin Pediatr* (Phila.), *11*:241–243, 1972.

166. Vinik, M., and Altman, D.H.: Congenital malignant tumors. *Cancer, 19*:967–979, 1966.

167. Bolande, R.P.: Benignity of neonatal tumors and concept of cancer repression in early life. *Am J Dis Child, 122*:12–14, 1971.

168. Birner, W.F.: Neuroblastoma as a cause of antenatal death. *Am J Obstet Gynecol, 82*: 1388–1391, 1961.

169. Beckwith, J.B., and Perrin, E.V.: In situ neuroblastomas: a contribution to the natural history of neural crest tumors. *Am J Pathol, 43*:1089–1104, 1963.

170. Guin, G.H., Gilbert, E.F., and Jones, B.: Incidental neuroblastoma in infants. *Am J Clin Pathol, 51*:126–136, 1969.

171. Moertel, C.G., Dockerty, M.B., and Baggenstoss, A.H.: Multiple primary malignant neoplasms. I. Introduction and presentation of data. *Cancer, 14*:221–230, 1961.

172. Moore, R., Tsukada, Y., Regelson, W., Pickren, J.W., and Bross, I.D.J.: Synchronous tumors in patients with multiple primary cancers. *Cancer, 18*:1423–1430, 1965.

173. Warren, S., and Gates, O.: Multiple primary malignant tumors. A survey of the literature and a statistical study. *Am J Cancer, 16*:1358–1414, 1932.

174. Spratt, J.S., Jr., and Hoag, M.G.: Incidence of multiple primary cancers per man-year of follow up. 20-year review from the Ellis Fischel State Cancer Hospital. *Ann Surg, 164*:775–784, 1966.

175. Kuehn, P.G., Beckett, R., and Reed, J.F.: Tissue specificity in multiple primary malignancies. A study of 460 cases. *Am J Surg, 111*:164–167, 1966.

176. Sahar, A., and Streifler, M.: Multiple intracranial tumors of diverse origin. Report

of a case with review of literature. *Neurochirurgia* (Stuttg), *9*:18–27, 1966.

177. Myerson, P.G.: Multiple tumors of the brain of diverse origin. *J Neuropathol Exp Neurol, 1*:406–415, 1942.

178. Solomon, A., Perret, G.E., and McCormick, W.F.: Multicentric gliomas of the cerebral and cerebellar hemispheres. Case report. *J Neurosurg, 31*:87–93, 1969.

179. O'Connell, J.E.A.: Intracranial meningiomata associated with other tumours involving the central nervous system. *Br J Surg, 48*:373–383, 1961.

180. Arai, H., Chichibu, M., Ikuta, F., and Oyake, Y.: Triple diverse multiple primary tumors in the nervous system: report of an autopsy case with special reference to their origins. *Brain Nerve* (Tokyo), *21*:1241–1249, 1969. (Jap)

181. Batzdorf, U., and Malamud, N.: The problem of multicentric gliomas. *J Neurosurg, 20:* 122–136, 1963.

182. Waga, S., Matsuda, M., Handa, H., Matsushima, M., and Ando, K.: Multiple meningiomas. Report of four cases. *J Neurosurg, 37*:348–351, 1972.

183. Daum, S., and Le Beau, J.: Un cas de méningiomatose. Discussion des rapports avec la neurofibromatose de Recklinghausen. *Rev Neurol* (Paris), *105*:349–353, 1961.

184. Wahl, R.W., and Dillard, S.H., Jr.: Multiple ganglioneuromas of the central nervous system. *Arch Pathol, 94*:158–164, 1972.

185. Madonick, M.J., Shapiro, J.H., and Torack, R.M.: Multiple diverse primary brain tumors. Report of a case with review of literature. *Neurology* (Minneap), *11*:430–435, 1961.

186. Bastian, F.O., and Parker, J.C., Jr.: A rare combination of multicentric gliomas: a problem of interpretation. *Am J Clin Pathol, 54*:839–844, 1970.

187. Elam, E.B., and McLaurin, R.L.: Multiple primary intracranial tumors. Case report. *J Neurosurg, 18*:388–392, 1961.

188. Whitcomb, B.B., and Tennant, R.: Brain tumors of diverse germinal origin arising in juxtaposition. Report of three cases. *J Neurosurg, 25*:194–198, 1966.

189. Fisher, R.G.: Intracranial meningioma followed by a malignant glioma. Case report. *J Neurosurg, 29*:83–86, 1968.

190. Batchelor, T.M., and Maun, M.E.: Congenital glycogenic tumors of the heart. *Arch Pathol, 39*:67–73, 1945.

191. Sorenson, B.F.: Multiple primary tumors of the brain and bowel. Case report. *J Neurosurg, 36*:93–96, 1972.

192. Dodge, H.W., Jr., Keith, H.M., and Campagna, M.J.: Intraspinal tumors in infants and children. *J Internat Coll Surgeons, 26*:199–215, 1956.

193. Lehar, T.J., and Heard, J.L.: Agammaglobulinemia and thymoma associated with nonthymic cancer. *Cancer, 25*:875–879, 1970.

194. Nicola, G.C., and Nizzoli, V.: Multiple intracranial tumours of diverse origin in the same patient. Report of a case. *J Neurol Sci, 4*:595–599, 1967.

195. McPhedran, R.S., and Tom, M.I.: Multiple primary intracranial tumors. A case report. *Neurology* (Minneap), *12*:524–528, 1962.

196. Greenhouse, A.: Pheochromocytoma and meningioma of the foramen magnum. *Ann Intern Med, 55*:124–127, 1961.

197. Wiesinger, H., Phipps, G.W., and Guerry, D., III.: Bilateral melanoma of the choroid associated with leukemia and meningioma. *Arch Ophthalmol, 62*:889–893, 1959.

198. Paches, A.I., and Khamitov, S.H.: On the combination of histogenetically different malignant tumours of the brain and parotid gland. *Vopr Onkol, 7*(5):85–88, 1961. (Rus)

199. Joslin, E.P., Lombard, H.L., Burrows, R.E., and Manning, M.D.: Diabetes and cancer. *N Engl J Med, 260*:486–488, 1959.

200. Kessler, I.I.: A genetic relationship between diabetes and cancer. *Lancet, 1*:218–220, 1970.

201. Kessler, I.I.: Cancer and diabetes mellitus. A review of the literature. *J Chronic Dis, 23*:579–600, 1971.

202. Kessler, I.I.: Cancer mortality among diabetics. *J Natl Cancer Inst, 44*:673–686, 1970.

203. Aronson, S.M., and Aronson, B.E.: Central nervous system in diabetes mellitus. Low-

ered frequency of certain intracranial neoplasms. *Arch Neurol, 12:*390–398, 1965.

204. Buckwalter, J.A., Turner, J.H., Gamber, H.H., Raterman, L., Soper, R.T., and Knowler, L.A.: Psychoses, intracranial neoplasms, and genetics. *Arch Neurol Psychiatry, 81:*480–485, 1959.

205. Selverstone, B., and Cooper, D.R.: Astrocytomas and ABO blood groups. *J Neurosurg, 18:*602–604, 1961.

206. Iraci, G., and Toffolo, G.G.: Frequenza dei gruppi ABO nei meningiomi. *Tumori, 50:* 473–475, 1964.

207. Pearce, K.M., and Yates, P.O.: Blood groups and brain tumours. *J Neurol Sci, 2:*434–441, 1965.

208. Strang, R.R., Tovi, D., and Lopez, J.: Astrocytomas and the ABO blood groups. *J Med Genet, 3:*274–275, 1966.

209. Yates, P.O.: Malignant glioma and ABO blood group. *Br Med J, 1:*310, 1964.

210. Carter, R.L., Hitchcock, E.R., and Sato, F.: Malignant glioma and ABO blood group. *Br Med J, 1:*122, 1964.

211. Garcia, J.H., Okazaki, H., and Aronson, S.M.: Blood-group frequencies and astrocytomata. *J Neurosurg, 20:*397–399, 1963.

212. Choi, N.W., Schuman, L.M., and Gullen, W.H.: Epidemiology of primary central nervous system neoplasms. II: Case-control study. *Am J Epidemiol, 91:*467–485, 1970.

213. McKhann, C.F.: Primary malignancy in patients undergoing immunosuppression for renal transplantation. A request for information. *Transplantation, 8:*209–212, 1969.

214. Sharma, B.K., Poticha, S.M., and Oyasu, R.: Reticulum cell sarcoma involving the cerebellum in a renal transplant recipient. *Transplantation, 13:*52–53, 1972.

215. Penn, I.: Malignant tumors in organ transplant recipients. In *Recent Results in Cancer Research,* 35. New York, Springer-Verlag, 1970.

216. Pierce, J.C., Madge, G.E., Lee, H.M., and Hume, D.M.: Lymphoma, a complication of renal allotransplantation in man. *JAMA, 219:*1593–1597, 1972.

217. Starzl, T.E., Penn, I., Putnam, C.W., Groth, C.G., and Halgrimson, C.G.: Iatrogenic alterations of immunologic surveillance in man and their influence on malignancy. *Transplant Rev, 7:*112–145, 1971.

218. Schneck, S.A., and Penn, I.: De-novo brain tumours in renal-transplant recipients. *Lancet, 1:*983–986, 1971.

219. Hirsch, M.S., Ellis, D.A., Black, P.H., Monaco, A.P., and Wood, M.L.: Leukemia virus activation during homograft rejection. *Science, 180:*500–502, 1973.

220. Allison, A.C.: Potentiation of viral carcinogenesis by immunosuppression. *Br Med J, 4:*419–420, 1970.

221. Penn, I., Halgrimson, C.G., and Starzl, T.E.: De novo malignant tumors in organ transplant recipients. *Transplantation Proc, 3:* 773–778, 1971.

222. Spencer, E.S.: Immunosuppression and cancer. *Lancet, 1:*777–778, 1969.

223. Cornelius, E.A.: Induction of tumors in neonatally thymectomized mice. *Transplantation, 12:*531–532, 1971.

224. Vessey, M.P., and Doll, R.: Thymectomy and cancer—a follow-up study. *Br J Cancer, 26:*53–58, 1972.

225. Futrell, J.W., Albright, N.L., and Myers, G.H., Jr.: Prevention of tumor growth in an "immunologically privileged site" by adoptive transfer of tumor-specific transplantation immunity. *J Surg Res, 12:*62–69, 1972.

226. Futrell, J.W.: Transplantation tumors and immunologically privileged sites. *JAMA, 220:*1130, 1972.

227. Yoffey, J.M., and Courtice, F.C.: *Lymphatics, Lymph and the Lymphomyeloid Complex.* New York, Acad Pr, 1970, p. 15.

228. Lipsmeyer, E.A.: Development of malignant cerebral lymphoma in a patient with systemic lupus erythematosus treated with immunosuppression. *Arthritis Rheum, 15:* 183–186, 1972.

229. Kinlen, L.J.: Malignancy and immunosuppression (abstract). *Proc R Soc Med, 65:* 242, 1972.

230. Smith, D.R., Hardman, J.M., and Earle, K.M.: Metastasizing neuroectodermal tumors of the central nervous system. *J Neurosurg, 31:*50–58, 1969.

231. Rubinstein, L.J.: Development of extracranial metastases from a malignant astrocytoma in the absence of previous craniotomy. *J Neurosurg, 26:*542–547, 1967.

232. Earle, K.M.: Metastatic and primary intracranial tumors of the adult male. *J Neuropathol Exp Neurol, 13:*448–454, 1954.

233. Wickremesinghe, H.R., and Yates, P.O.: Immunological properties of neoplastic neural tissues. *Br J Cancer, 25:*711–720, 1971.

234. Catalano, L.W., Jr., Harter, D.H., and Hsu, K.C.: Common antigen in meningioma-derived cell cultures. *Science, 175:*180–182, 1972.

235. Trouillas, P.: Immunologie des tumeurs cérébrales: l'antigéne carcino-foetal glial. *Ann Inst Pasteur, 122:*819–828, 1972.

236. Trouillas, P.: Carcino-fetal antigen in glial tumours. *Lancet, 2:*552, 1971.

237. O'Conor, G.T., Tatarinov, Y.S., Abelev, G.I., and Uriel, J.: A collaborative study for the evaluation of a serologic test for primary liver cancer. *Cancer, 25:*1091–1098, 1970.

238. Gold, P.: The model of colonic cancer in the study of human tumor-specific antigens. In Burdette, W.J., (Ed.): *Carcinoma of the Colon and Antecedent Epithelium.* Springfield, Thomas, 1970, pp. 131–142.

239. Zamcheck, N., Moore, T.L., Dhar, P., and Kupchik, H.: Immunologic diagnosis and prognosis of human digestive-tract cancer: carcinoembryonic antigens. *N Engl J Med, 286:*83–86, 1972.

240. Herschman, H.R.: S-100 protein accumulation in developing animals and cell cultures. *UCLA Forum Med Sci, 14:*491–498, 1971.

241. Pfeiffer, S.E., Kornblith, P.L., Cares, H.L., Seals, J., and Levine, L.: S-100 protein in human acoustic neurinomas. *Brain Res, 41:*187–193, 1972.

242. Haglid, K.G., and Carlsson, C.A.: An immunological study of some human brain tumours concerning the brain specific protein S_{100}. *Neurochirurgia* (Stuttg), *14:*24–27, 1971.

243. Wechsler, W., Pfeiffer, S.E., Swenberg, J.A., and Koestner, A.: S 100 protein in experimental rat tumors of the central and peripheral nervous system. *Naturwissenschaften, 59:*370–371, 1972.

244. Benda, P., Someda, K., Messer, J., and Sweet, W.H.: Morphological and immunochemical studies of rat glial tumors and clonal strains propagated in culture. *J Neurosurg, 34:*310–323, 1971.

245. Uozumi, T., and Ryan, R.J.: Isolation, amino acid composition, and radioimmunoassay of human brain S 100 protein. *Mayo Clin Proc, 48:*50–56, 1973.

246. Mahaley, M.S., Jr.: Immunologic aspects of the growth and development of human and experimental brain tumors. In Kirsch, W.M., Grossi-Paoletti, E., and Paoletti, P. (Eds.): *The Experimental Biology of Brain Tumors.* Springfield, Thomas, 1972, pp. 561–573.

247. Mahaley, M.S., Jr.: Immunological studies with human gliomas. *J Neurosurg, 34:*458–459, 1971.

248. Wilkins, R.H.: Effects on cell growth by a serum fraction from patients with central nervous system neoplasms. *J Neuropathol Exp Neurol, 22:*677–694, 1963.

249. Mitts, M.G., and Walker, A.E.: Autoimmune response to malignant glial tumors. Preliminary observations. *Neurology* (Minneap), *15:*474–476, 1965.

250. Ridley, A., and Cavanagh, J.B.: Lymphocytic infiltration in gliomas: evidence of possible host resistance. *Brain, 94:*117–124, 1971.

251. Lauder, I., and Aherne, W.: The significance of lymphocytic infiltration in neuroblastoma. *Br J Cancer, 26:*321–330, 1972.

252. Everson, T.C.: Spontaneous regression of cancer. *Ann NY Acad Sci, 114:*721–735, 1964.

253. Gross, R.E., Farber, S., and Martin, L.W.: Neuroblastoma sympatheticum. A study and report of 217 cases. *Pediatrics, 23:*1179–1191, 1959.

254. Dalforno, S., and Ramella Gigliardi, M.: Maturazione di metastasi di neuroblastoma con trasformazione in ganglioneuroma. *Cancro, 21:*669–675, 1960.

255. D'Angio, G.J., Evans, A.E., and Koop, C.E.: Special pattern of widespread neuroblas-

toma with a favourable prognosis. *Lancet,* 1:1046–1049, 1971.

256. Harrington, W.J.: Curable forms of disseminated cancer. *Adv Intern Med, 15:* 317–337, 1969.

257. Eyre-Brook, A.L., and Hewer, T.F.: Spontaneous disappearance of neuroblastoma with maturation to ganglioneuroma. *J Bone Joint Surg* (Br), *44B:*886–890, 1962.

258. Karsgaard, A.T.: Spontaneous regression of retinoblastoma. A report of two cases. *Can J Ophthalmol, 6:*218–222, 1971.

259. Hunter, W.S.: Unexpected regressed retinoblastoma. *Can J Ophthalmol, 3:*376–380, 1968.

260. Swami Mehra, K., and Banerji, C.: Spontaneous regression of retinoblastoma. *Br J Ophthalmol, 49:*381–382, 1965.

261. Boniuk, M., and Girard, L.J.: Spontaneous regression of bilateral retinoblastoma. *Trans Am Acad Ophthalmol Otolaryngol, 73:*194–198, 1969.

262. Margolis, J., and West, D.: Spontaneous regression of malignant disease: report of three cases. *J Am Geriatr Soc, 15:*251–253, 1967.

263. Kidd, J.G.: Does the host react against his own cancer cells? *Cancer Res, 21:*1170–1183, 1961.

264. Hellström, I.E., Hellström, K.E., Pierce, G.E., and Bill, A.H.: Demonstration of cell-bound and humoral immunity against neuroblastoma cells. *Proc Natl Acad Sci USA, 60:*1231–1238, 1968.

265. Hellström, I., and Hellström, K.E.: Some aspects of the immune defense against cancer. II. *In vitro* studies on human tumors. *Cancer, 28:*1269–1271, 1971.

266. Hellström, I.E., Hellström, K.E., and Pierce, G.E.: Cell-bound immune reactions against tumor specific transplantation antigens. *Can Cancer Conf, 8:*425–442, 1969.

267. Hellström, I., Hellström, K.E., Bill, A.H., Pierce, G.E., and Yang, J.P.S.: Studies on cellular immunity to human neuroblastoma cells. *Int J Cancer, 6:*172–188, 1970.

268. Hellström, K.E., and Hellström, I.: Some aspects of the cellular and humoral immune response to tumour antigens. *Triangle, 11:*23–28, 1972.

269. Levy, N.L., Mahaley, M.S., Jr., and Day, E.D.: *In vitro* demonstration of cell-mediated immunity to human brain tumors. *Cancer Res, 32:*477–482, 1972.

270. Feiring, E.H., and Foer, W.H.: Meningioma following radium therapy. Case report. *J Neurosurg, 29.*192–194, 1968.

271. Munk, J., Peyser, E., and Gruszkiewicz, J.: Radiation induced intracranial meningiomas. *Clin Radiol, 20:*90–94, 1969.

272. Beller, A.J., Feinsod, M., and Sahar, A.: The possible relationship between small dose irradiation to the scalp and intracranial meningiomas. *Neurochirurgia* (Stuttg), *15:* 135–143, 1972.

273. Kyle, R.H., Oler, A., Lasser, E.C., and Rosomoff, H.L.: Meningioma induced by thorium dioxide. *N Engl J Med, 268:*80–82, 1963.

274. Noetzli, M., and Malamud, N.: Postirradiation fibrosarcoma of the brain. *Cancer, 15:* 617–622, 1962.

275. Donohue, W.L., Jaffe, F.A., and Rewcastle, N.B.: Radiation-induced neurofibromata. *Cancer, 20:*589–595, 1967.

276. Goldberg, M.B., Sheline, G.E., and Malamud, N.: Malignant intracranial neoplasms following radiation therapy for acromegaly. *Radiology, 80:*465–470, 1963.

277. Mann, I., Yates, P.C., and Ainslie, J.P.: Unusual case of double primary orbital tumour. *Br J Ophthalmol, 37:*758–762, 1953.

278. Waltz, T.A., and Brownell, B.: Sarcoma: a possible late result of effective radiation therapy for pituitary adenoma. *J Neurosurg, 24:*901–907, 1966.

279. MacMahon, B.: Prenatal X-ray exposure and childhood cancer. *J Natl Cancer Inst, 28:* 1173–1191, 1962.

280. MacMahon, B., and Hutchison, G.B.: Prenatal X-ray and childhood cancer: a review. *Acta Un Int Contra Cancr, 20:*1172–1174, 1964.

281. Stewart, A., and Kneale, G.W.: Changes in the cancer risk associated with obstetric radiography. *Lancet, 1:*104–107, 1968.

282. Pifer, J.W., Hempelmann, L.H., Dodge, H.J., and Hodges, F.J., II.: Neoplasms in the Ann Arbor series of thymus-irradiated

children; a second survey. *Am J Roentgenol Radium Ther Nucl Med, 103:*13–18, 1968.

283. Walker, D.L., Padgett, B.L., ZuRhein, G.M., Albert, A.E., and Marsh, R.F.: Human papovavirus (JC): induction of brain tumors in hamsters. *Science, 181:*674–676, 1973.

284. Bastian, F.O.: Papova-like virus particles in a human brain tumor. *Lab Invest, 25:*169–175, 1971.

285. Trouillas, P.: Antigène d'un virus oncogène à A.R.N. dans les gliomes humains. Sa relation avec les antigènes carcino-embryonnaires. *Nouv Presse Méd, 1:*1979–1982, 1972.

286. Walshe, F.: Head injuries as a factor in the aetiology of intracranial meningioma. *Lancet, 2:*993–996, 1961.

287. Cushing, H., and Eisenhardt, L.: *Meningiomas.* Springfield, Thomas, 1938. Reprinted 1969, pp. 71–73.

288. Walsh, J., Gye, R., and Connelley, T.J.: Meningioma: a late complication of head injury. *Med J Aust, 1:*906–908, 1969.

289. Piazza, G.: Meningioma endocranico da corpo estraneo. *Riv Otoneurooftalmol, 42:* 411–421, 1967.

290. Lanigan, J.P.: Can a head injury cause a meningioma? *J Ir Med Assoc, 56:*12–13, 1965.

291. Schmidt, H., and Jaquet, G.-H.: Meningeomentstehung um Fremdkörper. *Zentralbl Neurochir, 24:*65–73, 1963.

292. Turner, O.A., and Laird, A.T.: Meningioma with traumatic etiology. Report of a case. *J Neurosurg, 24:*96–98, 1966.

293. Zülch, K.J.: *Brain Tumors. Their Biology and Pathology,* 2nd Am Ed. New York, Springer, 1965, pp. 51–58.

294. Levin, V.A., Shapiro, W.R., Clancy, T.P., and Oliverio, V.T.: The uptake, distribution, and antitumor activity of 1-(2-chloroethyl)-3-cyclohexyl-1-nitrosourea in the murine glioma. *Cancer Res, 30:*2451–2455, 1970.

295. Hansen, H.H., and Muggia, F.M.: Treatment of malignant brain tumors with nitrosoureas. *Cancer Chemother Rep, 55:*99–100, part 1, 1971.

296. Shapiro, W.R., Ausman, J.I., and Rall, D.P.: Studies on the chemotherapy of experimental brain tumors: evaluation of 1,3-bis (2-chloroethyl)-1-nitrosourea, cyclophosphamide, mithramycin, and methotrexate. *Cancer Res, 30:*2401–2413, 1970.

297. Broder, L.E., and Rall, D.P.: Chemotherapy of brain tumors. *Prog Exp Tumor Res, 17:* 373–399, 1972.

298. Mancuso, T.F.: Tumors of the central nervous system. Industrial considerations. *Acta Un Int Contra Cancr, 19:*488–489, 1963.

299. Brooks, W.H.: Geographic clustering of brain tumors in Kentucky. *Cancer, 30:*923–926, 1972.

300. Schuman, L.M., Choi, N.W., and Gullen, W.H.: Relationship of central nervous system neoplasms to Toxoplasma gondii infection. *Am J Public Health, 57:*848–856, 1967.

301. Jänisch, W., and Werner, G.: Polares Spongioblastom und Toxoplasmose bei einem Totgeborenen. *Dtsch Z Nervenheilkd, 185:* 403–410, 1963.

302. Rieger, H.: Die Toxoplasmose als vermutlich mutagener Faktor. *Albrecht von Graefes Arch Klin Ophthalmol, 170:*223–234, 1966.

303. Polstorff, F.: Lues connata und mediobasales Gangliogliom bei einem neunjährigen Jungen. *Zentralbl Allg Pathol, 101:*380–386, 1960.

304. McKusick, V.A.: *Mendelian Inheritance in Man.* 3rd Ed. Baltimore, Johns Hopkins Press, 1971.

305. Papatestas, A.E., Osserman, K.E., and Kark, A.E.: The relationship between thymus and oncogenesis. A study of the incidence of non-thymic malignancy in myasthenia gravis. *Br J Cancer, 25:*635–645, 1971.

306. Field, E.J.: Role of viral infection and autoimmunity in aetiology and pathogenesis of multiple sclerosis. *Lancet, 1:*295–297, 1973.

307. Barbosa, L.H., and Hamilton, R.: Virological studies with multiple-sclerosis brain tissues. *Lancet, 1:*1415–1417, 1973.

308. Weiner, L.P., Johnson, R.T., and Herndon, R.M.: Viral infections and demyelinating

diseases. *N Engl J Med, 288*:1103–1110, 1973.

309. Mathews, T., and Moossy, J.: Mixed glioma, multiple sclerosis, and Charcot-Marie-Tooth disease. *Arch Neurol, 27*:263–268, 1972.

310. Boyazis, R.M., Martin, L., Bouteille, M., Guazzi, G.C., and Manacorda, A.: Images histochimiques et ultrastructurales dans un cas de sclérose en plaques associée à un spongioblastome. *Riv Patol Nerv Ment, 88*:1–20, 1967.

311. Barnard, R.O., and Jellinek, E.H.: Multiple sclerosis with amyotrophy complicated by oligodendroglioma. History of recurrent herpes zoster. *J Neurol Sci, 5*:441–455, 1967.

312. Brihaye, J., Périer, O., and Sténuit, J.: Multiple sclerosis associated with a cerebral glioma. *J Neuropathol Exp Neurol, 22*:128–137, 1963.

313. Raaf, J., and Kernohan, J.W.: Relation of abnormal collections of cells in posterior medullary velum of cerebellum to origin of medulloblastoma. *Arch Neurol Psychiatry, 52*:163–169, 1944.

314. Miller, R.W.: Relation between cancer and congenital defects in man. *N Engl J Med, 275*:87–93, 1966.

315. Miller, R.W.: Relation between cancer and congenital defects: an epidemiologic evaluation. *J Natl Cancer Inst, 40*:1079–1085, 1968.

316. Kobayashi, N., Furukawa, T., and Takatsu, T.: Congenital anomalies in children with malignancy. *Paediatria Univ Tokyo, 16*:31–37, 1968.

317. Miller, R.W.: Relation between cancer and congenital malformations. The value of small series, with a note on pineal tumors in native and migrant Japanese. *Isr J Med Sci, 7*:1461–1464, 1971.

318. Fraumeni, J.F., Jr.: Constitutional disorders of man predisposing to leukemia and lymphoma. *Natl Cancer Inst Monogr, 32*:221–232, 1969.

319. Duckett, S., Claireaux, A.E., and Pearse, A.G.E.: Histoenzymatic study of fetal medulloblastoma with associated congenital malformations. *Neurology* (Minneap), *16*:283–287, 1966.

320. Molz, G., and Biswas, R.K.: Konnataler Hirntumor: Ependymom der Großhirnmarklager bei einem Frühgeborenen. *Zentralbl Allg Pathol, 115*:439–444, 1972.

321. Reisman, M., Goldenberg, E.D., and Gordon, J.: Congenital heart disease and neuroblastoma. Case report and brief comment. *Am J Dis Child, 111*:308–310, 1966.

322. Sy, W.M., and Edmonson, J.H.: The developmental defects associated with neuroblastoma–etiologic implications. *Cancer, 22*:234–238, 1968.

323. Mitgang, R.N.: Teratoma occurring within a myelomeningocele. *J Neurosurg, 37*:448–451, 1972.

324. Love, J.G.: Delayed malignant development of a congenital teratoma with spina bifida. Case report. *J Neurosurg, 29*:532–534, 1968.

325. Gitlin, G., and Behar, A.J.: Meningeal angiomatosis, arhinencephaly, agenesis of the corpus callosum and large hamartoma of the brain, with neoplasia, in an infant having bilateral nasal proboscis. *Acta Anat* (Basel), *41*:56–79, 1960.

326. Heffner, R.R., Jr., Porro, R.S., and Deck, M.D.F.: Benign astrocytoma associated with arteriovenous malformation. *J Neurosurg, 35*:229–233, 1971.

327. Hubbell, D.V., Vogel, P.J., and Abbott, K.H.: Multiple brain tumors: glioblastoma multiforme associated with an arteriovenous angiomatous malformation. *Bull Los Angeles Neurol Soc, 26*:212–216, 1961.

328. Krieger, A.J.: A vascular malformation of the spinal cord in association with a cauda equina ependymoma. *Vasc Surg, 6*:167–172, 1972.

329. Warren, G.C.: Intracranial arteriovenous malformation, pulmonary arteriovenous fistula, and malignant glioma in the same patient. *J Neurosurg, 30*:618–621, 1969.

330. Taktikos, A.: Association of retinoblastoma with mental defect and other pathological manifestations. *Br J Ophthalmol, 48*:495–498, 1964.

331. Vidal, O.R., Damel, A., and Cordero Funes, J.: Dermatoglyphics in retinoblastoma. *J Génét Hum, 17*:99–106, 1969.

332. Miller, R.W., Fraumeni, J.F., Jr., and Hill,

J.A.: Neuroblastoma: epidemiologic approach to its origin. *Am J Dis Child, 115:* 253–261, 1968.

333. Lennox, B.: Sex chromatin in tumours. In Overzier, C., (Ed.): *Intersexuality.* New York, Acad Pr, 1963, pp. 462–473.

334. Frezza, M., Perona, G., Vettore, L., and De Sandre, G.: Cerebropatia familiare con presenza di un piccolo extracromosoma metacentrico. *Folia Hered Pathol* (Milano), *15:*107–114, 1966.

335. Emery, J.L., and Lendon, R.G.: Lipomas of the cauda equina and other fatty tumours related to neurospinal dysraphism. *Dev Med Child Neurol* (Suppl.), *20:*62–70, 1969.

336. Fraumeni, J.F., Jr., and Miller, R.W.: Adrenocortical neoplasms with hemihypertrophy, brain tumors, and other disorders. *J Pediatr, 70:*129–138, 1967.

337. Koch, G.: Genetic aspects of the phakomatoses. In Vinken, P.J., and Bruyn, G.W., (Eds.): *Handbook of Clinical Neurology,* Amsterdam, North-Holland Publishing Co., 1972, Vol. 14, pp. 488–561.

338. Van der Hoeve, J.: Les phakomatoses de Bourneville, de Recklinghausen et de von Hippel-Lindau. *J Belge Neurol Psychiatr, 33:*752–762, 1933.

339. Yakovlev, P.I., and Guthrie, R.H.: Congenital ectodermoses (neurocutaneous syndromes) in epileptic patients. *Arch Neurol Psychiatry, 26:*1145–1194, 1931.

340. Van Bogaert, L.: Neuropathologie générale des phacomatoses et de quelques dystrophies neuro-cutanées moins bien connues, chez l'enfant. *Bibl Paediatr, 76:*349–386, 1961.

341. Musger, A.: Was sind Phakomatosen? Versuch einer Zusammenstellung und Einteilung jener Entwicklungsanomalien, die heute als Phakomatosen bezeichnet werden können. *Hautarzt, 15:*151–156, 1964.

342. Herbst, B.A., and Cohen, M.E.: Linea nevus sebaceus. A neurocutaneous syndrome associated with infantile spasms. *Arch Neurol, 24:*317–322, 1971.

343. Chao, D.H.: Congenital neurocutaneous syndromes in childhood. I. Neurofibromatosis. *J Pediatr, 55:*189–199, 1959.

344. Chapman, R.C., Kemp, V.E., and Taliaferro,

I.: Pheochromocytoma associated with multiple neurofibromatosis and intracranial hemangioma. *Am J Med, 26:*883–890, 1959.

345. Hermans, E.H.: A fifth phacomatosis. Naevus epitheliomatodes multiplex. *Dermatologica, 127:*216–218, 1963.

346. Randazzo, S.D., and Greppi, C.: Contributo allo studio della malattia di Bourneville-Pringle (a proposito di un caso associato a neurofibromatosi di Recklinghausen). *Minerva Dermatologica, 39:*316–326, 1964.

347. Sánchez Sicilia, L., Oliva Aldámiz, H., Castro Torres, A., and Hernando Avendaño, L.: Asociación de esclerosis tuberosa, neurofibromatosis y riñones poliquisticos. *Rev Clin Esp, 108:*311–318, 1968.

348. Schull, W.J., and Crowe, F.W.: Neurocutaneous syndromes in the M kindred. A case of simultaneous occurrence of tuberous sclerosis and neurofibromatosis. *Neurology* (Minneap), *3:*904–909, 1953.

349. Gluszcz, A., and Lach, B.: Melanoblastosis diffusa meningocerebralis i choroba Sturge-Webera. *Neuropatol Pol, 8:*97–108, 1970.

350. Solomon, L.M., and Bolat, I.H.: Adenoma sebaceum in encephalofacial angiomatosis (Sturge-Weber syndrome). *Acta Derm Venereol* (Stockh), *52:*386–388, 1972.

351. Willis, R.A.: The hamartomatous syndromes: their clinical, pathological and fundamental aspects. *Med J Aust, 1:*827–833, 1965.

352. Crowe, F.W., Schull, W.J., and Neel, J.V.: *A Clinical, Pathological, and Genetic Study of Multiple Neurofibromatosis.* Springfield, Thomas, 1956.

353. Retif, J.: Syringomyélie et phacomatose. Etude anatomoclinique de deux observations de maladie de von Recklinghausen et d'une observation de maladie de von Hippel-Lindau, associées à une syringomyélie. *Acta Neurol Belg, 64:*832–851, 1964.

354. Heffner, R.R., Jr.: Hydromyelia in von Recklinghausen's disease with neurofibrosarcoma. *Conn Med, 33:*311–313, 1969.

355. Sammons, B.P., and Thomas, D.F.: Extensive lumbar meningocele associated with neurofibromatosis. *Am J Roentgenol Radium Ther Nucl Med, 81:*1021–1025, 1959.

356. Booth, A.E.: Lateral thoracic meningocele. *J Neurol Neurosurg Psychiatry, 32*:111–115, 1969.

357. Zacks, A.: Atlanto-occipital fusion, basilar impression, and block vertebrae associated with intraspinal neurofibroma, meningocele, and von Recklinghausen's disease. *Radiology, 75*:223–231, 1960.

358. Miles, J., Pennybacker, J., and Sheldon, P.: Intrathoracic meningocele. Its development and association with neurofibromatosis. *J Neurol Neurosurg Psychiatry, 32*:99–110, 1969.

359. Rosman, N.P., and Pearce, J.: The brain in multiple neurofibromatosis (von Recklinghausen's disease): a suggested neuropathological basis for the associated mental defect. *Brain, 90*:829–838, 1967.

360. Magbagbeola, J.A.O.: Abnormal responses to muscle relaxants in a patient with von Recklinghausen's disease (multiple neurofibromatosis). *Br J Anaesth, 42*:710, 1970.

361. Norman, M.E.: Neurofibromatosis in a family. *Am J Dis Child, 123*:159–160, 1972.

362. Barson, A.J., and Cole, F.M.: Neurofibromatosis with congenital malformation of the spinal cord. *J Neurol Neurosurg Psychiatry, 30*:71–74, 1967.

363. Pearce, J.: The central nervous system pathology in multiple neurofibromatosis. *Neurology* (Minneap), *17*:691–697, 1967.

364. Crome, L.: A case of central neurofibromatosis. *Arch Dis Child, 37*:640–651, 1962.

365. Reubi, F.: Neurofibromatose et lésions vasculaires. *Schweiz Med Wochenschr, 75*:463–465, 1945.

366. Reubi, F.: Les vaisseaux et les glandes endocrines dans la neurofibromatose. Le syndrome sympathicotonique dans la maladie de Recklinghausen. *Schweiz Z Pathol Bakteriol, 7*:168–236, 1944.

367. Halpern, M., and Currarino, G.: Vascular lesions causing hypertension in neurofibromatosis. *N Engl J Med, 273*:248–252, 1965.

368. Smith, C.J., Hatch, F.E., Johnson, J.G., and Kelly, B.J.: Renal artery dysplasia as a cause of hypertension in neurofibromatosis. *Arch Intern Med, 125*:1022–1026, 1970.

369. Ganner, E.: Eine Patientin mit Translokation 46, XX, t(Dq–; Bq+) und Neurofibromatose, Schwachsinn sowie Aortenisthmusstenose. *Schweiz Med Wochenschr, 99*:182–186, 1969.

370. Barbieri, G.: Morbo cutaneo di Recklinghausen e criptorchidismo. *Rass Int Clin Ter, 40*:659–666, 1960.

371. Corkill, A.G.L., and Ross, C.F.: A case of neurofibromatosis complicated by medulloblastoma, neurogenic sarcoma, and radiation-induced carcinoma of thyroid. *J Neurol Neurosurg Psychiatry, 32*:43–47, 1969.

372. Heard, G.: Malignant disease in von Recklinghausen's neurofibromatosis. *Proc R Soc Med, 56*:502–503, 1963.

373. Knight, W.A., III, Murphy, W.K., and Gottlieb, J.A.: Neurofibromatosis associated with malignant neurofibromas. *Arch Dermatol, 107*:747–750, 1973.

374. Knudson, A.G., Jr., and Amromin, G.D.: Neuroblastoma and ganglioneuroma in a child with multiple neurofibromatosis. *Cancer, 19*:1032–1037, 1966.

375. Adamski, A., Witoszyński, S., and Zengteler, G.: Embryonal ganglioma in adults. A rare coincidence with neurofibromatosis. *Wiad Lek, 19*:453–457, 1966. (Pol)

376. Sinclair, J.E., and Yang, Y.H.: Ganglioneuromata of the spine associated with von Recklinghausen's disease. *J Neurosurg, 18*:115–119, 1961.

377. Schönebeck, J., and Ljungberg, O.: Recklinghausen's disease: a multifacetted syndrome. *Acta Pathol Microbiol Scand*, (A) *78*:437–442, 1970.

378. McWhirter, W.R., Savage, D.C.L., and Williams, B.M.: Neurofibromatosis with leukaemia. *Br Med J, 4*:114–115, 1971.

379. Fraumeni, J.F., Jr.: Neurofibromatosis and childhood leukaemia. *Br Med J, 4*:489–490, 1971.

380. Waleszkowski, J., and Hajdukiewicz, Z.: Recklinghausen's disease with involvement of the central nervous system. *Neuropatol Pol, 9*:165–169, 1971. (Pol)

381. Davidson, K.C.: Cranial and intracranial lesions in neurofibromatosis. *Am J Roent-*

genol Radium Ther Nucl Med, 98:550–556, 1966.

382. Rodriguez, H.A., and Berthrong, M.: Multiple primary intracranial tumors in von Recklinghausen's neurofibromatosis. *Arch Neurol*, 14:467–475, 1966.

383. Jamieson, K.G.: Multiple intracranial tumours in neurofibromatosis: report of a case. *Aust NZ J Surg*, 38:51–54, 1968.

384. Haberland, C., and Brumlik, J.: Palatal myoclonus associated with cerebellar neoplasm in von Recklinghausen's disease (a clinicopathologic study). *Psychiatr Neurol* (Basel), 154:209–229, 1967.

385. Nager, G.T.: Association of bilateral VIIIth nerve tumors with meningiomas in von Recklinghausen's disease. *Laryngoscope*, 74:1220–1261, 1964.

386. Pendefunda, Gh., Nemteanu, E., Oprisan, C., and Gherasimescu, Gh. Multiple intracavitary neurinomas associated with meningiomatosis, a variant of Recklinghausen's disease. *Neurol Psihiatr Neurochir*, 14:123–129, 1969. (Rum)

387. Lazorthes, G., Anduze-Acher, H., Amaral-Gomes, F., and Karkous, F.: Les méningiomes multiples, les méningiomatoses et les méningiomes associés à d'autres tumeurs nerveuses. *Neurochirurgie*, 6:156–160, 1960.

388. Lee, D.K., and Abbott, M.L.: Familial central nervous system neoplasia. Case report of a family with von Recklinghausen's neurofibromatosis. *Arch Neurol*, 20:154–160, 1969.

389. Paillas, J.-E., Bonnal, J., Legre, J., and Combalbert, A.: Des méningiomes multiples a la méningiomatose en plaques au cours de la maladie de Recklinghausen. *Presse Med*, 69:2604–2606, 1961.

390. Hitselberger, W.E., and Hughes, R.L.: Bilateral acoustic tumors and neurofibromatosis. *Arch Otolaryngol*, 88:700–711, 1968.

391. Kramer, W.: Lesions of the central nervous system in multiple neurofibromatosis. *Psychiatr Neurol Neurochir*, 74:349–368, 1971.

392. Brady, W.J.: Brain stem gliomas causing hydrocephalus in twins with von Recklinghausen's disease. *J Neuropathol Exp Neurol*, 21:555–565, 1962.

393. Taylor, P.E.: Encapsulated glioma of the Sylvian fissure associated with neurofibromatosis. Report of a case with histopathological comparison of surgical lesion and autopsy specimen following recurrence. *J Neuropathol Exp Neurol*, 21:566–578, 1962.

394. Pavićević, R., and Jekić, B.: Glioblastoma multiform in the course of Recklinghausen disease. *Srp Arh Celok Lek*, 97:1381–1386, 1969. (Ser)

395. Terao, H., Tsukamoto, Y., and Sano, K.: Intracranial tumors associated with von Recklinghausen's disease. *Brain Nerve* (Tokyo), 19:1235–1245, 1967. (Jap)

396. Araki, C.: Von Recklinghausen's disease and glioma of brain. *Jap J Clin Med*, 29:1939–1943, 1971. (Jap)

397. Janny, P., Montrieul, B., and Hurth, M.: Les tumeurs gliales au cours de la maladie de Recklinghausen. *Maroc Med*, 42:902–904, 1963.

398. Babchin, I.S., and Krivosheina, Yu.P.: Clinical forms of central neurofibromatosis. *Zh Nevropatol Psikhiatr*, 68:481–486, 1968. (Rus)

399. Noeske, K., and Sandritter, W.: XIII. Neurofibromatose (von Recklinghausen) mit ungewöhnlichen malignen Tumoren. *Med Welt*, 30:1693–1694, 1965.

400. Nakajima, T., Okumura, Y., Kanai, N., Fujii, C., Fujiyama, T., and Mogami, H.: V. Recklinghausen's disease; a case of multiple neurilemmomatosis with spinal meningioma. *Brain Nerve*, 23:91–94, 1971. (Jap)

401. Arroyo, H., Aubert, L., and Daumas, B.: Neurofibromatose, méningiome et syndrome de Richter. *Mars Med*, 107:491–492, 1970.

402. Masheter, H.C.: Phaeochromocytoma, astrocytoma, and neurofibromatosis in one patient. *Br Med J*, 2:1518, 1963.

403. Roberts, A.H.: Association of a phaeochromocytoma and cerebral gliosarcoma with neurofibromatosis. *Br J Surg*, 54:78–79, 1967.

404. Barnard, R.O., and Lang, E.R.: Cerebral and cerebellar gliomas in a case of von Recklinghausen's disease with adrenal phaeo-

chromocytomas. *J Neurosurg, 21:*506–511, 1964.

405. Skrzypczak, J.: Neurofibromatosis Recklinghausen mit Phäochromozytom des Nebennierenmarks und Großhirnspongioblastom. *Dtsch Gesundheitsw, 26:*2173–2175, 1971.

406. Tsubota, Y., Takeshita, M., Goto, I., Hori, S., Tsuchiya, M., Katsuki, S., Shigemi, U., and Tanaka, K.: Case of neurofibromatosis with adrenal pheochromocytoma and cerebral astrocytoma. Case report. *J Jap Soc Intern Med, 59:*255–262, 1970.

407. Saran, N., and Winter, F.C.: Bilateral gliomas of the optic discs associated with neurofibromatosis. *Am J Ophthalmol, 64:*607–612, 1967.

408. Davis, F.A.: Primary tumors of the optic nerve (a phenomenon of Recklinghausen's disease). A clinical and pathologic study with a report of five cases and a review of the literature. *Arch Ophthalmol, 23:*735–821 and 957–1018, 1940.

409. Nordmann, J., Brini, A., and Philippides, D.: Gliome du nerf optique et naevi de l'iris (maladie de von Recklinghausen). *Bull Soc Ophtalmol Fr, 70:*132–135, 1970.

410. Vallat, M., Bioulac, B., Banayan, A., Vital, C., and Pouyanne, H.: Gliomes du chiasma et phacomatoses. A propos de deux cas. *Bord Med, 5:*645–650, 1972.

411. Nordmann, J., and Brini, A.: Von Recklinghausen's disease and melanoma of the uvea. *Br J Ophthalmol, 54:*641–648, 1970.

412. Fialkow, P.J., Sagebiel, R.W., Gartler, S.M., and Rimoin, D.L.: Multiple cell origin of hereditary neurofibromas. *N Engl J Med, 284:*298–300, 1971.

413. Dörstelmann, D., Kerschensteiner, M., Markus, E., and Sturm, K.W.: Chorea Huntington und Neurofibromatosis v. Recklinghausen. Beobachtung von kombiniertem Auftreten über zwei Generationen in einer Chorea-Sippe. *Z Neurol, 199:*39–45, 1971.

414. Gardner, W.J., and Frazier, C.H.: Bilateral acoustic neurofibromas. A clinical study and field survey of a family of five generations with bilateral deafness in thirty-eight members. *Arch Neurol Psychiatry, 23:*266–300, 1930.

415. Gardner, W.J., and Turner, O.: Bilateral acoustic neurofibromas. Further clinical and pathologic data on hereditary deafness and Recklinghausen's disease. *Arch Neurol Psychiatry, 44:*76–99, 1940.

416. Young, D.F., Eldridge, R., and Gardner, W.J.: Bilateral acoustic neuroma in a large kindred. *JAMA, 214:*347–353, 1970.

417. Bundey, S., and Evans, K.: Tuberous sclerosis: a genetic study. *J Neurol Neurosurg Psychiatry, 32:*591–603, 1969.

418. Ross, A.T., and Dickerson, W.W.: Tuberous sclerosis. *Arch Neurol Psychiatry, 50:* 233–257, 1943.

419. Dickerson, W.W.: Familial occurrence of tuberous sclerosis. *Arch Neurol Psychiatry, 65:*683–702, 1951.

420. Nickel, W.R., and Reed, W.B.: Tuberous sclerosis. Special reference to the microscopic alterations in the cutaneous hamartomas. *Arch Dermatol, 85:*209–224, 1962.

421. Garron, L.K., and Spencer, W.H.: Retinal glioneuroma associated with tuberous sclerosis. *Trans Am Acad Ophthalmol Otolaryngol, 68:*1018–1021, 1964.

422. Borromei, A., and Capelli, A.: Contributo alla conoscenza dei tumori intraventricolari cerebrali nella sclerosi tuberosa. Presentazione di un caso con considerazioni embriologiche ed istopatologiche. *Arch Ital Anat Istol Patol, 43:*302–314, 1970.

423. Juul Jensen, K.E.: Hjernetumorer ved tuberøs sklerose. *Nord Med, 86:*1219, 1971.

424. De Divitiis, E., Mattioli, G., and Puca, F.M.: Sclerosi tuberosa e tumore intraventricolare. *Rass Neuropsichiatr, 20:*302–309, 1966.

425. Haberland, C., and Perou, M.: Glioma with nuclear inclusions in tuberose sclerosis. *Acta Neuropathol* (Berlin), *16:*73–76, 1970.

426. Rudnick, P.A., Hoshino, N., Kitaoka, T., and Miura, M.: Tuberous sclerosis complex and astrocytoma. Report of a case with successful removal of the neoplasm. *JAMA,178:*73–75, 1961.

427. Bollati, A., and Caneschi, S.: Un caso di associazione di tumore intraventricolare e morbo di Bourneville. *G Psichiatr Neuropatol, 97:*339–349, 1969.

428. Escalona Zapata, J.: El astrocitoma gigantocelular subependimario y su relación con

la esclerosis tuberosa. *Trab Inst Cajal Invest Biol, 55:*173–192, 1963.

429. Cooper, J.R.: Brain tumors in hereditary multiple system hamartomatosis (tuberous sclerosis). *J Neurosurg, 34:*194–202, 1971.

430. MacCarty, W.C., Jr., and Russell, D.G.: Tuberous sclerosis. Report of a case with ependymoma. *Radiology, 71:*833–839, 1958.

431. Davis, R.L., and Nelson, E.: Unilateral ganglioglioma in a tuberosclerotic brain. *J Neuropathol Exp Neurol, 20:*571–581, 1961.

432. Kapp, J.P., Paulson, G.W., and Odom, G.L.: Brain tumors with tuberous sclerosis. *J Neurosurg, 26:*191–202, 1967.

433. Melmon, K.L., and Rosen, S.W.: Lindau's disease. Review of the literature and study of a large kindred. *Am J Med, 36:*595–617, 1964.

434. Lindau, A.: Studien über Kleinhirncysten. Bau, Pathogenese und Beziehungen zur Angiomatosis retinae. *Acta Pathol Microbiol Scand,* Vol. 3, suppl. 1, 1926.

435. McIntosh Nicol, A.A.: Lindau's disease in five generations. *Ann Hum Genet, 22:*7–15, 1957.

436. Richards, R.D., Mebust, W.K., and Schimke, R.N.: A prospective study on von Hippel-Lindau disease. *J Urol, 110:*27–30, 1973.

437. Tonning, H.O., Warren, R.F., and Barrie, H.J.: Familial haemangiomata of the cerebellum. Report of three cases in a family of four. *J Neurosurg, 9:*124–132, 1952.

438. Shokeir, M.H.K.: Von Hippel-Lindau syndrome: a report on three kindreds. *J Med Genet, 7:*155–157, 1970.

439. Jain, I.S., Das, K.C., and Mahajan, B.C.: Von Hippel-Lindau disease. A chromosomal study. *J All India Ophthalmol Soc, 17:*1–7, 1969.

440. Kobayashi, M., and Shimada, K.: Chromosome studies on ocular diseases. *Acta Ophthal Jap, 70:*1752–1763, 1966. (Jap)

441. Silver, M.L., and Hennigar, G.: Cerebellar hemangioma (hemangioblastoma). A clinicopathological review of 40 cases. *J Neurosurg, 9:*484–494, 1952.

442. Archer, C.R., Roberson, G.H., and Taveras,

J.M.: Posterior medullary hemangioblastoma. *Radiology, 103:*323–328, 1972.

443. Banerjee, T., and Hunt, W.E.: A case of spinal cord hemangioblastoma and review of the literature. *Am Surg, 38:*460–464, 1972.

444. Otenasek, F.J., and Silver, M.L.: Spinal hemangioma (hemangioblastoma) in Lindau's disease. Report of six cases in a single family. *J Neurosurg, 18:*295–300, 1961.

445. Hoff, J.T., and Ray, B.S.: Cerebral hemangioblastoma occurring in a patient with von Hippel-Lindau disease. *J Neurosurg, 28:*365–368, 1968.

446. Wright, R.L.: Familial von Hippel-Lindau's disease. Case report. *J Neurosurg, 30:*281–285, 1969.

447. Chapman, R.C., and Diaz-Perez, R.: Pheochromocytoma associated with cerebellar hemangioblastoma. Familial occurrence. *JAMA, 182:*1014–1017, 1962.

448. Mulholland, S.G., Atuk, N.O., and Walzak, M.P.: Familial pheochromocytoma associated with cerebellar hemangioblastoma. *JAMA, 207:*1709–1711, 1969.

449. Nibbelink, D.W., Peters, B.H., and McCormick, W.F.: On the association of pheochromocytoma and cerebellar hemangioblastoma. *Neurology* (Minneap), *19:*455–460, 1969.

450. Christoferson, L.A., Gustafson, M.B., and Petersen, A.G.: Von Hippel-Lindau's disease. *JAMA, 178:*280–282, 1961.

451. Grossman, M.O., and Kesert, B.H.: Familial incidence of tumors of the brain. Cerebellar hemangioblastoma. *Arch Neurol Psychiatry, 52:*327–328, 1944.

452. Adams, J.E.: Familial hemangioblastoma of the cerebellum. Pedigree of two families. *J Neurosurg, 10:*421–423, 1953.

453. Bonebrake, R.A., and Siqueira, E.B.: The familial occurrence of solitary hemangioblastoma of the cerebellum. *Neurology* (Minneap), *14:*733–743, 1964.

454. Fornatto, L., Portaleone, P., and Schiffer, D.: Sulla comparsa familiare dell'angioblastoma cerebellare solitario e sui suoi rapporti con il complesso von Hippel-Lindau. *Acta Neurol* (Napoli), *27:*286–290, 1972.

455. Wilkins, R.H., and Brody, I.A.: Neurological

classics. XXV. Sturge-Weber syndrome. *Arch Neurol, 21:*554–555, 1969.

456. Wiel, H.J. van der: *Inheritance of Glioma.* Amsterdam, Elsevier, 1959.

457. Hamanaka, Y., Mori, S., Kanoh, M., Uozumi, T., Matsuoka, K., Inoue, E., Yokoi, H., and Yoshitatsu, S.: A case of bilateral Sturge-Weber's disease with a plexus papilloma at the left lateral ventricle. *Brain Nerve* (Tokyo), *22:*99–103, 1970. (Jap)

458. Noran, H.H.: Intracranial vascular tumors and malformations. *Arch Pathol, 39:*393–416, 1945.

459. Osetowska, E., and Janowska, K.: Un cas d'idiotie amaurotique juvénile avec une angiomatose méningo-cérébrale non-calcifiante. *J Neurol Sci, 4:*131–140, 1966.

460. Wolf, P.A., Rosman, N.P., and New, P.F.J.: Multiple small cryptic venous angiomas of the brain mimicking cerebral metastases. A clinical, pathological, and angiographic study. *Neurology* (Minneap), *17:* 491–501, 1967.

461. Bech, K., and Jensen, O.A.: On the frequency of co-existing racemose haemangiomata of the retina and brain. *Acta Psychiatr Scand, 36:*47–56, 1961.

462. Gass, J.D.M.: Cavernous hemangioma of the retina. A neuro-oculo-cutaneous syndrome. *Am J Ophthalmol, 71:*799–814, 1971.

463. Heffner, R.R., Jr., and Solitare, G.B.: Hereditary haemorrhagic telangiectasia: neuropathological observations. *J Neurol Neurosurg Psychiatry, 32:*604–608, 1969.

464. Fine, R.D.: Angioma racemosum venosum of spinal cord with segmentally related angiomatous lesions of skin and forearm. *J Neurosurg, 18:*546–550, 1961.

465. Bergstrand, A., Höök, O., and Lidvall, H.: Vascular malformations of the spinal cord. *Acta Neurol Scand, 40:*169–183, 1964.

466. Hooft, C., Deloore, G., Van Bogaert, L., and Guazzi, G.C.: Sudanophilic leucodystrophy with meningeal angiomatosis in two brothers: infantile form of diffuse sclerosis with meningeal angiomatosis. *J Neurol Sci, 2:*30–51, 1965.

467. Bruens, J.H., Guazzi, G.C., and Martin, J.J.: Infantile form of meningeal angiomatosis with sudanophilic leucodystrophy associated with complex abiotrophies. Study of a second family. *J Neurol Sci, 7:*417–425, 1968.

468. Hermans, E.H., Grosfeld, J.C.M., and Spaas, J.A.J.: The fifth phacomatosis. *Dermatologica, 130:*446 476, 1965.

469. Wallace, D.C., Murphy, K.J., Kelly, L., and Ward, W.H.: The basal cell naevus syndrome. Report of a family with anosmia and a case of hypogonadotrophic hypopituitarism. *J Med Genet, 10:*30–33, 1973.

470. Gorlin, R.J., Vickers, R.A., Kelln, E., and Williamson, J.J.: The multiple basal-cell nevi syndrome. An analysis of a syndrome consisting of multiple nevoid basal-cell carcinoma, jaw cysts, skeletal anomalies, medulloblastoma, and hyporesponsiveness to parathormone. *Cancer, 18:*89–104, 1965.

471. Hermans, E.H.: A fifth phacomatosis, naevus epitheliomatodes multiplex. *Acta Leiden, 33:*89–91, 1964–5.

472. Herzberg, J.J., and Wiskemann, A.: Die fünfte Phakomatose. Basalzellnaevus mit familiärer Belastung und Medulloblastom. *Dermatologica, 126:*106–123, 1963.

473. Neblett, C.R., Waltz, T.A., and Anderson, D.E.: Neurological involvement in the nevoid basal cell carcinoma syndrome. *J Neurosurg, 35:*577–584, 1971.

474. Graham, J.K., McJimsey, B.A., and Hardin, J.C., Jr.: Nevoid basal cell carcinoma syndrome. *Arch Otolaryngol, 87:*72–77, 1968.

475. Kedem, A., Even-Paz, Z., and Freund, M.: Basal cell nevus syndrome associated with malignant melanoma of the iris. *Dermatologica, 140:*99–106, 1970.

476. Happle, R., Mehrle, G., Sander, L.Z., and Höhn, H.: Basalzellnävus-Syndrom mit Retinopathia pigmentosa, rezidivierender Glaskörperblutung und Chromosomenveränderungen. *Arch Dermatol Forsch, 241:*96–114, 1971.

477. Happle, R., and Kupferschmid, A.: A further case of basal cell nevus syndrome and structural chromosome abnormalities. *Humangenetik, 15:*287–288, 1972.

478. Slaughter, J.C., Hardman, J.M., Kempe, L.G., and Earle, K.M.: Neurocutaneous mela-

nosis and leptomeningeal melanomatosis in children. *Arch Pathol, 88:*298–304, 1969.

479. Hoffman, H.J., and Freeman, A.: Primary malignant leptomeningeal melanoma in association with giant hairy nevi. Report of two cases. *J Neurosurg, 26:*62–71, 1967. *26:*62–71, 1967.

480. Mathew, N.T., Mathai, K.V., and Bhakthaviziam, A.: Giant hairy naevi and leptomeningeal primary malignant melanoma. *Neurol India, 18:*113–115, 1970.

481. Williams, H.I.: Primary malignant meningeal melanoma associated with benign hairy naevi. *J Pathol, 99:*171–172, 1969.

482. Sobajima, Y., Uchiyama, T., and Kudo, H.: An autopsy case of mélanose neurocutanée (Touraine). *Acta Pathol Jap, 21:* 553–562, 1971.

483. Chatelain, R., De Rougemont, J., Tommasi, M., Barge, M., and Martin, H.: Mélanose neurocutanée (observation anatomo-clinique). *J Med Lyon, 50:*1325–1334, 1969.

484. Dailly, R., Forthomme, J., Samson, M., Tayot, J., Clement, J.-Ch., and Morin, Cl.: Mélanose neuro-cutanée a évolution tumorale. Une observation anatomo-clinique. *Presse Med, 73:*2867–2872, 1965.

485. Wieczorek, V., Waldmann, K.-D., Teweleit, H.-D., and Hoffmeyer, O.: Melano-Phakomatose vom Typus der Mélanoblastose neurocutanée Touraine unter Berücksichtigung der Liquorzytologie. *Dtsch Gesundheitsw, 27:*987–991, 1972.

486. Morris, L.L., and Danta, G.: Malignant cerebral melanoma complicating giant pigmented naevus: a case report. *J Neurol Neurosurg Psychiatry, 31:*628–632, 1968.

487. Hjelt, L., and Vilska, J.: Malignant meningeal melanoma in a 3-year-old boy. A case report. *Ann Paediatr Fenn, 12:*246–250, 1966.

488. Tveten, L.: Primary meningeal melanosis. A clinico-pathological report of two cases. *Acta Pathol Microbiol Scand, 63:*1–10, 1965.

489. Deshpande, D.H., Dastur, H.M., and Pandya, S.K.: Primary melanoma of the leptomeninges. *Neurol India, 18:*107–112, 1970.

490. Beresford, H.R.: Melanoma of the nervous system. Treatment with corticosteroids and radiation. *Neurology* (Minneap), *19:* 59–65, 1969.

491. Bouton, J.: Primary melanoma of the leptomeninges. *J Clin Pathol, 11:*122–127, 1958.

492. Pappenheim, E., and Bhattacharji, S.K.: Primary melanoma of the central nervous system. *Arch Neurol, 7:*101–113, 1962.

493. Tolnai, G., Campbell, J.S., Hill, D.P., Peterson, E.W., Hudson, A.J., and Luney, F.W.: Primary malignant melanomatosis of leptomeninges. *Arch Neurol, 15:*404–409, 1966.

494. Salm, R.: Primary malignant melanoma of the cerebellum. *J Pathol Bacteriol, 94:*196–200, 1967.

495. Becker, S.M., Emanuele, S.J., and Sami, A.W.: Primary melanoma of the leptomeninges of the spinal cord. A case report and review of the literature. *J Med Soc NJ, 67:*271–275, 1970.

496. Gibson, J.B., Burrows, D., and Weir, W.P.: Primary melanoma of the meninges. *J Pathol Bacteriol, 74:*419–438, 1957.

497. Lewis, M.G.: Melanoma and pigmentation of the leptomeninges in Ugandan Africans. *J Clin Pathol, 22:*183–186, 1969.

498. Krabbe, K.H., and Bartels, E.D.: *La Lipomatose Circonscrite Multiple.* Copenhaven, Einar Munksgaard, 1944.

499. Haberland, C., and Perou, M.: Encephalocraniocutaneous lipomatosis. A new example of ectomesodermal dysgenesis. *Arch Neurol, 22:*144–155, 1970.

500. Meyerson, L.B.: Nevus unius lateralis, brain tumor, and diencephalic syndrome. *Arch Dermatol, 95:*501–504, 1967.

501. Gatti, R.A., and Good, R.A.: Occurrence of malignancy in immunodeficiency diseases. A literature review. *Cancer, 28:*89–98, 1971.

502. Waldmann, T.A., Strober, W., and Blaese, R.M.: Immunodeficiency disease and malignancy. Various immunologic deficiencies of man and the role of immune processes in the control of malignant disease. *Ann Intern Med, 77:*605–628, 1972.

503. Liebow, A.A., Carrington, C.R.B., and Fried-

man, P.J.: Lymphomatoid granulomatosis. *Hum Pathol, 3*:457–558, 1972.

504. Shuster, J., Hart, Z., Stimson, C.W., Brough,
     A.J., and Poulik, M.D.: Ataxia telangi-
     ectasia with cerebellar tumor. *Pediatrics,
     37*:776–786, 1966.

505. Young, R.R., Austen, K.F., and Moser,
     H.W.: Ataxia-telangiectasia and the thy-
     mus. *Trans Am Neurol Assoc, 89*:28–29,
     1964.

506. Solitare, G.B.: Louis-Bar's syndrome (ataxia-
     telangiectasia). Anatomic considerations
     with emphasis on neuropathologic ob-
     servations. *Neurology* (Minneap), *18*:
     1180–1186, 1968.

507. German, J.: Genes which increase chromo-
     somal instability in somatic cells and
     predispose to cancer. *Prog Med Genet, 8*:
     61–101, 1972.

508. McFarlin, D.E., Strober, W., and Waldmann,
     T.A.: Ataxia-telangiectasia. *Medicine* (Bal-
     timore), *51*:281–314, 1972.

509. Baldini, M.G.: The Wiskott-Aldrich syn-
     drome. *Birth defects: original article series,
     8*:151–157, 1972.

510. Brand, M.M., and Marinkovich, V.A.: Pri-
     mary malignant reticulosis of the brain in
     Wiskott-Aldrich syndrome. Report of a
     case. *Arch Dis Child, 44*:536–542, 1969.

511. ten Bensel, R.W., Stadlan, E.M., and Krivit,
     W.: The development of malignancy in the
     course of the Aldrich syndrome. *J Pediatr,
     68*:761–767, 1966.

512. Good, R.A.: Relations between immunity and
     malignancy. *Proc Natl Acad Sci USA, 69*:
     1026–1032, 1972.

513. Good, R.A., and Finstad, J.: Essential rela-
     tionship between the lymphoid system,
     immunity, and malignancy. *Natl Cancer
     Inst Monogr, 31*:41–58, 1969.

514. Adams, J.H., and Jackson, J.M.: Intracere-
     bral tumours of reticular tissue: the prob-
     lem of microgliomatosis and reticulo-
     endothelial sarcomas of the brain. *J Pathol
     Bacteriol, 91*:369–381, 1966.

515. Gunderson, C.H., Henry, J., and Malamud,
     N.: Plasma globulin determinations in
     patients with microglioma. Report of five
     cases. *J Neurosurg, 35*:406–415, 1971.

516. Jensen, R.D., and Miller, R.W.: Retinoblas-

toma: epidemiologic characteristics. *N
Engl J Med, 285*:307–311, 1971.

517. Hoefnagel, D., McIntyre, O.R., Storrs, R.C.,
     Sullivan, P.B., and Maurer, L.H.: Retino-
     blastoma followed by acute lymphoblastic
     leukaemia. *Lancet, 1*:725, 1973.

518. Levene, M.,: Congenital retinoblastoma and
     sarcoma botryoides of the vagina. *Cancer,
     13*:532–537, 1960.

519. Von Hagen, K.O., and Barrows, H.S.: Fa-
     milial pheochromocytoma with ependy-
     moma of the spinal cord. Case report and
     review of the literature. *J Neurosurg, 20*:
     600–604, 1963.

520. Turcot, J., Després, J.-P., and St. Pierre, F.:
     Malignant tumors of the central nervous
     system associated with familial polyposis
     of the colon: report of two cases. *Dis Colon
     Rectum, 2*:465–468, 1959.

521. Baughman, F.A., Jr., List, C.F., Williams,
     J.R., Muldoon, J.P., Segarra, J.M., and
     Volkel, J.S.: The glioma-polyposis syn-
     drome. *N Engl J Med, 281*:1345–1346,
     1969.

522. Yaffee, H.S.: Gastric polyposis and soft
     tissue tumors. *Arch Dermatol, 89*:806–
     808, 1964.

523. Davis, M., and Dorfman, J.: Gaucher's dis-
     ease associated with a cerebral astrocy-
     toma. A case report involving an adult.
     Am Practit, 12:673–677, 1961.

524. Hueper, W.C.: Macromolecular agents as
     benign and malignant cell proliferants.
     Natl Cancer Inst Monogr, 14:357–377,
     1964.

525. Hueper, W.C.: Carcinogenic studies on water-
     soluble and insoluble macromolecules.
     Arch Pathol, 67:589–617, 1959.

526. Page, L.K.: The concurrence of osteitis de-
     formans and acoustic neurinoma. *Am J
     Med, 53*:697–700, 1972.

527. Cristi, G., Dettori, P., Gaist, G., and Scialfa,
     G.: Su un caso di meningioma associato
     a morbo di Paget. *Riv Otoneurooftalmol,
     44*:593–599, 1969.

528. Legré, J., Pitot, G., and Serratrice, G.: Glio-
     blastome hémisphérique et maladie de
     Paget. *Rev Otoneuroophtalmol, 31*:423–
     424, 1959.

529. Thannhauser, S.J.: Werner's syndrome (pro-

geria of the adult) and Rothmund's syndrome: two types of closely related heredofamilial atrophic dermatoses with juvenile cataracts and endocrine features; a critical study with five new cases. *Ann Intern Med, 23*:559–626, 1945.

530. Rosen, R.S., Cimini, R., and Coblentz, D.: Werner's syndrome. *Br J Radiol, 43*:193–198, 1970.

531. Degreef, H.: The Werner syndrome. *Dermatologica, 142*:45–49, 1971.

532. Reichel, W., Garcia-Bunuel, R., and Dilallo, J.: Progeria and Werner's syndrome as models for the study of normal human aging. *J Am Geriatr Soc, 19*:369–375, 1971.

533. Epstein, C.J., Martin, G.M., Schultz, A.L., and Motulsky, A.G.: Werner's syndrome. *Medicine* (Baltimore), *45*:177–221, 1966.

534. Stecker, E., and Gardner, H.A.: Werner's syndrome. *Lancet, 2*:1317, 1970.

535. Fuldauer, M.L., and Eggink, S.J.: A propos d'un cas de démence présénile (maladie d'Alzheimer) compliqué de tumeur cérébrale. *Psychiatr Neurol Neurochir, 63*:47–56, 1960.

536. Rubinstein, J.H.: Broad thumb-hallux syndrome. Int Congress Pediatr, Vienna, separatum, Verlag Wiener Med Akad, pp. 471–476, 1971.

537. Simpson, N.E., and Brissenden, J.E.: The Rubinstein-Taybi syndrome: familial and dermatoglyphic data. *Am J Hum Genet, 25*:225–229, 1973.

538. Rice, J.S., and Fischer, D.S.: Blue rubber-bleb nevus syndrome. *Arch Dermatol, 86*:503–511, 1962.

539. Carleton, A., Elkington, J.St.C., Greenfield, J.G., and Robb-Smith, A.H.T.: Maffucci's syndrome. *QJ Med,* New series, *11*:203–228, 1942.

540. Ashenhurst, E.M.: Dyschondroplasia with hemangioma (Maffucci's syndrome). Report of a case complicated by brain tumor. *Arch Neurol, 2*:552–555, 1960.

541. Sakurane, H.F., Sugai, T., and Saito, T.: The association of blue rubber bleb nevus and Maffucci's syndrome. *Arch Dermatol, 95*:28–36, 1967.

542. Decker, R.E., and Wei, W.C.: Thoracic cord compression from multiple hereditary exostoses associated with cerebellar astrocytoma. Case report. *J Neurosurg, 30*:310–312, 1969.

543. Poser, C.M.: *The Relationship Between Syringomyelia and Neoplasm.* Springfield, Thomas, 1956.

544. Ferry, D.J., Hardman, J.M., and Earle, K.M.: Syringomyelia and intramedullary neoplasms. *Med Ann DC, 38*:363–365, 1969.

545. Kosary, I.Z., Braham, J., Shaked, I., and Tadmor, R.: Cervical syringomyelia associated with occipital meningioma. *Neurology* (Minneap), *19*:1127–1130, 1969.

546. Epstein, L.I., Bixler, D., and Bennett, J.E.: An incident of familial cancer including 3 cases of osteogenic sarcoma. *Cancer, 25*:889–891, 1970.

547. Walker, M.D., Rumack, B.H., and Rosenblum, M.L.: Malignant central nervous system tumor and other neoplasms in a large family. *Neurology* (Minneap), *21*:440–441, 1971.

548. Li, F.P., and Fraumeni, J.F., Jr.: Soft-tissue sarcomas, breast cancer, and other neoplasms. A familial syndrome? *Ann Intern Med, 71*:747–752, 1969.

549. Li, F.P., and Fraumeni, J.F., Jr.: Rhabdomyosarcoma in children: epidemiologic study and identification of a familial cancer syndrome. *J Natl Cancer Inst, 43*:1365–1373, 1969.

550. Lynch, H.T., Krush, A.J., Harlan, W.L., and Sharp, E.A.: Association of soft tissue sarcoma, leukemia, and brain tumors in families affected with breast cancer. *Am Surg, 39*:199–206, 1973.

551. Miller, R.W.: Deaths from childhood leukemia and solid tumors among twins and other sibs in the United States, 1960–67. *J Natl Cancer Inst, 46*:203–209, 1971.

552. Lynch, H.T., and Krush, A.J.: Cancer family "G" revisited: 1895–1970. *Cancer, 27*:1505–1511, 1971.

553. Lynch, H.T., and Krush, A.J.: Carcinoma of the breast and ovary in three families. *Surg Gynecol Obstet, 133*:644–648, 1971.

554. Cannon, M.M., and Leavell, B.S.: Multiple cancer types in one family. *Cancer, 19*:538–540, 1966.

555. Bottomley, R.H., Trainer, A.L., and Condit,

P.T.: Chromosome studies in a "cancer family." *Cancer, 28*:519–528, 1971.

556. Chen, W.Y., Crittenden, L.B., Mantel, N., and Cameron, W.R.: Site distribution of cancer deaths in husband-wife and sibling pairs. *J Natl Cancer Inst, 27*:875–886, 1961.

557. Marshall, S.: Connubial cancer: coincidence vs. contagion. *JAMA, 218*:1831–1832, 1971.

558. Swift, M.: Fanconi's anaemia in the genetics of neoplasia. *Nature, 230*:370–373, 1971.

559. Swift, M., Zimmerman, D., and McDonough, E.R.: Squamous cell carcinomas in Fanconi's anemia. *JAMA, 216*:325–326, 1971.

560. Jackson, J.F.: Ataxia telangiectasia. In Lynch, H.T., (Ed.): *Skin, Heredity, and Malignant Neoplasms.* Flushing, Med Exam, 1972, pp. 94–103.

561. Lynch, H.T., Krush, A.J., Mulcahy, G.M., and Reed, W.B.: Familial occurrences of a variety of premalignant diseases and uncommon malignant neoplasms. *Cancer, 33*:1474–1479, 1974.

562. Lynch, H.T.: *Hereditary Factors in Carcinoma.* In *Recent Results in Cancer Research, 12.* New York, Springer-Verlag, 1967.

563. Lynch, H.T.: Genetic factors in carcinoma. *Med Clin North Am, 53*:923–939, 1969.

564. Knudson, A.G., Jr., Strong, L.C., and Anderson, D.E.: Heredity and cancer in man. *Progr Med Genet, 9*:113–158, 1973.

565. Strong, L.C.: Genetic concept for the origin of cancer: historical review. *Ann NY Acad Sci, 71*:810–838, 1958.

566. Heston, W.E.: Genetic factors in the etiology of cancer. *Cancer Res, 25*:1320–1326, 1965.

567. Jarvik, L.F., and Falek, A.: Cancer rates in aging twins. *Am J Hum Genet, 13*:413–422, 1961.

568. Oliver, C.P.: Studies on human cancer families. *Ann NY Acad Sci, 71*:1198–1212, 1958.

569. Aita, J.A.: Genetic aspects of tumors of the nervous system. In Lynch, H.T., (Ed.): *Hereditary Factors in Carcinoma, in Recent Results in Cancer Research, 12.* New York, Springer-Verlag, 1967, pp. 86–110.

570. Pratt, R.T.C.: *The Genetics of Neurological Disorders.* London, Oxford U Pr, 1967, pp. 93–97.

571. Wilkins, R.H.: Genetic factors related to the induction and hereditary transmission of primary intracranial neoplasms. In Kirsch, W.M., Grossi-Paoletti, E., and Paoletti, P., (Eds.): *The Experimental Biology of Brain Tumors.* Springfield, Thomas, 1972, pp. 551–560.

572. Metzel, E.: Uber die familiär gehäuften Gliome. *Archiv Psychiatr Zeitschrift ges Neurol, 204*:537–555, 1963.

573. Zülch, K.J.: *Brain Tumors. Their Biology and Pathology,* 2nd Am Ed. New York, Springer, 1965, pp. 45–50.

574. Manuelidis, E.E.: Genetics of glioblastomas. In Minckler, J., (Ed.): *Pathology of the Nervous System.* New York, McGraw-Hill, 1972, vol. 3, pp. 2917–2926.

575. Kjellin, K., Müller, R., and Åström, K.E.: The occurrence of brain tumors in several members of a family. *J Neuropathol Exp Neurol, 19*:528–537, 1960.

576. Koch, G., and Middendorf, E.: Vorkommen von Glioblastoma multiforme bei 3 Schwestern im Alter von 50 bis 54 Jahren (neuere Betrachtungen zur Ätiologie dysontogenetischer Geschwülste). *Med Welt, 2*:2541–2544, 1960.

577. Fairburn, B., and Urich, H.: Malignant gliomas occurring in identical twins. *J Neurol Neurosurg Psychiatry, 34*:718–722, 1971.

578. Kaufman, H.H., and Brisman, R.: Familial gliomas. Report of four cases. *J Neurosurg, 37*:110–112, 1972.

579. Symonds, C.: Disease of mind and disorder of brain. *Br Med J, 2*:1–5, 1960.

580. Grosz, K., and Plaschkes, S.J.: The occurrence of cerebral tumors in a brother and sister. *Isr Med J, 19*:302–305, 1960.

581. Armstrong, R.M., and Hanson, C.W.: Familial gliomas. *Neurology* (Minneap), *19*:1061–1063, 1969.

582. Parkinson, D., and Hall, C.W.: Oligodendrogliomas. Simultaneous appearance in frontal lobes of siblings. *J Neurosurg, 19*:424–426, 1962.

583. Belamaric, J., and Chau, A.S.: Medulloblastoma in newborn sisters. Report of two cases. *J Neurosurg, 30*:76–79, 1969.

584. Bickerstaff, E.R., Connolly, R.C., and Woolf,

A.L.: Cerebellar medulloblastoma occurring in brothers. *Acta Neuropathol* (Berl), *8:*104–107, 1967.

585. Joynt, R.J., and Perret, G.E.: Meningiomas in a mother and daughter. Cases without evidence of neurofibromatosis. *Neurology* (Minneap), *11:*164–165, 1961.

586. Joynt, R.J., and Perret, G.E.: Familial meningiomas. *J Neurol Neurosurg Psychiatry, 28:*163–164, 1965.

587. Gaist, G., and Piazza, G.: Meningiomas in two members of the same family (with no evidence of neurofibromatosis). *J Neurosurg, 16:*110–113, 1959.

588. Sahar, A.: Familial occurrence of meningiomas. *J Neurosurg, 23:*444–445, 1965.

589. Wagman, A.D., Weiss, E.K., and Riggs, H.E.: Hyperplasia of the skull associated with intra-osseous meningioma in the absence of gross tumor. Report of three cases. *J Neuropathol Exp Neurol, 19:*111–115, 1960.

590. Grunert, V., Horcajada, J., and Sunder-Plassmann, M.: Familiäres Auftreten intrakranieller Meningeome. *Wien Med Wochenschr, 120:*807–808, 1970.

591. Bromowicz, J., Araszkiewicz, H., and Kinderman, B.: Familial occurrence of neoplasms of the central nervous system. *Neurol Neurochir Pol, 5:*721–725, 1971. (Pol)

592. Komminoth, R., Woringer, E., Baumgartner, J., Braun, J.P., and Le Maistre, D.: Papillome intraventriculaire familial. Caractéristiques angiographiques. *Neurochirurgie, 11:*267–272, 1965.

593. Chateau, R., de Rougemont, J., Groslambert, R., Barge, M., Pasqlier, B., and Faure, H.: A propos des tumeurs cérébrales familiales (méningiome fibroblastique et hémangioblastome solitaire du cervelet). *J Med Lyon, 52:*675–678, 1971.

594. Myers, R.N., Austin, G.M., Walker, A.E., and Gallagher, J.P.: Solitary spinal cord tumors occurring in multiple members of a family. *J Neurosurg, 17:*783–787, 1960.

595. Blaauw, G., and Schenk, V.W.D.: Cervical cord tumor in two haemophiliac brothers. *J Neurol Sci, 14:*409–416, 1971.

596. Bergland, R.M.: Congenital intraspinal extradural cyst. Report of three cases in one family. *J Neurosurg, 28:*495–499, 1968.

597. Clark, J.V.: Familial occurrence of cavernous angiomata of the brain. *J Neurol Neurosurg Psychiatry, 33:*871–876, 1970.

598. Hardy, P.C., and Nesbit, M.E., Jr.: Familial neuroblastoma: report of a kindred with a high incidence of infantile tumors. *J Pediatr, 80:*74–77, 1972.

599. Feingold, M., Gheradi, G.J., and Simons, C.: Familial neuroblastoma and trisomy 13. *Am J Dis Child, 121:*451, 1971.

600. Chatten, J., and Voorhess, M.L.: Familial neuroblastoma. Report of a kindred with multiple disorders, including neuroblastomas in four siblings. *N Engl J Med, 277:*1230–1236, 1967.

601. Wong, K.-Y., Hanenson, I.B., and Lampkin, B.C.: Familial neuroblastoma. *Am J Dis Child, 121:*415–416, 1971.

602. Griffin, M.E., and Bolande, R.P.: Familial neuroblastoma with regression and maturation to ganglioneurofibroma. *Pediatrics, 43:*377–382, 1969.

603. Ullrich, R.: Sympathikogoniome und Vererblichkeit maligner Geschwülste. *Schweiz Med Wochenschr, 100:*749–751, 1970.

604. Koch, G.: Beitrag zur Erblichkeit der Hirngeschwülste (Vorläufige Mitteilung). *Acta Genet Med Gemellol* (Roma), *3:*170–191, 1954.

605. Norris, F.D., and Jackson, E.W.: Childhood cancer deaths in California-born twins. A further report on types of cancer found. *Cancer, 25:*212–218, 1970.

606. Harvald, B., and Hauge, M.: Heredity of cancer elucidated by a study of unselected twins. *JAMA, 186:*749–753, 1963.

607. Miller, R.W.: Deaths from childhood cancer in sibs. *N Engl J Med, 279:*122–126, 1968.

608. Harvald, B., and Hauge, M.: On the heredity of glioblastoma. *J Natl Cancer Inst., 17:*289–296, 1956.

609. Hauge, M., and Harvald, B.: Studies in the etiology of intracranial tumours. *Acta Psychiatr Neurol Scand, 35:*163–170, 1960.

610. Hauge, M., and Harvald, B.: Genetics in intracranial tumours. *Acta Genet, 7:*573–591, 1957.

611. De Weerdt, C.J., and Schut, T.: Some aspects of heredity of brain tumours. *Psychiatr Neurol Neurochir, 75:*293–298, 1972.

612. Metzel, E.: Betrachtungen zur Genetik der

familiären Gliome. *Acta Genet Med Gemellol* (Roma), *13:*124–131, 1964.

613. Pass, K.E.: Erbpathologische Untersuchungen in Familien von Hirntumorkranken. *Z Gesamte Neurol Psychiatr, 161:*204–211, 1938.

614. Nowell, P.C.. Chromosome changes in primary tumors. *Progr Exp Tumor Res, 7:* 83–103, 1965.

615. Miles, C.P.: Chromosomal alterations in cancer. *Med Clin North Am, 50:*875–885, 1966.

616. Zang, K.D., and Singer, H.: The cytogenetics of human tumors. *Angew Chem* (Engl), *7:* 709–718, 1968.

617. Sandberg, A.A., and Hossfeld, D.K.: Chromosomal abnormalities in human neoplasia. *Annu Rev Med, 21:*379–408, 1970.

618. de Grouchy, J., and de Nava, C.: A chromosomal theory of carcinogenesis. *Ann Intern Med, 69:*381–391, 1968.

619. Porter, I.H., Benedict, W.F., Brown, C.D., and Paul, B.: Recent advances in molecular pathology: a review. Some aspects of chromosome changes in cancer. *Exp Mol Pathol, 11:*340–367, 1969.

620. O'Riordan, M.L., Langlands, A.O., and Harnden, D.G.: Further studies on the frequency of constitutional chromosome abnormalities in patients with malignant disease. *Eur J Cancer, 8:*373–379, 1972.

621. Nowell, P.C., and Morris, H.P.: Chromosomes of "minimal deviation" hepatomas: a further report on diploid tumors. *Cancer Res, 29:*969–970, 1969.

622. Källén, B., and Levan, A.: Chromosomes in man, with special reference to neuropathological disorders. In Tedeschi, C.G., (Ed.): *Neuropathology: Methods and Diagnosis.* Boston, Little, Brown, 1970, pp. 547–582.

623. Bicknell, J.M.: Chromosome studies of human brain tumors. *Neurology* (Minneap), *17:*485–490, 1967.

624. Mark, J.: Chromosomal characteristics of neurogenic tumors in children. *Acta Cytol* (Baltimore), *14:*510–518, 1970.

625. Cox, D.: Chromosome studies in 12 solid tumours from children. *Br J Cancer, 22:* 402–414, 1968.

626. Conen, P.E., and Falk, R.E.: Chromosome studies on cultured tumors of nervous tissue origin. *Acta Cytol* (Baltimore), *11:* 86–91, 1967.

627. Singer, H., and Zang, K.D.: Cytologische und cytogenetische Untersuchungen an Hirntumoren. I. Die Chromosomenpathologie des menschlichen Meningeoms. *Humangenetik, 9:*172–184, 1970.

628. Zang, K.D., and Singer, H.: Chromosomal constitution of meningiomas. *Nature* (Lond), *216:*84–85, 1967.

629. Mark, J.: Chromosomal patterns in human meningiomas. *Eur J Cancer, 6:*489–498, 1970.

630. Zankl, H., and Zang, K.D.: Cytological and cytogenetical studies on brain tumors. IV. Identification of the missing G chromosome in human meningiomas as no. 22 by fluorescence technique. *Humangenetik, 14:* 167–169, 1972.

631. Zankl, H., and Zang, K.D.: Cytological and cytogenetical studies on brain tumors. III. Ph¹-like chromosomes in human meningiomas. *Humangenetik, 12:*42–49, 1971.

632. Zankl, H., Singer, H., and Zang, K.D.: Cytological and cytogenetical studies on brain tumors. II. Hyperdiploidy, a rare event in human primary meningiomas. *Humangenetik, 11:*253–257, 1971.

633. Mark, J.: Two benign intracranial human tumours with an abnormal chromosomal picture. *Acta Neuropathol* (Berl), *14:*174–184, 1969.

634. Mark, J.: Chromosomal aberrations and their relation to malignancy in meningiomas: a meningioma with ring chromosomes. *Acta Pathol Microbiol Scand* (A) *79:*193–200, 1971.

635. Hansteen, I.-L.: Chromosome studies in glial tumours. *Eur J Cancer, 3:*183–191, 1967.

636. Lubs, H.A., Jr., and Salmon, J.H.: The chromosomal complement of human solid tumors. II. Karyotypes of glial tumors. *J Neurosurg, 22:*160–168, 1965.

637. Wilson, C.B., Kaufmann, L., and Barker, M.: Chromosome analysis of glioblastoma multiforme. *Neurology* (Minneap), *20:* 821–828, 1970.

638. Mark, J., and Granberg, I.: The chromosomal aberration of double-minutes in three gliomas. *Acta Neuropathol* (Berl), *16*:194–204, 1970.

639. Kucheria, K.: Double minute chromatin bodies in a sub-ependymal glioma. *Br J Cancer, 22*:696–697, 1968.

640. Lubs, H.A., Jr., Salmon, J.H., and Flanigan, S.: Studies of a glial tumor with multiple minute chromosomes. *Cancer, 19*:591–599, 1966.

641. Levan, A., Manolov, G., and Clifford, P.: Chromosomes of a human neuroblastoma: a new case with accessory minute chromosomes. *J Natl Cancer Inst, 41*:1377–1387, 1968.

642. Sandberg, A.A., Sakurai, M., and Holdsworth, R.N.: Chromosomes and causation of human cancer and leukemia. VIII. DMS chromosomes in a neuroblastoma. *Cancer, 29*:1671–1679, 1972.

643. Brewster, D.J., and Garrett, J.V.: Chromosome abnormalities in neuroblastoma. *J Clin Pathol, 18*:167–169, 1965.

644. Wakonig-Vaartaja, T., Helson, L., Baren, A., Koss, L.G., and Murphy, M.L.: Cytogenetic observations in children with neuroblastoma. *Pediatrics, 47*:839–843, 1971.

645. Whang-Peng, J., and Bennett, J.M.: Cytogenic studies in metastatic neuroblastoma. *Am J Dis Child, 115*:703–708, 1968.

646. Makino, S., Sofuni, T., and Mitani, M.: Cytological studies on tumors. XLIII. A chromosome condition in effusion cells from a patient with neuroblastoma. *Gann, 56*:127–133, 1965.

647. Nakagomi, H.: Cytogenetic studies in pediatrics. Report 1. Chromosomes in childhood malignancies. *Acta Paediatr Jap, 69*:651–667, 1965. (Jap)

648. Gagnon, J., Dupal, M.-F., and Katyk-Longtin, N.: Anomalies chromosomiques dans une observation de sympathome congénital. *Rev Can Biol, 21*:145–155, 1962.

649. Donner, L., and Bubeník, J.: Minute chromatin bodies in two mouse tumours induced in vivo by Rous sarcoma virus. *Folia Biol* (Praha), *14*:86–88, 1968.

650. Mitelman, F., Levan, G., and Mark, J.: The origin of double-minutes in a Rous rat sarcoma. *Acta Pathol Microbiol Scand,* (A), *80*:428–429, 1972.

651. Olinici, C.D.: Double minute chromatin bodies in a case of ovarian ascitic carcinoma. *Br J Cancer, 25*:350–353, 1971.

652. Granberg, I., and Mark, J.: The chromosomal aberration of double-minutes in a human embryonic rhabdomyosarcoma. *Acta Cytol* (Baltimore), *15*:42–45, 1971.

653. Cox, D., Yuncken, C., and Spriggs, A.I.: Minute chromatin bodies in malignant tumours of childhood. *Lancet, 2*:55–58, 1965.

654. Mark, J.: Chromosomal analysis of a human retinoblastoma. *Acta Ophthalmol* (Kbh), *48*:124–135, 1970.

655. Shimada, K., Oda, I., and Kobayashi, M.: Chromosome studies in retinoblastoma. Report 1. On the frequent incidence of the tumor cells in tetraploid range. *Acta Soc Ophthalmol Jap, 71*:2014–2019, 1967. (Jap)

656. Mark, J.: Chromosomal characteristics of secondary human brain tumours. *Eur J Cancer, 8*:399–407, 1972.

657. Viale, G.L.: Transfer RNA and transfer RNA methylase in human brain tumors. *Cancer Res, 31*:605–608, 1971.

658. Mintz, B., Custer, R.P., and Donnelly, A.J.: Genetic diseases and developmental defects analyzed in allophenic mice. *Int Rev Exp Pathol, 10*:143–179, 1971.

659. Fumagalli, R., and Paoletti, P.: Sterol test for human brain tumors: relationship with different oncotypes. *Neurology* (Minneap), *21*:1149–1156, 1971.

660. Knudson, A.G., Jr., and Strong, L.C.: Mutation and cancer: neuroblastoma and pheochromocytoma. *Am J Hum Genet, 24*:514–532, 1972.

CHAPTER 18

HEREDITY AND COLON CANCER

HENRY T. LYNCH, JANE LYNCH, AND HODA GUIRGIS

Introduction

ADENOCARCINOMA OF THE colon is the most commonly occurring visceral malignant neoplasm in the United States, accounting for nearly 1,000 deaths per week.[1] The first report of successful surgical excision of a cancer of the rectum occurred in 1833,[2] and since then substantial progress has been achieved with this therapeutic modality. The control of this lesion will undoubtedly be aided significantly when cancer detection programs by physicians lead toward the recognition of earlier cases,[3] and educational programs for the layman concentrate on recognition of early signs and symptoms of cancer. However, slightly more than half of the victims of intestinal cancer continue to die of their disease each year in spite of efforts toward improved surgical control and cancer detection campaigns. It is hoped that newer methods of cancer detection might improve survival statistics. One of the more promising of these is the production of carcinoembryonic antigen (CEA) by carcinomas arising in the endodermally-derived epithelium of the digestive tract. This antigen was first described by Gold and his associates in 1965;[4,5] later, they developed a radioimmunoassay for detecting the presence of CEA in blood serum.[6] This antigen is also found in cancers arising in the esophagus, stomach, duodenum, small bowel, pancreas, breast and lung, though it is found in higher concentrations in cancers arising in the colon.[6] It is present in the fetus during the first two trimesters of pregnancy and is also found in the mother during that time. It disappears during and after the third trimester of pregnancy. The antigen has not been found in benign tumors of the digestive tract, in nondigestive tumors, nor in cancer that has metastasized to the digestive tract. These facts have led to the conclusion that the antigen arises primarily from endodermal cancer.[7]

Although Moore and associates found a high degree of reliability in detection of cancer of the colon utilizing CEA they also found that the antigen was less specific than originally thought since they found positive tests in alcoholic liver disease, alcoholic pancreatic disease and carcinoma of the lung.[7] Nugent and Hansen[8] found 36 percent false negative results utilizing CEA assay and concluded that more experience with this assay will be necessary before valid conclusions can be drawn.

The magnitude and seriousness of colon cancer is such that every possible measure should be employed for earlier detection with a goal of improved cancer control. Cancer genetics harbors a potentially powerful cancer control tool which could be applied profitably in several hereditary colon cancer problems including familial polyposis coli and Gardner's syndrome. Therefore, in this chapter, we shall delineate a number of types of colon cancer in which hereditary factors play a part.

Genetics and Colon Cancer

In considering the role of hereditary factors in colon cancer, one must differentiate carefully between so-called sporadic occurrences, site specific colon cancer in the absence of distinguishing clinical signs consistent with cancer predisposing diseases, i.e. ulcerative colitis, or syndromes, familial colon cancer in association with malignant neoplasms such as breast cancer, and the several specific genetic syndromes in which colon malignancy is manifested.

Table 18-I provides a listing including the important clinical features and mode of inheritance (when this is known) of the several clinical disorders which are associated with adenocarcinoma of the colon. One

TABLE 18-I
COLON CANCER IN HEREDITARY DISORDERS

Syndrome	Mode of Inheritance	Anatomical Location and Pathology of Polyps or Cancer or Both	Associated Clinical Features
Familial Polyposis Coli	Autosomal Dominant	Colon, adenomatous polyps	None
Gardner's Syndrome	Autosomal Dominant	Colon, adenomatous polyps; adenomatous polyps may occasionally be found in the small intestine and stomach	Soft tissue (sebaceous cysts, fibromas) and bone lesions (osteomas of manible, sphenoid, and maxilla). Rare occurrences thyroid carcinoma and retroperitoneal sarcoma.
Peutz-Jeghers Syndrome	Autosomal Dominant	Entire gastrointestinal tract, except esophagus, harbors polyps which may show malignant degeneration (cancer issue remains controversial in spite of recent documentation). Hamartomas of muscularis mucosa.	Melanin spots of oral and vaginal mucosa and distal portions of fingers. Ovarian cancer excess.
Solitary Polyps	Possible Autosomal Dominant	Colon	None
Ulcerative Colitis	Possible Autosomal Dominant in Certain Families	Colon	Occasionally arthritis, systemic manifestations, and psychological aberrations.
Juvenile Polyposis Coli	Autosomal Dominant	Hamartomatous polyps of colon; increased occurrence of adenomatous polyps and adenocarcinoma in relatives; connective tissue abnormality.	None
Cancer Family Syndrome	Possible Autosomal Dominant	Colon	Various adenocarcinomas, particularly of endometrium; multiple primary malignant neoplasms; early age at onset of cancer.
Turcot's Syndrome	Autosomal Recessive	Colon and central nervous system; adenomatous polyps.	None
Generalized Gastrointestinal Juvenile Polyposis	Not Established	Stomach, small and large bowel.	None.
Generalized Gastrointestinal Adenomatous Polyposis	Possible Autosomal Dominant	Stomach, small and large bowel; adenomatous polyps.	Desmoid reported.
Cronkite-Canada Syndrome	No known familial reports	Stomach, small and large bowel; adenomatous polyps.	Skin pigmentation, atrophy of nails, hypoproteinemia.
Familial Combined Breast and Colon Cancer	Possible Autosomal Dominant	Colon and breast.	None.

notes that subclassifications of these disorders may be made readily, i.e. one might
group colon cancer with the so-called polyposis syndromes and thereby include familial
polyposis coli in the absence of other associated physical stigmata, or it may be
grouped with those disorders which have
such distinguishing phenotypic signs as those
which occur in Gardner's syndrome, Peutz-
Jegher's syndrome, Turcut's syndrome, Old-
field's syndrome, Gorlin's syndrome, and the
Cronkhite-Canada syndrome. In turn, we
may conveniently subclassify colon cancer
in terms of several other clinical syndromes
with hereditary etiology in the absence of
polyposis coli, such as the cancer family
syndrome (see Chapter 19), and in association with breast cancer in certain families
(see Chapter 20). Finally, increased incidences of adenocarcinoma of the colon may
occur in certain families on a site-specific
basis, occasionally associated with multiple
primary malignant neoplasms, and transmitted in certain incidences in an autosomal dominant pattern.

Polyposis Coli Syndromes

Adenomatous polyps in familial polyposis
coli and in the several syndromes that are
associated with polyposis coli, do not appear
to differ histologically from the type of
solitary adenomatous polyps frequently
found in adults. The individual adenomatous polyps in polyposis coli appear to be
subject to the same frequency of malignant
transformation as the isolated discrete
polyps. However, the inordinately high colon
cancer risk in patients with multiple polyposis coli is seemingly in direct proportion
to the presence of vast numbers of polyps.
Fortunately, it is relatively simple to make
a diagnosis of familial polyposis coli, particularly when the physician is aware of its
presence in other members of a family.[9]

We shall outline briefly some of the important clinical characteristics of the above-
named syndromes and provide evidence for
the role of heredity in these disorders.

Familial Polyposis Coli

The familial nature of polyposis coli was
first recognized by Cripps in 1882[10] and
was reaffirmed by Lockhart-Mummery in
1925[11] and later by Dukes.[12] An autosomal dominant mode of inheritance was
established by Cockayne in 1927.[13] The
disease is characterized by the occurrence
of numerous adenomatous polyps which
may *carpet* the entire colon and rectum.
The propensity for neoplastic transformation to adenocarcinoma in these polyps is
exceedingly high. Indeed, it is estimated that
40 percent of patients with polyposis already
will show evidence of cancer when first seen
by a physician and that 50 percent of these
patients will develop cancer by age 30.[14]

While the colon and rectum are the major
sites for polyps in familial polyposis coli, it
is not generally appreciated that adenomatous polyps may also occur in the upper
gastrointestinal tract. Morson[15] stated categorically that polyps do *not* occur in the
stomach or small bowel in familial polyposis
coli. He based this conviction on his experience and that of others at St. Mark's
Hospital. However, on rare occasions, patients with familial polyposis coli have been
known to have polyps involving the upper
gastrointestinal tract. For example, Hoffman
and Goligher[16] described three cases of
familial polyposis coli in which both the
stomach and small bowel contained adenomatous polyps: 1) a 20-year-old male with
multiple polyposis coli had multiple polyps
in the antrum of the stomach and the duodenum, confirmed by gastroscopy. No other
member of the family had evidence of familial
polyposis coli. This patient had no signs of
Gardner's syndrome; 2) the father of an

18-year-old female with familial polyposis coli died of carcinoma of the large intestine secondary to polyposis coli. Two of her brothers also had familial polyposis coli. The patient had many small polyps in the stomach but none in the small intestine. This observation was confirmed by gastroscopy. None of her relatives showed any features of Gardner's syndrome; and 3) a 24-year-old male presented initially because of swelling in his jaw, at which time radiologic examination revealed multiple osteomas of the mandible and melorheostosis of both fibulae.[16] He also had many sebaceous cysts on his face and trunk. The patient had multiple polyps of the rectum. At gastroscopy, multiple sessile polyps were seen in the antrum of the stomach. Because of the osteomas and sebaceous cysts, Gardner's syndrome was considered. The authors[16] reviewed the world literature for cases of familial polyposis coli showing concurrent gastric and small intestinal polyps. They found 14 references on the subject and in 8 of these reports, patients showed features of Gardner's syndrome.

The frequency with which polyps of the upper gastrointestinal tract occur in patients with familial polyposis coli is not known. This information is evidently unavailable at the present time since thorough examination of the entire gastrointestinal tract in patients with familial polyposis coli would be necessary in order to prove this association, and this is not carried out routinely. However, in Gardner's syndrome, the association of polyposis coli with upper gastrointestinal tract polyps has been well known and indeed Gardner himself[17] reported occasional examples of stomach polyps in this syndrome, and McKusick[18] also stated that adenomatous polyps may occur in any area of the gastrointestinal tract in patients with Gardner's syndrome. Finally, Duncan, *et al.*,[19] in their literature review, found 83 patients with Gardner's syndrome of whom approx-

imately 10 to 12 percent had concurrent polyps involving small bowel, including the duodenum. It is not known how frequently patients with familial polyposis coli and concurrent polyps of the upper gastrointestinal tract develop cancer of the upper gastrointestinal tract. Malignant lesions have been reported in patients with duodenal polyposis;[19-21] and a single report revealed that a 16-year-old boy had polyposis coli and died of carcinoma of the stomach.[22]

Because of our meager knowledge concerning upper gastrointestinal polyposis and malignant degeneration in patients with familial polyposis coli, it is difficult to establish guidelines for managing patients with familial polyposis coli. However, Duncan[19] recommends a barium meal in addition to proctosigmoidoscopy and a barium enema. All patients found to have polyps of the upper gastrointestinal tract should then be more critically evaluated and whenever possible, simple removal of polyps of the upper gastrointestinal tract should be performed. In one of the patients reported by Hoffman and Goligher[16] polypectomy through a gastrotomy incision was performed. However, this same patient developed additional polyps 18 months after this procedure. These authors concluded that the only means of preventing the occurrence of polyposis of the stomach in such a patient would be through radical surgery, but they were reluctant to recommend prophylactic total gastrectomy because of mortality and morbidity statistics. Therefore, they prefer to keep such patients under close observation.

Gardner's Syndrome

In 1912, Devic and Bussy[23] described a woman with multiple polyposis of the colon, sebaceous cysts of the scalp, subcutaneous lipomas, and osteomas of the mandible. Several isolated cases have been reported which were somewhat similar to that of Devic and Bussy.[24-26] Eldon Gardner was the first scientist to characterize these findings as a hereditary syndrome[17,26,27] and to show that it was an autosomal dominantly inherited disorder which included the combination of polyposis coli,[28,29] osteomas,[30,31] and cutaneous manifestations.[17] By 1967, approximately 118 cases of this syndrome had been reported in the world literature.[32]

Watne[33] has provided some of the most recent descriptions of the syndrome, many of these having been based upon his own study of several large unrelated kindreds. Figure 18-1 depicts the genealogy of 4 of these unrelated families with Gardner's syndrome.

Diagnostic features of the syndrome vary widely when families are carefully studied. Sebaceous cysts of the skin represent the most common soft-tissue tumors in this syndrome. Indeed, Gardner and Richards[17] have emphasized the relationship between the sebaceous cysts and polyps of the colon. The occurrence of large cysts around the face and neck are considered an important clinical characteristic of the syndrome (Fig. 18-2).

The most frequently observed bone abnormalities in Gardner's syndrome are benign osteomatoses. These comprise dense, bony proliferations, variable in size, which may involve almost all areas of the skeletal system (Figs. 18-3 and 18-4). Localized cortical thickening of the long tubular bones was the most common abnormality found in a bone survey of Gardner's syndrome families.[34] The frontal bone was the most frequent site of osteoma in the skull. Dental abnormalities have also been described including supernumerary and unerupted teeth.

Any patient who develops soft-tissue tumors and/or osteomas, and who has a family history of Gardner's syndrome, should undergo a careful evaluation of the colon for the presence of polyps. In Watne's experience, polyps in adults have never been diagnosed by barium enema which were not also visible at proctoscopy. However, he has observed the reverse situation in children in whom polyps have been identified only by barium enema after the identification of soft-tissue and bony tumors. On the other hand, individuals with a family history of Gardner's syndrome have been found to have soft-tissue tumors and no other manifestation of the disease when they reached the fourth and fifth decades of life.[33]

Gardner's syndrome should be searched for in children of an affected parent since colon polyps have been identified in 16 patients under the age of 15. In one report,[35] multiple colon polyps were observed in a four month old infant. These polyps showed the same characteristics in terms of biologic behavior and location as those polyps found in patients with simple familial polyposis coli. Thus, the polyps are most prevalent in the rectum, but they may also be scattered throughout the remainder of the colon predominantly at one or both colon flexures. The disease may start with one or several polyps and progress to carpet the entire colon with adenomatous polyps. Figure 18-5 shows a gross specimen of the colon from a patient with Gardner's syndrome. It is believed that there is a 100 percent potential for malignant degeneration of polyps in these patients if they are untreated just as has been postulated for simple multiple polyposis coli.[33] When cancers develop, they are typical adenocarcinomas and are often multiple. One such patient[7] developed five synchronous colon carcinomas at age 14 and four years later developed adenocarcinoma of the Ampulla of Vater; and 13 years following his initial colon surgery, he developed a transitional cell carcinoma of the bladder.

Other lesions in Gardner's syndrome have included anaplastic carcinoma of the mandible,[37] and fibrous tumor of the parotid

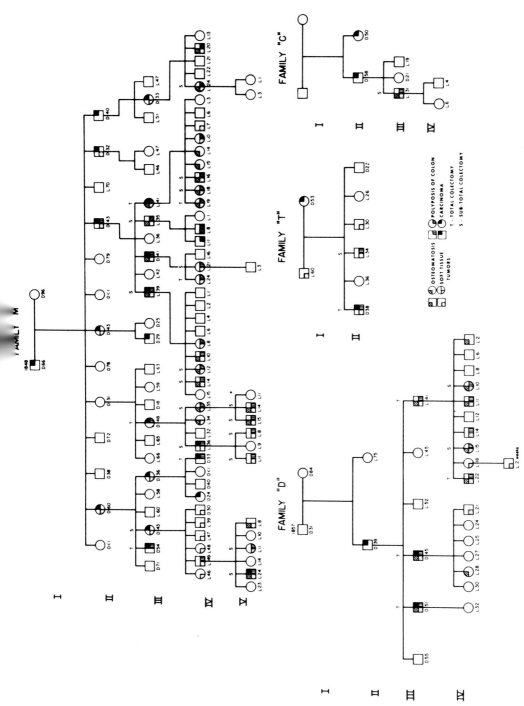

Figure 18–1. Watne's pedigree of four families with Gardner's syndrome (with permission of A. Watne, M.D.).

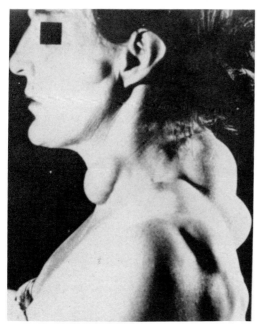

Figure 18–2. Large cysts of the face and neck in Gardner's syndrome. (Permission for republication of this figure was granted by Alvin Watne, M.D.).

gland in a 9-year-old patient.[38] Camiel and associates[39] reported pigmented nevi in one of their patients with the syndrome who had developed thyroid carcinoma nine years prior to the diagnosis of Gardner's syndrome. This patient's father had colorectal polyposis and a brain tumor. Retroperitoneal fibrosis and fibrodysplasias have also been described in Gardner's syndrome.[33] The retroperitoneal fibrosis and development of desmoid tumors and fibrosarcomas following colon surgery have posed a serious complication and are a significant aspect of Gardner's syndrome.[33] Surgery is the treatment of choice for these tumors; radiation has not proved to be of any value.[40] To treat colonic polyposis, Watne recommends subtotal colectomy with ileoproctostomy immediately upon diagnosis, dependent, of course, upon the degree of involvement and the dependability of the patient. Watne has never observed spontaneous regression of

the colon polyps without some type of surgical intervention.[33] When the rectum is extensively involved with polyps and/or cancer, or there is no regression of rectal polyps following ileoproctostomy. Total proctocolectomy with ileostomy is strongly recommended.

Turcot's Syndrome

Turcot, *et al.*[41] described a brother and sister with polyposis of the colon which progressed to adenocarcinoma. Autopsy examination of the boy at age 18 revealed medulloblastoma invading the medulla spinalis in addition to polyposis. Autopsy examination of his sister at age 21 revealed a glioblastoma of the left frontal lobe and a small chromophobe adenoma of the hypo-

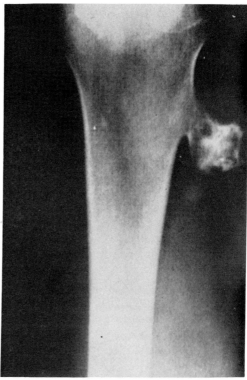

Figure 18–3. Benign osteoma in Gardner's syndrome.

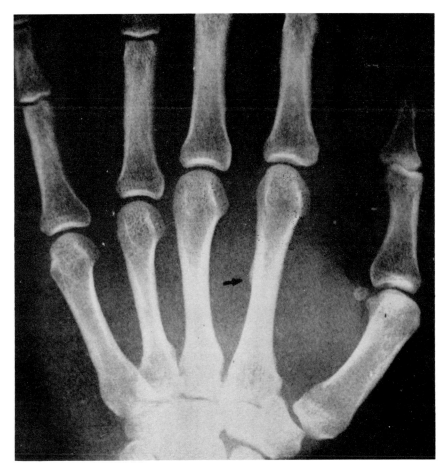

Figure 18–4. Benign osteoma in Gardner's syndrome.

physis. There was no evidence of gastro-intestinal or central nervous system disorders in other relatives.

A second family was reported by Baughman and associates.[42] The family comprised a sibship of six (2 boys and 4 girls). A 12-year-old girl presented with a history of seizure, frontal headache, and diarrhea. Her father was age 47 and her mother, 41. There was no consanguinity. Her sisters were ages 21, 6, and 5 years and her brothers were ages 25 and 12. This girl had a single café-au-lait spot on her back and a pigmented nevus on her right leg. Neurologic examination indicated the presence of an intra-cranial mass lesion. Sigmoidoscopy disclosed 2 polyps in the rectal amulla; one of these was a villous adenoma located 10 cm above the anal ring. She died, and at autopsy a larger polyp showed villous hyperplasia and clusters of atypical cells invading the muscularis mucosa. Brain sections revealed a well circumscribed, infiltrating tumor of the white matter of both hemispheres. Histological diagnosis revealed glioblastoma multiforme. The tumor seemed to be multicentric since there was also an increased number of hyperchromatic glial cells in the medulla and in sections from the dorsal spinal cord.

Her 25-year-old brother was admitted to the hospital with seizures and progressive right hemiparesis. Five years previously, he had undergone surgery for carcinoma of the colon. Pigmented nevi were abundant over the back and abdomen. Brain scan and left carotid arteriogram revealed a tumor of the left temporal lobe. He died and at autopsy approximately 2 dozen polyps, 5 to 30 mm in diameter were found in the colon and rectum. Two of the polyps were examined. One showed polypoid hyperplasia and the other malignant change with formation of signet cells invading the stump. Brain sections disclosed an infiltrating tumor beginning at the level of the head of the caudate nucleus and spreading through the isthmus of the temporal lobe and into the

white matter of the temporal lobe proper. The histologic diagnosis was glioblastoma multiforme.

A 12-year-old brother was hospitalized for convulsions and headache. Four café-au-lait spots were noted. At craniotomy there was a subcortical, grayish-red cystic tumor. The histologic diagnosis was glioblastoma multiforme. He died at home and an autopsy was not performed. During his life, he had never received diagnostic examinations of the bowel.

A 21-year-old sister was hospitalized following two generalized seizures. An electro-encephalogram showed slow and sharp activity from the left hemisphere and a brain scan indicated a left posterior frontal tumor. This was partially resected and a histologic

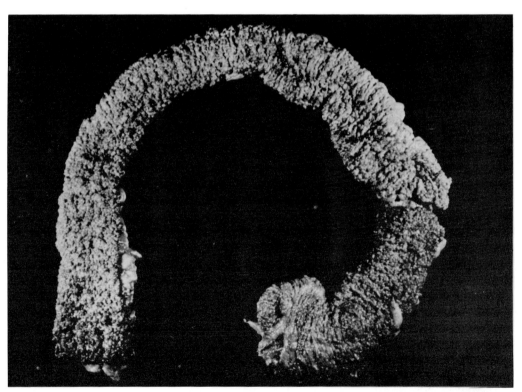

Figure 18–5. A section of a gross specimen of colon carpeted with polyps in polyposis coli.

diagnosis was made of glioblastoma multiforme. Sigmoidoscopy revealed two tiny polyps but no other details were reported.

Medical history of 76 family members through 5 generations indicated only one case of brain tumor. This was a posterior fossa ependymoma in a three-year-old girl who was a maternal second cousin of the siblings. No additional cases of polyposis and no occurrences of neurofibromatosis were reported in this family.

In summary, three of four affected siblings showed concurrent glioma and polyposis while the fourth had only a glioma.

Findings in Turcot's[41] family and that of Baughman, *et al.*[42] are consistent with an autosomal recessive factor. Similarities between these two families include the occurrence of gliomas, polyposis coli, similar age of onset, and the fact that neither brain tumors nor colonic polyps appeared in the parents of either of these sibships.

Peutz-Jeghers Syndrome

The cardinal features of this disorder include intestinal polyposis and a distinctive type of melanin pigmentation of the oral mucosa, occasionally the vaginal mucosa, and the distal portions of the fingers (Fig. 18–6). Intestinal polyps may be found at any level of the gastrointestinal tract, exclusive of the esophagus. About 36 percent of the polyps are found in the colon and rectum. The polyps have usually been considered hamartomas and the question of malignant change in them has been controversial. In a review of the subject, Lynch[43] was able to document several cases of metastatic adenocarcinoma arising from malignant polyps in patients with this disease. A woman was reported recently in whom adenocarcinoma was resected from a polyp in the transverse colon.[44] Ovarian cancer

may also occur in the syndrome[45] (See Chapt. 23).

It is interesting that polyposis of the colon is an integral component of the several disorders mentioned. McKusick[18] concludes that these conditions are probably nonallelic and represent distinct genetic entities.

Juvenile Polyposis Coli

Juvenile polyposis coli is an inherited disorder (autosomal dominant) wherein colon polyps are believed to represent hamartomatous structures and are not thought to be precancerous.[46,47] However, an increased frequency of colorectal cancer and adenomatous polyposis coli in relatives of probands with juvenile polyposis coli has occurred in several families.[47] The gross appearance of polyps in juvenile polyposis coli may be strikingly similar to those found in adenomatous polyps in the several multiple adenomatous polyposis syndromes. Histologic examination is therefore mandatory in order to make a critical differentiation.

The presenting symptom in juvenile polyposis coli has almost invariably been rectal bleeding. The average age of onset has been three to six years; however, this has shown considerable variability. In occasional patients bleeding may be accompanied by protrusion of a polyp through the anus. Pink or red-stained mucous following a bowel movement is also a frequent finding. Intussusception of a polyp(s) with obstruction occurs rarely. Polyps may also slough giving rise to consternation in some patients.

Treatment of juvenile polyposis coli is conservative, as opposed to therapy in adenomatous polyposis coli problems. Gathright and Coffer[47a] strongly believe that radical removal of the colon is not indicated since malignant degeneration does not occur in the polyps associated with juvenile polyposis coli.

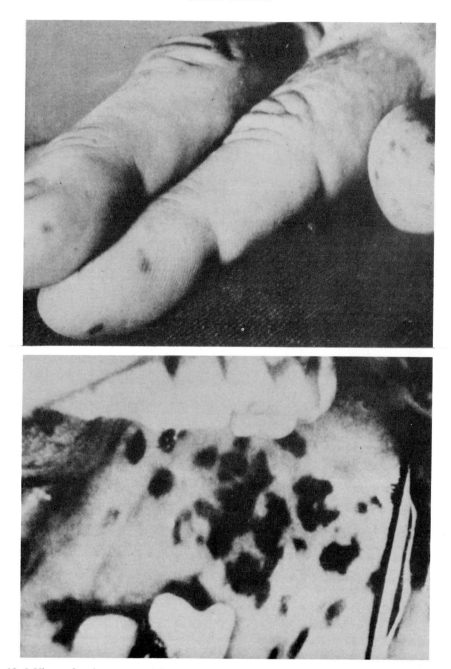

Figure 18–6. Views of oral mucosa and fingers of a patient with Peutz-Jeghers syndrome. Reprinted by permission of The Williams and Wilkins Company, from Butterworth and Strean: *Clinical Genodermatology.*

Generalized Gastrointestinal Adenomatous Polyposis

Adenomatous polyps involving the entire gastrointestinal tract and in the absence of other distinguishing phenotypic signs are rare. An autosomal dominant mode of inheritance has been suggested and cancer has been shown to be associated with this condition, though the exact relationship is not known. Yonemoto, *et al.*[48] reported three patients with generalized polyposis involving the entire gastrointestinal tract; an invasive carcinoma of the rectum was found in one of these patients.

Generalized adenomatous polyposis of the entire gastrointestinal tract differs from familial polyposis coli by virtue of the fact that polyps are not restricted to the colon and rectum. However, the disease is similar in that the polyps are adenomatous and the genetic mechanism appears to be the same, namely, that of an autosomal dominant factor. This condition is more rare than familial polyposis coli. Although the polyps in generalized adenomatous polyposis involve the entire gastrointestinal tract, there have been no reports of carcinoma developing in the stomach or small bowel, though, as mentioned, there is documentation of carcinoma of the rectum.

Cronkhite-Canada Syndrome

In the differential diagnosis of the polyposis coli syndromes, one must consider the relatively rarely occurring condition known as the Cronkhite-Canada syndrome. This syndrome comprises generalized gastrointestinal polyposis, pigmentation of the skin, loss or atrophy of the fingernails and toenails, alopecia, and hypoproteinemia.[49-54]

To date, the family history in patients with this disorder has been essentially negative. However, we must remember that only a relatively small number of cases have been described since the syndrome was first identified by Cronkhite and Canada in 1955.[49]

Hypoproteinemia is a frequent finding and labeled albumin studies have confirmed a protein-losing enteropathy.

The polyps described in this syndrome are adenomatous and are present throughout the entire gastrointestinal tract. Malignant transformation has not been reported in this disorder in spite of the fact that the polyps are adenomatous and not hamartomatous.

The mortality rate is high; death is usually secondary to malabsorption with associated cachexia. There is no specific treatment program, though recently Takahata, *et al.*[50] reported a rather dramatic clinical improvement manifested by cessation of diarrhea, increase of serum protein, and disappearance of pigmentation with regrowth of scalp hair, fingernails and toenails following the administration of 30 mg of prednisone daily.

Significance of Polyps of the Gastrointestinal Tract

The genetic significance of colon polyps may be clearcut in certain situations such as classicsl familial polyposis coli or it may be more complex as in other syndromes. One might ask the question, "How many polyps are necessary for one to make the diagnosis of familial polyposis coli? Is the family history invariably positive in patients predisposed to familial polyposis coli?" Unfortunately, there are no definitive answers to these important questions. For example, polyps of the colon are relatively common and it has been estimated that among patients over 35 years of age undergoing sigmoidoscopy as part of a routine examination, approximately 5 percent will show one or more polyps of the colon. However, authorities differ concerning the possibility of malignant transformation of polyps. Concerning hereditary aspects of discrete polyps, as opposed to myriad polyps carpeting the colon in polyposis coli, it should be noted that Woolf, *et al.*[54] found an incidence of 45.4 percent of discrete polyps in a single large family as opposed to the mentioned 5 percent occurrence in the general population. In addition, the pattern of inheritance in this family was consistent with a dominant factor. While findings of this type do not answer fully some of the questions we have raised, they certainly indicate that more study will be necessary in order to delineate more clearly the problems of phenotypic variability in the pattern and distribution of colon polyps as well as their etiologic considerations. One will more likely find fewer polyps in younger patients who may be destined later to develop the full-blown picture of familial polyposis coli and some of these may lack a positive family history of this disease. Findings in such patients may represent new mutations. A negative family history would, therefore, be misleading in such cases.

The important point in this discussion is that patients with familial adenomatous polyposis coli and/or conditions associated with it are highly susceptible to carcinoma of the colon (virtually 100 percent will develop colon cancer by age 50 unless a colectomy is performed), whereas patients with isolated or only several polyps, but lacking the true picture of familial adenomatous polyposis coli, will have a cancer risk which is significantly less, and therefore should not have to undergo the more radical surgical approach of colectomy. However, for sound medical management they should be followed closely, and depending upon the size and location of the polyps, it may be prudent to remove specific polyps surgically (see below).

Treatment of Patients with Gastrointestinal Polyps

The primary treatment of patients with familial polyposis coli is surgical removal of the colon once the diagnosis has been established. However, the choice of the specific surgical approach is controversial.[33] Some feel strongly that total colectomy is the best approach in the management of this disease. However, others favor subtotal colectomy and fulguration of the rectal stump for the prevention of cancer in this remaining portion of the colon. With respect to the latter operation, it has been suggested that no more than 10 cm of the rectum should remain. This amount of rectum would be sufficient for adequate rectal functioning. The major point in limiting the amount of rectum remaining is the fact that the shorter the stump, the less area requiring fulguration; there is evidence suggesting that a shorter rectal stump is associated with more frequent polyp regression; in turn this may be a factor inhibiting carcinomatous transformation.[55]

Carcinoma of the Colon in Conditions that are Not Associated with Multiple Polyposis of the Colon

Solitary Colon Polyps

One or more polyps of the rectum and colon, as opposed to myriad polyps in familial polyposis coli, occur in approximately 5 percent of individuals over 35 years of age. As mentioned, the malignant potential of these polyps has been a controversial issue.[56] It is not clear how often the development of solitary polyps of the colon and rectum may result from hereditary etiology. However, as mentioned in a study of one kindred with the condition and a high incidence of adenocarcinoma of the colon, Woolf, *et al.*[54,57] found solitary polyps in 25 (45%) of the adult members of one generation. Polyps also were found in relatives in the direct line of descent through several generations. The findings were consistent with an autosomal dominant mode of inheritance.

Carcinoma of the Colon in the Absence of Polyps

Adenocarcinoma of the colon in the absence of colon polyps or associated malignant neoplasms has been shown to occur frequently in certain families. Interestingly, the age at onset of malignant disease in these kindreds frequently is lower than that found in the general population.[58-61] Some of these families actually may be examples of the cancer family syndrome (see Chapter 19) Moertel, *et al.*[62] found an earlier age at onset of adenocarcinoma in relatives in a large series of patients with multiple primary malignant neoplasms of the colon (polyposis coli excluded); however, the overall frequency of adenocarcinoma in the relatives of these patients was not increased significantly over that in control groups.

Ulcerative Colitis

Ulcerative colitis results from an inflammatory reaction affecting the mucosa and submucosa of the colon and/or the rectum; so far as is known, it is not directly due to invasion of these tissues by viruses, bacteria, or parasites. Clinically, the patients initially emit an inflammatory exudate consisting of blood, pus, fibrin, or combinations of these materials which are excreted into the lumen of the bowel and may be mixed with unformed stool or may coat the normal stool, or it may even be excreted solely as an exudate. This disorder may involve the colon diffusely or it may be limited to the proximal colon at variable distances, i.e. so-called idiopathic proctocolitis. Mucosal alterations of the bowel frequently occur. In the majority of circumstances, ulcerative colitis is a chronic relapsing disease with cardinal initial symptoms consisting of diarrhea and bright red blood in the stool. However, as more is learned about this disease, one begins to appreciate the fact that an increasing spectrum of systemic manifesta-tions may be observed. These include abdominal pain, weight loss, fever, vomiting, hepatic lesions (Laennec's cirrhosis, biliary cirrhosis), renal lesions (renal lithiasis), eye lesions (uveitis and corneal ulcer), oral lesions (aphthous stomatitis, gingivitis, and pyostomatitis vegetans), cutaneous lesions (pyogenic toxic erythema, urticaria, erythema nodosum, erythema multiforme, and pyoderma gangrenosum), joint lesions (arthralgias, rheumatoid spondylitis, and so-called *colitic* arthritis), blood abnormalities, blood loss anemia, or anemia due to nutritional defects, fever, *toxicity*, drugs, etc., including coagulation defects with a tendency to hemorrhage which may result from vitamin K or C deficiency, and psychiatric abnormalities including neurotic manifestations, toxic, psychosis, depression, and schizophrenic episodes.[63] Etiology and pathogenesis of this disease, including the variety of manifestations remain an enigma, though autoimmune factors have received considerable attention recently.[63]

While carcinoma of the colon does not represent the most common complication of this disease, it occurs with sufficient frequency to warn both patient and physician about this ominous possibility.[64,65] Specifically, the cancer risk in patients with localized forms of ulcerative colitis such as occurs in idiopathic proctitis is small and probably is no greater than that found in the general population.[66] However, in patients with total or near total involvement of the colon, the risk for cancer may be exceedingly high and appears to correlate closely with the duration of the disease. For example, during the first ten years of symptoms of ulcerative colitis, the cancer risk is low and is in the order of approximately 0.4 percent per annum. However, after this decade, the annual risk rises sharply to 2 percent per annum during the second decade and to 5 percent per annum for the remainder of the patient's life.[65] Because of this cancer risk prophylactic colectomy is performed by many physicians who are concerned about cancer prevention in patients who have manifested this disease for a long period of time.

While etiology of ulcerative colitis is not clear, hereditary factors appear to be significant in some families.[67-74]

In support of a genetic etiology of ulcerative colitis, seven sets of monozygotic twins[69-72] have been recorded who have shown concordance for this disease. In addition, ulcerative colitis has never been reported in one monozygotic twin without its appearance in the other twin.

There is also abundant evidence for the occurrence of ulcerative colitis in more than one member of a family. For example, Sanford[68] reviewed the records of 143 proven cases of ulcerative colitis in two hospitals in Spokane, Washington, and found 7 patients (4.9%) having nine relatives with ulcerative colitis making a total of 16 cases in 7 families. Seven other patients with ulcerative colitis had relatives with an unknown type of gastrointestinal disease and it was believed that several of these relatives had ulcerative colitis though it could not be proven. Recently, Morris[67] described a kindred in which 8 patients had ulcerative colitis in three generations. His literature review disclosed 160 families in which ulcerative colitis had occurred in more than 1 relative. An autosomal dominant mode of inheritance was suggested. Other reports in the literature describe a familial incidence of ulcerative colitis ranging from the estimate of Sanford of 5 percent to as high as 11.3 percent reported by Paulley.[74] This incidence of ulcerative colitis in families is significantly in excess of the estimated incidence of 0.7 percent in controls as obtained in the study by Binder[75] who incidentally also found a familial incidence of 5.3 percent. Of further interest is the association of ulcerative colitis with ankylosing spondylitis which is also known to have a hereditary etiology in certain families.[76] It was of interest that both of the twins reported by Sanford[69] had ankylosing spondylitis; and in his study of hospital records of patients with ulcerative colitis in Spokane, he found that 16 percent of the patients had x-ray evidence of spondylitis. There is also supporting evidence of hereditary etiology for ulcerative colitis which shows a variable distribution in certain ethnic groups.[77] For example, the Bedouin Arabs[69] and the New Zealand Maoris[78] rarely manifest the disease even when living under conditions similar to Anglo-Saxons and Jews, who, incidentally, have the highest incidence of this disease. Regardless of the etiology, all patients with ulcerative colitis should be followed carefully for the possible development of adenocarcinoma of the colon.

A Genetic Study of Colon Cancer Probands *

We have discussed a number of genetic and presumptive genetic disorders with colon cancer association and now we would like to describe our own research involving a retrospective and prospective series of colon cancer probands.

Medical records were reviewed of all patients who received a diagnosis of adenocarcinoma of the colon at the Omaha Veterans Administration Hospital from 1951 to 1969 (209 probands). Whenever possible, all living probands were interviewed in their homes. When pertinent information was in doubt, these patients were excluded from the study. Only those patients whose tumor and family histories were considered to be reliable were included. This resulted in 98 patients in a retrospective series.

The prospective phase of our study began in 1969 with a review of the medical records and interviews with each new patient who

*Portions of this material are published by permission of the Editor, *Archives of Surgery* (Lynch, H. T., *et al., Arch Surg 106*:669–675, 1973.

was admitted to hospital with histologically verified adenocarcinoma of the colon. Each patient in the prospective series was matched with a patient of the same age and sex with a diagnosis other than cancer who was admitted to the same hospital at approximately the same time. The same procedures were followed for evaluation of these control patients as were employed for the prospective experimental group. All available first degree relatives of both experimental and control patients were interviewed whenever possible. Special attention was given to the evaluation of all histologic varieties of cancer including multiple primary malignant neoplasms. Genealogy was documented as completely as possible. Secondary sources, in addition to physician and hospital records, included records from bureaus of vital statistics, historical archives, and genealogical societies. Verification of family history, however, was less complete for some of the patients in the retrospective series because of difficulty in locating certain close relatives. This is one of the major shortcomings of retrospective studies in genetics.

Statistical analysis was performed on the following parameters:

1. The total number of first-degree relatives in each family was determined and the range and mean were calculated for the prospective, control, and retrospective groups.
2. Age at diagnosis and distribution by age in both prospective and retrospective studies were determined and expressed as frequency distribution curves.
3. The frequency distribution of all histologic varieties of cancer present in first-degree relatives was compiled and the differences between experimental and control groups were evaluated for significance based upon chi-square tests.
4. The families were divided according to the total number of cancers in each

family and the respective percentages were calculated.
5. Data were tabulated for first degree relatives in families which contained 2 or more relatives with cancer in a search for possible familial associations between different types of cancer: 1) when the subjects affected were restricted to sibships (sibs only affected), 2) vertically transmitted (parent-child affected), and 3) both (parent and sibs).
6. A sex-ratio analysis was determined with respect to tumor occurrence in first degree relatives.

Results

Data analysis was based upon the medical histories of probands and their first-degree relatives in the two experimental groups and one control group. The first experimental group included 98 probands with colon cancer (histologically verified) who were studied retrospectively. The number of relatives in these families ranged from 3 to 43 members with a mean of 6.0. The second experimental group included 50 probands with diagnoses of colon cancer (histologically verified) and their first-degree relatives who were studied prospectively. The number of subjects in these families ranged from 3 to 24 with a mean of 9.4. This group was matched with 50 control subjects and their first degree relatives who were also studied prospectively. The number of members in these families ranged from 4 to 18 with a mean of 9.2.

The age distribution at diagnosis of colonic cancer in members of the retrospective and prospective groups are shown in Figures 18–7 and 18–8. The results show no difference between the groups with respect to age at diagnosis. A maximum number of patients was diagnosed between the ages of 60 and 80 with a mean age of 64.8.

The frequency distribution of all histo-

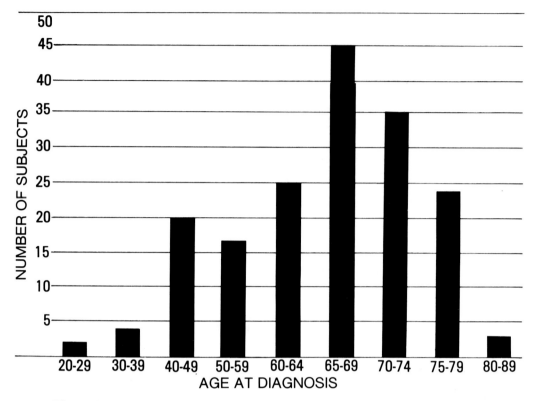

Figure 18–7. Frequency distribution curve of age at diagnosis in the retrospective group.

logical varieties of cancer present in first degree relatives of probands from the prospective probrand group and the control group is shown in Figure 18–9.

Colon cancer was found in 23 first degree relatives of the 98 colon cancer probands in the retrospective series and in 15 first degree relatives of the 50 colon cancer probands in the prospective series. In turn, only 3 cases of colon cancer were found in the control group (Table 18-II). A comparison of the prospective and control groups revealed an increase in the frequency of colon cancer ($P < 0.01$) and breast cancer ($P < 0.05$) in the first degree relatives of the experimental group.

The number of families in the experimental and control groups with different frequencies of cancer, excluding colon cancer,

in the first degree relatives is shown in Table 18-III.

An increased frequency of multiple primary malignancies was found in the experimental group compared with the control group ($P < 0.001$) as shown in Table 18-IV. Consanguinity was absent in both the proband and control groups.

The histological types of cancer are recorded for first degree relatives of probands in each family in the prospective and retrospective groups in Tables 18-V to 18-IX and summarized in Table 18-X. We have classified these families into three groups: 1) families in which only sibs were affected and none of the parents or grandchildren were affected, 2) those in which one or both parents and only one child were affected, and 3) those in which one or both parents and more than one child, and in some cases also grandchildren, were affected.

There was no significant difference concerning cancer of all sites between the two proband groups and the control group. When the number of occurrences of colon and breast cancer was compared between the experimental and control groups, there was a significant difference ($P < 0.05$). The familial association of colon and breast cancer has also been verified in a study of 34 families, ascertained originally for breast cancer, among whom gastrointestinal cancer was observed in 22 families with colon cancer the most frequently associated malignant neoplasm in 14 of these families.[79] A control group was not utilized in this series of 34 breast cancer families. In the present colon cancer study, however, an association is demonstrated when the data are compared with a control group.

Comment

These data are consistent with findings by Macklin[60] and others[59,61] who clearly demonstrated an increased frequency of colon cancer in close relatives of colon cancer probands when compared with control families. However, we have extended our data and, comparing the probands' families with controls, we have shown other possible combinations of differing histologic varieties of cancer. Thus, among first degree relatives of colon cancer probands, breast cancer appears to be the most frequently associated malignant neoplasm ($P < 0.05$). It should also be

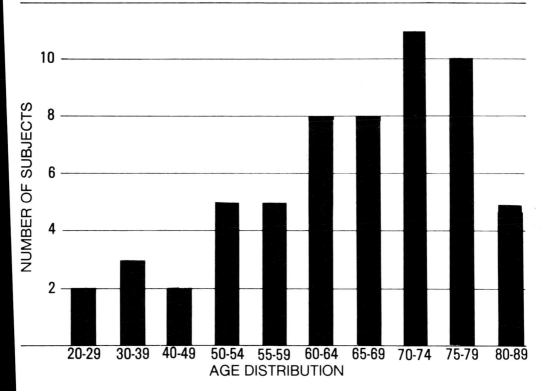

Figure 18–8. Frequency distribution curve of age at diagnosis in the prospective group.

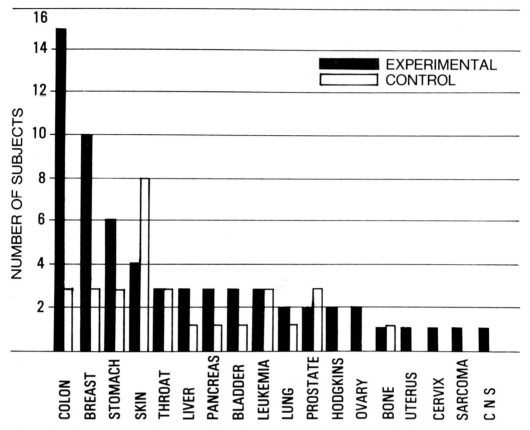

Figure 18–9. Frequency distribution of all histologic varieties of cancer present in first degree relatives of prospective and control groups.

noted that in a review of a large series of multiple primary malignant neoplasms, colon cancer was the most frequently occurring extra primary malignant neoplasm associated with breast cancer.[80]

We found no significant association of colon cancer with any other histologic varieties of cancer. Ours is a limited series; a much larger series of patients might show other tumor associations.

TABLE 18-II
COLON CANCER IN PROSPECTIVE AND
RETROSPECTIVE OVAH STUDY

	No. Colon Cancer Retro-spective	No. Colon Cancer Pro-spective	No. Colon Cancer Control
Total No. Proband	98	50	—
Total Colon	121	65	3
(First Degree Relative + Proband)			
Colon Cancer	23	15	3
(Only in Family)			

TABLE 18-III
FREQUENCY OF CANCER IN FIRST DEGREE
RELATIVES IN A RETROSPECTIVE AND
PROSPECTIVE STUDY OF COLONIC CANCER

First Degree Relatives with Cancer other than Colon	Retro-spective (98)		Prospective (48)		Control (48)	
	No.	%	No.	%	No.	%
1 Cancer	54	55.1	12	25.0	17	35.4
2 Cancers	21	21.4	8	16.7	6	12.5
3 Cancers	6	6.1	1	2.1	—	—
4 Cancers	8	8.2	2	4.2	1	2.1
5–10 Cancers	1	1.1	—	—	—	—

TABLE 18-IV
PERCENTAGES OF COLON AND MULTIPLE
CANCERS IN THE TWO EXPERIMENTAL
AND CONTROL GROUPS

Study	Colon Cancer		Other Cancers		Multiple	
	No.	%	No.	%	No.	%
Retrospective	23	13.9	142	86.1	18	18.4
Prospective	15	21.4	55	78.6	8	16.7
Control	3	10.3	26	89.7	1	2.1

Analysis of familial combinations in the colon cancer proband series has shown 25 sibships with two or more members affected with colon cancer in the retrospective series, and 5 in the prospective series, and only 2 in the control series. Parent and offspring combinations were affected with colon cancer in 24 families of the retrospective series, and in 8 families of the prospective series. Only 4 families with such a combination were found in the control series. Finally, parents and two or more siblings were affected in 16 families in the retrospective series, and in 9 families in the prospective series, while the control series showed only one.

Our data are consistent with the observation that the phenomenon of colon cancer is associated with multiple etiologies. Thus, in certain families, colon cancer is restricted to sibships with both parents free of this disease and in others the disease is manifested in parents and offspring. In considering the complexity of colon cancer, with variable but often late age of onset, it is impossible to state categorically that the parents in some of these families would not have developed the condition if they had lived long enough. Furthermore, we are unable to evaluate their true risk for the disease, since we do

TABLE 18-V
RETROSPECTIVE GROUP
(Parent–Child Only)

Family No.	Parents		Children			
			Males Affected		Females Affected	
	Father	Mother	Affected	Total No.	Affected	Total No.
5	Colon 59	Endometrial 64	Colon 65	1		1
15	Unknown 60		Colon 48	4		1
21	Colon 86		Colon 55	2		
31		Colon 37	Colon 44	2		1
61	Unknown 60		Colon 44	6		2
			Lung 55			
68	Colon 79		Colon 43	1		3
70		Unknown 68	Multiple	5		4
			Colon 65			
			Lung 74			
72	Stomach 60		Colon 65	1		
74	Skin 74		Colon 77	2		1
77	Unknown		Colon 65	4		
79	Bladder		Colon 67	1		1
92	Unknown 84		Colon 62	1		2
96		Liver 59	Colon 55	1		
110	Bladder 66		Colon 60	1		
112	Unknown		Colon 69	1		
137		Stomach 62	Colon 40	1		
152		Unknown 84	Colon 66	2		2
154	Throat		Colon 73	1		
169			Colon 77	3		2
170		Liver 60	Colon 74	4		2
179		Breast 65	Colon 67			
185	Hodgkin's		Colon 45	1		
190	Stomach		Colon 71	1		
245		Breast 72	Colon 72	1		1

not have a reliable genetic marker available to ascertain risk status. The absence of consanguinity is not sufficient to dismiss the possible involvement of recessive factors,

TABLE 18-VI
SIBS ONLY
(Retrospective Group)

Family No.	Males Affected — Affected	Total No.	Females Affected — Affected	Total No.
1	Colon 64 Throat 47	4		1
7	Colon 60 Unknown	2	Skin Lung 77	7
9	Colon 54	2	Breast	1
13	Colon 72 Colon	4		1
14	Colon Unknown	2		
40	Colon 66	1	Stomach	1
42	Colon 77 Lung 65	5		1
60	Colon 68 Unknown	2		
82	Colon 51 Skin	2		
88	Multiple Colon 77 Lip 78 Stomach	7		3
89	Colon 62	4	Esophagus 53	2
95	Colon 75 Prostate 74	5		3
115	Multiple Colon 75 Skin 69 Skin 78	3	Neck Female Organs	4
129	Colon 76 Bone Leukemia	7	Neck	5
130	Colon 74 Leukemia 70	3		
139	Colon 69 Prostate 65	3		1
147	Colon 74 Prostate 59	2		1
151	Colon 67 Throat 65	6		2
153	Colon 70 Esophagus 60	5		4
176	Colon 68 Leukemia 70	2		
189	Colon 47	2	Leukemia	3
205	Colon 68	3	Breast 57	3
224	Colon 76 Stomach 74	3		
39	Colon 67 Colon 59	3		
45	Colon 43 Throat 63 Stomach 70	8		6

since colon cancer is relatively common in our population.

The finding of parent-child involvement with colon cancer is consistent with a familial factor transmitted from one generation to the next. This association could involve factors that are gene-transmitted, nongenetic factors such as virus, diet, or other carcinogenic factors, or a combination of the different factors. In one of the families described in this series, several generations were affected with colon cancer, multiple primary cancers, and early age of onset with overall findings consistent with the cancer family syndrome which we consider to be under the influence of an autosomal dominant gene.[81]

The epidemiology of colon cancer is exceedingly complex. This discussion is concerned primarily with the role of genetic factors in diatheses for colon cancer, although both genetic and nongenetic factors must be considered. For example, Burkitt[82] has emphasized the importance of dietary factors in the evolution of carcinoma of the colon and rectum, basing his hypothesis on studies from Africa and other parts of the world, where the frequency of colon cancer appears to show marked variations which parallel populations showing characteristic dietary patterns. Accordingly, areas of low colon cancer incidence tended to be associated with high residue diet and, conversely, those areas showing a high frequency of colon cancer had low residue diets. It was also of interest that diverticular disease of the colon also occurred more frequently among individuals exposed to a low residue diet.[82]

Other factors of importance in colon cancer include bile acids and coliform bacteria, all of which may be interrelated with the dietary factor. Thus, dietary fiber was shown to regulate the speed of transit, bulk, and consistency of stools. Burkitt reasoned that it would be more likely that carcinogens produced by the action of abnormal bacterial flora when held for a prolonged period in a concentrated form in contact with the bowel mucosa may account for the high incidence of colon cancer in the more economically developed countries where low residue diet is so popular. Bacterial flora are capable of producing many secondary bile acids which are found in the colon,[83,84] a fact alluded to first in 1941 by Druckery[85] when he demonstrated the association of bacterial flora with cancer. It would be valuable to see if familial factors are operative in context with these environmental factors and thereby predisposing members of certain colon cancer prone families differentially to these exogenous agents.

Unfortunately, there have been no genetic studies of which we are aware wherein special attention has been given to the interactions with some of these nongenetic factors. We believe it is essential, for the full elucidation of colon cancer etiology, that host factors be appraised with due consideration to their interaction with such environmental factors as diet, bile acids, and bacterial flora.

TABLE 18-VII
SIBS AND PARENTS
(Retrospective Group)

	Parents		Children			
			Males Affected		Females Affected	
Family No.	Father	Mother	Affected	Total No.	Affected	Total No.
17		Stomach	Colon 64	2		2
29	Liver 72		Colon 62	2	Endometrial 50	3
56	Colon 65		Colon 70 Stomach 56 Lung	9	Hodgkin's Stomach Stomach	8
58		Stomach 64	Colon 66	3	Stomach 46	1
73	Prostate 72		Colon 65 Leukemia 73	2		2
109	Stomach 71	Stomach 71	Colon 67	4	Endometrial 57	4
118		Throat	Colon 67 Pancreas	4		2
126		Unknown 84	Colon 66 Unknown 60		Unknown 80 Breast 43	
128		Throat 80	Colon 66 Leukemia	3		2
142		Colon 55	Colon 51 Unknown	6	Leukemia	8
143		Unknown	Colon 76 Epiglottis 67	3	Stomach	1
175		Stomach	Colon 74 Stomach	4		1
198	Leukemia		Colon 66 Unknown Prostate	4	Leukemia	3
202			Colon 67 Hodgkin's 37 Throat 59	4		3
171			Colon 64 Prostate 65	2		
32			Colon 71	2	Endometrial 85	
145	Skin 66	Leukemia 72	Colon 62	2		3
26	Rectal 59		Colon 69	1	Unknown	2
105		Unknown 85	Colon 56 Skin 67 Colon 70	4		2

A large-scale prospective study of colon cancer prone families with matched controls might clarify these etiologies. In addition to their implication for carcinogenesis, genetic studies also harbor a potential for cancer control through the recognition of relatives at high risk for the development of colon cancer, and in certain circumstances, for the development of breast cancer.

Thus, it is possible that the gene(s) pre-

TABLE 18-VIII
PARENT-CHILD ONLY
(Prospective Groups)

	Parents		Children			
			Males Affected		Females Affected	
Family No.	Father	Mother	Affected	Total No.	Affected	Total No.
64	Prostate 72		Colon 71	3		2
65		Skin 89	Colon 57	0		3
106	Multiple Bladder 71 Colon 73	Lung 66	Multiple Colon 62 Skin 63	3		3
167	Colon 81		Colon 72	5		
183		Colon	Colon 70	6		3
209		Stomach 75	Colon 57	2		3
216	Kidney		Colon 49 Colon 52 Lung 52			
		SIBS ONLY				
3			Colon 66 Bladder 68 Lung 65	6		5
4			Colon 66 Leukemia 69	3		3
116			Colon 75	3	Colon 80	3
146			Colon 79 Lung 51	9		2
255			Colon 55 Bladder 81	7		2
		SIBS AND PARENTS				
16	Bladder 84		Colon 50 Skin 69	5	Unknown	2
81		Colon 78	Colon 54	3	Breast 65 Colon 62	3
114		Hodgkin's 71	Colon 64 Skin 64 Colon	5		2
164	Multiple 60 Pancreas Liver Stomach		Colon 57	5	Colon 29 Colon 31	2
187	Stomach 84		Colon 71	10	Breast Stomach	4
207		Breast 65	Colon 62 Liver	6		3
220	Leukemia 80	Breast 67	Colon 71 Stomach 54 Leukemia 24	10	Reticulum Cell Sarcoma	3
221	Colon 44 Colon 56	Breast	Colon 33 Cecum Pancreas Colon 27	7	Colon 40	4
229	Bone 55		Colon 82 Liver 45	5	Colon 45	3

disposing to cancer may cause a mutation in a particular cell which may render this specific cell susceptible to malignant transformation through interaction with a carcinogen(s) such as an oncogenic virus.

Prognosis in Hereditary Colon Cancer

Familial polyposis coli as well as the several hereditary syndromes with polyposis of the colon are diseases which predispose to colon cancer at an unusually young age. Johnson, et al.[86] reported in 1959 on 27 patients with familial polyposis of the colon and rectum who developed adenocarcinoma of the colon or rectum before the age of 30. Only 4 of the patients who were under 20 years of age survived more than 10 years. O'Brien[87] reported on fewer than 200 patients who had contracted carcinoma of the colon under 20 years of age of whom only three survived 5 years or longer. Recently, Ferguson and Obi[88] described 6 patients with adenocarcinoma of the colon who were 25 years of age or younger, only one of whom survived more than seven years. Data on prognosis

for persons who develop hereditary colon cancer at later ages is extremely limited.

Thus, we see from these data the extremely grave prognosis for young patients who develop adenocarcinoma of the colon or rectum. Therefore, we should make every attempt to diagnose this disease as early as possible and when one finds a family history of familial polyposis coli, or colon cancer in other conditions lacking polyposis coli such as the cancer family syndrome, it should be possible through an increased index of suspicion to search for an earlier diagnosis. In the case of polyposis coli, once the diagnosis has been established, one should proceed with colectomy prophylactically and thereby avoid the consequence of adenocarcinoma in a young patient.

General Epidemiologic Considerations and Summary

While the main thrust of this chapter has been to delineate the role of hereditary factors in colon cancer, we must not lose sight of the fact that numerous other epi-

TABLE 18-IX
PARENT-CHILD ONLY
(Control Group)

Family No.	Parents		Children			
			Males Affected		Females Affected	
	Father	Mother	Affected	Total No.	Affected	Total No.
C 65		Endometrial 70	Leukemia	4		3
C212		Skin 32	Liver	5		2
C207	Brain 75		Lip 65	2		2
C177	Skin		Skin	2		1
C164		Breast 77	Lung 55	8		6
			SIBS ONLY			
C 4			Colon 64	5	Endometrial 35	4
			Colon 69			
C255			Spine 60	9	Spleen 72	3
			Prostate 72		Colon 72	
			SIBS AND PARENTS			
C206		Skin 78	Prostate 66	9		2
			Prostate 68			
			Prostate 81			

TABLE 18-X
SUMMARY OF HISTORY OF CANCER IN
FIRST DEGREE RELATIVES IN THE TWO
EXPERIMENTAL AND CONTROL GROUPS

Study	Sibs Only		Parent-Child Only		Sibs & Parent-Child	
	No.	%	No.	%	No.	%
Prospective (No. = 50)	5	10	8	16	9	18
Control (No. = 50)	2	4	4	8	1	2
Retrospective (No. = 98)	25	25	24	24	16	16
Prospective/Retrospective (No. = 148)	30	20	32	21	25	17

demiologic issues have been under consideration in the etiology of human colon cancer. The problem, nevertheless, remains unclear, though we believe that eventually an interaction between host or genetic factors and nongenetic factors will be found. For example, Burkitt[82] has emphasized the importance of dietary factors in the evolution of carcinoma of the colon and rectum, basing his hypothesis on studies from Africa and other parts of the world where dietary habits vary considerably and interestingly, where the frequency of colon cancer appears to show marked variations which parallel populations showing certain dietary patterns, i.e. low residue diet was associated with an increased frequency of colon cancer and contrariwise, a high residue diet was found to be associated with a low frequency of colon cancer. Dietary factors in interaction with bile acids and bacteria may also be of importance in colon cancer etiology. However, we still need to study heredity to see if those individuals who develop cancer, though following a certain diet, also have a familial predilection for this disease. In certain other situations, such as familial polyposis coli, heredity is more clear; however, certain clinical features of these syndromes, including associated physical stigmata and the spectrum of extra-colonic malignant neoplasms require clarification. For example, Smith and Kern[89] have described a family with multiple polyposis of the colon in association with papillary carcinoma of the thyroid. They made an extensive review of the literature and discovered many other malignant neoplasms in addition to those involving the thyroid and brain, in association with familial polyposis coli. These included malignant melanoma, periampullary malignancy, adenomatosis and juvenile polyposis of the stomach and small intestine, multiple endocrine adenomatosis, endometrial carcinoma, prostatic carcinoma, papillary bladder tumor, and chromophobe adenoma. Their review suggested that the frequency of extra-colonic neoplasms may be increased in familial multiple polyposis coli. However, one must evaluate these findings with caution since many of these observations represent single case reports and therefore the alleged associations could be due to chance factors alone. Needed is the study of a large series of families with familial polyposis coli wherein meticulous documentation is made of all varieties of cancer. This would help solve the issue of multiple genotypes and phenotypes in the so-called familial polyposis syndromes. In other clinical problems such as ulcerative colitis, heredity plays a variable role and cancer development is dependent upon such factors as activity and chronicity of the disease. Much more work will be necessary to help elucidate more fully the etiologic problems involved in the colon cancer mystery.

REFERENCES

1. Cancer Facts and Figures, New York, American Cancer Society, Inc. 1972, p. 7.
2. Lisfranc, J.: Sur L'Excision de la Partie Inférieure du Rectum devenue Carcinomateuse. *Mem Acad R Med Belg, 3:*291–302, 1833.
3. Gilbertsen, V.A.: The earlier diagnosis of adenocarcinoma of the large intestine: a report of 1,884 cases, including five-year follow-up survival data, results of surgery for the disease, and effect on survival prognosis of treatment earlier in the development of the disease. *Cancer, 27:*143–149, 1971.
4. Gold, P., and Freemand, S.O.: Demonstration of tumor-specific antigens in human colonic carcinomata by immunological tolerance and absorption techniques. *J Exp Med, 121:*439–462, 1965.
5. Gold, P., and Freemand, S.O.: Specific carcinoembryonic antigens of the human digestive system. *J Exp Med, 122:*467–481, 1965.
6. Thomson, D.M.P., Krupey, J., Freedman, S.O., and Gold, P.: The radioimmunoassay of circulating carcinoembryonic antigen of the human digestive system. *Proc Natl Acad Sci USA, 64:*161–167, 1969.
7. Moore, T.L., Kupchik, H.Z., Marcon, U., and Samcheck, N.: Carcinoembryonic antigen assay in cancer of the colon and pancreas and other digestive tract disorders. *Am J Dig Dis, 16:*1–7, 1971.
8. Nugent, F.W., and Hansen, E.R.: Radioimmunoassay of carcinoembryonic antigen as a diagnostic test for cancer of the colon: a preliminary report. *Lahey Clinic Found Bull, 20:*85–88, 1971.
9. Belleau, R., and Braasch, J.W.: Genetics and polyposis. *Med Clin N Am, 50:*379–392, 1966.
10. Cripps, H.: Two cases of disseminated polyps of rectum. *Tr Path Soc London, 33:*165–168, 1881–1882.
11. Lockhart-Mummery, P.: Cancer and heredity. *Lancet, 1:*427–429, 1925.
12. Dukes, C.E.: Familial intestinal polyposis. *Ann R Coll Surg Engl, 10:*293–304, 1952.
13. Cockayne, E.A.: Heredity in relation to cancer. *Cancer Rev, 2:*337–347, 1927.
14. Warren, S., and Gates, O.: Multiple primary malignant tumors: a survey of the literature and statistical study. *Cancer, 16:*1358–1414, 1932.
15. Morson, B.C.: *Diseases of the Colon, Rectum and Anus.* London, Heinemann, 1969.
16. Hoffman, C.C., and Goligher, J.C.: Polyposis of the stomach and small intestine in association with familial polyposis coli. *Br J Surg, 58:*126–128, 1971.
17. Gardner, E.J., and Richards, R.C.: Multiple cutaneous and subcutaneous lesions occurring simultaneously with hereditary polyposis and osteomatosis. *Am J Hum Genet, 5:*139–147, 1953.
18. McKusick, V.A.: Genetic factors in intestinal polyposis *JAMA, 182:*271–277, 1962.
19. Duncan, B.R., Dohner, V.A., and Priest, J.H.: The Gardner syndrome: need for early diagnosis. *J Pediatr, 72:*497–505, 1968.
20. Cabot, R.C.: Presentation of case #21061: in case records of the Massachusetts general hospital. *New Engl J Med, 212:*263–268, 1935.
21. MacDonald, J.M., Davis, W.C., Crago, H.R., and Berk, A.D.: Gardner's syndrome and periampullary malignancy. *Am J Surg, 113:*425–430, 1967.
22. Murphy, E.S., Mireles, M.V., and Beltrán, A.O.: Familial polyposis of the colon and gastric carcinoma: concurrent conditions in a 16-year-old boy. *JAMA, 179:*1026–1028, 1962.
23. Devic, A., and Bussy: Un Cas de Polypose adénomateuse Généralisée à tout L'Intestin. *Arch Mal App Digest, 6:*278–299, 1912.
24. Fitzgerald, G.M.: Multiple composite odontomes coincidental with other tumorous conditions. Report of a case. *J Am Dent Assoc, 30:*1408–1417, 1943.
25. Guptill, P.: Familial polyposis of the colon: two families, five cases. *Surgery, 22:*286–304, 1947.
26. Gardner, E.J.: Follow-up study of family group exhibiting dominant inheritance for

syndrome including intestinal polyps, osteomas, fibromas and epiderman cysts. *Am J Hum Genet, 14:*376–390, 1962.

27. Gardner, E.J.: Inherited multiple neoplasia syndrome. Genetics today. *Proc XI Intern Cong Genet, 1:*287, 1963.

28. Gardner, E.J., and Stephens, F.E.: Cancer of the lower digestive tract in one family group. *Am J Hum Genet, 2:*41–48, 1950.

29. Gardner, E.J.: A genetic and clinical study of intestinal polyposis, a predisposing factor for carcinoma of the colon and rectum. *Am J Hum Genet, 3:*167–176, 1951.

30. Gardner, E.J., and Plenk, H.P.: Hereditary pattern for multiple osteomas in a family group. *Am J Hum Genet, 4:*31–36, 1952.

31. Plenk, H.P., and Gardner, E.J.: Osteomatosis (leontiasis ossea): hereditary disease of membranous bone formation associated in one family with polyposis of the colon. *Radiology, 62:*830–840, 1954.

32. MacDonald, J.M., Davis, W.C., Crago, H.R., and Berk, A.D.: Gardner's syndrome and periampullary malignancy. *Am J Surg, 113:*425–430, 1967.

33. Watne, A.: Gardner's Syndrome. In Lynch, H.T. (Ed.): *Skin, Heredity, and Malignant Neoplasms.* New York, Med Ex, 1972, Chapt. 10, p. 299.

34. Chang, C.H., Piatt, E.D., Thomas, K.E., and Watne, A.L.: Bone abnormalities in Gardner's syndrome. *Am J Roentgen, 103:*645–652, 1968.

35. Le Fevre, H.W., Jr., and Jacques, T.G.: Multiple polyposis in an infant of four months. *Am J Surg, 81:*90–91, 1951.

36. Capps, W.G., Jr., Lewis, M.I., and Gassaniga, D.A.: Carcinoma of the colon, ampulla of vater and urinary bladder associated with familial multiple polyposis: a case report. *Dis Colon Rectum, 11:*298–305, 1968.

37. Fader, M., Kline, S.N., Spatz, S.S., and Zubrow, H.J.: Gardner's syndrome (intestinal polyposis, osteomas, sebaceous cysts) and a new dental discovery. *Oral Surg, 15:*153–172, 1962.

38. O'Brien, J.P., and Wels, P.: The synchronous occurrence of benign fibrous tissue neoplasia in hereditary adenosis of the colon and rectum. *NY J Med, 55:*1877–1880, 1955.

39. Camiel, M.R., Mulé, J.E., Alexander, L.L., and Benninghoff, D.L.: Association of thyroid carcinoma with Gardner's syndrome in siblings. *New Engl J Med, 278:*1056 1058, 1968.

40. Schweitzer, R.J., and Robbins, G.F.: A desmoid tumor of multicentric origin. *Arch Surg, 80:*489–494, 1960.

41. Turcot, J., Despres, J.P., and St. Pierre, F.: Malignant tumors of the central nervous system associated with familial polyposis of the colon: report of two cases. *Dis Colon Rectum, 2:*465–468, 1959.

42. Baughman, F.A., List, C.F., Williams, J.R., Muldoon, J.P., Segarra, J.M., and Volkel, J.S.: The Glioma-Polyposis syndrome. *New Engl J Med, 281:*1345–1346, 1969.

43. Lynch, H.T.: Hereditary factors in carcinoma. In Rentchnik, P. (Ed.): *Recent Advances in Cancer Research.* Berlin, Springer-Verlag, 1967, Vol. 12.

44. Humphries, A.L., Shepherd, M.H., and Peters, H.J.: Peutz-Jeghers syndrome with colonic adenocarcinoma and ovarian tumor. *JAMA, 197:*296–298, 1966.

45. Christian, D.D.: Ovarian tumors: an extension of the Peutz-Jeghers syndrome. *Am J Obstet Gynecol, 111:*529–534, 1971.

46. Morson, B.C.: Some peculiarities in the histology of intestinal polyps. *Dis Colon Rectum, 5:*337–344, 1962.

47. Veale, A.M.O., McColl, I., Bussey, H.J.R., and Morson, B.C.: Juvenile polyposis coli. *J Med Genet, 3:*1–16, 1966.

47a. Gathright, J.B., Jr., and Coffer, T.W., Jr.: Familial incidence of juvenile polyposis coli, *Surg Gynec and Obstet, 138:*185–188, 1974.

48. Yonemoto, R.H., Slayback, J.B., Byron, R.L., and Rosen, R.B.: Familial polyposis of the entire gastrointestinal tract. *Arch Surg, 99:*427–434, 1969.

49. Cronkhite, L.W., and Canada, W.J.: Generalized gastrointestinal polyposis. An unusual syndrome of polyposis, pigmentation, alopecia and onychotrophia. *New Engl J Med, 252:*1011–1015, 1955.

50. Takahata, J., Okubo, K., Komeda, T., Kono,

T., and Fukui, I.: Generalized gastrointestinal polyposis associated with ectodermal changes and protein-losing enteropathy with a dramatic response to prednisolone. *Digestion, 5:*153–161, 1972.

51. Gomes Da Cruz, G.M.: Generalized gastrointestinal polyposis. An unusual syndrome of adenomatous polyposis, alopecia, onychotrophia. *Am J Gastroenterology, 47:* 504–510, 1967.

52. Jarnum, S., and Jensen, H.: Diffuse gastrointestinal polyposis with ectodermal changes. *Gastroenterology, 50:*107–118, 1966.

53. Johnston, M.M., Vosburgh, J.W., Wiens, A.T., and Walsh, G.C.: Gastrointestinal polyposis associated with alopecia, pigmentation and atrophy of the fingernails and toenails. *Ann Intern Med, 56:*935–940, 1962.

54. Woolf, C.M., Richards, R.C., and Gardner, E.J.: Occasional Discrete polyps of the colon and rectum showing an inherited tendency in a kindred. *Cancer, 8:*403–408, 1955.

55. Schnug, G.E.: Familial polyposis of the colon. *Am Surg, 37:*449–454, 1971.

56. Rider, J.A., Kirsner, J.B., Moeller, H.C., and Palmer, W.L.: Polyps of the colon and rectum; their incidence and relationship to carcinoma. *Am J Med, 16:*555–564, 1954.

57. Richard, R.C., and Woolf, C.M.: Solitary polyps of the colon and rectum: a study of inherited tendency. *Am Surg, 22:*287–294, 1956.

58. Ceulemans, G.: Incidence familiale multiple du cancer du rectum. *J Int Coll Surg (Bull), 30:*649–652, 1958.

59. Kluge, T.: Familial cancer of the colon. *Acta Chir Scand, 127:*392–398, 1964.

60. Macklin, M.T.: Inheritance of cancer of the stomach and large intestine in man. *J Natl Cancer Inst, 24:*551–571, 1960.

61. Peltokallio, P., and Peltokallio, V.: Relationship of familial factors to carcinoma of the colon. *Dis Colon Rectum, 9:*367–370, 1966.

62. Moertel, C.G., Bargen, J.A., and Dockerty, M.B.: Multiple carcinomas of the large intestine. *Gastroenterology, 34:*85–98, 1958.

63. Nugent, F.W., and Rudolph, N.E.: Extra-

colonic manifestations of chronic ulcerative colitis. *Med Clin North Am, 50:*529–534, 1966.

64. Welch, C.E., and Hedberg, S.E.: Colonic cancer in ulcerative colitis and idiopathic colonic cancer. *JAMA, 191:*815–818. 1965.

65. de Dombal, F.T., Watts, J.McK., Watkinson, G., and Goligher, J.C.: Local complications of ulcerative colitis: stricture, pseudopolyposis, and carcinoma of colon and rectum. *Br Med J, 1:*442–447, 1966.

66. MacDougall, I.P.M.: The cancer risk in ulcerative colitis. *Lancet, 2:*655–658, 1964.

67. Morris, P.J.: Familial ulcerative colitis, *GUT, 6:*176–178, 1965.

68. Kirsner, J.B., and Spencer, J.A.: Familial occurrences of ulcerative colitis, regional enteritis and ileocolitis. *Ann Intern Med, 59:*133–144, 1963.

69. Sanford, G.E.: Genetic implications in ulcerative colitis. *Am Surg, 37:*512–517, (August), 1971.

70. Bacon, H.E.: *Ulcerative Colitis.* Philadelphia, Lippincott, 1958.

71. Lyons, C.K., and Postlethwait, R.W.: Chronic ulcerative colitis in twins. *Gastroenterology, 10:*545–550, 1948.

72. Moltke, O.: Familial occurrence of nonspecific suppurative coloproctitis. *Acta Med Scand* [Suppl]. *77:*426–432, 1936.

73. Webb, L.R., Jr.: The occurrence of chronic ulcerative colitis in twin males. *Gastroenterology, 15:*523–524, 1950.

74. Paulley, J.W.: Ulcerative colitis, a study of 173 cases. *Gastroenterology, 16:*556–576, 1950.

75. Binder, V., Weeke, E., Olsen, J.H., Anthonisen, P., and Riis, P.: A genetic study of ulcerative colitis. *Scand J Gastroenterol, 1:*49–56, 1966.

76. Hersh, A.H., Strecher, R.M., and Solomon, W.M., et al.: Heredity in ankylosing spondylitis. *Am J Hu Genet, 2:*391–408, 1950.

77. Billinghurst, J.R., and Welchman, J.M.: Idiopathic ulcerative colitis in the African: a report of four cases. *Br Med J, 1:*211–213, 1966.

78. Wigley, R.D., and MacLaurin, B.P.: A study of ulcerative colitis in New Zealand, show-

ing a low incidence in Maoris. *Br Med J,* *2:*228–231, 1962.

79. Lynch, H.T., Krush, A.J., Lemon, H.M., Kaplan, A.R., Condit, P.T., and Bottomley, R.H.: Tumor variations in families with breast cancer. *JAMA, 222:*1631–1635, 1972.

80. Schoenburg, B.S., Greenberg, R.W., and Eisenberg, H.: Occurrence of certain multiple primary cancers in females. *J Natl Cancer Inst, 43:*15–32, 1969.

81. Lynch, H.T., Swartz, M.J., Lynch, J.S., and Krush, A.J.: A family study of adenocarcinoma of the colon and multiple primary cancer. *Surg Gynecol Obstet, 134:*781–786, 1972.

82. Burkitt, D.P.: Epidemiology of cancer of the colon and rectum. *Cancer, 28:*3–13, 1971.

83. Wynder, E.L., and Shigamatsu, T.: Environmental factors of cancer of the colon and rectum. *Cancer, 20:*1520–1561, 1967.

84. Synder, E.L., Kajitani, T., Ishikawa, S., Dodo, H., and Takano, A.: Environmental factors of cancer of the colon and rectum, II. Japanese epidemiological data. *Cancer, 23:* 1210–1220, 1969.

85. Druckrey, H., Richter, R., and Vienthaler, R.: Sur Endogenen Entstehung krebserrengender Stoffe beim Menschen. *Klin Wochenschr, 20:*781, 1941.

86. Johnson, J.W., Judd, E.S., and Dahlin, D.C.: Malignant neoplasms of the colon and rectum in young persons. *Arch Surg, 79:* 365–372, 1959.

87. O'Brien, S.E.: Carcinoma of the colon in childhood and adolescence. *Can Med Assoc J, 96:*1217–1219, 1967.

88. Ferguson, E., Jr., and Obi, L.J.: Carcinoma of the colon and rectum in patients up to 25 years of age. *Am Surg, 37:*181–189, 1971.

89. Smith, W.G., and Kern, B.B.: The nature of the mutation in familial multiple polyposis: papillary carcinoma of the thyroid, brain tumors, and familial multiple polyposis. *Dis Colon Rectum, 16:*264–271, 1973.

CHAPTER 19

CANCER FAMILY SYNDROME

HENRY T. LYNCH, ANNE J. KRUSH, ROBERT J. THOMAS AND JANE LYNCH

Introduction

THE TERM *cancer* is generic and embodies a variety of clinical conditions and/or syndromes stemming from specific pathological aberrations peculiar to the several histological varieties of cancer. This would therefore include such phenomena as the totipotential characteristics of individual cancer cells, such as oat cell cancer of the lung in which a potential exists for producing a variety of endocrine-like syndromes. In turn, a wide array of etiologic factors may be implicated in the development of any particular form of cancer. The complexity of these etiological problems seems staggering when a clinical investigator studies a particular patient and attempts to analyze critically the etiologic roles of endogenous and exogenous factors. This problem is magnified even further when specific pathologic aberrations are considered with associated clinical conditions in his patient as well as in his patient's close relatives. When reliable markers are lacking, as in the case of the cancer family syndrome, the problem becomes particularly difficult.

Any investigation pertaining to etiology must necessarily involve the securing of detailed medical and epidemiological data from a variety of sources; it is mandatory that every possible effort be made to obtain pathological verification of specific malignant neoplasms. All of these findings are in turn correlated with genealogy in the particular family.[1] Of course, difficulties may be encountered at every turn, i.e. in-complete, lost, or destroyed medical records, *unavailable* records because of incorrect addresses, deaths from unknown causes, occasionally a frank reticence on the part of the patient to cooperate in the studies, and many other unpredictable human obstacles. These problems notwithstanding, occasionally scientists are assisted in their efforts by the work of previous clinical investigators, some of whom have already accumulated extensive and precise information about patients and their relatives and have preserved it so that subsequent generations of clinicians might continue these studies.[2,3,4]

Criteria for the Cancer Family Syndrome

During the past 10 years, our genetics group has had an opportunity to investigate a number of families with the cancer family syndrome both retrospectively and prospectively. These families are unrelated and are widely dispersed geographically. This syndrome is characterized as follows: 1) increased occurrence of adenocarcinoma, primarily of colon and endometrium; 2) increased frequency of multiple primary malignant neoplasms (approximately 20%); 3) early age of onset of cancer as opposed to the average age of occurrence of that specific malignancy in the general population; and 4) vertical transmission of cancer consistent with an autosomal dominant inheritance pattern. Genealogy, medical history, and verification of tumor pathology have been secured so far as possible. During the course of study, cancer has continued to occur relentlessly (see discussion of this issue under section dealing with Family N).

Several additional families with findings consistent with the definition of the cancer family syndrome have been studied in different areas of the world. These have included two families from Switzerland,[5,6] one from England,[7] and one from Virginia.[8] Undoubtedly, many other families with findings consistent with this syndrome are being evaluated daily in medical practice but often are not recognized, primarily because of the difficulty in establishing this diagnosis. Specifically, the diagnosis must be based upon a detailed medical and genetic history including histologic confirmation of cancer, since, at this time, there are no known distinguishing physical or laboratory markers for this syndrome.

Cancer Families

Family "G" of Warthin

We are fortunate in having available to us a family which has been under investigation for 75 years. This family is known in the literature as Family "G" of Warthin. A study of the family was initiated in 1895 by the late Aldred Warthin, M.D.,[2,3] former Chairman of Pathology at the University of Michigan School of Medicine. We shall present this family in detail and will provide additional supporting evidence from our studies of several other families which exhibit all of the clinical features of the cancer family syndrome.

Warthin first published a detailed report of Family "G" in 1913.[2] He later updated the kindred in 1925.[3] His colleagues, Hauser and Weller, updated the family in 1936.[4] The fourth evaluation of the kindred was begun by Weller in 1955, but was not completed due to his death.

In 1965, through the kindness of A. J. French, M.D., Chairman of the Department of Pathology at the University of Michigan School of Medicine, and Margery W. Shaw, M.D., formerly at the University of Michigan (now at the M.D. Anderson Hospital and Tumor Institute in Houston, Texas), all of the records were made available to us including Warthin's original observations in 1895 and Dr. Weller's more recent work on the kindred. Our medical and genealogical search was particularly fruitful since a large number of kindred members have remained residents of the Ann Arbor area, and for the most part have been willing to participate in our studies. We have also received considerable assistance from the physicians of the Ann Arbor members of the family, several of whom initiated personal contact with surviving members of the family and other family physicians in order that we might secure medical and genealogic information.

The pedigree of Family "G"[9] is now extensive (more than 842 descendants), and, for purposes of clarity, we shall present the cancer-prone and cancer-resistant descendants of the progenitor as separate family lines or branches. Thus, Figure 19–1 shows the progenitor (Generation I) and his 10 children (Generation II), with all the progeny of 9 of the 10 branches placed in Generations III-VIII (Fig. 19–1A, 19–1B, 19–1C, 19–1D, 19–1E, 19–1F, 19–1G, 19–1H, 19–1I). In turn Tables 19-I through 19-VIII comprise tumor registries for each branch of the kindred. Table 19-IX is a registry of cancer of specific anatomic sites in the 10 branches of Family "G".

Cancer occurred in the descendants of two of the progeny who, themselves, did not develop cancer (Fig. 19–1, II-D, who died at age 26 in childbirth, and II-E, and Tables 19-III and 19-IV). Branches A, B, D, F, G, H, and I were noteworthy for increased incidences of adenocarcinomas, predominantly adenocarcinoma of the colon (48 members) and endometrium (18 members), Tables 19-I–19-III, 19-V–19-IX, and Figs. 19–1A, 19–1B, 19–1D, 19–1F, 19–1G, 19–1H, and 19–1I). Branch E (Table 19-IV and Fig. 19-1E) had a complete absence of cancer until several years ago when chronic lymphocytic leukemia and lymphosarcoma appeared in 3 of 7 members of a sibship.

Interestingly, several members of Branches A, B, G, H, and I also developed chronic lymphocytic leukemia, sarcomas, and brain tumors (Tables 19-I, 19-II, 19-VI–19-IX).

One hundred and thirteen cancers occurred in 95 individuals in this family, 13 of whom had multiple primary malignant neoplasms (14%), (Table 19-IX). Nineteen developed cancer before age 40. Age 40 or over was taken as an arbitrary age for cancer risk. When only those family members who developed cancer after the age of 40 are considered, it is seen that the percent of members at risk for cancer who developed cancer varies considerably (20–62%) among the several branches (Tables 19-I–19-VIII). The average cancer incidence in the cancer susceptible branches was 35 percent. Finally, of 35 members in Branch C, 20 have reached the age of 40 without developing cancer. The

TABLE 19-I
TUMOR REGISTRY FOR BRANCH A

Pedigree No.	Sex	Site	Age at Diagnosis
II-A	F	Endometrium	
III-4	F	Endometrium	
III-5	M	Stomach	
III-7	F	Endometrium	42
III-8	M	Round cell sarcoma of colon	51
III-11	F	Site unknown	
IV-4	M	Lymphatic leukemia	
IV-8	F	Breast	58
IV-15	F	Colon	73
IV-16	F	Breast	
IV-17	F	Colon	78
V-9	F	Colon	51
Total number of members, all ages			171
Number of members who reached age 40 without cancer			43
Total number with cancer			12
Number who developed cancer after age 40			12 (22%)

other 15 members either have not yet reached the age of 40, or died of a disease or condition other than cancer before the age of 40.

In 72 of the 95 patients with cancer (76%), a parent in the direct genetic line also manifested cancer. Exceptions to this occurred in 8 cases wherein a patient with cancer had a parent in the direct genetic line who survived to age 40 or over and allegedly never developed cancer. Further

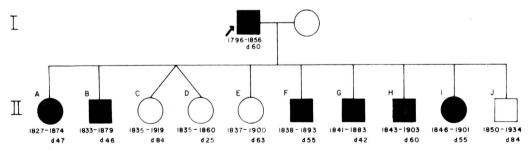

Figure 19–1. Because of the large size of Family G (more than 842 descendants), cancer-prone and cancer resistant descendants of the progenitor will be presented as separate figures representing specific family lines or branches. Figure 19–1 depicts the progenitor (Generation I) and has 10 children (Generation II). The progeny of 9 of the 10 branches will be indicated in Generations III to VIII in Figures 19–1A, 1B, 1C, 1D, 1F, 1G, 1H, and 1I. To facilitate cross reference to tumor registries for these specific branches, Tables 19-1 through 19-VIII will comprise tumor registries for each branch of the kindred. Table 19-IX is a registry of specific anatomic sites in the 10 branches of Family G.

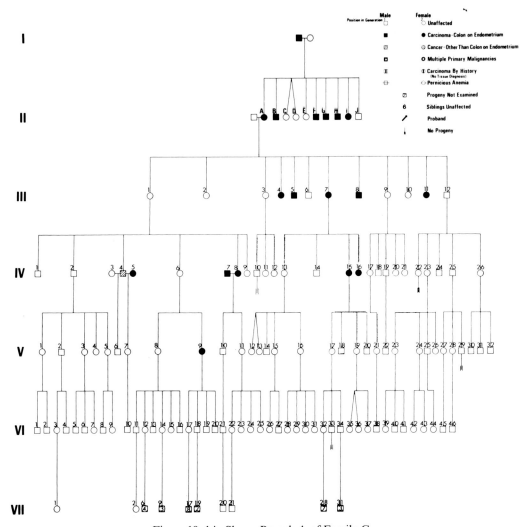

Figure 19–1A. Shows Branch A of Family G.

analysis of each of the 8 cases revealed that the medical data were incomplete in 7, obviating complete exclusion of the occurrence of cancer in these individuals. In one case, the parent with cancer was not in the direct genetic line.

Cancer was present in one or more members of 41 sibships in 8 of the 10 branches of the kindred (Table 19-X). The number of generations involved varied from 2 to 5

(including the progenitor). Expressing these findings in terms of the total number of 41 sibships with cancer, 25 of 41 sibships (69%) exhibited cancer in 2 or more generations.

Analysis of cancer by sex showed a sex ratio which was essentially one-to-one with 47 males and 48 females affected. This finding is completely in accord with an autosomal, as opposed to sex-linked, inheritance pattern.

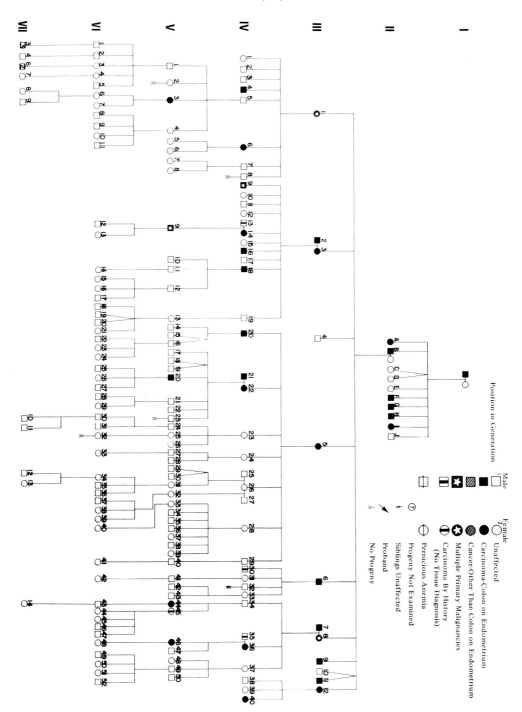

Figure 19–1B. Shows Branch B of Family G.

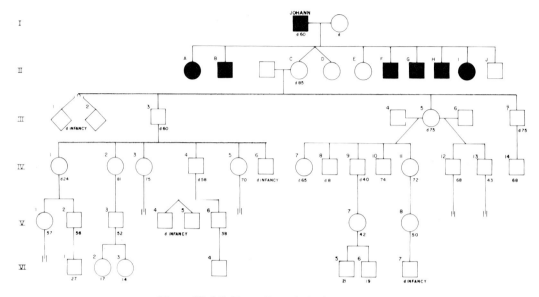

Figure 19–1C. Shows Branch C of Family G.

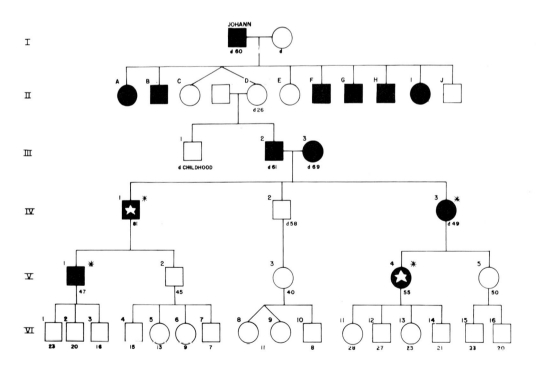

Figure 19–1D. Shows Branch D of Family G.

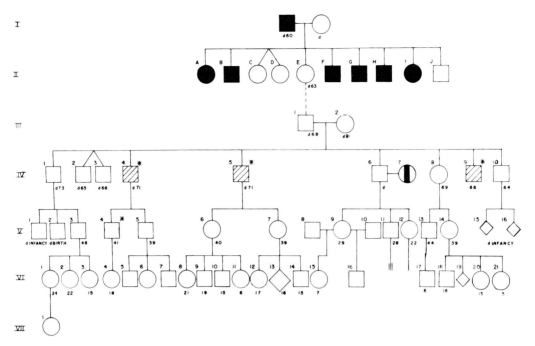

Figure 19–1E. Shows Branch E of Family G.

A striking observation was that malignant neoplasms have consistently occurred in relatives who, on genetic grounds, would be expected to be at risk; this phenomnon has been consistent with dominant transmission as demonstrated in sibships having a parent affected and the number of individuals affected in cancer-prone sibships. Variation in affected versus nonaffected in some of the cancer-prone sibships can be explained on the basis of mathematical probabilities which are consistent with biological variations in segregation ratios in any genetic setting. If our hypothesis of autosomal dominance is valid, a closer approximation to the true 50 percent of affected individuals would be expected if a larger number of families of this type could be ascertained. Consanguinity was absent throughout this entire family.

An excess of adenocarcinomas has occurred in this family, particularly those of the colon and the endometrium (Table 19-IX), but, of unusual interest, have been the increased occurrences of leukemia, lymphoma, and sarcoma in Branch E of this kindred with 3 occurrences among its 46 members. This concurrence of reticuloendothelial and mesodermal neoplasms is in sharp distinction to the overwhelming predominance of adenocarcinoma typically encountered in the cancer family syndrome as recently described in 6 families.[10] In the total family and considering *all* ages, seven members in 3 generations have developed sarcoma, leukemia, and/or brain tumors. Two others have received a diagnosis of splenomegaly and are being followed for the possible future development of hematopoietic malignancy.

In the family described here, an unusually early age at onset of cancer has been documented in a number of relatives, although the average age of onset of cancer throughout the family could not be determined with sufficient accuracy to make this percentage

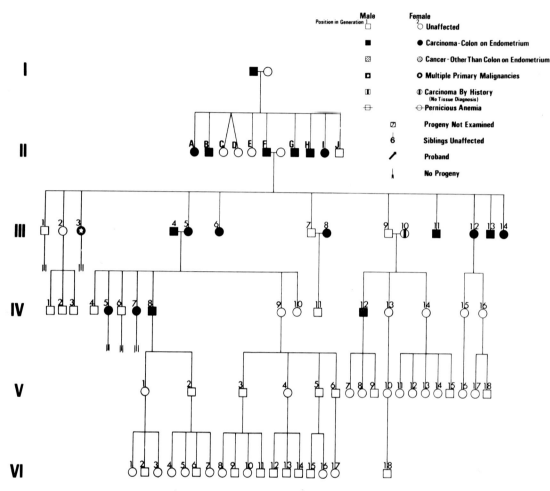

Figure 19–1F. Shows Branch F of Family G.

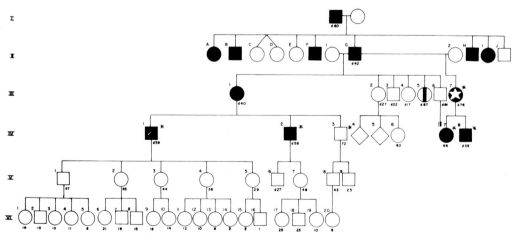

Figure 19–1G. Shows Branch G of Family G.

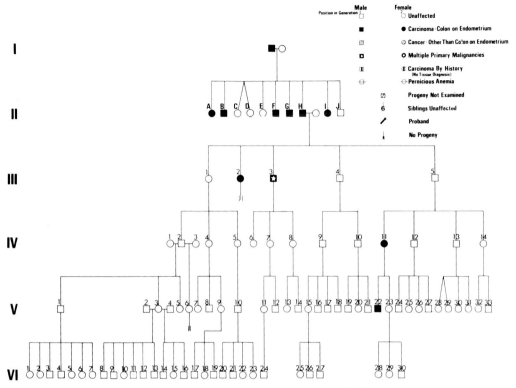

Figure 19–1H. Shows Branch H of Family G.

meaningful. Thus, a major differentiating factor between Family "G" and the cancer family syndrome is the occurrences of sarcomas, brain tumors, and leukemia in branch E that was cancer-free for two generations prior to these occurrences. This appearance of sarcoma, brain tumors and leukemia could be fortuitous and thereby unassociated with the cancer family syndrome. It might also result from acquisition of new genetic material from marriages into Family G or may be an additional example of expressivity of this cancer prone diathesis.

Another aspect of our study of Family G now involves the initiation of studies of a large branch of the family which remained in Germany after the progenitor of the 9 United States branches had emigrated. To date only one member has been found to have had a diagnosis of cancer (pancreas). However, these studies are in only a pre-liminary stage at this time. It will be of interest to determine what effect the geographic and dietary, etc. differences may have on the incidence of cancer in this kindred.

Family "N"

The propositus (No. U-117770) (Fig. 19–2–19–6) was studied at the Omaha Veterans Administration Hospital where he died at age 44 from adrenocortical carcinoma.[11]

Because of the large size of family "N" Figures 19–2 to 19–6 have been constructed in order to reflect more clearly genealogy and cancer occurrences.

The proband's medical history revealed that many of his immediate relatives had had cancer and that although they lived in a wide geographic area (Fig. 19–7), many resided in the State of Missouri. A study of the family was made in accor-

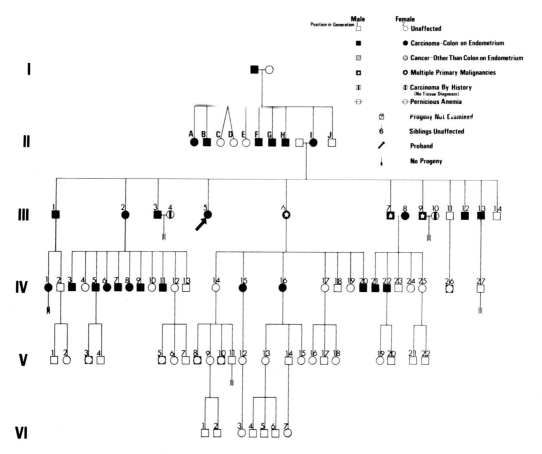

Figure 19–1I. Shows Branch I of Family G.

dance with the same methods as those involved in the study of Family "G". In addition, several field trips were made to the area where many of the relatives resided. Clinical facilities were kindly donated by a private physician who had cared for some of the affected members of the family. Complete histories and physical examinations, including pelvic examinations, cervical cytology, and proctosigmoidoscopy, were performed on 44 individuals. When lesions were accessible to surgical biopsy, appropriate tissue was obtained. Blood was obtained for ABO typing, hemoglobin, hematocrit, and cell indices.

Analysis of the pedigree showed 40 individuals with carcinoma, which occurred through four generations. The proband had twelve siblings and, of these, six have had diagnoses of carcinoma (Fig. 19–4, V-127, V-130, V-132, V-136, V-144, V-148) with four of these six affected individuals showing separate multiple primary malignant neoplasms (Fig. 19–4, V-127, V-130, V-132, V-148). The histologic types of carcinoma in his siblings included carcinoma of the lip, stomach, colon, endometrium, and kidney.

Of the four showing multiple primary carcinomas, the combinations included colon and skin (Fig. 19–4, V-127), stomach and

TABLE 19-II
TUMOR REGISTRY FOR BRANCH B

Pedigree No.	Sex	Site	Age at Diagnosis
II-B	M	Stomach	
III-1	F	Endometrium and colon	42,54*
III-3	F	Stomach	43
III-5	F	Basal cell	68,89*
III-6	M	Colon	82
III-8	F	Basal cell	75
		Endometrium	60*
III-9	M	Brain tumor	53
III-11	M	Prostate	63
III-12	F	Colon	39
IV-4	M	Stomach	25
IV-6	F	Endometrium	
IV-9	M	Squamous cell (skin)	62
		Prostate	66*
IV-14	F	Endometrium	41
IV-16	M	Colon	30
IV-18	M	Colon	37
IV-20	M	Colon	74
IV-22	F	Colon	60
IV-30	M	Colon	20
IV-36	F	Colon	76
IV-40	F	Colon	65
V-3	F	Colon	
V-9	M	Two, colon	49*
V-20	M	Colon	
V-44	F	Ovary	27
V-45	F	Colon	
V-46	F	Colon	
Total number of members, all ages			158
Number of members who reached age 40 without cancer			43
Total number with cancer			26
Number who developed cancer after age 40			20 (32%)

*Multiple primary malignant neoplasms.

TABLE 19-III
TUMOR REGISTRY FOR BRANCH D

Pedigree No.	Sex	Site	Age at Diagnosis
III-2	M	Colon	49
IV-1	M	Three, colon	54,63,65*
IV-3	F	Colon	48
V-1	M	Colon	41
V-4	F	Thyroid	35*
		Lung	
Total number of members, all ages			27
Number of members who reached age 40 without cancer			4
Total number with cancer			5
Number who developed cancer after age 40			4 (50%)

*Malignant primary malignant neoplasms.

TABLE 19-IV
TUMOR REGISTRY FOR BRANCH E

Pedigree No.	Sex	Site	Age at Diagnosis
IV-4	M	Chronic lymphocytic leukemia	70
IV-5	M	Lymphosarcoma	69
IV-9	M	Lymphosarcoma	63
Total number of members, all ages			46
Number of members who reached age 40 without cancer			12
Total number with cancer (hematopoietic)			3
Number who developed cancer after age 40			3 (20%)

TABLE 19-V
TUMOR REGISTRY FOR BRANCH F

Pedigree No.	Sex	Site	Age at Diagnosis
II-F	M	Colon	
III-3	F	Endometrium	*
		Two, colon	78,82
III-5	F	Endometrium	before age 60
III-6	F	Breast	
III-11	M	Colon	
III-12	F	Endometrium	
III-13	M	Colon	79
III-14	F	Endometrium	
IV-5	F	Endometrium	77
IV-7	F	Basal cell	65
IV-8	M	Lung	60
IV-12	M	Colon	57
IV-16	F	Liver	
Total number of members			64
Number of members who reached age 40 without cancer			14
Number with cancer			13
Number who developed cancer after age 40			13 (48%)

colon (Fig. 19–4, V-148), uterus and ovary (Fig. 19–4, V-130), carcinoma of the cervix and four primary colon carcinomas (Fig. 19–4, V-132). The proband's mother (Fig. 19–4, IV-41) died at age 51 from carcinoma (unconfirmed) and his maternal grandmother (Fig. 19–4, III-8) died at age 31 from metastatic carcinoma (unconfirmed). His father (Fig. 19–4, IV-42) died at age 70 and was known not to have had cancer. However, his paternal grandmother (Fig. 19–5, III-10) died at age 81 from carcinoma of the larynx (unconfirmed). A maternal first cousin of the proband (Fig. 19–4, V-86) had two primary carcinomas (colon and endometrium). Her mother (Fig. 19–4, IV-30) died

TABLE 19-VI
TUMOR REGISTRY FOR BRANCH G

Pedigree No.	Sex	Site	Age at Diagnosis
II-G	M	Colon	
III-1	F	Endometrium	38
III 5	F	Colon	
III-7	F	Endometrium	55
		two, colon	60,69
		stomach	76*
IV-1	M	Gastric fibrosarcoma	
IV-2	M	Colon	58
IV-7	F	Colon	
IV-8	M	Colon	37
IV-16			
Total number of members			43
Number of members who reached age 40 without cancer			8
Total number with cancer			8
Number who developed cancer after age 40			6 (43%)

*Multiple primary malignant neoplasms.

TABLE 19-VII
TUMOR REGISTRY FOR BRANCH H

Pedigree No.	Sex	Site	Age at Diagnosis
II-H	M	Stomach	
III-2	F	Endometrium	43
III-3	M	Colon	77
		Ureter	77* (at autopsy)
IV-11	F	Breast	47
V-22	M	Brain	22
Total number of members			78
Number of members who reached age 40 without cancer			14
Total number with cancer			5
Number who developed cancer after age 40			4 (22%)

*Multiple primary malignant neoplasms.

at age 61 from carcinoma of the colon. She had two children with carcinoma. Of these, one (Fig. 19–4, V-91) died at age 31 from carcinoma; the second is still alive but has had a diagnosis of squamous cell carcinoma of the skin, and carcinoma of the breast, and is under treatment for diabetes mellitus (Fig. 19–4, V-84).

Thirteen of the 44 family members who were examined had blood group A, and, of the five with a history of a malignant neoplasm, all had blood group A. Two of these five had multiple primary tumors.

There was no evidence of consanguinity in this family.

Our medical genetic investigation of Family "N" has been continuous since 1966. During this interval twenty-three family members have received diagnoses of cancer. Four of these 23 individuals developed a second primary malignant lesion (Fig. 19–3, V-38, Fig. 19–3, V-57, Fig. 19–4, V-132, and Fig. 19–4, V-136). Two other individuals developed two additional malignant lesions during this period (Fig. 19–4, V-84, and Fig. 19–4, V-110) (Table 19-XI).

Family "M"

The propositus (Fig. 19–8, IV-1) (No. 945482) was studied at the University Hos-

TABLE 19-VIII
TUMOR REGISTRY FOR BRANCH I

Pedigree No.	Sex	Site	Age at Diagnosis
II-I	F	Endometrium	
III-1	M	Colon	
III-2	F	Liver	58
III-3	M	Colon	
III-5	F	Endometrium	46
III-6	F	Endometrium	55
		Colon	57*
III-7	M	Colon	51
		Pancreas	51*
III-9	M	Skin	before age 72
		Seminoma	86
		Squamous cell	85
		plasmacytoma sternum	85*
III-12	M	Stomach	28
III-13	M	Bladder	76
IV-1	F	Colon	
IV-3	M	Colon	26
IV-5	M	Stomach	
IV-6	F	Pituitary	50
IV-7	M	Colon	33
IV-8	F	Colon	
IV-9	M	Not specified	
IV-11	M	Colon	49
IV-15	F	Colon	45
IV-16	F	Colon	37
IV-20	M	Pancreas	48
IV-21	M	Colon	24
IV-22	M	Colon	50
Total number of members			61
Number of members who reached age 40 without cancer			11
Total number with cancer			23
Number who developed cancer after age 40			18 (62%)

*Multiple primary malignant neoplasms.

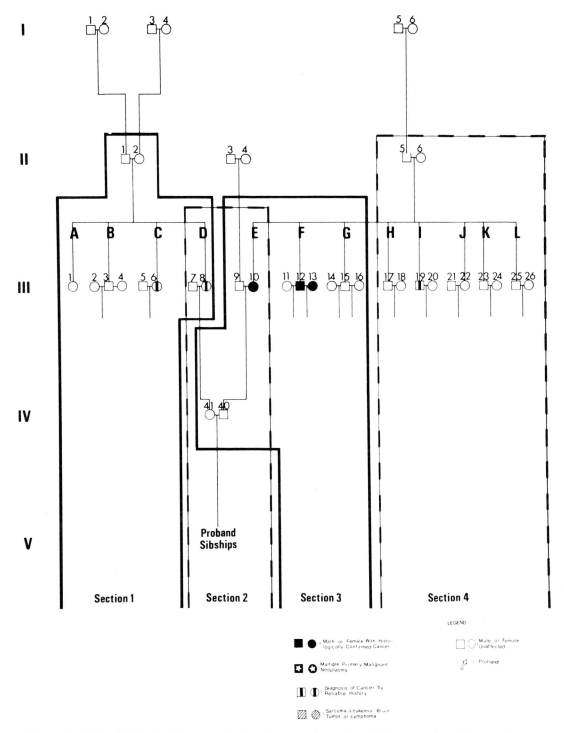

Figure 19–2. Family N, showing transmission of cancer through multiple generations. Please refer to Legend, which will indicate histologic verification of adenocarcinoma, multiple primary malignant neoplasms with histologic verification, and carcinoma verified by reliable history. Because of the large size of this family it has been necessary to continue branches of the family as sections in Figures 19–3, 19–4, 19–5, and 19–6. By permission, Lynch, H.T., *Arch Int Med, 134*:931, 1974.

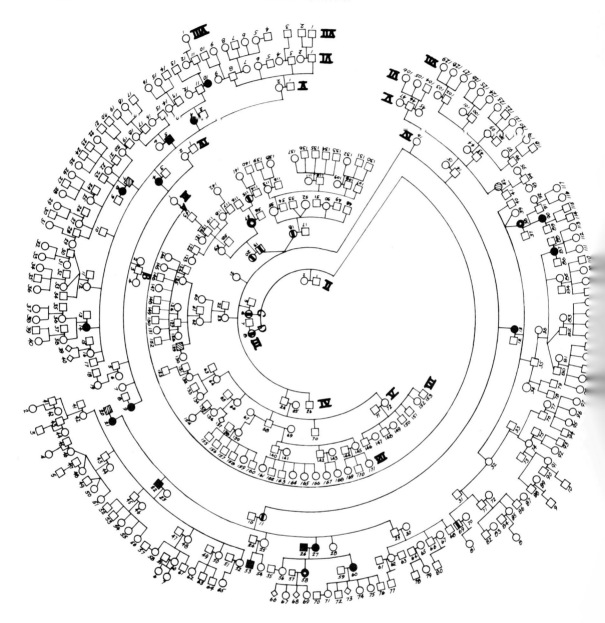

Figure 19–3. Family N presented as Section 1 shows Branches A, B, C, and D.

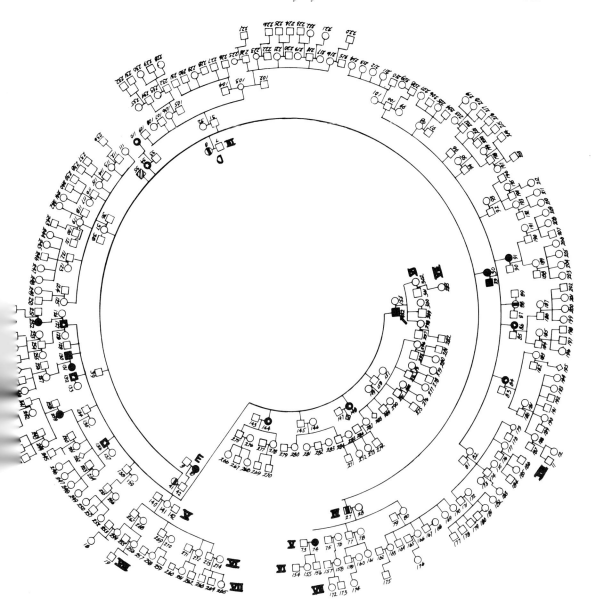

Figure 19–4. Continuation of Family N as Section 2 shows Branches D and E forming proband sibships and progeny.

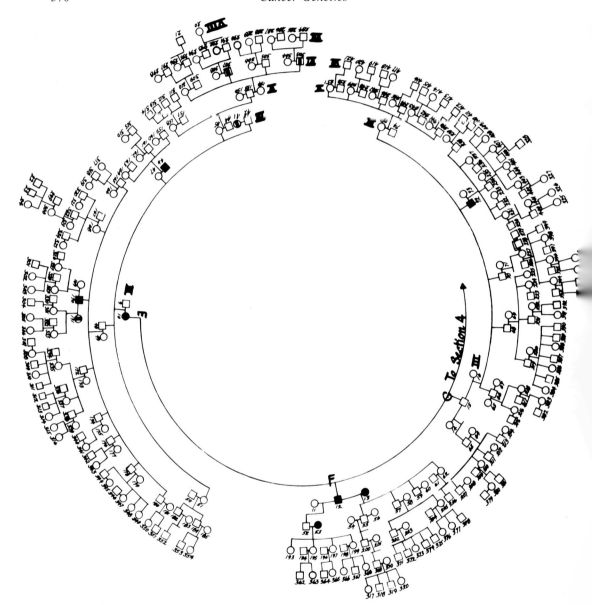

Figure 19–5. Continuation of Family N as Section 3 shows Branches E, F, and G. In the numbering sequence in Generation IV, numbers 186–192 are vacant, and in Generation V numbers 355–361 are vacant.

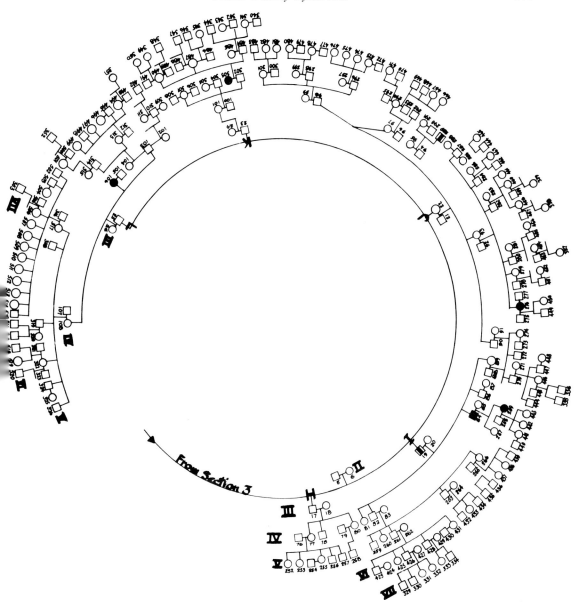

Figure 19–6. Continuation of Family N as Section 4 shows Branches H, I, J, K, and L.

TABLE 19-IX
REGISTRY OF CANCER OF SPECIFIC ANATOMIC SITES BY FAMILY BRANCHES

Site	A	B	C	D	E	F	G	H	I	J	Total
Colon	3	16	—	6	—	6	7	1	13	—	52+
Endometrium	3	4	—	—	—	5	2	1	3	—	18
Stomach	1	3	—	—	—	—	1	1	2	—	8
Breast	2	—	—	—	—	1	—	1	—	—	4
Skin											
Basal cell	—	2	—	—	—	1	—	—	1	—	4
Squamous cell	—	1	—	—	—	—	—	—	1	—	2
Transitional cell bladder	—	—	—	—	—	—	—	—	1	—	1
Transitional cell ureter	—	—	—	—	—	—	—	1	—	—	1
Prostate	—	2	—	—	—	—	—	—	—	—	2
Liver	—	—	—	—	—	1	—	—	1	—	2
Ovary	—	1	—	—	—	—	—	—	—	—	1
Thyroid	—	—	—	1	—	—	—	—	—	—	1
Lung	—	—	—	1	—	1	—	—	—	—	2
Chromophobe adenoma of pituitary	—	—	—	—	—	—	—	—	1	—	1
Pancreas	—	—	—	—	—	—	—	—	2	—	2
Site unknown	1	—	—	—	—	—	—	—	1	—	2
Sarcoma*	1	—	—	—	2	—	1	—	1	—	5
Plasmacytoma-sternum	—	—	—	—	—	—	—	—	1	—	1
Lymphocytic leukemia	1	—	—	—	1	—	—	—	—	—	2
Brain tumor	—	1	—	—	—	—	—	1	—	—	2
Total	12	30	—	8	3	15	11	6	28	—	113+

*Sarcoma of several anatomic sites.
+ 95 patients had cancer, and 13 of these had multiple primary malignant neoplasms.

pital, Ann Arbor, Michigan, where she died at age 36 from metastatic carcinoma of the breast. After a strong family history of carcinoma was elicited, as in the families above, questionnaires were sent to members of the family.[11] Histologic confirmation of carcinoma was made through physicians' records and pathology reports from several hospitals. In addition, cytogenetic studies were performed on the proband prior to her death. They included karyotype analyses of leukocytes from two peripheral blood cultures, skin from her leg and from her pituitary gland following its surgical ablation for palliative reasons. The findings, from karyotyping each of these tissues, were normal. Pedigree analysis (Fig. 19–8) showed that malignant neoplasms were present in 18 individuals and were transmitted through two and probably three generations (Generation II having diagnoses by reliable history) (Fig. 19–8, II-1, carcinoma of the lip; II-2, II-4, II-5, and II-8, carcinoma of the colon).

The proband's mother (Fig. 19–8, III-1) had a confirmed carcinoma of the endometrium. She had ten siblings and of these seven had histologically confirmed carcinoma and one had a diagnosis of "intestinal cancer" by history and died at age 20. Four siblings had multiple primary cancers which included the following combinations: carcinoma of the colon, uterus, and ovary (Fig. 19–8,

TABLE 19-X
NUMBER OF SIBSHIPS WITH CANCER IN:

Branch	Number of Sibships with Cancer	2 Generations	3 Gen.	4 Gen.	5 Gen.
A	5	—	1	1	—
B	13	—	1	6	3
C	0	—	—	—	—
D	4	—	2	—	—
E	1	—	—	—	—
F	4	—	1	2	—
G	4	—	—	2	—
H	4	1	1	—	—
I	6	—	—	4	—
J	0	—	—	—	—
Totals	41	1	6	15	3

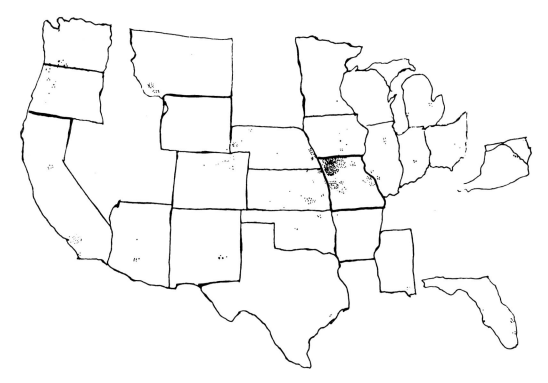

Figure 19–7. Diagrammatic map of the United States wherein dots indicated patients from Family N with the Cancer Family Syndrome. Note the concentration of relatives in the Midwest, particularly in northwestern Missouri.

III-3), three primary colon carcinomas (Fig. 19–8, III-5), carcinoma of the pancreas and uterus (Fig. 19–8, III-7), and carcinoma of the lip and colon (Fig. 19–8, III-8), (Table 19-XII). Again, note the large variety of malignant neoplasms in this family which included adenocarcinoma of the breast, carcinoma of the lip, duodenum, colon, pancreas, endometrium, and ovary. In addition, a history of diabetes mellitus, hypertension obesity, and rheumatoid arthritis occurred in many affected as well as unaffected members of the kindred. Consanguinity was absent in this family.

Family "O"

In Family "O" (Fig. 19–9), adenocarcinoma of the colon occurred in four generations. The proband (Fig. 19–9, III-4) was 64 years old in 1966 when this family was ascertained. He had received treatment for carcinoma of the ascending colon at age 22, a second primary carcinoma of the transverse colon at age 46, and three squamous cell cancers of the hands at age 59, 62, and 63. The proband was one of five siblings, all of whom had received treatment for carcinoma. His oldest sister, (Fig. 19–9, III-1) age 73, had four separate primary carcinomas of the colon at age 47, 54, 61, and 69. A second sister, (Fig. 19–9, III-2) age 69, had a diagnosis of endometrial carcinoma at age 53 and a secondary primary carcinoma of the colon at age 73. Two brothers (Fig. 19–9, III-3 and III-5) died at ages 30 and 35, respectively, of carcinoma of the colon (by reliable history). A

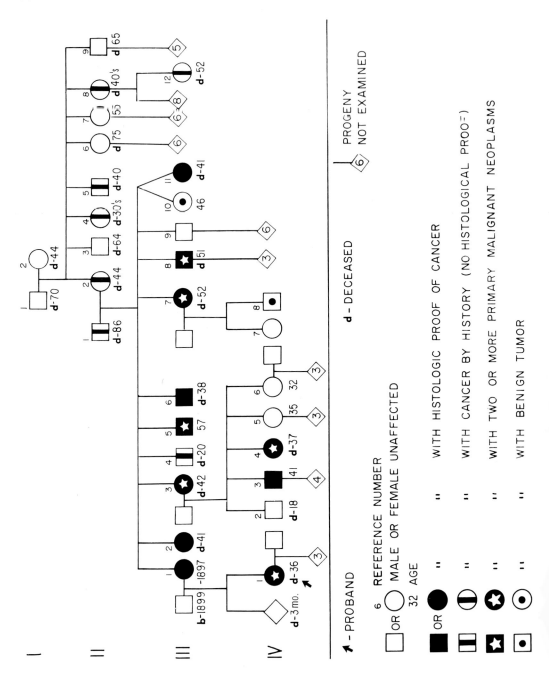

Figure 19–8. Pedigree of Cancer Family M.

daughter of one of these brothers (Fig. 19–9, IV-1) died at age 32 of carcinoma of the colon. The proband's mother (Fig. 19–99, II-3) died at age 74 of carcinoma of the colon. One of her sisters (Fig. 19–9, II-1) died of carcinoma of the kidneys (reliable history); a second sister (Fig. 19 8, II-4) died of carcinoma of an unknown site, and her father (Fig. 19–9, I-1), a brother (Fig. 19–9, II-5), and one of his children (Fig. 19–9, III-7) all died of colon carcinoma (reliable history).

Family "P"

Of eight members of Family "P" (Fig. 19–10) with diagnoses of carcinoma, four had adenocarcinoma of the colon in two consecutive generations. Two had multiple primary malignant neoplasms, one of which was a colon malignancy in each case.

The proband (Fig. 19–10, III-10) was a 63-year-old white woman who had been in good health until the age of 38 when she received a diagnosis of squamous cell carcinoma of the uterine cervix. The cervix was removed surgically and Roentgen X-ray therapy was administered postoperatively. At age 40, grade II adenocarcinoma of the endometrium was detected. The patient was treated by hysterectomy and further Roentgen X-ray therapy. Approximately eight months later, she underwent a surgical pro-

TABLE 19-XI
NEW TUMORS ASCERTAINED IN FAMILY N SINCE 1966 (See Figs. 19-3 to 19-6)

Pedigree Number	Birthdate	Tumor	Age at Diagnosis	Date of Ascertainment
V-21	1895	Bladder	76	1971
V-5	1894	Prostate	78	1972
VI-53	1926	Basal Cell—Nose	44	1971
VI-58	1924	Breast	46	1972
		Endometrium	46	1972
		Stomach	47	1972
VI-69	1920	Colon**	d50	1972
VI-87	1942	*In Situ* Cervix	27	1973
V-38	1914	Endometrium	38	*
		Colon	58	1973
V-42	1903	Hodgkin's Disease	33 d65	1968
V-57	1915	Endometrium	49	*
		Kidney, Ureter, Bladder	57	1973
V-4	1893	Breast	78	1973
V-7	1898	Astrocytoma	69	1968
V-59	1922	Endometrium	43	1966
V-84	1906	Carcinoma of Left Cheek	56	*
		Squamous Cell, Finger	63	1970
		Breast	63	1970
V-110	1914	Endometrium	36	*
		Colon	50	*
		Stomach	53	1968
		Bladder	54	1968
V-139	1902	Colon (Cecum)	56	*
		Carcinoma of Lower Lip	48	*
		Sigmoid Colon	66	1968
V-132	1904	Left Kidney	60	*
		Pancreas	67	1971
VI-304	1923	Face (Skin)**	54	1971
V-170	1910	Larynx	59	1972
IV-72	1894	Lung	75	1971
V-269	1924	Breast	48	1973
V-276	1908	Basal Cell	58	1967
VI-184	1932	Colon	42	1974
VI-60	1930	Endometrium	44	1974

* = Previously ascertained.
** = By reliable history.

TABLE 19-XII
REGISTRY OF MALIGNANT NEOPLASMS IN FAMILY M

Pedigree Index No.	Age	Sex	Lip	Duodenum	Colon	Pancreas	Uterus	Ovary	Stomach	Breast	Unknown
II-1	D86	M	--	...	...	...	...	...	...	...	...
II-2	D44	F	...	...	--	...	...	...	...	...	...
II-4	D30	F	...		--	...	...	...	...	...	...
II-5	D40	M	...	...	--	...	...	...	...	...	...
II-8	D40	F	...	...	--	...	...	...	...	...	...
III-1	68	F	...	...	...	...	+ 52	...	...	...	...
III-2	D41	F	...	...	...	...	...	...	+ 39	...	...
III-3	D42	F	...	...	+ 41	...	+ 42	+ 39	...	...	...
III-4	D20	M	...	...	...	...	...	...	...	...	-- 20
III-5	57	M	...	...	+ + + 42 45 56	...	...	...	...	...	...
III-6	D38	M	...	+ 38	...	...	...	...	...	...	...
III-7	D52	F	...	...	...	+ 52	+ 45	...	...	...	...
III-8	D51	M	+ 50	...	+ 36	...	...	...	...	...	...
III-11	D41	F	...	...	...	...	+ 38	...	...	...	...
III-12	D52	F	...	...	...	...	...	...	...	...	--
IV-1	⬈D36	F	...	...	...	...	...	...	...	+ + 33 35	...
IV-3	41	M	...	...	+ 32	...	...	...	...	...	...
IV-4	D37	F	...	...	+ 37	...	+ 28	+ 28	...	...	...

⬈ = proband; + = tissue confirmation; -- = no tissue confirmation.
Numbers set below + and -- signs indicate the age at which the lesion was discovered.

TABLE 19-XIII
REGISTRY OF NEOPLASMS IN FAMILY "P"

Pedigree No.	Age	Sex	Colon	Endometrium	Cervix	Brain	Unknown Primary	Ovary	Lymphosarcoma
I-1	*D?	M	...	...	...	...	--	...	...
II-2	D49	F	...	--	...	...	...	...	...
II-6	D52	M	+ 51	...	...	...	...	...	...
III-5	D50	F	...	...	...	+ 49	...	...	...
III-8	D47	F	+ 46	...	...	...	...	...	...
III-10	⬈63	F	+ + 60, 60	+ 40	-- 38	...	...	+ 40	...
III-12	D42	F	...	+ 42	...	...	...	...	+ 42
III-14	D44	F	-- 36	...	...	...	...	...	...

+ = histologically confirmed; -- = by history; *D = age at death; ⬈ = proband.

cedure for papillary carcinoma of the left ovary; both ovaries were removed. At age 57, a polyp of the colon was removed through the proctoscope at the level of 17 cm. It proved to be a benign adenoma. At age 60, she underwent an abdomino-perineal resection at which time a polyp from the sigmoid colon proved to be a well-differentiated mucinous adenocarcinoma invading but not piercing the muscular wall. Several small lymph nodes were examined but showed no abnormalities. Several months later, the patient noted blood in her stools, and anoscopy revealed a suspicious lesion. This biopsied lesion proved to be a grade II adenocarcinoma of the rectum. The patient underwent a second abdominoperineal resection; a permanent colostomy was con-

structed. Sections from the surgical specimen showed a transition from squamous epithelium into a zone composed of a poorly differentiated adenocarcinoma which was not mucin secreting and which appeared to arise primarily at the pectinate line. From this malignant epithelium, there was an abrupt transition into normal rectal-type mucosa. Superficial invasion into the underlying muscle was present but no tumor was found at the excised margins. This lesion was independently reviewed by several pathologists and was found to be a separate primary malignant neoplasm arising at the pectinate line.

The patient made a complete recovery. She had a total of five primary malignant neoplasms. She leads a vigorous and active

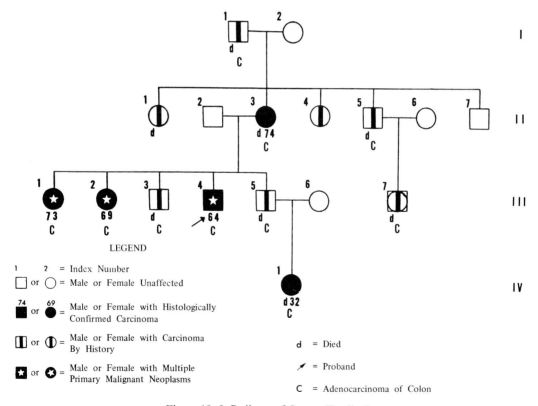

Figure 19–9. Pedigree of Cancer Family O.

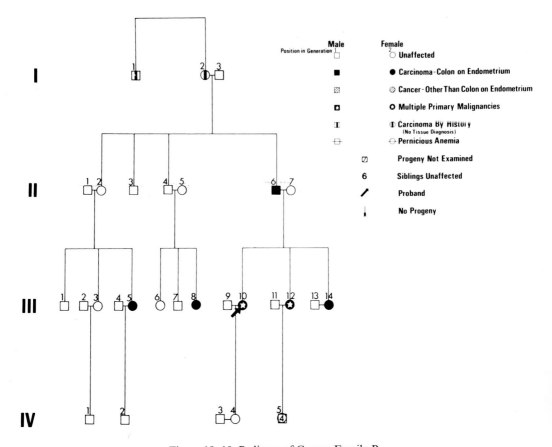

Figure 19–10. Pedigree of Cancer Family P.

TABLE 19-XIV
REGISTRY OF NEOPLASMS IN FAMILY "Q"

Age	Sex	Colon	Endometrium	Lip	Lung	Malignant-Carcinoid Tumor
D33	F	33*	...	...	...	...
D42	F	42+	...	...	...	...
D34	M	34*	...	...	...	...
43	M	40+	...	...	...	...
D47	F	44+	47+	...	...	...
50	M	48+, 49+	...	...	...	...
D52	M	...	...	46+	52+	...
D45	F	43+	42+	...	...	42+
D42	M	40+	...	...	...	...
43	M	41 ‖	...	...	...	...

* = malignancy by history.
+ = malignancy histologically confirmed.

life, travels widely and has accepted her many cancer problems with amazing equanimity. The results of physical examination at age 63, with the exception of a palpable thyroid isthmus and several surgical scars, were entirely normal.

The patient's family history was noteworthy for the presence of malignant neoplasms in her first degree relatives (Fig. 19–10 and Table 19-XIII).

Family "Q"

Family "Q" (Table 19-XIV) consists of 52 individuals, of whom ten have had malignant neoplasms. Eight individuals had carcinoma of the colon, two had endo-metrial carcinoma, and three individuals had multiple primary malignancies, two of whom had the combination of endometrial and colon carcinoma.

The proband was a white married woman who had been in good health until age 42, when she underwent a resection of the transverse colon for a tumor that proved histologically to be a malignant carcinoid. Six months later a diagnosis of adenocarcinoma of the endometrium was established. She underwent radium implantation and external radiation therapy, followed by panhysterectomy approximately two months later. About four months following the diagnosis of endometrial carcinoma, she underwent a surgical resection for the third primary

TABLE 19-XV
TUMOR REGISTRY OF FAMILY "S"

Pedigree Index	Age	Sex	Colon	Breast	Endometrium	Stomach	Pancreas	Vulva	Bladder	Cervix	Unknown
I-4	D64	F	...	...	−− −−	...	...	...	...	...	...
II-3	D74	F	...	...	...	...	+ 73	...	...	...	...
II-5	D67	F	+ + 56 56	...	...	...	...	...	...	...	...
II-6	D71	F	...	...	...	...	+ 71	...	...	...	...
II-7	D52	M	−−	...	...	...	...	...	...	...	...
II-10	D56	F	...	...	...	+ 54	...	...	...	...	...
II-11	65	M	+ 44	...	...	...	...	...	+ 64	...	...
III-2	56	F	...	+ 42	...	...	...	...	...	+ 49	...
III-3	64	M	+ + 44 56	...	...	...	...	...	...	...	...
III-5	D57	F	+ 56	...	+ 40	...	...	...	...	...	...
III-6	?	F	−−	...	...	...	...	...	...	...	...
III-7	?	F	...	...	...	...	...	...	...	...	−−
III-8	D21	F	...	−−	...	...	...	...	...	...	...
IV-1	↗35	M	+ + 33 33	...	...	...	+ 35	...	...	...	...
IV-2	D41	M	+ 37	...	...	...	...	...	...	...	...
IV-5	38	F	+ 29	...	...	...	...	...	...	...	...
IV-7	31	F	+ 27	...	...	...	...	...	...	...	...

↗ = proband.
+ = tissue confirmation.
−− = no tissue confirmation.
sub. no. = age lesion discovered.
D = died.
? = unknown age.

malignancy, adenocarcinoma of the recto-sigmoid.

This patient was a nonsmoker and used alcohol infrequently. There were no known unusual environmental exposures. She was gravida 4, para 3, and had experienced one miscarriage. The family history was striking for the presence of malignant neoplasms (Table 19-XIV).

A physical examination during her last hospitalization showed the patient to be normotensive. She was 5'6" tall and weighed 120 lbs. There were cystic lesions of the breast, pectus excavatum, mild thoracic scoliosis, and a left inguinal mass that subsequently proved to be carcinoma of the rectosigmoid colon. The remainder of the physical examination was within normal limits.

An endocrine evaluation revealed normal thyroid and adrenal function; the latter evaluation included a normal response to metyrapone-suppression studies. A mammogram of the breast revealed bilateral fibrocystic disease.

The remainder of the laboratory work, including liver function studies and blood glucose levels, was within normal limits. The patient did well for several months after her last hospitalization but then began a downhill course and died at age 45. Autopsy revealed generalized carcinomatosis.

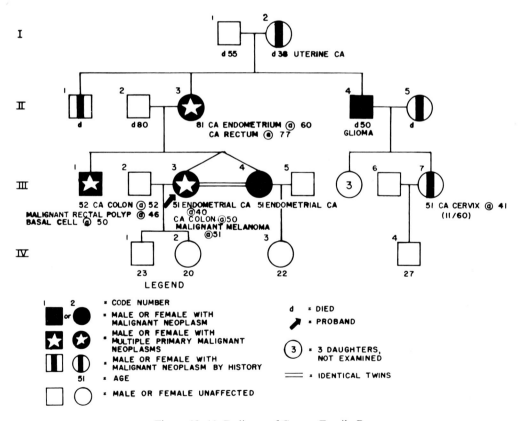

Figure 19–11. Pedigree of Cancer Family R.

Family "R"

The proband (Fig. 19–11, III-3) was a 51-year-old white woman of English ancestry who had received a diagnosis of endometrial carcinoma at age 40 in 1958. Cancer control implications[12] were found in this family as follows: In 1968, because of the occurrence of adenocarcinoma of the colon in her 52-year-old brother (Fig. 19–11, III-1) (see below), this patient requested that her physician perform appropriate diagnostic studies on her colon even though she was completely asymptomatic. This request was prompted primarily by the fact that cancer was unusually prevalent in her family. Findings on proctosigmoidoscopy and barium enema revealed the presence of an early adenocarcinoma of the transverse colon and a colectomy was successfully performed. The patient is surviving at this time one year following surgery. However, she had a *malignant mole* removed at age 51.

The proband's identical twin sister, (Fig. 19–11, III-4) had been completely asymptomatic at age 40 in 1968, but requested an evaluation of her uterus because of the occurrence of endometrial carcinoma in her co-twin. A diagnosis of early endometrial carcinoma was established and a hysterectomy was successfully performed. The patient was surviving 2 years after this surgery. When her twin sister developed adenocarcinoma of the colon in 1968, the patient requested that her physician perform a sigmoidoscopic examination. This examination was negative and she continues to receive regular follow-up rectal examinations.

The proband's brother (Fig. 19–11, III-1) had a malignant rectal polyp removed by surgery at age 46; a basal cell carcinoma of the integument at the eyebrow and temple was removed at age 50. He subsequently developed a change in bowel habits and rectal bleeding, and was found to have adenocarcinoma of the colon at the age of 52 in 1968. A colectomy was successfully performed and he was surviving one year after surgery.

Other members of the family have received diagnoses as follows: The mother (Fig. 19–11, II-3) had endometrial carcinoma at age 70 in 1948 and adenocarcinoma of the rectum in 1956 at age 77. She was living at age 81, four years post surgery. A maternal uncle (Fig. 19–11, II-1) died of cancer, unconfirmed and the primary site not known. Another maternal uncle (Fig. 19–11, II-4) developed an intracranial glioma at age 49 in 1941, and died at age 50. A maternal first cousin (Fig. 19–11, III-7) was diagnosed as having *in situ* carcinoma of the uterine cervix. The maternal grandmother (Fig. 19–8, I-2) died at age 38 of endometrial carcinoma (by history).

The homozygosity of the twins in this kindred has been established primarily on the basis of physical characteristics and blood group antigens. The physicians involved in this family, including the patients themselves, emphasize the striking similarities between them. For example, the following is a quotation from one of the twin sisters:

> As far as my sister and I being identical, you can be assured we definitely are. My mother's doctor did tell her that. My sister and I still look very much alike even though we are now 51, and in earlier years we were very hard to tell apart. We have the same red hair, blue eyes, and physical features . . . our weight has just about stayed the same; our eyes have always seemed to need the same correction in glasses, etc.— even our teeth are the same . . .

Major blood group antigens in the sisters were identical. However, skin transplantations and other more refined measures for identifying zygosity have not been performed.

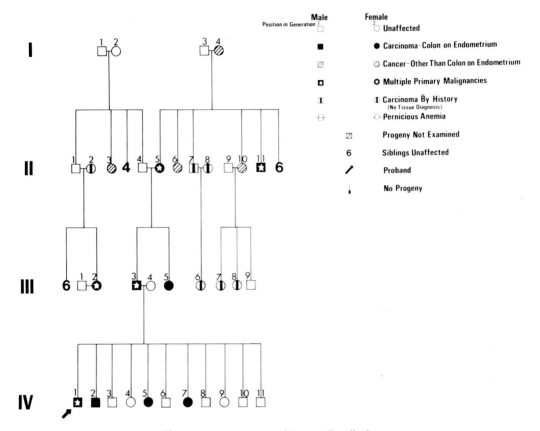

Figure 19–12. Pedigree of Cancer Family S.

Family "S"

The proband, (Fig. 19–12, and Table 19-XV, IV-1) (#V.A. 508-36-5373) a 35-year-old white male presented at the Omaha Veterans Administration Hospital with a previous history of two primary colon carcinomas.[13] At this admission a third primary cancer (pancreatic carcinoma) was identified. More than one hundred family members have been ascertained.

This patient was first hospitalized in January, 1969, with a complaint of bright red pararectal bleeding. This was of abrupt onset and was not associated with any weight loss. A proctoscopy and barium enema examination were performed which demonstrated an annular lesion in the descending colon. At subsequent laparotomy, an adenocarcinoma was removed and an end-to-end colonic anastomosis was performed. There was no further difficulty until April, 1969, when jaundice developed. At this second laparotomy a hard mass was found in the head of the pancreas but was not resected. Rather, a choledochojejunostomy was performed which relieved the jaundice. During the same operation, on palpation of the cecum, another tumor was found and was resected. This was thought to be a second primary lesion. Following recovery from surgery, he had no further difficulties until November of 1970 when he developed some abdominal cramps. A serum amylase of 300 somogyi units was noted. An upper GI series demonstrated no tumor. The gall bladder was not visualized following an oral cholecystoscopy.

His fourth hospitalization was in December, 1970; admission was for continuing abdominal cramps, a weight loss of 17 pounds and recurrent jaundice. An upper GI demonstrated invasion of the duodenum by a malignant process which represented a marked change from the upper GI in November. At laparotomy, a pancreatico-duodenostomy with gastro-jejunostomy, choledojejunotomy, and a pancreatico-jejunotomy were performed. The pancreatic tumor was not metastatic but was felt to be a primary carcinoma of the head of the pancreas which was considered to be a third gastro-intestinal primary lesion in this patient. He died about six months later.

TABLE 19-XVI
DIFFERENTIAL DIAGNOSIS OF CANCER FAMILY SYNDROME

	Cancer Family Syndrome	Familial Polyposis Coli	Gardner's Syndrome	Turcot's Syndrome	Adenocarcinoma Colon	Endometrial Cancer
Adenocarcinoma Colon	+	+	+	+	+	+
Endometrial Carcinoma	+	−	−	−	−	+
Multiple Primary Malignant Neoplasms	+	+	+	+	+	−
Early Age at Onset	+	+	+	+	+	+
Genetics	D	D	D	R	Er	Er
Associated Signs:						
Dermatological	−	−	+	+	−	−
Skeletal	−	−	+	−	−	−
Endocrinological	−	−	+	−	−	−
Other	−	−	+	−	−	−
Associated Malignant Neoplasms	+	−	+	+	−	−

	Breast Cancer	Gastric Cancer	Leukemia Sarcoma & Brain Tumors	Hereditary Endocrine Adenomatosis	Zollinger-Ellison Syndrome	Multiple Mucosal Neuroma Syndrome
Adenocarcinoma Colon	−	−	−	−	−	−
Endometrial Carcinoma	−	−	−	−	−	−
Multiple Primary Malignant Neoplasms	+	−	+	+	+	+
Early Age at Onset	+	+	+	+	+	+
Genetics	Er	Er	Er	D	D	D
Associated Signs:						
Dermatological	−	−	−	Poss.	Poss.	+
Skeletal	−	−	−	−	−	−
Endocrinological	−	−	−	+	+	+
Other	−	−	−	+	+	+
Associated Malignant Neoplasma	+,−	−	+	+	+	+

D = Dominant   Er = Empiric risk.
R = Recessive   Poss. = Possible.

Detailed medical history revealed the presence of carcinoma in several of the proband's relatives. Cancer was histologically verified in three generations and ascertained by reliable history in a fourth generation. Table 19-XVI provides a tumor registry designating anatomic site of carcinoma in each member of the family with approximate age at onset of cancer. Of the total kindred of 193 members, 33 blood relatives developed cancer (17%). Colon carcinoma occurred in 15 members of the family. This represents 8 percent when all 193 family members are considered and 45 percent when only members with cancer are considered. When considering only the proband's paternal grandmother's (Fig. 19-12, II-5) side of the family in which all of the colon cancer is concentrated, and excluding the paternal grandfather's (Fig. 19-12, II-4) side of the family, then 10 members developed this lesion. Fifteen members of this branch of the family had cancer of all sites. Breast cancer occurred in 3 members as did carcinoma of the pancreas. All other tumors (endometrial, stomach, vulva, bladder, and cervix) occurred in only one member each.

Multiple primary malignant neoplasms occurred in 8 family members in 3 generations in the total family of 193 (4%) (Table 19-XV and Fig. 19-12, II-5, II-11, III-3, III-5, and IV-1). Colon carcinoma was one of the primary malignant lesions in five of these patients. One patient developed breast and uterine cervical carcinomas. When considering the paternal grandmother's side, then five members had multiple primary malignant neoplasms and in each case one was of the colon. When considering only those members in the total family with cancer, then six of 17 members with cancer developed multiple primary malignant neoplasms.

Socioeconomic factors in the family revealed a consistent pattern of lower middle class laboring and general nonprofessional occupations. The majority of the family members live in small rural towns in western Nebraska though they do not live on farms.

Consanguinity was absent in the family.

Biological Studies

It will be important to search for underlying biological determinants which may be related to cancer predisposition in these families. Such investigations have been initiated, involving numerous collaborators and concerning such factors as HL-A, serum proteins, viral antibodies, SV-40 viral transformation of fibroblasts, cytogenetics, and dermatoglyphics.

Initial cytogenic surveys of cultured peripheral-blood leukocytes from members of Family "N" have indicated the possibility of a rare familial aberration. Each of three members of the family—two female cancer survivors and one of the two females with currently-undetermined cancer susceptibility —includes a minority cell line characterized by an enlarged satellite in one of the D chromosomes. The etiology and any possible pathological relevance of such a mosaicism are unknown. The familial occurrence of such a rare abnormality, and its association with familial malignancy, are provocative and suggest the possibility of associated familial malignancy diathesis with other familial biological characteristics. In addition HL-A haplotype 2–12 showed a significant association ($p < 0.01$) with members of cancer prone as opposed to cancer free branches of Family N. Eleven of twelve family members with cancer in branches C and D (Fig. 19-2–19-4) actually HL-A typed had 2-12 and the single exception showing cancer and another haplotype is a child of a family member with 2-12. In Family G a significant increase in SV-40 viral transformation of fibroblasts was observed ($p < 0.02$) in patients with a high genetic cancer risk as opposed to those at low cancer risk. These studies are currently being expanded, but presently should be evaluated with caution.

Discussion

A relatively complete description of a clinical syndrome should facilitate not only its diagnosis but also comphrehension of its etiology and pathogenesis. The first step in the process is descriptive. This, in fact, has been the primary object of this chapter. It is entirely possible that subsequent investigations may modify significantly certain aspects of this description and indeed the "syndrome" in its present context may even in due time be subdivided into two or more distinct cancer genetic syndromes with the discovery of separate genotypic mechanisms, i.e. due to distinctly separate mutant genes, polygenic inheritance factors and/or modifying genes in specific families. For example, a definite problem at the present time concerns the classification of Family "G" because of the sudden appearance of sarcoma and leukemia in one branch of the family which of course diverges from the previously stated criteria for the cancer family syndrome wherein leukemia and sarcoma were not identified. Thus several questions come immediately to the fore. Does Family "G" represent a separate hereditary cancer syndrome with additional features of sarcoma and leukemia? Or is it the same syndrome but through benefit of more complete ascertainment have we merely elucidated a full clinical expression of the cancer family syndrome which now includes sarcoma and leukemia? This reasoning would suggest that other families classified under the heading of "cancer family syndrome" might have a similar potential for the development of sarcoma and leukemia, given the appropriate malignant hematopoietic stimuli. Or could a combination of modifying genes react with different exogenous car-

cinogenic factors as might have occurred in the specific sarcoma-leukemia-prone branch of Family "G", thereby enhancing a susceptibility to hematopoietic cancer?

The line of reasoning advanced above may well explain not only the possible differences and subsequent classification of the cancer family syndrome but might also explain some of the existing controversies concerning classification of other hereditary cancer syndromes, i.e. the Zollinger-Ellison syndrome, the hereditary multiple endocrine adenomatosis syndrome and the multiple mucosal neuroma syndrome. The discovery of biochemical, cytogenetic or other constitutional factors and/or markers could enhance significantly our understanding of differences or common denominators in these hereditary cancer syndromes. We believe that short of such discoveries, painstaking efforts involved in the compilation and documentation of medical and genealogical findings in cancer prone families will lead toward increased comprehension of these phenomena.

Our working hypothesis proposes that an individual's genetic endowment is an important determinant in susceptibility to environmental carcinogens. Liability or proneness to cancer is a function of interacting environmental and genetic factors. These factors operate in differing orders of magnitude depending upon the individual's specific genetic and environmental circumstances. Thus, when environmental factors are more significant, the relative effects of hereditary factors will be less significant. Families that are cancer resistant or cancer-prone may be associated with environments which are not strikingly different from each other. However, a major differentiating variable may be genetic factors. Thus, an individual's predisposition or resistance to a particular disease process depends upon that individual's genetic norm or range of reaction and the environmental factors interacting with his genotype. A genetic factor may be manifested only by appropriate genotype-environment combinations. A gene's harmfulness or usefulness is determined by the bearer's environment. In the case of Family N, wherein a reliable biochemical, cytogenetic or clinical marker is lacking, we must infer genetic risk from analysis of the pedigree.

Our cytogenetic studies of Family "N" are preliminary and must be evaluated cautiously. However, should we confirm these observations on other relatives in Family "N", as well as in some of our other families, we may find a marker for this complex problem.

Differential Diagnosis

In the differential diagnosis of the cancer family syndrome the clinician must consider an increasingly large number of hereditary cancer problems because of the increased occurrence of cancer of the colon, endometrium, stomach, and other adenocarcinomas. He must analyze critically the several distinct hereditary settings in which these particular hereditary neoplasms may occur on a site-specific hereditary basis. For example, the polyposis coli syndromes, including familial polyposis coli, Gardner's syndrome and Turcot's syndrome may be readily excluded by confirming the absence of multiple colonic polyps in patients suspected of manifesting the cancer family syndrome. However, difficulties will arise in differentiating site-specific colon cancer from the cancer family syndrome. For example, site-specific hereditary occurrences of adenocarcinoma of the colon have been infrequently reported and it is the belief of these writers that a more detailed search for cancer in families suspected of showing a site-specific increased occurrence of adenocarcinoma of the colon might reveal examples

of the cancer family syndrome. This very situation occurred in our study of Family "S". At the beginning of our genetic study, we thought the cancer occurrences in this family represented hereditary site-specific adenocarcinoma of the colon. However, detailed investigation of the family revealed occurrences of endometrial carcinoma and we now feel that this family should be classified as the cancer family syndrome. Indeed, this family depicts some of the differential diagnostic problems in the classification of this syndrome.

We have also accumulated evidence that endometrial carcinoma may occur in excess on a site-specific basis in a pattern consistent with dominant inheritance in certain kindreds (Chapt. 23). Just as more intensive studies of site-specific colon carcinoma families have disclosed the presence of endometrial carcinoma, so might similar findings occur in so-called endometrial carcinoma families, some of which could also manifest the cancer family syndrome. Finally, endometrial carcinoma has been found to occur frequently in patients with the Stein-Leventhal syndrome, a condition in which several kindreds have been described as following a dominant inheritance pattern.

Adenocarcinoma of the stomach is known to have an increased incidence in many families, empirical risk figures showing a three-fold greater risk to first degree relatives of stomach cancer probands over that in the general population (Chapt. 23). In addition, some families have shown increased occurrences of adenocarcinoma of the stomach in several generations (consistent with autosomal dominant inheritance). Again, as in adenocarcinoma of the colon and endometrium, we must consider the possibility that, with a more detailed medical genetic study, certain families with increased incidence of stomach carcinoma might also be found to have colon and endometrial carcinoma and multiple primary cancers and thereby later be classified as showing the cancer family syndrome.

Other hereditary cancer syndromes, including multiple hereditary endocrine adenomatosis, the Zollinger-Ellison syndrome, the multiple mucosal neuroma syndrome, and other disorders manifesting an increased familial occurrence of adenocarcinoma, will automatically be considered in the differential diagnosis of the cancer family syndrome (Table 19-XVI). However, in most cases, these conditions can be easily differentiated by virtue of certain specific clinical characteristics, i.e. extremely high gastric acidity, atypical peptic ulceration, insulinoma, and endocrine neoplasms (parathyroid, pituitary, adrenal) in the Zollinger-Ellison syndrome which, incidentally may also be considered under the following classifications: 1) multiple endocrine adenomatoses type 1; 2) adenoma-peptic ulcer syndrome; and 3) Wermer's syndrome; on the other hand, café-au-lait spots, mucosal neuromas, pheochromocytoma, and medullary thyroid cancer characterize the multiple mucosal neuroma syndrome.

Finally, as in the case of adenocarcinoma of the endometrium and stomach, families with malignant neoplasms of other specific anatomic organs or systems, i.e. carcinoma of the breast, kidney, as well as sarcoma and leukemia, must be considered as possible candidates for the cancer family syndrome. Additional studies of these families might indeed reveal in certain circumstances an overall pattern of adenocarcinoma of the colon, endometrium, multiple primary malignant neoplasms, and early age of onset, although the particular investigators may have been impressed initially with the aforementioned site-specific lesions, i.e. carcinoma of the breast, kidneys, etc.

It should now be clear that making a diagnosis of the cancer family syndrome in any particular family may be exceedingly difficult since it requires an enormous amount of genealogic and medical documentation. This problem is compounded by the complexity of the cancer problem, i.e. the relatively late age of onset, occasional difficulties in establishing a specific cancer diagnosis, as well as by the social and emotional problems engendered by the presence of cancer in the patient and/or his family, which causes fear and denial and thereby poses obstacles to the retrieval of precise information. However, it will behoove the clinician to search meticulously for this disease since the cancer control implications may be rewarding to the physician and family alike.

Finally, since relatively few families with this condition have been described in the medical literature, it is important for cancer epidemiologists, medical geneticists, clinical oncologists, and practicing physicians to search for and report additional families in which the cancer family syndrome has been well documented.

REFERENCES

1. Lynch, H.T.: Hereditary factors in carcinoma. In Rentchnick, P., (Ed.): *Recent Results in Cancer Research*. New York, Springer Verlag, 1967, Vol. 12, pp. 186.

2. Warthin, A.S.: Heredity with reference to carcinoma. *Arch Intern Med, 12:*546–555, 1913.

3. Warthin, A.S.: The further study of a cancer family. *J Cancer Res, 9:*279–286, 1925.

4. Hauser, I.J., and Weller, C.V.: A further report on the cancer family of Warthin. *Am J Cancer, 27:*434–449, 1936.

5. Bieler, V., and Heim, U.: Doppelkarzinom bei Geschwistern Familiäre Häufung von Genital-und Intestinalkarzinomen. *Schweiz Med Wochenschr, 95:*496–497, 1965.

6. Heinzelmann, F.: Über eine Krebsfamilie. Ein Beitrag zur Frage der Heredität des Colonkarzinoms. *Helv Chir Acta, 31:*316–324, 1964.

7. Savage, D.: A family history of uterine and gastrointestinal cancer. *Br Med J, 2:*341–343, 1956.

8. Cannon, M.M., and Leavell, B.S.: Multiple cancer types in one family. *Cancer, 19:*538–540, 1966.

9. Lynch, H.T., and Krush, A.J.: Cancer family "G" revisited: 1895–1970. *Cancer, 27:*1505–1511, 1971.

10. Lynch, H.T., and Krush, A.J.: Heredity and adenocarcinoma of the colon. *Gastroenterology, 53:*517–527, 1967.

11. Lynch, H.T., Shaw, M.W., Magnuson, C.W., Larsen, A.L., and Krush, A.J.: Hereditary factors in cancer: study of two large midwestern kindreds. *Arch Intern Med, 117:*206–212, 1966.

12. Lynch, H.T., and Krush, A.J.: The cancer family syndrome and cancer control. *Surg Gynecol Obstet, 132:*247–250, 1971.

13. Lynch, H.T., Swartz, M.J., Lynch, J.S., and Krush, A.J.: Adenocarcinoma of the colon and multiple primary cancer: a family study. *Surg Gynecol Obstet, 134:*781–786, 1972.

CHAPTER 20

GENETIC FACTORS IN BREAST CANCER

HENRY T. LYNCH, HODA GUIRGIS, JANE LYNCH, CAROL KRAFT AND ROBERT THOMAS

Introduction

UNFORTUNATELY, BREAST CANCER is extremely common in the United States, accounting for 22 percent of all cancer in women and it ranks highest as the cancer killer of American women. In spite of steady progress in surgical and radiotherapeutic approaches to this disorder, a relatively constant trend of mortality has persisted during the past 25 years. Undoubtedly, under the existing therapeutic circumstances, the best hope for improvement in morbidity and mortality from this disease lies in its earlier detection. An, emphasis upon the utilization of mammography, thermography, xeroradiography, periodic breast examinations by physicians and of equal importance, a sensible practice of self-breast examination, should materially help to improve the prognosis of this disease. A valuable adjunct to the physician's cancer control program should be the identification of patients at unusually high risk for this diease in his practice. This includes any patient who has already had a single breast cancer, patients with chronic cystic mastitis, patients who are nulliparous or whose first pregnancy occurred after age thirty, and patients with a positive family history of breast cancer among first or second degree relatives.

Epidemiology of Breast Cancer

Literature on the epidemiology of breast cancer in animals and in man is more numerous than for any other malignant neoplasm. However, in spite of these extensive investigations, a surprisingly small amount of effort has been expended to control this cancer in man.[1]

Age at first pregnancy has a consistent relationship to breast cancer risk. The breast cancer risk in women who have had their first child before age 20 is about one-third that for those whose first delivery occurs at age 35 or older.[1-4] In order to be afforded protection against development of breast cancer, it is now believed that the first pregnancy must occur before age 30 and interestingly, women who do not become pregnant until age 30 have a risk for breast cancer which appears to exceed that for nulliparous women. Subsequent and even multiple births seems to have little additive effect so far as protection from breast cancer is concerned.[2] This protection also appears to be afforded only by a full-term pregnancy and it appears to be lasting. It can be suggested that young women are at an increased risk for development of breast cancer but events at the first full-term pregnancy, in some way, alter the susceptibility to tumor induction through endocrine or other unknown factors.[2] Stated another way, the women who first becomes pregnant late in the reproductive cycle (after age 30) are more likely to have undergone tumor induction prior to this late pregnancy.

Lactation as a factor in reducing the risk for breast cancer has been a popular hypothesis for approximately 50 years.[1] However, those international studies which have appraised the role of lactation have found no consistent difference in breast cancer risk between breast cancer patients and controls[5] with one exception, namely, in Japan, where lactation seemingly provides a protective effect.[6]

Endocrine factors have long been considered to play an important role in the etiology of breast cancer.[7,8] Oophorectomy affords a lowered risk for breast cancer[9] and a reduced risk appears to be present among women who have had a surgical menopause prior to age 40.[10,11] The reduction in breast cancer risk appears to be slight in the first 10 years following oophorectomy but appears to persist for the remainder of the patient's life. Breast cancer risk appears to be increased with early menarche[3,12] and women with a later natural menopause also appear to be at an increased risk for breast cancer.[12] One study reported that women with a natural menopause at age 55 or older have twice the breast cancer risk as those women whose menopause occurred before age 45.[13]

Studies of adrenal steroids have been inconclusive.[14-16] The prospective cohort study on the Island of Guernsey, which is based on 24 hour urine collections for steroid analysis collected from approximately 5,000 women, may in due time provide insight into this problem.[17] Preliminary findings on 27 women who had developed breast cancer since the study began, when compared with unaffected women, have shown a low excretion of androgen metabolites, particularly etiocholanolone.[18] However, since these findings are based on only 27 breast cancer patients, they must be evaluated cautiously.

Estrogens and their possible etiologic role in human breast cancer have been evaluated extensively in experimental animals and through clinical studies.[7,8] Specifically, Lemon has called attention to the ratio of estriol to other estrogen fractions, and has concluded that when this ratio is low, patients have a greater risk for the development of breast cancer.[7,8] However, there is not universal agreement about these observations.[19]

Prolactin has been investigated but as in the estrogen studies the results are not conclusive.[20]

Progesterone has also been considered to be of etiologic importance in breast cancer, particularly with respect to its ability to oppose estrogen activity.[21] Anovular cycles appear to be associated with a paucity of progesterone production. Grattarola[22] observed a high frequency of anovular cycles in young breast cancer patients.

The incidence of breast cancer varies throughout the world with the rates as much as six times higher in North America and Europe than in many parts of Asia and Africa. Intermediate rates for breast cancer appear to occur in southern European and South American countries.[23] Migrant studies hold promise for greater elucidation of this problem. For instance, Japanese women who have migrated to the United States have rates of breast cancer which are higher than those for women who remain in Japan,[24] while in Hawaii the rates for descendants of Chinese and Japanese individuals who have lived in this area two or three generations are of the same order as those for Caucasians in the same area of the same age.[25]

Viruses and Human Breast Cancer

Knowledge about viruses in human breast cancer has been accured rapidly in recent years heralded by the significant work of Moore and his associates in 1971.[26] They concluded that "the similarities between adenocarcinoma of the breast in mice and women are too extensive to be coincidental;

... human breast cancer may also be a viral disease." These comments were based on their finding of virus-like particles morphologically indistinguishable from the Bittner agent, the so-called mammary tumor virus of mice, in specimens of human milk. Specifically, Moore and his colleagues found a high prevalence (39%) of these virus-like particles in the milk of Parsi women in Bombay, India. These individuals are known to have a significantly higher frequency of mammary cancer than their non-Parsi peers from Bombay and other parts of India. Additional evidence was obtained from a similar collection of milk from women in the United States without a family history of breast cancer, approximately 5 percent of whom showed the viral-like particles. However, in a small group of 10 American women whose family history was positive for breast cancer, the prevalence of virus-like particles rose to 60 percent.

Schlom, Spiegelman, and Moore[27] observed that particles from human milk contained reverse-transcriptase activity. This particular enzyme is also described as RNA-dependent or RNA-directed DNA polymerase which was found to catalyze the synthesis of DNA from the template provided by viral RNA.[28,29] DNA thus produced has a base-sequence complementary to the viral RNA which will hybridize with RNA molecules showing the same base sequence. This newly synthesized DNA can be used as a specific probe in search for the presence of complementary or viral RNA. Significantly, reverse-transcriptase activity has now been observed in several groups of oncogenic RNA viruses including the murine mammary tumor virus.[30] Reverse-transcriptase activity was also found in four of thirteen samples of human milk and significantly, these were the same four samples from which viral-like particles were observed.[27] However, Spiegelman and his co-workers urged caution in the evaluation of these data by calling attention to the fact that reverse-transcriptase cannot be taken as proof of oncogenic potential since it has also been shown to be present in viruses which have not been proved to be oncogenic. Nevertheless, it provides additional insight into the similarities between the particles found in human milk and the Bittner virus.

A recent editorial on the subject of viruses and breast cancer[31] summarizes some of the information gained from pioneering efforts which indicate that:

a majority of human breast tumors contain RNA which is complementary to the DNA of a known mammary tumor virus but not to the DNA of other oncogenic RNA viruses. The extent of their homology is unknown (the recent work with the Moloney sarcoma virus suggests that it could be quite extensive[32]) and the critical hybridization experiments using DNA synthesized by human milk virus have yet to be performed. The presence of complementary RNA in mammary carcinoma must presumably indicate the replication of human-milk virus but one cannot exclude the possibility that the virus replicates in the cancer cells because they are cancer and not vice versa.

The possibility that an oncogenic agent is transmitted through the mother's milk, similar to the situation of the Bittner mammary agent in mice, has unfortunately led to wide publicity recommending that mothers with a family history of breast cancer should not breast feed their daughters because of the possibility of an attendant risk for development of breast cancer through the transmission of an oncogenic virus in their milk.[33] However, Miller and Fraumeni,[34] reviewing the epidemiologic data on this problem, have concluded that they could not unequivocally support the belief that breast cancer is related to breast feeding.

Therefore, we admonish the reader to realize that we are faced with an exceedingly complex problem involving viruses, family history of breast cancer, and many other epidemiologic factors. The final answer may not be simple but rather it may involve factors much more complex than the individual components which have been theorized as causes of breast cancer. In short, "What is the significance of the interactions of all of these known and presently unknown epidemiologic factors of human breast cancer in context with a genotypically breast cancer-prone patient?"

Genetics

Historically, the first significant report on the genetics of breast cancer was that of the famed French surgeon, Paul Broca, published in 1866.[35] He traced the cause of death of 38 members of his wife's family through five generations between 1788 and 1856. Interestingly, 10 of the 24 women in this family died of breast cancer, and with

great wisdom, he documented all *other* malignant neoplasms which included an excess of cancer of the gastrointestinal tract. He was concerned about the possibility of the inheritance of a general cancer diathesis in the family (Fig. 20–1). Numerous reports of familial concentrations of breast cancer have been documented in the literature since the Broca report.[36,37]

In spite of long-standing genetic and epidemiologic interest in this disease, its etiology remains an enigma. For more than half a century, with minor exceptions, this disease was considered to be hereditary and transmitted on a site-specific basis. It was generally presumed that first degree relatives of breast cancer probands had an approximately two to four-fold increased empiric risk for developing a similar lesion.[36] Recently, however, evidence indicates that breast cancer might be associated with *other* malignant neoplasms in certain families, thus suggesting the possibility of differing etiologic factors. For example, Li and Fraumeni[38] have described breast cancer occurrences in four families having soft-

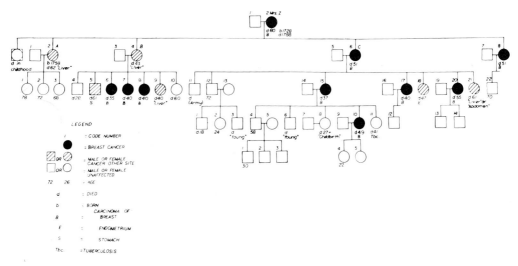

Figure 20–1. This is a pedigree of a breast cancer family which we constructed based upon findings of Broca published in 1869. This represents the *first* detailed study of familial breast cancer and interestingly it shows an increased frequency of gastrointestinal tract cancers in addition to breast cancer.

tissue sarcomas, leukemia, and lymphoma. Recently Lynch and Krush have described three families with breast cancer in association with ovarian cancer[39] and several families showing breast cancer in association with colonic cancer.[40] Finally, other studies have demonstrated additional characteristics associated with breast cancer in certain families: 1) increased occurrences of bilateral breast cancers;[41] 2) a breast cancer family showing a variety of histological types of malignant neoplasms;[42] and 3) breast cancer associated with other medical and/or cancerous problems, but not necessarily on a hereditary basis. These associations have included thyroid disease, including goiter and thyroid cancer,[43] acute myelocytic leukemia,[44] salivary gland cancer,[45] endometrial carcinoma,[46] ovarian cancer (mentioned above),[39] colonic cancer,[47] and Klinefelter's syndrome.[48]

From this review we note that several associations must be considered in evaluating genetic studies in breast cancer families. In addition, when certain determinants such as comparisons of premenopausal and postmenopausal diagnoses and unilateral and bilateral cancer within families were assessed, Anderson showed even greater variations in breast cancer risk to first degree relatives of breast cancer probands.[49] Specifically, Anderson compared breast cancer patients who had family histories of breast cancer, with controls consisting of cancer patients with family histories of malignant neoplasms other than breast cancer. He found that first degree relatives of breast cancer patients, excluding the affected initial patients, manifested a two to three-fold higher breast cancer frequency than that reported in the literature.[50] However, the risks increased from 1.8 to 3.1 for relatives of patients who had breast cancer diagnoses during their premenopausal period but there was no significant increased risk to relatives of patients in whom the diagnosis of breast

cancer was established during the postmenopausal period. Striking differences were found when patients with unilateral breast cancer were compared with patients with bilateral breast cancer; in the latter case, the risk for the relatives was five times that for controls; and if she were both premenopausal and had bilateral breast cancer the risk to relatives increased to nine-fold. In contrast, the risk to relatives of patients with unilateral disease, whether or not it was premenopausal or postmenopausal, ranged from 1.2 to 1.8 which is only slightly higher than the control values. Finally, relatives of patients with bilateral breast cancer manifested a nine-fold higher risk of bilateral breast cancer than among relatives of patients with unilateral breast cancer. Thus, Anderson concluded that genetic factors appear to be more important in patients with early onset and bilateral breast cancer than in patients with late onset and unilateral breast cancer. However, Anderson failed to record *other* histologic varieties of cancer in his study. This is unfortunate, since data by Li and Fraumeni[38] and Lynch and associates[39,51,52] showed clearly that other malignant neoplasms may be associated significantly in certain breast cancer families.

The observations enumerated above demonstrate that studies of breast cancer etiology should include observations concerning a wide variety of parameters including: 1) the geographic area; 2) demographic considerations such as socio-economic, religious, racial and ethnic factors, and parity; 3) family background (genetics) including the relative age of onset (premenopausal vs. postmenopausal) and the presence of unilateral or bilateral disease; and 4) the presence of other histologic varieties of cancer within the families.

The genetics of breast cancer are exceedingly complex since a variety of extra-genetic factors already enumerated, in particular, the pregnancy history of the individual undoubtedly plays a significant role in the development of this lesion.[53] The influence of parity, a factor mentioned frequently in this chapter, was documented by Macklin[37] who differentiated the relative roles of genetics and parity in relatives of breast cancer probands. Another potentially important extragenetic factor now receiving increasing attention concerns the use of drugs which could be carcinogenic. For example, Gould and associates[54] described carcinoma of the breast in three women taking hormonal contraceptives. These lesions were described with both lobular and ductal components, common secretory activity and conspicuous mucopolysaccharides in the stroma of the involved lobules and around the neoplastic ducts. In addition, the lesions were pleiomorphic, diffuse and contained abundant lymphocytic infiltration. They reviewed an extensive literature giving histologic features of uterine and mammary lesions diagnosed in women who were taking hormonal contraceptives and emphasized the fact that a precise cause-and-effect relationship has not been elucidated. One must keep in mind the fact that about seven million women are taking hormonal contraceptives. Therefore, chance factors could account for some of the histologic observations of tumors in these women. However, these authors concluded that in the light of the possible stimulating effect of estrogens and/or progestins on the growth of some breast neoplasms, physicians should be cautious when prescribing these medications to patients who may be at risk for the development of mammary carcinomas. Such high risk patients would include those with cystic mastopathy and those with a strong family history of breast cancer.

In spite of this interest in breast cancer genetics, surprisingly little attention has been given to familial occurrence of breast cancer, including its association with other malignant neoplasms in a sampling from the general population. We shall present our data on this subject and we will discuss several family investigations where genetic factors appear to affect differentially the occurrence of breast cancer and/or other malignant neoplasms in the families.

Familial Breast Cancer in a Normal Population*

Family histories of cancer of all anatomic sites were evaluated in more than 4,000 consecutive persons who underwent either routine cancer screening examinations in a mobile multiphasic cancer detection unit (group I [Omaha], all ages considered, 3261 patients) or were seen as part of a breast-milk study (group II [Detroit], women 45 years or younger, 1058 patients), from which 2,044 maternal and paternal lineages were studied. These investigations were conducted independently at the two medical centers. Our data will be assembled so that lineages with single breast cancer occurrences may be compared with lineages showing two or more occurrences. Certain of these lineages will have varying combinations of other histologic varieties of cancer.

Description of groups I and II

Approximately 94 percent of group I members were Caucasian (equal numbers of the remaining 6% were composed of American Indians and Negroes). Most of the members of this group were rural dwellers with a wide range of socio-economic and occupational backgrounds. This group included men and women with age range of 20 to 88. The total number of men was 1,079. There were 650 men over the age of 45 and 329 age 45 or under. The total number of women was 2,182. Of these 1,368 were over age 45 and 814 were under 45 years of age.

*Portions of this material by permission of *Cancer*.

Group II was composed entirely of Caucasian women, primarily urban dwellers, with socio-economic and occupational backgrounds somewhat similar to group I. Patients in group II were in the age range of 20 to 45 years.

Detailed questionnaires and interviews were employed for data gathering at the two centers. In Omaha (group I) the family history of cancer was verified primarily by interviews with the original patient and a detailed questionnaire. In Detroit (group II) verifications consisted of a reliable history from two members of the same family, hospital records, pathology reports, and death certificates.

Data Management

In order to make appropriate comparisons between groups I and II, age considered, those under age 45 in group I, and all members in group II (all were under age 45)

were assembled into paternal and maternal lineages as follows: paternal and maternal family histories of cancer were recorded separately, and were treated as two units. Therefore, each patient under 45 years of age (from groups I and II) generated a) one unit including mother, maternal grandmother, maternal grandfather, maternal aunts and uncles, and b) one unit including father, paternal grandmother, paternal grandfather, and paternal aunts and uncles. The family history of those probands over 45 years of age (from group I only) was recorded as mother, father, proband, and sibs of the proband. Therefore, each proband over 45 years of age generated only one unit. All units are called lineages, and each unit will include two generations (See Fig. 20–2). The mean number of subjects in lineages for group I was 6.6 and for group II was 6.7.

The results are shown in Tables 20-I, 20-II, and 20-III and Figures 20–2 to 20–7. It is of

TABLE 20-I
DISTRIBUTION OF PARTICIPANTS IN OMAHA AND DETROIT TO THE
NUMBER OF CANCERS IN THE FAMILY

Category	Group I Participants		Group II Participants	
	Number	*Percent*	*Number*	*Percent*
No History of Cancer	1520	46.6	470	46.6
History of a Single Cancer	1082	33.2	296	29.3
History of Multiple Cancers	659	20.2	243	24.1
Total	3261	100.0	1009	100.0

TABLE 20-II
THE OCCURRENCE OF BREAST AND OTHER CANCERS IN LINEAGES OF PARTICIPANTS

	Group I No. of Lineages Involved 1244		Group II No. of Lineages Involved 2044	
	Number	*Percent*	*Number*	*Percent*
1 breast cancer and no other cancer	59	4.7	84	4.1
1 breast cancer + 1 other cancer	35	2.8	58	2.8
1 breast cancer + 2 other cancers	12	1.0	5	0.2
1 breast cancer + 3 other cancers	2	0.2	3	0.1
2 breast cancers and no other cancers	7	0.6	6	0.3
2 breast cancers + 1 other cancer	1	0.1	7	0.3
2 breast cancers + 2 other cancers	2	0.2	3	0.1

TABLE 20-III
EXPECTED AND OBSERVED FAMILIAL ASSOCIATION OF
BREAST CANCER WITH OTHER CANCERS

Cancer Site	Group I			Group II			Groups I & II		
	Expected	Observed	P	Expected	Observed	P	Expected	Observed	P
Prostate	0.88	17	0.005	2.55	7	0.25	3.43	24	0.005
Ovary	2.54	6	0.50	1.23	4	0.75	3.77	10	0.25
Brain	3.66	6	0.9	0.82	3	0.75	4.48	9	0.50
Skin	17.81	26	0.25	4.92	11	0.25	22.73	37	0.10
Cervix	3.10	2	0.9	4.35	10	0.25	7.45	12	0.5
Endometrium	10.89	10	0.9	2.62	8	0.25	13.51	18	0.75
Colon	22.03	24	0.75	9.44	16	0.25	31.47	40	0.50
Breast	25.44	33	0.50	13.80	16	0.90	39.24	49	0.50
Lung	10.24	10	—	5.43	7	0.90	15.67	17	0.90
Stomach	15.21	12	0.75	4.18	9	0.25	19.39	21	0.75
Leukemia	6.01	4	0.75	1.97	2	0.9	7.98	6	0.9

interest that Table 20-I and Figure 20–3 show that approximately one half of all families (maternal and paternal lineages together) studied do not manifest any evidence of cancer. In 33.2 percent of group I families and 29.3 percent of group II families, cancer occurred in one first degree relative; two or more first degree relatives had cancer in 20.2 percent of families in group I and 24.1 percent in group II. Comparison of the results of the cancer histories of group I and group II show great similarity, though ascertained independently at the two medical centers. This same observation holds for practically all statistical categories in this study, regardless of the specific histologic variety of cancer or the specific age category analyzed.

Data with respect to breast cancer occurrences in groups I and II show that approximately 9.1 percent of all lineages in group I have a single member with breast cancer, and 7.4 percent of all lineages in group II have a single member with breast cancer. These figures define a circumstance where a single member has carcinoma of the breast but where other members may have cancers of other anatomic sites. In both groups I and II, approximately 0.7 percent of all lineages screened have two or more first degree relatives with breast cancer. Findings

show that the ratio of single (sporadic) to multiple breast cancer is 13.0 to 1.0 in group I, and in group II the ratio is 10.6 to 1.0. When groups I and II are combined the ratio is 11.8 to 1.0.

Table 20-II shows the occurrence of breast cancers and other cancers in lineages of probands screened in groups I and II. This table shows the distribution of families according to occurrence of breast cancer and other cancers, and it indicates the similarity between groups I and II.

Table 20-III and Figures 20–4, 20–5, and 20–6 show the expected and observed associations of breast and other varieties of cancer in lineages in groups I and II, and the two groups combined. These observations were obtained on the basis of calculating the expected values for each association and by multiplying the proportion of lineages with one or more breast cancers by the proportion of lineages that had one or more other varieties of cancer, wherein each histologic variety of cancer was considered separately. The observed values for each association was obtained by computing the actual number of the lineages that had combinations of breast and each other variety of cancer.

As can be seen in Table 20-III, there are multiple associations identified between breast cancer and other histologic varieties of cancer. The highest expected and observed familial association identified was between cancers of the breast and breast, and breast and colon in groups I and II. Nevertheless, the difference between observed and expected values for these lesions were not statistically significant. However, a statistically significant difference between observed and expected values was found in the familial association of cancers of the breast and prostate $p < 0.005$ in group I, $p < 0.25$ in group II, and $p < 0.005$ when the two groups were combined.

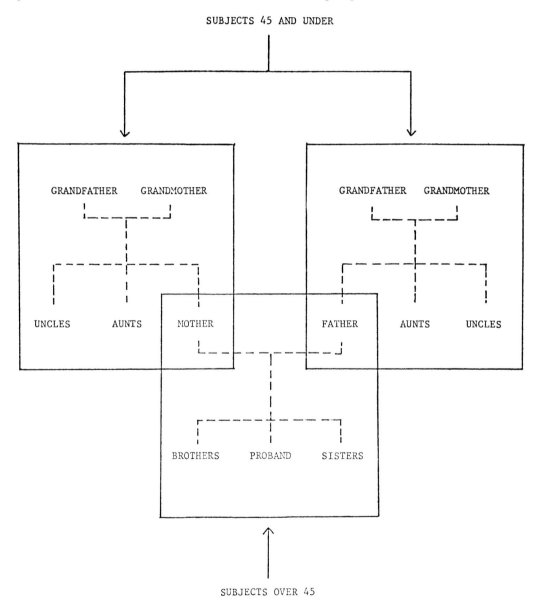

Figure 20–2. Lineages generated from families of participants under and over 45 years of age.

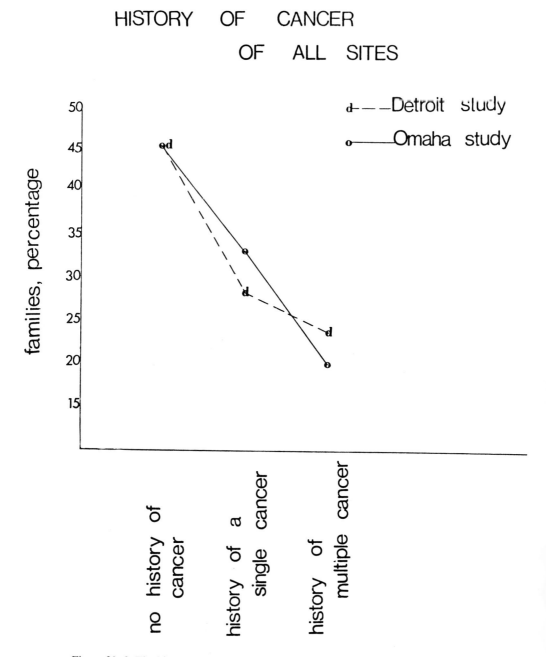

Figure 20–3. The history of cancer of all sites in families studied in groups I and II.

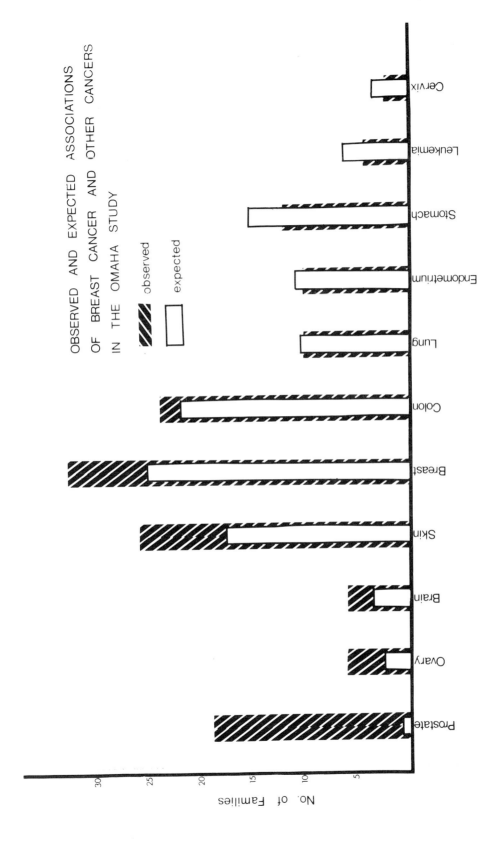

Figure 20–4. Familial association between breast cancer and other histologic varieties of cancer in Omaha group. Shown are the expected versus the observed associations in the several histologic varieties of cancer.

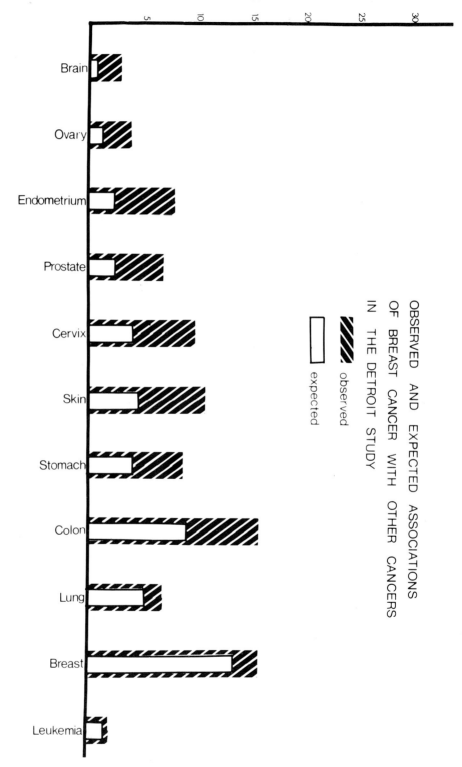

No. of Families

OBSERVED AND EXPECTED ASSOCIATIONS OF BREAST CANCER WITH OTHER CANCERS IN THE DETROIT STUDY

observed

expected

Brain
Ovary
Endometrium
Prostate
Cervix
Skin
Stomach
Colon
Lung
Breast
Leukemia

Figure 20–5. Familial association between breast cancer and other histologic varieties of cancer in Detroit group. Shown are the expected versus the observed associations in the several histologic varieties of cancer.

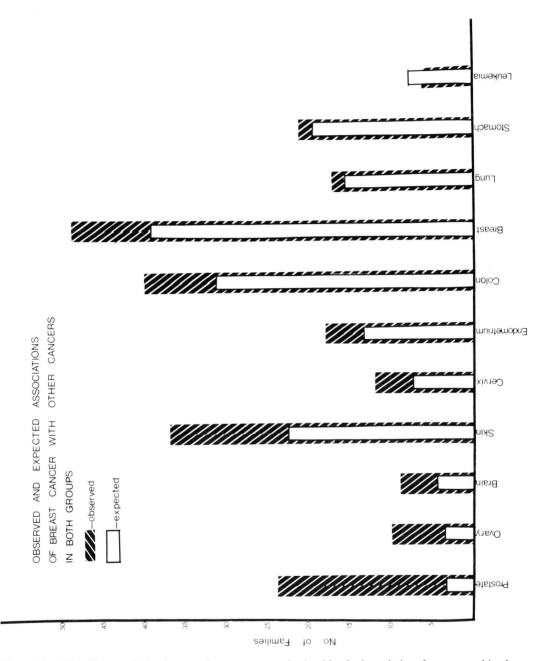

Figure 20–6. Familial association between breast cancer and other histologic varieties of cancer combined for both the Omaha and Detroit populations. As in Figures 20–4 and 20–5, the expected versus observed cancer associations have been calculated.

Comment

A major limitation to our understanding of cancer genetics in general and breast cancer genetics in particular has been a deficit of studies concerning familial occurrence in normal populations. In order to fill this gap, we have collected data on family histories involving cancer in normal individuals from two different areas of the United States. The similarities of findings from the two centers lend support to the reliability and validity of the methods employed in their gathering and management. An interesting observation from these data is that approximately one half of all the families (maternal and paternal lineages together) studied showed an absence of cancer (all sites) in first degree relatives. On the other hand, only approximately 7 percent of all families studied showed a marked predominance (three or more cancers among first degree relatives) of cancer (all sites). These observations reveal a lack of uniformity in cancer distribution in families, and suggest that some of the families may be relatively cancer resistant while others may be relatively cancer prone. Nonuniformity of cancer distribution is observed repeatedly when specific histologic varieties of cancer are studied in different areas of the world. While the overall frequency of cancer of specific anatomic sites varies from country to country and continent to continent, the overall frequency of cancer of all anatomic sites in the normal population remains remarkably similar. However, worldwide cancer statistics do not reflect variation of cancer incidence in individual families, although strain differences in cancer frequency are well known at the infrahuman level.[55] Certain strains of mice are cancer resistant, while others are remarkably cancer prone.[56,57] Preliminary investigations by Lynch and Krush have shown that certain kindreds have a reduced frequency of cancer

(1% or less) while other families were classified as cancer prone with rates of cancer exceeding 40 percent.[58]

When interpreting results in Table 20-II, it is important to realize that the findings are restricted to first degree relatives. In addition, breast cancer must be considered in context with its association with other varieties of cancer. We have therefore assembled the data to reflect a spectrum of cancer associations. Thus breast cancer as a single reported neoplasm occurs in 4.7 percent of the lineages in group I and 4.1-percent of group II while breast cancer in association with multiple cancers (three other cancers) occurs in a very small percent (0.2%, group I and 0.1% in group II) of families. Finally, Table 20-II shows very few lineages in the entire population of groups I and II where two patients with breast cancer and other associated malignant neoplasms are observed. These lineages, rare as they may be, may nevertheless be considered at unusually high familial cancer risk and should be studied in greater detail through extending the pedigrees to include second and third degree relatives. This should define more clearly the specific familial cancer syndromes.

A significant departure was found to exist between expected and observed values for familial associations between carcinoma of the breast and prostate, (Table 20-III and Fig. 20-7), colon, ovary, endometrium, brain, and skin in lineages in groups I and II. However, when subjected to conservative statistical correction of P values the only familial association which maintained statistical significance was found between carcinoma of the breast and prostate in group I. However, statistical significance was maintained when groups I and II were combined (p < 0.005). *Only for Prostate*

A unifying characteristic in the association between breast and prostate cancer is that each of these organs is the target of

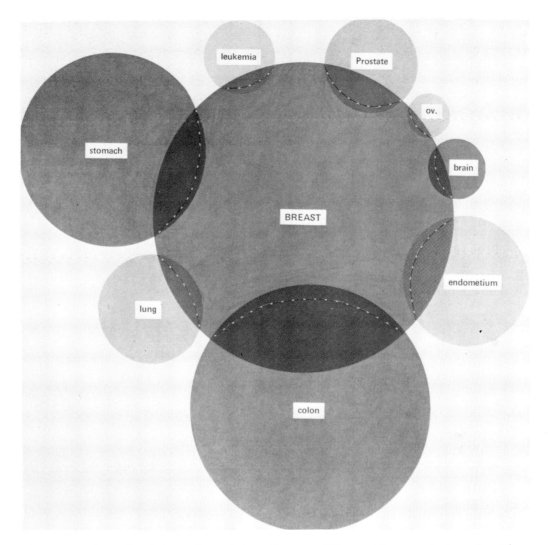

Figure 20–7. Expected and observed associations of cancers of the prostate, ovary, brain, endometrium, colon, lung and stomach with breast cancer in families studied.

gonadal hormones. It is possible that hereditary factors in these circumstances may involve specific variations in either hormone productions, chemical alterations, or possibly they may involve the target organ per se, i.e. aberrations in the response to hormones due to receptor defects. Possibly *both* mechanisms and/or their interactions may be of etiologic importance.

These observations reflect a trend with respect to familial associations between breast and several differing histological varieties of cancer. They indicate the need for expansion of this particular approach in an epidemiological study of breast cancer in that the data developed and analyzed would harbor a powerful potential for the study of carcinogenesis as well as for cancer con-

TABLE 20-IV
A LISTING OF ALL HISTOLOGIC VARIETIES OF CANCER OCCURRING IN
34 BREAST CANCER FAMILIES

Anatomical Site	Number of Families	Number of Individuals 32 Years & Over	Number of Males	Number of Females	Number Affected	Percent of 221 Affected Individuals in 34 Families
Breast	34	655	309	346	112	50.6
Gastrointestinal Tract	22	491	244	247	47	21.2
Prostate	7	121	60	61	8	3.6
Lung	6	108	48	60	7	3.2
Ovary	5	81	30	51	7	3.2
Endometrium	5	194	102	92	6	2.7
Skin	6	153	73	80	6	2.7
Sarcoma	4	79	37	42	6	2.7
Brain	5	125	65	60	5	2.2
Cervix	3	45	16	29	4	1.8
Leukemia	3	49	19	30	3	1.8
Other (1 or 2 families each)	8	255	116	109	10	4.5
Total					221	

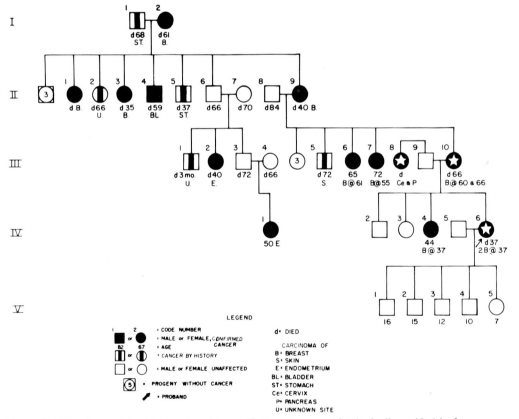

Figure 20–8. Pedigree of family showing site specific breast cancer histologically verified in four generations. Note the occurrence of multiple primary (bilateral) breast cancers as noted by the star symptoms. By permission, Lynch, H.T., *et al.*, *JAMA, 222:*1631, 1972.

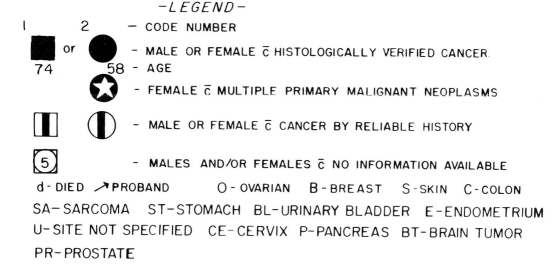

-LEGEND-

	2	– CODE NUMBER
■ or ●	– MALE OR FEMALE c̄ HISTOLOGICALLY VERIFIED CANCER.
74 58	– AGE
★	– FEMALE c̄ MULTIPLE PRIMARY MALIGNANT NEOPLASMS
▯ ⏻	– MALE OR FEMALE c̄ CANCER BY RELIABLE HISTORY
⑤	– MALES AND/OR FEMALES c̄ NO INFORMATION AVAILABLE

d- DIED ➚PROBAND   O - OVARIAN   B - BREAST   S - SKIN   C - COLON

SA− SARCOMA   ST−STOMACH   BL−URINARY BLADDER   E−ENDOMETRIUM

U−SITE NOT SPECIFIED   CE−CERVIX   P−PANCREAS   BT−BRAIN TUMOR

PR−PROSTATE

Figure 20–8A. Legend for this and subsequent pedigrees.

trol through the elucidation of familial cancer associations in breast cancer prone families.

Background for Data Collection of Extended Family Studies*

The following clinical material is based upon our study of 34 breast cancer families during a ten-year period. The criterion for the selection of a breast cancer family is that two or more first degree relatives had received a diagnosis of breast cancer. Histological verification was sought for all malignant neoplasms in relatives, and genealogies were documented by a variety of sources. To increase the precision of genetic analysis the medical data was restricted to first and second degree relatives aged 32 and over (for cancer age correction purposes).

Results of these studies are recorded according to cancer distribution and the specific families will be presented in the following

*By permission, Lynch, H.T., *et al., JAMA, 222:* 1631, 1972.

order: 1) site-specific breast cancer; 2) breast cancer associated with cancer of the gastro-intestinal system; 3) breast cancer associated with ovarian cancer; and 4) breast cancer associated with sarcoma, leukemia, and brain tumors. Table 20-IV provides a listing of all malignant neoplasms found in the 34 families (309 males and 346 females).

Site-specific Breast Cancer

Breast cancer occurring on a site-specific basis and not associated with an excess of other malignant neoplasms or of other anatomic sites is depicted in Fig. 20–8. This lesion was histologically verified in 8 women through 4 generations. Bilateral breast cancer was histologically verified in two women in two generations. The ratio of affected to unaffected with breast cancer (3 out of 6 women in generation II; 3 out of 6 women in generation III; and 2 out of 3 women in generation IV) is compatible with the 1:1 ratio for a dominant gene.

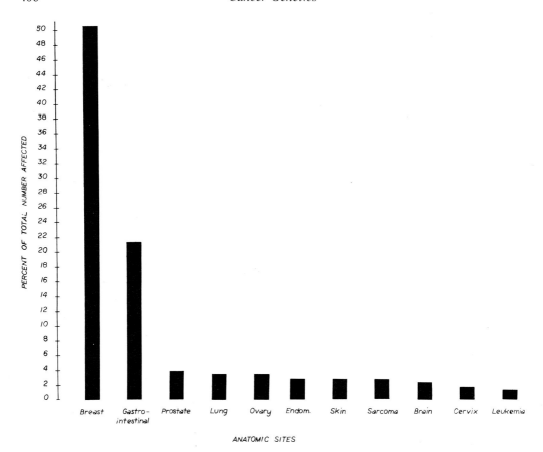

Figure 20–9. Histogram depicting the relative frequency of gastrointestinal tract cancer in 34 breast cancer families.

Breast Cancer Associated with Adenocarcinoma of the Gastrointestinal System

Findings in 34 Families

In 22 families, comprising 491 individuals (244 males and 247 females), one or more members of each family had a diagnosis of gastrointestinal tract cancer (Table 20-IV).

Figure 20–9 is a histogram which depicts the frequency of cancer of specific anatomic sites in the 34 breast cancer families.

Table 20-V depicts the number of affected individuals in each of the 22 families by the anatomic site of gastrointestinal tract cancer. The most frequently occurring cancer in this group was cancer of the colon which occurred in one or more members in 14 families (25 individuals affected).

Figure 20–10 is a histogram depicting the distribution of each type of gastrointestinal tract cancer in the 22 families. Note that colonic cancer was the most frequent tumor followed by carcinoma of the stomach and pancreas. These findings must be appraised in light of the fact that when both sexes are considered, carcinoma of the colon is the most common visceral tumor in man. Analysis of the distribution of cancer of the gastro-

TABLE 20-V
THIS TABLE DEPICTS THE NUMBER OF INDIVIDUALS AFFECTED IN EACH OF THE
22 FAMILIES ACCORDING TO ANATOMIC SITE OF GASTROINTESTINAL CANCER

Cancer Sites	Number of Families	Total Number of Individuals (Age 32 & Over)	Number Affected	Percentage of Affected
Breast	22	491	75	15.2
Colon	14	335	25	7.4
Stomach	7	123	12	9.7
Pancreas	4	96	4	4.1
Gallbladder	2	25	2	8.0
Liver	3	50	3	6.0
Esophagus	1	7	1	14.2

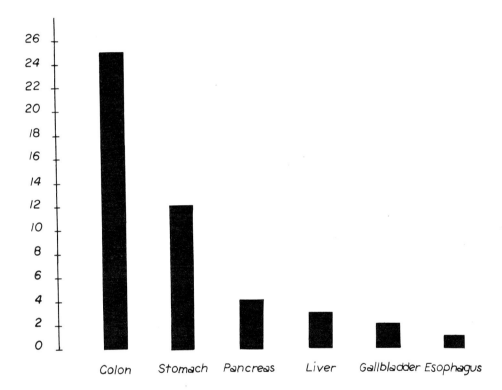

Figure 20–10. Histogram depicting the relative frequency of gastrointestinal cancer by specific anatomic site in 22 breast cancer families.

intestinal tract in these 22 families revealed equal distribution among men and women.

Multiple primary malignancies occurred in 19 individuals.

The age at diagnosis of breast cancer ranged from 32 to 84 (the average age was 54.4). The age at diagnosis of gastrointestinal cancer ranged from 37 to 87 (the average age was 62.2) (Fig. 20–11).

In analyzing the pedigrees of the 22 families with gastrointestinal tract cancer, it was found that breast cancer was transmitted through two or more generations in 16 families and occurred in one generation

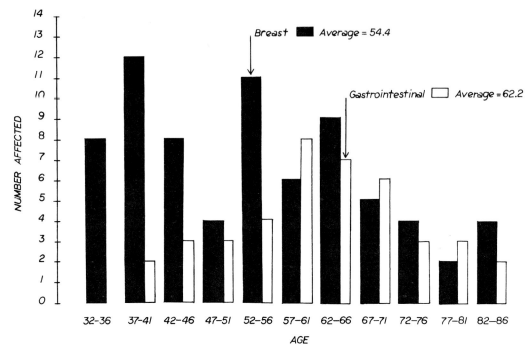

Figure 20–11. Histogram depicting the age at diagnosis of cancer of the breast and gastrointestinal tract in 22 families.

in six families. Gastrointestinal tract cancer was transmitted through two or more generations in nine families and was present in one generation in 13 families.

Family Study

The propositus, (Fig. 20–12, III-2) a 73-year-old white woman, was ascertained at her own initiation because of her concern about the multiple occurrences of cancer in her family. The patient gave a history of having had a uterine suspension and appendectomy at age 46 and a cholecystectomy four years later. She had had a prolonged history of allergic rhinitis. She was gravida 3, para 1, abortus 2. In 1952, at the age of 56, she noted a small scaling lesion in her left breast which cleared and then recurred during a two-month period prompting her to visit her physician. A biopsy was im-

mediately performed and revealed Paget's disease of the left breast; subsequently she had a radical mastectomy.

Physical findings, except for moderate obesity, were noncontributory and she survives, in reasonably good health.

The family history was of extreme interest and is shown in detail in Table 20-VI and Figure 20–12. Cancer has occurred in four generations. Note that eight of thirteen siblings have had histologically verified diagnoses of cancer, three of whom had multiple primary malignant neoplasms (Fig. 20–12, III-3, cutaneous malignant melanoma at age 63 and breast carcinoma at age 66; III-4, breast cancer at age 63 and colon cancer at age 63; and III-8, endometrial carcinoma at age 56 and carcinoma of the colon at age 56). Six members in three generations received diagnoses of colonic carcinoma, four of these being in the proband's sibship.

TABLE 20-VI
TUMOR REGISTRY OF FAMILY SHOWN IN FIGURE 20–12 WHICH IS NOTEWORTHY FOR AN
EXCESS OF CANCER OF THE BREAST, GASTROINTESTINAL TRACT AND
MULTIPLE PRIMARY MALIGNANT NEOPLASMS

Pedigree No.	Sex	Age	Breast	Cancer of Colon	Endometrium	Pancreas	Kidney	Melanoma (cutaneous)
I-1	M	d64		−				
II-2	F	d80			− ?	− ?		
II-3	F	d84	+35					
II-4	M	d37		+37				
III-2	↗F	73	+56					
III-3	F	d70	+66					+63
III-4	F	64	+63	+63				
III-5	M	d61		+60				
III-6	M	d73		+67				
III-7	M	d69					+67	
III-8	F	d56		+56	+56			
III-9	M	d46		+46				
IV-4	F	44	+43					

+ = histologically confirmed diagnosis.
− = diagnosis by history.
↗ = proband.

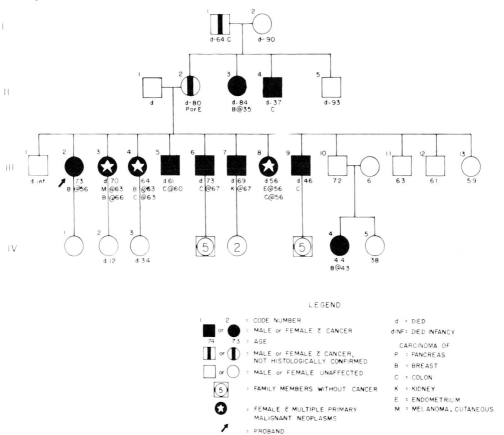

Figure 20–12. Pedigree of family with combined breast and colon cancer and multiple primary cancers. Note that cancer has occurred in four generations of this family.

Breast Cancer Associated with Ovarian Carcinoma

The following is a detailed medical genetic evaluation of three kindreds showing an association of breast and ovarian carcinoma.

Family A

The proband, (Fig. 20–13, III-3), was a 55-year-old woman hospitalized with carcinoma of the ovary (papillary scirrhous carcinoma, histologically confirmed). Her mother (Fig. 20–13, II-2) died at the age of 76, also with a diagnosis of metastatic carcinoma of the ovary (histologically confirmed). Of eight maternal aunts and uncles of the proband, four aunts died of breast cancer (one histologically verified, Fig. 20–13, II-4; and three on a reliable history, Fig. 20–13, II-5, II-9, II-11), between the ages of 50 and 70. Another maternal aunt

is living at age 78 (Fig. 20–13, II-7), having undergone surgery for adenocarcinoma of the colon at age 73 (histologically verified). Of four daughters of one of the proband's maternal aunts (who died of breast cancer at age 59, Fig. 20–13, II-4), one (Fig. 20–13, III-4), had two primary malignant neoplasms, a sarcoma of the finger at age 32 (reliable history), and bronchogeneic carcinoma at age 43 (histologically confirmed), resulting in her death. A second daughter (Fig. 20–13, III-5), died of breast cancer (reliable history) at age 40, and a third (Fig. 20–13, III-6), died of breast cancer at age 50 (reliable history). The only daughter (Fig. 20–13, III-10) of a maternal aunt (Fig. 20–13, II-9), who had also had a diagnosis of breast cancer) developed cancer of the right breast at age 43 and died of metastatic carcinoma of the left breast at age 45 (histologically confirmed).

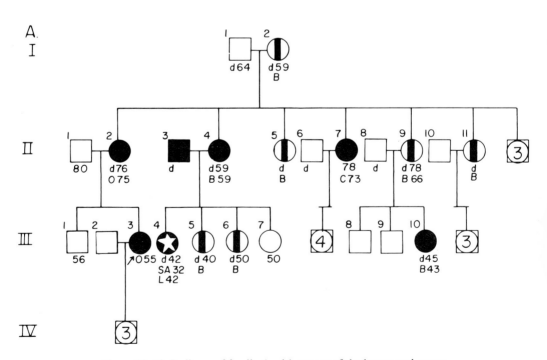

Figure 20–13. Pedigree of family A with cancer of the breast and ovary.

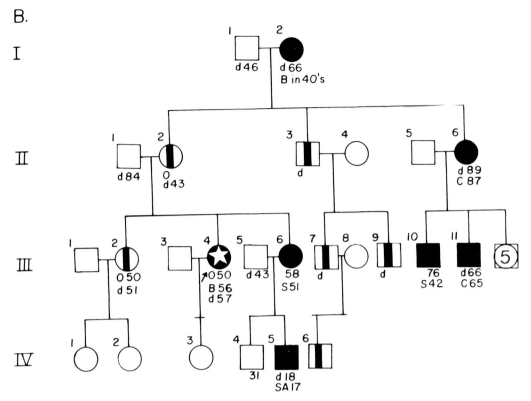

Figure 20–14. Pedigree of family B showing cancer of the breast and ovary.

Family B

The proband (Fig. 20–14, III-4), underwent a panhysterectomy at the age of 50 for Grade IV papillary adenocarcinoma of the left ovary (histologically confirmed), with extension to the right ovary and visceral peritoneum. Six years later, she underwent a right radical mastectomy for an infiltrating ductal carcinoma (histologically confirmed) thus manifesting two distinct primary carcinomas. She died at the age of 57. The proband's mother (Fig. 20–14, II-2), died at the age of 43 of ovarian cancer (reliable history). The proband's maternal grandmother (Fig. 20–14, I-2) lived to *old age,* but many years earlier had received surgery for

breast cancer (histologically confirmed), from which she recovered completely.

The proband's two sisters (Fig. 20–14, III-2, III-6), both developed cancer. One (Fig. 20–14, III-2), died of ovarian cancer at the age of 51 (reliable history). The second sister (Fig. 20–14, III-6), requested and received a prophylactic panhysterectomy at the age of 47 because of the strong family history of cancer. Since that time, she has received treatment for a basal cell carcinoma of the nose. Her son (Fig. 20–14, IV-5), died at the age of 19 of sarcoma of the left tibia which metastasized to the lungs (histologically confirmed).

The proband's maternal uncle (Fig. 20–14, II-3), and maternal aunt (Fig. 20–14, II-6), each had diagnoses of cancer. The uncle died of cancer of an unknown site in 1957 (reliable history). His two sons (Fig. 20–14, III-7, III-9), and a grandson (Fig. 20–14, IV-6), also have had diagnoses of cancer (reliable history), but complete information of type and site is not yet available. The aunt (Fig. 20–14, II-6), was treated for carcinoma of the rectum at age 87 (histologically confirmed), and died of a CVA at age 89. Of her 7 children, two sons (Fig. 20–14, III-10, III-11), developed cancer (histologically confirmed), one a skin cancer in his early forties. A second son received surgery for adenocarcinoma of the cecum at the age of 65, but died of obstructive pulmonary disease at age 66.

Family C

The proband (Fig. 20–15, II-2) underwent a left radical mastectomy at the age of 44 for carcinoma of the breast (histologically confirmed). Because of the high incidence of breast cancer in this patient's family, a right simple mastectomy was performed soon afterward. A basal cell carcinoma of the skin of the right chest wall was excised at age 45 (histologically confirmed). At the age of 50 following symptoms of left lower quadrant pain, she underwent surgery for adenocarcinoma of both ovaries with metastases (papillary scirrhous cystadenocarcinoma). She died at the age of 53. The proband's mother (Fig. 20–15, I-3) died at age 52 of breast cancer (histologically confirmed). Two maternal aunts (Fig. 20–15, I-4, and I-5) both died of breast cancer, one at age 48 (age not given for I-5) (both histologically confirmed). A paternal aunt (Fig. 20–15, I-1) of the proband died at age 49 of breast carcinoma (histologically confirmed). One sister of the proband (Fig. 20-15, II-3) died of breast cancer at age 34

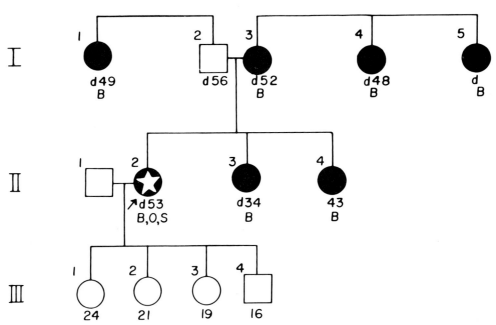

Figure 20–15. Pedigree of family C showing cancer of breast and ovary. Note that the proband has had 3 separate primary cancers (all histologically confirmed, namely, cancer of the breast, ovary, and sarcoma, indicated by S in this particular pedigree).

TABLE 20-VII
DATA FROM 34 BREAST CANCER FAMILIES SHOWING FINDINGS IN ELEVEN OF THESE
FAMILIES WHERE SARCOMA, LEUKEMIA AND BRAIN TUMORS WERE ALSO FOUND.
PROBABILITY RATES FOR COMPARABLE CANCERS IN NEW YORK STATE ARE LISTED

No. of Families	Males[1]	Females[1]	Total[1]	Breast Cancer	Number with Malignant Neoplasms			Prevalence Rate	New York State Probability Rate
					(Sarcoma)	(Leukemia)	(Brain Tumor)		
34	323	398	721	109	—	—	—	27.4%[2]	5.93%
11[3]	121	154	275	34	10	6	5	—	—
5	62	78	140	(17)	10	—	—	1.3%[4]	0.53%
4	46	69	115	(10)	—	6	—	0.83%	0.69%
5	53	61	114	(15)	—	—	5	0.69%	0.27%

[1] First and second degree relatives (includes proband, parents, children, grandparents, grandchildren, aunts, uncles, nephews, and nieces).
[2] This figure is based on consideration of females only in this series.
[3] The families with sarcoma, leukemia, or brain tumor.
[4] These percents are based on the total sample of 721 persons.

(histologically confirmed). A second sister (Fig. 20–15, II-4) was living at age 43, having received a diagnosis of breast cancer with metastases to the lungs (histologically confirmed). The proband's husband's mother (not shown on Fig. 20–15) received a diagnosis of breast cancer at age 73 (histologically confirmed). She is living at age 81. The proband had three daughters, now aged 24, 21 and 19 (Fig. 20-15, III-1, III-2, III-3). Because of the intense concentration of breast cancer on both maternal and paternal sides, the gynecologist recommended simple mastectomy for each of these young women as they reached the early twenties, assuming that no better course of action could be found to prevent breast cancer before they reached this age.

Breast Cancer Associated with Sarcoma, Leukemia, and Brain Tumors

Recent evidence has suggested a new hereditary syndrome in breast cancer families which includes an increased frequency of brain tumors, leukemia, and sarcoma among family members. Because of this association, we have elected to present our data on these malignancies collectively. Findings were as follows: eleven of the 34 breast cancer families have had sarcoma, leukemia, and brain tumors diagnosed among their members (Table 20-VII). Three of these families had a combination of two of these malignancies in association with breast cancer. Observed values for each group of tumors (breast cancer, sarcoma, leukemia, and brain tumors) were compared with values from the Cancer Control Program of the New York State Health Department (These statistics are for New York State but exclude New York City). The New York State values for these lesions are based on the probability of developing cancer from birth to death, whereas, in our series, many individuals are living who have not yet developed a malignant lesion but are at risk for developing one. Therefore, our values are lower than they would be if probabilities of developing a malignant lesion were ascertained for their entire lives. If one excludes the two breast cancer patients in each family, which are part of the criteria for inclusion in the series, then 41 of the relatives have received a diagnosis of breast cancer (of 330 women relatives) or 12.4 percent, which is still much higher than the New York State probability rate of 5.93 percent.

Sarcoma occurred in ten family members in five families for a prevalence rate of 1.3 percent, whereas, the New York State proba-

TABLE 20-VIII
TUMOR REGISTRY OF ELEVEN FAMILIES SHOWING VARYING AGGREGATIONS OF
BREAST CANCER, SARCOMA, LEUKEMIA, AND BRAIN TUMORS

Family Number	Sex	Age or Age at Death	Sarcoma	Leukemia	Brain Tumor	Breast Cancer
1*	M	d42	—	—	+39	—
	F	47	—	—	—	+38
	F	d36	—	—	—	+35
2	M	d37	—	—	+37	—
	M	d43	—	+	—	—
	F	d29	—	—	—	+
	F	d24	—	—	—	+
	F	d30	—	—	—	+
3	M	d30	—	—	+	—
	M	d36	+	—	—	—
	F	d45	—	—	—	+18
	F	d34	—	—	—	+
	F	d39	—	—	—	+34
4	M	d51	—	—	+	—
	F	d39	—	—	—	+32 +35
	F	51	—	—	—	+45
	F	72	—	—	—	+66
	F	d—	—	—	—	+
5	F	d71	—	—	+	—
	F	d40	—	—	—	+
	F	61	—	—	—	+58
	F	d49	—	—	—	+44
6*	M	47	+	—	—	—
	F	d10	+	—	—	—
	F	d17	+	—	—	—
	M	d10	—	+	—	—
	F	d47	—	+	—	+
	F	d15	—	+	—	—
	F	d53	—	—	—	+
7	M	d38	+22 +38	—	—	—
	M	d16	+	—	—	—
	M	d23	+	—	—	—
	F	d18	+	—	—	—
	F	d43	—	—	—	+
	F	d42	—	—	—	+
8	F	d42	+32	—	—	—
	F	d40	—	—	—	+
	F	d50	—	—	—	+
	F	d59	—	—	—	+
	F	d59	—	—	—	+
	F	d70+	—	—	—	+
	F	d45	—	—	—	+45
	F	d50+	—	—	—	+
	F	d—	—	—	—	+
9	M	d19	+	—	—	—
	F	d57	—	—	—	+56
	F	d66	—	—	—	+
10	M	d60+	—	+	—	—
	F	d76	—	—	—	+73
	F	d—	—	—	—	+ +
11	F	d74	—	+74	—	+67
	F	71	—	—	—	+62
	F	60	—	—	—	+47

*One member of family had a diagnosis of adrenal cortex carcinoma.

bility rate was 0.53 percent. Leukemia occurred in six individuals in four families. The prevalence rate was 0.83 percent as compared to a probability rate of 0.68 percent in New York State. Brain tumors occurred in five individuals in five families for a prevalence rate of 0.69 percent which was higher than the New York State rate of 0.27 percent (Table 20-VII). All of these percentages are higher than the New York probability rates, considering a total of 21 incidences of sarcoma, leukemia, and brain tumors among 274 members of 11 families. Since these 11 families were selected from a series of 34 families because of the incidence of one of the three types of cancer, this leaves ten cases (instead of 21) among 264 individuals (instead of 275) in 11 families for a combined incidence rate of 3.8 percent (also higher than the combined figure for New York State).

Because of the limitations with respect to both the number of families evaluated and the number of relatives at risk per family, it is clear that not all of the possible associations of tumors will be found in each family group (Table 20-VIII).

Family Study

Figure 20–16 presents the pedigree of two of the 11 families which were combined (Probands are III-10 and III-19) since they are two of ten branches of a large kindred in which four branches or family units had two or more first or second degree relatives with breast cancer and the mentioned associated malignant neoplasms in other family members. Twenty-one individuals among 60 members in five generations have received diagnoses of malignant neoplasms. Of these, six women in four generations developed breast cancer. Of these six, one (IV-11) had both breast cancer and myeloblastic leukemia. One other relative (III-12) had

multiple primary malignant neoplasms—a bronchogenic carcinoma of the lung (age 61), and leiomyosarcoma (at age 47). Sarcoma affected four members; leukemia affected three; brain tumors occurred in two persons; other malignant tumors included carcinoma of the colon (one), prostatic carcinoma (one), Hodgkin's disease (one), and adrenocortical tumor (one).

Discussion of Family Data

An individual's genotype determines his norm or range of reaction to the various environmental influences. The etiology of a malignant lesion in any particular individual may be appraised in terms of the combination of constitutional predisposition and precipitating influences. Multiple etiologies and multiple morbidity risks are masked by associating a specific lesion with a single morbidity risk figure derived from studies of heterogeneous populations. The families with affected individuals comprise both high-risk families with multiple familial index cases and low-risk families with only sporadic index cases. In our study of families with patients affected with breast cancer, we selected the available high-risk or familial cases, deliberately decreasing the heterogeneity of our sample by omitting the low-risk or sporadic families. Therefore, the 34 families in our study are more likely to involve primary familial factors, including genetically transmitted constitutional diffferences, in the etiologies of their breast cancers, compared to families of a random cross-section of breast cancer patients. The present study was designed to investigate the relative familiality of malignant lesions at several sites in the families selected for familial breast cancer.

Interpretation of our data should be approached with caution, because of the obvious possibilities for bias involved in

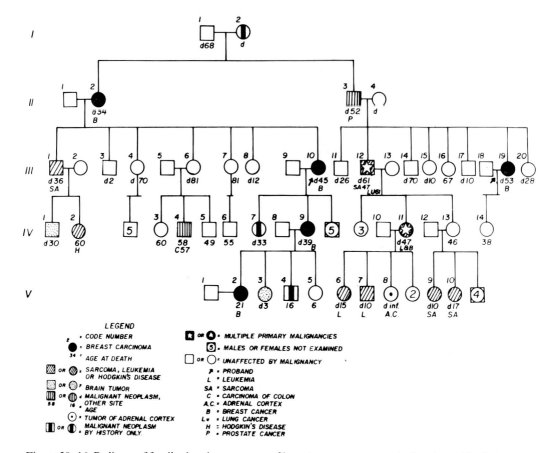

Figure 20–16. Pedigree of family showing an excess of breast cancer, sarcoma, leukemia, and brain tumors.

having selected *families of interest* for the study. We cannot exclude the possibility that such bias may have led to some distortion, but this issue can be resolved with future accumulation of additional data from families with increased incidences of breast cancer among their members. Such reports should include careful compilations of the genealogies, as well as documentation of the associated neoplasms.

The objectives of our studies were to provide extensive genealogies of families with breast cancer and to document associated neoplasms from which we have structured the following hypotheses:

1. Multiple etiologies are involved in breast cancer.

2. In some families, there appear to be associations between etiological factors for breast cancer and those for cancer of another anatomic site.

3. Selected families, from a series of kindreds characterized by familial breast cancer, suggest the occurrence of associated familial factors for increased risk of malignancy involving respectively: breast, colon, endometrium, stomach, ovary, brain tumors, leukemia, and sarcoma.

Therefore, we conclude that the test of a biological hypothesis is the determination of its consistency with empirical facts. The present pedigree data suggest that selected kindreds with familial breast cancer may be affected with familial factors that are etiologically associated with malignancies at other sites. The malignancies implicated as possibly being associated with familial breast cancer in different pedigrees are predominantly breast, breast and colon, breast and endometrium, breast and stomach, breast and ovary, and the new syndrome of sarcoma/leukemia/and brain tumors.

Klinefelter's Syndrome and Breast Cancer

Carcinoma of the male breast is an exceedingly rare malignant neoplasm accounting for approximately one case of breast cancer in men for every 100 cases in women. Jackson and associates[59] were the first to recognize an association between Klinefelter's syndrome and breast cancer. Specifically, these authors studied 21 cases of carcinoma of the breast in men and found 3 of these patients to be chromatin positive and to have abnormal sex chromosomes consistent with Klinefelter's syndrome. Recently, Harnden and associates[60] surveyed 150 cases of carcinoma of the breast in men and found that 5 of these individuals were chromatin positive. Cytogenetic studies were performed in three of these patients with findings com-

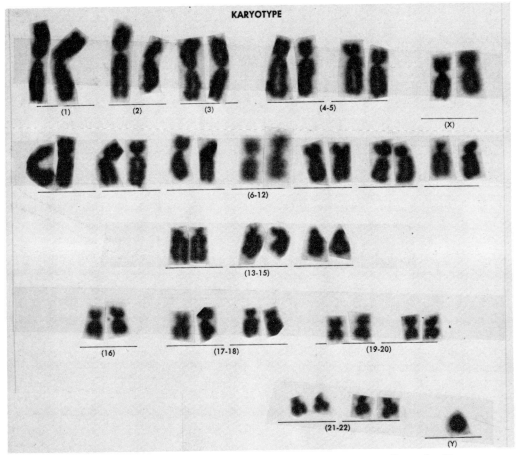

Figure 20–17. Karyotype of a man with Klinefelter's syndrome who has had a diagnosis of breast cancer.

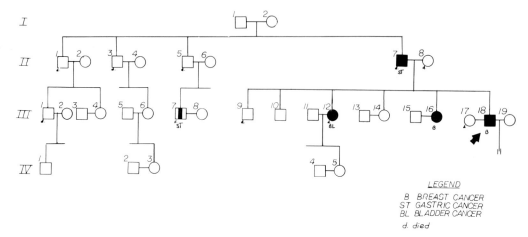

Figure 20–18. Pedigree of the family of a man with Klinefelter's syndrome and a history of breast cancer.

pletely consistent with the diagnosis of Klinefelter's syndrome. In the remaining two patients, cytogenetic studies have not been performed, but the clinical findings were completely consistent with the diagnosis of Klinefelter's syndrome. Finally, Nadel and Koss[61] studied 16 men with carcinoma of the breast, but found no evidence of chromatin positive individuals in this particular group. Harnden and associate[60] combined the findings from these studies and calculated that the incidence of chromatin positive men among the studied cases of breast cancer in men was 37.6 per thousand. This is contrasted with the finding of chromatin positive men showing a frequency of 1.9 per thousand newborn males.[62] This is a highly significant increase.

To date we are not aware of any medical genetic studies which have been carried out on families of male breast cancer patients. Recently, we were afforded an opportunity to make such a study on a 55-year-old white male who had a breast cancer diagnosis in 1972 and reported this later to the local newspaper because he wished to warn other *men* that breast cancer is not confined to women. When he responded to our letter of inquiry, it was learned that in 1951 he had had a testicular biopsy with "findings consistent with Klinefelter's syndrome." We have completed cytogenetic studies on this man who has an XXY karyotype, confirming the Klinefelter's diagnosis (Fig. 20–17). A preliminary study of his family indicates that one sister has had histologically verified breast cancer. A second sister had a diagnosis of cancer of the bladder (histologically verified), and his father had cancer of the stomach (histologically verified) (Fig. 20–18).

Our interest in determing the number of men with breast cancer in our own area led us to document the total number of male breast cancer cases in the city of Omaha during the last 15 years (1957–1972). Six men in a total male population of 187,618 in Omaha were found to have had this diagnosis. Of interest, also, is the fact that in this preliminary study, the fathers of two probands had died of gastrointestinal cancer, the mother of one died of cancer (site unknown) and in one case a sister of the proband had received a diagnosis of breast cancer and her mother a diagnosis of cancer (site unknown). Only one proband in this series had received a cytogenetic study which revealed that he was a normal XY male.

Cytogenetics and Breast Cancer

Cytogenetic studies to date have not been rewarding so far as identifying consistent chromosomal aberrations in breast cancer patients or in their close relatives who are at an increased risk for this disease. For example, in a preliminary study,[63] the possibility was considered that there might be an excess of chromosomally abnormal women with breast cancer. However, in a survey of 228 women with breast cancer, only four abnormal chromosomal constitutions were found. The possibility that there might be an excess of chromosomally abnormal female patients with breast cancer diagnosed at an early age was considered but was not confirmed when their study was extended to an additional 328 women with breast cancer. In addition, this group studied eight women from families with a high frequency of breast cancer and all of these patients were found to have normal chromosomal findings.[64]

Genetic Markers and Breast Cancer

No consistent genetic marker for breast cancer has been verified. However, Petrakis[65] studied cerumen (ear wax) in Japanese Americans from California who manifested breast cancer. A genetic dimorphism in human cerumen has been identified. Specifically, it has been shown that cerumen occurs in two phenotypic forms, wet (sticky) and dry. The quality of cerumen appears to be controlled by a single pair of genes in which the allele for the sticky trait is dominant to the allele for the dry. To date, no method has been developed to distinguish the homozygous wet type from the heterozygous form. In his review Petrakis has shown that races vary widely in their frequencies of alleles for wet and dry cerumen. He studied cerumen in order to determine whether there might

be an association between wet cerumen and rates of breast cancer in diverse population groups. He considered that such an association might be plausible in that ceruminous, mammary and certain axillary sweat glands are histologically of the apocrine type, and their secretions are biochemically similar. He studied ear wax in 31 California Japanese women with histologically verified breast cancer, and compared these with an additional 54 Japanese women without breast cancer (control group). The findings showed that breast cancer in this pilot retrospective study of individual Japanese cancer patients correlated with the presence of wet cerumen (9 out of 31, or 29 percent of the Japanese breast cancer patients had wet cerumen while in the control group 9 out of 52 or 17% had wet cerumen). He concluded that Japanese women with wet cerumen had an approximately two-fold increased relative risk of developing breast cancer. There was a suggestion that "the association of wet cerumen and cancer rates may be due to the action of a pleiotropic allele, affecting the apocrine system (ceruminous, mammary, and axillary apocrine sweat glands), the fat depots, and possibly other systems, which in turn may affect susceptibility to breast cancer." While preliminary, these observations merit further studies in differing population groups, and indeed within individual breast cancer prone families.

Florid Papillomatosis of the Nipple

In the differential diagnosis of hereditary disease affecting the breast, one should consider florid papillomatosis of the nipple in the light of a recent report indicating the occurrence of this lesion in a mother and her daughter. The most frequent tumor involving the nipple is Paget's disease with underlying duct cell carcinoma. However, in 1955, Jones[66] described florid papillomatosis of the nipple, a benign tumor which clinically shows many similarities to Paget's disease of the nipple. The first familial report of the disease was recorded by Mendelbaum,[67] who described the lesion in a mother and daughter.

Florid papillomatosis is apparently a rare lesion affecting the nipple and is referred to in the European literature as well as by the Armed Forces Institute of Pathology as "adenomatosis of the nipple."[68] To date the lesion has been described in one man.[69] This lesion differs from the more common papillomas of the breast in that it is located more superficially on the breast; in addition, simple papillomas are infrequently associated with an enlargement and ulceration of the nipple, a finding common in florid papillomatosis. Finally, in florid papillomatosis, the nipple may be enlarged, ulcerated, encrusted, and a serosanguineous discharge may occur.[67] It must be differentiated from Paget's disease by histologic evaluation. Since Mendelbaum[67] was the first to report the familial nature of this condition. It certainly should be looked for in patients and their families and evaluated appropriately.

Summary and Conclusions

The complexity of the genetics of breast cancer appears to be increasing significantly as investigators search for and identify familial associations of different malignant neoplasms in breast cancer prone families. The particular familial contexts with specific patterns of tumor associations are becoming more clearly apparent, particularly when painstaking efforts are given to the problem of verification of all histologic varieties of cancer in the families. For example, our own group is conducting a study of a large kindred manifesting the previously described syndrome of carcinoma of the breast, sarcoma, leukemia and brain tumors through four generations. Concordance-discordance analysis has revealed findings remarkably consistent with an autosomal dominant pattern of genetic transmission. Interestingly, breast cancers have occurred at an unusually young age: 23, 25, and 29. Brain tumors have occurred in six members of the family. Cutaneous abnormalities consistent with diseases such as neurofibromatosis, which might explain the excess occurrence of brain tumors in this family, could not be found (see Fig. 17–1).

The above family, as well as others are being studied for any correlation between HL-A antigens or haplotypes, SV-40 viral transformation of skin fibroblasts, cytogenetics, viral antibodies, genetic polymorphs, and endocrinologic studies (including urinary and blood steroids). We hope that these studies may lead to better methods for identification of patients at high risk for breast cancer, and that they might provide insight into the pathogenesis of this disease.

Finally, we conclude that breast cancer etiology is heterogeneous. Certain occurrences of this disease appear to be sporadic due possibly to fresh gene mutations, unknown environmental influences, and/or the interaction of these events. Differing tumor associations appear in some breast cancer prone families and are manifested in definite patterns suggesting cancer genetic syndromes. Considerably more work will be required to document and analyze the inheritance patterns in these particular cancer settings. Most importantly, investigators must continue to be cognizant of the myriad endogenous and exogenous factors which may assume etiologic importance in these families.

REFERENCES

1. MacMahon, B., Lin, T.M., Lowe, C.R., Mirra, A.P., Ravnihar, T., Salber, E.J., Trichopoulos, D., Valaoras, V.G., and Yuasa, S.: Lactation and cancer of the breast: a summary of an international study. *Bull WHO, 42:*185–194, 1970.

2. MacMahon, B., Cole, P., Lin, T.M., Lowe, C.R., Mirra, A.P., Ravnihar, B., Salber, E.J., Valaoras, V.G., and Yuasa, S.: Age at first birth and breast cancer risk. *Bull WHO, 43:*209–221, 1970.

3. Lowe, C.R., and MacMahon, B.: Breast cancer and reproductive history of women in South Wales. *Lancet, 1:*153–156, 1970.

4. Mirra, A.P., Cole, P., and MacMahon, B.: Breast cancer in an area of high parity: Säo Paulo, Brazil. *Cancer Res, 31:*77–83, 1971.

5. Levin, M.L., Sheehe, P.R., Graham, S., and Glidewell, O.: Lactation and menstrual function as related to cancer of the breast. *Am J Public Health, 54:*580–587, 1964.

6. Kamoi, M.: Statistical study on relation between breast cancer and lactation period. *Tohoku J Exp Med, 72:*59–65, 1960.

7. Lemon, H.M., Wotiz, H.H., Parsons, L., and Mozden, P.J.: Reduced estriol excretion in patients with breast cancer prior to endocrine therapy. *JAMA, 196:*1128–1136, 1966.

8. Lemon, H.M.: Endocrine influences on human mammary cancer formation: a critique. *Cancer, 23:*781–790, 1969.

9. Lilienfeld, A.M.: The relationship of cancer of the female breast to artificial menopause and marital status. *Cancer, 9:*927–934, 1956.

10. Hirayama, T., and Wynder, E.L.: A study of the epidemiology of cancer of the breast. II. The influence of hysterectomy. *Cancer, 15:*28–38, 1962.

11. Feinleib, M.: Breast cancer and artificial menopause. A cohort study. *J Natl Cancer Inst, 41:*315–329, 1968.

12. Valaoras, V.G., MacMahon, B., Trichopoulos, D., and Polychronopoulous, A.: Lactation and reproductive histories of breast cancer patients in greater Athens,1965–1967. *Int J Cancer, 4:*350–363, 1969.

13. Trichopoulos, D., MacMahon, B., and Cole, P.: The menopause and breast cancer risk. *J Natl Cancer Inst, 48:*605–613, 1972.

14. Bulbrook, R.D., Hayward, J.L., Spicer, C.C., and Thomas, B.S.: Abnormal excretion of urinary steroids by women with early breast cancer. *Lancet, 2:*1238–1240, 1962.

15. Bulbrook, R.D., and Hayward, J.L.: Discriminants and breast cancer (letter to the editor), *Lancet, 1:*1161, 1969.

16. Stern, E., Hopkins, C.E., Weiner, J.M., and Marmorston, J.: Hormone excretion patterns in patients with breast cancer and prostate cancer are abnormal. *Science, 145:* 716–719, 1964.

17. Bulbrook, R.D., and Hayward, J.L.: Abnormal urinary steroid excretion and subsequent breast cancer. A prospective study in the island of Guernsey. *Lancet, 1:*519–522, 1967.

18. Bulbrook, R.D., Hayward, J.L., and Spicer, C.C.: Relation between urinary androgen and corticoid excretion and subsequent breast cancer. *Lancet, 2:*395–398, 1971.

19. Grönroos, M., and Aho, A.J.: Estrogen metabolism in post-menopausal women with primary and recurrent breast cancer. *Eur J Cancer, 4:*523–527, 1968.

20. Turkington, R.W., Underwood, L.E., and Van Wyk, J.J.: Elevated serum prolactin levels after pituitary-stalk section in man. *New Engl J Med, 285:*707–710, 1971.

21. Poel, W.E.: Progesterone enhancement of mammary tumor development as a model of co-carcinogenesis. *Br J Cancer, 22:* 867–873, 1968.

22. Grattarola, R.: The premenstrual endometrial pattern of women with breast cancer. *Cancer, 17:*1119–1122, 1964.

23. Doll, R.: *Prevention of Cancer. Pointers from Epidemiology.* Nuffield Provincial Hospitals Trust, London, Chicago, Aldine, 1967.

24. Haenszel, W., and Kurihara, M.: Studies of Japanese migrants. I. Mortality from cancer and other diseases among Japanese in the

United States. *J Natl Cancer Inst, 40*:43–68, 1968.

25. Doll, R., Muir, C., and Waterhouse, J.: *Cancer Incidence in Five Continents. A Technical Report.* 1966 International Union Against Cancer, Berlin, Springer-Verlag, 1970, Vol. 2.

26. Moore, D.H., Charney, J., Kramarsky, B., Lasfargues, E.Y., Sarkhar, N.H., Brennan, M.J., Burrows, J.H., Sirsat, S.M., Paymaster, J.C., and Vaidya, A.B.: Search for a human breast cancer virus. *Nature, 229:* 611–614, 1971.

27. Schlom, J., Spiegelman, S., and Moore, D.: RNA-dependent DNA polymerase activity in virus-like particles isolated from human milk. *Nature, 231*:97–100, 1971.

28. Editorial: Long-acting thyroid stimulator (L.A.T.S.). *Lancet, 2*:349–350, 1970.

29. Temin, H.M.: RNA-directed DNA synthesis. *Sci Am, 226*:25–33, 1972.

30. Spiegelman, S., Burny, A., Das, M.R., Keydar, J., Schlom, J., Travenick, M., and Watson, K.: Characterization of the products of RNA-directed DNA polymerases in oncogenic RNA viruses. *Nature, 227*:563–567, 1970.

31. Editorial: Viruses and human breast cancer. *Lancet, 1*:359–360, 1972.

32. Green, M., Rokutanda, H., and Rokutanda, M.: Virus-specific RNA in cells transformed by RNA tumor viruses. *Nature (New Biol), 230*:229–232, 1971.

33. Wade, N.: Scientists and the press: cancer scare story that wasn't. *Science, 174*:679–680, 1971.

34. Miller, R.W., and Fraumeni, J.F.: Does breast feeding increase the child's risk of breast cancer? *Pediatrics, 49*:645–646, 1972.

35. Broca, P.P.: *Traite' des Tumeurs.* P. Asselin, Paris, 1866–1869, Vol. 1 and 2.

36. Lynch, H.T.: *Hereditary Factors in Carcinoma.* In *Recent Results in Cancer Research.* Berlin, Springer-Verlag, 1967, pp. 186.

37. Macklin, M.T.: Comparison of the number of breast cancer deaths observed in relatives of breast cancer patients, and the number expected on the basis of mortality rates. *J Natl Cancer Inst, 22*:927–951, 1959.

38. Li, F.P., and Fraumeni, J.F., Jr.: Soft-tissue sarcomas, breast cancer, and other neoplasms: a familial syndrome. *Ann Intern Med, 71*:747–752, 1969.

39. Lynch, H.T., and Krush, A.J.: Carcinoma of the breast and ovary in three families. *Surg Gynecol Obstet, 133*:644–648, 1971.

40. Lynch, H.T., Krush, A.J., and Guirgis, H.: Genetic factors in families with combined gastrointestinal and breast cancer. *Am J Gastroenterology, 1*:31–40, 1973.

41. Cady, B.: Familial bilateral cancer of the breast. *Ann Surg, 172*:264–272, 1970.

42. Stephens, F.E., Gardner, E.J., and Woolf, C.M.: A recheck of kindred 107, which has shown a high frequency of breast cancer. *Cancer, 11*:967–972, 1958.

43. Schottenfeld, D.: The relationship of breast cancer to thyroid disease. *J Chronic Dis, 21*:303–313, 1968.

44. Carey, R.W., Holland, J.F., Sheehe, P.R., and Graham, S.: Association of cancer of the breast and acute myelocytic leukemia. *Cancer, 20*:1080–1088, 1967.

45. Moertel, C.G., and Elveback, L.R.: The association between salivary gland cancer and breast cancer. *JAMA, 210*:306–308, 1969.

46. Schottenfeld, D., and Berg, J.W.: Incidence of multiple primary cancers. IV. Cancers of the female breast and genital organs. *J Natl Cancer Inst, 46*:161–170, 1971.

47. Schottenfeld, D., Berg, J.W., and Vitsky, B.: Incidence of multiple primary cancers. II. Index cancers arising in the stomach and lower digestive system. *J Natl Cancer Inst, 43*:77–86, 1969.

48. Dodge, O.G., Jackson, A.W., and Muldal, S.: Breast cancer and interstitial-cell tumor in a patient with Klinefelter's syndrome. *Cancer, 24*:1027–1032, 1969.

49. Anderson, D.E.: A genetic study of human breast cancer. *J Natl Cancer Inst, 48:* 1029–1034, 1972.

50. Lynch, H.T., and Krush, A.J.: Genetic predictability in breast cancer risk. *Arch Surg, 103*:84–88, 1971.

51. Lynch, H.T., Krush, A.J., Harlan, W.L., and Sharp, E.A.: Association of breast cancer,

soft tissue sarcoma, leukemia, and brain tumors in breast cancer families. *Am Surg, 39:*199–206, 1973.

52. Lynch, H.T., Krush, A.J., Lemon, H.M., Kaplan, A.R., Condit, P.T., and Bottomley, R.H.: Tumor variations in families with breast cancer. *JAMA, 222:*1631–1635, 1972.

53. Lemon, H.M.: Abnormal estrogen metabolism and tissue estrogen receptor proteins in breast cancer. *Cancer, 25:*423–435, 1970.

54. Gould, V.E., Wolff, M., and Mottet, N.K.: Morphologic features of mammary carcinomas in women taking hormonal contraceptives. *Am J Clin Pathol, 57:*139–143, 1972.

55. Lynch, H.T.: *Hereditary Factors in Carcinoma.* New York, Springer-Verlag, 1967.

56. Jacobs, B.B.: Growth of tumors in allogenic hosts after organ culture explanation. II. Tumor host interactions. *J Natl Cancer Inst, 42:*537–543, 1969.

57. Stern, K., and Goldfeder, A.: Radiation studies on mice of an inbred tumor-resistant strain. VI. Immune responses to heterologous red cells of nonirradiated and radiated mice. *Intl Arch Allergy Appl Immunol, 35:*504–513, 1969.

58. Lynch, H.T., Krush, A.J., and Kaplan, A.R.: Cancer frequency variations among and within families. *Acta Genet Med Gemellol, 81:*53–65, 1972.

59. Jackson, A.W., Muldal, S., Ockey, C.H., and O'Connor, P.J.: Carcinoma of male breast in association with the Klinefelter's syndrome. *Br Med J, 1:*223–225, 1965.

60. Harnden, D.G., Maclean, N., and Langlands, A.O.: Carcinoma of the breast and Klinefelter's syndrome. *J Med Genet, 8:*460–461, 1971.

61. Nadel, M., and Koss, L.G.: Klinefelter's syndrome and male breast cancer. *Lancet, 2:*366, 1967.

62. Court-Brown, W.M., Harnden, D.G., Jacobs, P.A., Maclean, N., and Mantle, D.J.: *Abnormalities of the Sex Chromosome Complement in Man.* Medical Research Council Special Report, No. 305, H.M.S.O., London, 1964.

63. Harnden, D.G., Langlands, A.O., McBeath, S., O'Riordan, M., and Faed, N.J.: The frequency of constitutional chromosome abnormalities in patients with malignant disease. *Eur J Cancer, 5:*605–614, 1969.

64. O'Riordan, M.L., Langlands, A.O., and Harnden, D.G.: Further studies on the frequency of constitutional chromosome abnormalities in patients with malignant disease. *Eur J Cancer, 8:*373–379, 1972.

65. Petrakis, N.L.: Cerumen genetics and human breast cancer. *Science, 173:*347–349, 1971.

66. Jones, D.B.: Florid papillomatosis of the nipple ducts. *Cancer, 8:*315–319, 1955.

67. Mendelbaum, I.: Familial florid papillomatosis of the nipple. *Ann Surg, 175:*254–256, 1972.

68. Handley, R.S., and Thackray, A.C.: Adenoma of nipple. *Br J Cancer, 16:*187–194, 1962.

69. Shapiro, L., and Karpas, C.M.: Florid papillomatosis of the nipple: first reported case in a male. *Am. Am J Clin Pathol, 44:*155–159, 1965.

CHAPTER 21

SKIN, HEREDITY, AND CANCER

———— Henry T. Lynch ————

THE HISTORY OF medicine reflects considerable interest by physicians in the skin. This is not surprising when one considers the accessibility of the integument to observation and examination. Indeed, our medical forebears were especially adept at the description and characterization of cutaneous manifestations of both primary and secondary skin diseases. Unfortunately, however, with the advent of modern diagnostic techniques, less attention has been given to the fine clinical details present in the skin on mere inspection, which when coupled with other findings from the physical examination, could provide important clues to the diagnosis of a variety of diseases, including skin cancer or the presence of cancer in underlying organs and viscera.[1-3] In his book published in 1947, Weiner,[4] a medical contemporary, called attention to the importance of the skin as a clue to internal manifestations of diseases and referred to these as *dermadrones,* to indicate the skin component of a particular syndrome which is known to be a manifestation of an internal disorder. Dr. Weiner expressed his disturbance at the lack of attention given to cutaneous manifestations by his physician colleagues and states: "And yet, it seems that the tremendous wealth of clinical observations on cutaneous phenomena accompanying internal disease, has, in our time, not found the attention it deserves." Unfortunately, in the more than 25 years since Dr. Weiner expressed his views on this problem, the situation has continued to exist to an even significantly greater degree. One need only make ward rounds with senior medical students, interns, or residents, and observe their approach to the diagnostic workup of a patient and he will soon see how readily they may gloss over the skin in their attempt to search for "laboratory clues" through use of clinical pathology and radiology. I contend that thoughtful reflection upon and examination of the integument could expedite the diagnostic process significantly in many circumstances. At the expense of belaboring this point, I call attention to the necessity for observing the skin critically because I hope to illustrate clearly in this chapter the fact that many skin signs could provide important clues to a cancer diagnosis particularly when these signs are correlated with the family history, detailed physical examination, *and* the use of diagnostic laboratories.

Figure 21–1 depicts schematically a sequence of events which we believe could prove of inestimable value to physicians in the overall problem of skin, cancer, and genetics. Specifically, we believe that critical evaluation of the skin when coupled with a carefully obtained family history, placing particular emphasis upon an inquiry for similar cutaneous findings in first and second degree relatives could in certain circumstances narrow the number of diagnostic possibilities and differential diagnosis of the particular patient. Thus, more prudent selection of laboratory studies could be made in order to arrive at a definitive diagnosis. This chain of events may seem a bit over-

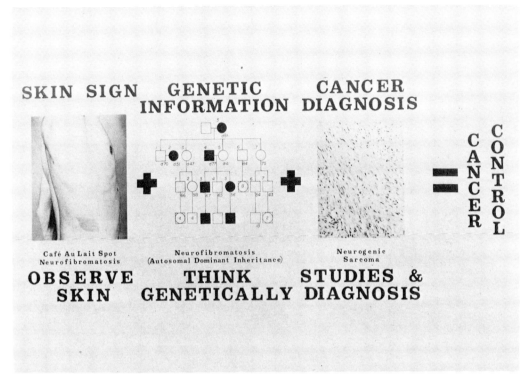

**SKIN SIGN   GENETIC   CANCER
INFORMATION DIAGNOSIS**

Café Au Lait Spot
Neurofibromatosis

Neurofibromatosis
(Autosomal Dominant Inheritance)

Neurogenic
Sarcoma

**OBSERVE   THINK   STUDIES &
SKIN   GENETICALLY DIAGNOSIS**

Figure 21–1. Diagrammatic formula for utilization of genetic information, physical signs, and diagnostic measures for cancer control. By permission, Lynch, H.T., *Skin, Heredity and Malignant Neoplasms*, New York City, Medical Examination Publishing Co.

simplified, but our own experience and that of many colleagues, indicates this to be a successful and rewarding approach to these problems.

In order to elucidate this subject further, we have prepared a series of tables (Tables 21-1–21-IV) which list cancerous and pre-cancerous diseases involving the skin which bespeak the presence of cancer in the skin or in underlying viscera. In each of these diseases, a familial or genetic etiology has been either verified or suggested, though perhaps not yet clearly delineated so far as the precise genetic mechanism is concerned. In addition, in some of these disorders, the association with cancer may not be clear-cut but the condition has nevertheless been included here because of active interest in a possible

cancer association. Diseases in this category include lupus erythematosis and scleroderma. In all events, the reader should weigh critically the existing evidence of genetic etiology and/or cancer association.

Many of the disorders mentioned in Tables 21-I to 21-IV are discussed in other contexts through this book. For example, diseases such as Fanconi's aplastic anemia, ataxia telangiectasia, and Wiskott-Aldrich syndrome are discussed by Drs. Gatti and Good in their chapter on immunology and cancer. In addition, these diseases are also discussed in the chapter by Drs. Dossik and Todaro on viruses and cancer. An entire group of skin diseases including neurofibromatosis, multiple nevoid basal cell carcinoma syndrome, and the multiple mucosal neuroma syndrome are discussed by Drs. Mulcahy and Harlan in their chapter on neurology, neuropathology, genetics, and cancer.

An attempt will be made throughout this presentation to provide a logical frame of reference for diagnosis, therapy and cancer control for these diseases through employing a keen appraisal of the skin in context with genetics and the family history.

Sunlight and Pigmentation

Genetic and environmental factors interact in the development of many forms of skin cancer. This is seen clearly by the fact that two major determinants in the production of skin cancer are: 1) the amount of ultraviolet light exposure and 2) the amount of natural pigmentation in the patient which of course is a function of his genetic make-up. When viewing races and their variations in pigmentation, we find that skin cancer occurs rarely in Negroes and other dark-complexioned races and ethnic groups. Conversely, skin cancer occurs most frequently in lightly pigmented individuals who also have an increased tendency to freckle rather than tan.[5,6]

The association of skin cancer with prolonged exposure to sunlight has been confirmed repeatedly by numerous investigators in different parts of the world.[5] It is generally accepted that wavelengths between 2800 and 3200 Å are primarily responsible for skin cancer formation and for phototoxic sunburn responses.[7] The factors affecting this fraction include the sun angle which is closely related to the time of day, the season of the year, and the latitude of exposure. In spite of the physical quantitative factors of solar radiation exposure of individuals at a given time residing in a specific area, one may sort out individuals differentially in any particular population who will be more likely to be at risk for the development of skin cancer.

It has been established that skin cancer occurs most frequently on areas which are more likely to receive sun exposure, namely the head, neck, arms, and hands. Skin cancer occurs more frequently in individuals of Nordic extraction with fair complexion, blue eyes, and blond or red hair. In addition, with a high degree of statistical significance, studies have shown that individuals of Celtic antecedents (Scotch, Irish, and Welsh) develop skin cancer more frequently than individuals of other ethnic origins. Silverstone's studies,[8,9] performed in 1964 in three different areas of Queensland, Australia, revealed a significantly greater number of skin tumors

TABLE 21-I
AUTOSOMAL DOMINANT INHERITANCE

Disorder	Skin Manifestations	Manifestations of Other Systems	Predominant Cancers
Neurofibromatosis	Café au lait spots, cutaneous neurofibromas, all sites, axillary freckle-like lesions, oral papillomatous tumors	Multiple congenital anomalies	Sarcoma, acoustic neuroma, pheochromocytoma
Gardner's Syndrome	Epidermoid inclusion cysts, sebaceous cysts, dermoid tumors	Osteomas, polyposis coli	Adenocarcinoma of the colon
Multiple Nevoid Basal Cell Carcinoma Syndrome	Multiple nevoid appearing basal cell carcinomas, benign cysts, hypokeratinized area of palms, "palmar pits," and soles	Jaw cysts, rib & vertebral anomalies, neurologic and ophthamologic anomalies, intracranial calcifications	Multiple basal cell carcinomas
Cutaneous Malignant Melanoma	Usually darkly and unevenly pigmented cutaneous growths, might be mistaken for junctional nevi	None	Cutaneous malignant melanoma

TABLE 21-I (CONTINUED)

Disorder	Skin Manifestations	Manifestations of Other Systems	Predominant Cancers
Tylosis & Esophageal Carcinoma (Keratosis Palmaris et Plantaris)	Tylosis of palms and soles	None	Esophageal Cancer
Tuberous Sclerosis	Adenoma sebaceum of Pringle, café au lait spots, periungle fibromata, shagreen patch, fibromatous plaques	Epilepsy, mental retardation, hamartomas in brain, kidneys, and heart	Intracranial neoplasms (astrocytomas, glioblastomas)
von Hippel-Lindau's	Vascular nevi of the face, angiomatosis of the retina, cystic lesions	Cerebellar angiomatosis	Hemangioblastoma of cerebellum, hypernephroma, & pheochromocytoma
Multiple Trichoepithelioma	Tumor derived from hair follicles (Brooke tumor) with predilection for the skin of the paranasal areas; usually appear near puberty	None	Rare examples of basal cell carcinoma, and trichochlamydocarcinoma; one case of anaplastic carcinoma with squamous differentiation
Porphyria Cutanea Tarda	Hyperpigmentation, scleroderma like changes, bullae, vessicles, sunlight sensitivity	During acute attacks, abdominal colic, motor paralysis, jaundice, and psychosis	Rare examples of basal cell carcinoma of skin and hepatoma*
Peutz-Jegher's Syndrome	Distinctive pigmentation (melanin spots) of nose, face, and distal portions of fingers, of mucous membranes and lip	Polyposis coli of intestinal tract except esophagus	Adenocarcinoma of duodenum and colon
Epidermolysis Bullosa Dystrophia (Congenital Traumatic Pemphigus)	Vesicles, bullae, epidermal cysts, extensor surfaces and sites exposed to trauma with disabling scarring	Bullae and ulcers of mucous membranes	Carcinoma of mucous membranes, multiple basal and squamous cell carcinoma of skin*
Kaposi's Sarcoma (Multiple Idiopathic Hemorrhagic Sarcoma of Kaposi)	Reddish, purplish, or bluish brown nodules, rubbery or firm consistency, often unilateral, predominantly on extremities along veins or lymphatics	Lesions may occur in gastrointestinal tract or genitalia	Sarcoma; high incidence of coexistent leukemia or lymphoma
Generalized Keratoacanthoma	Red macules with rapid progression to papules and nodules; circular, firm, pearly rolled, notched rim surrounding an umbilicated crater; may show exceedingly rapid involution	None	Rare occurrences of squamous cell carcinoma*
Pachynychia Congenita	Thickening of the nails, subungal hyperkeratosis, keratoderma of the palms and soles	Occasionally may encounter hyperhidrosis, abnormalities of hair, teeth, and bone development, bulla formation, and mental deficiency	Carcinoma of mucous membranes
Syndrome of Bilateral Pheochromocytoma; Medullary Thyroid Carcinoma and Multiple Neuromas	True neuromas which may occur on the eyelids, lips, tongue or the nasal and laryngeal mucosae	Parathyroid adenomas, hypertension secondary to pheochromocytoma	Pheochromocytoma (often bilateral) medullary thyroid carcinoma
Multiple Self-healing Squamous Epithelioma	Cutaneous lesions characterized as red macules and papules which enlarge, become ulcerated and eventually heal leaving deep pitted scars. Areas include face, ears, arms, thighs and legs	Lymphatic infiltration of anal and oral area	Squamous cell carcinoma of skin, anal and oral mucosa

* Rare, but nevertheless definite, cancer association.

TABLE 21-II
AUTOSOMAL RECESSIVE INHERITANCE

Disorders	Skin Manifestations	Manifestations of Other Systems	Predominant Cancers
Xeroderma Pigmentosum	Dry, scaling, hyperpigmentation and freckling, hyperkeratosis, and telangiectasia, basal and squamous cell carcinoma	Multi-system involvement	Basal and squamous cell carcinoma of skin and malignant melanoma
Werner's Syndrome (Progeria of the Adult)	Premature aging of the skin, scleroderma-like findings, loss of subcutaneous fat, greying of the hair, baldness	Juvenile cataract, diabetes mellitus, hypogonadism, short stature, arteriosclerosis	Sarcomas, meningiomas
Ataxia-Telangiectasia (Louis-Bar Syndrome)	Oculocutaneous telangiectasia temporal and nasal area of conjunctive, also of butterfly areas, ears, antecubital, popliteal, dorsum of hands and feet; telangiectasia are venous	Cerebellar ataxia, mental and growth retardation, recurrent sinopulmonary infection; lymphopenia; deficiency in developing delayed hypersensitivity (gamma-A globulin defect)	Acute leukemia and lymphoma
Bloom's Syndrome (Congenital Telangiectatic Erythema and stunted growth)	Congenital telangiectatic erythema of face "butterfly distribution," photosensitivity; occasionally, café au lait spots, ichthyosis, acanthosis nigricans, hypertrichosis and lichen pilaris	Short stature, fine featured face, dolicocephalic head	Acute leukemia
Chediak-Higashi Syndrome	Semi-albinism, hyperpigmentary response to sunlight, excessive sweating	Hematologic (anomalous intracellular granulations); retinal albinism, photophobia, recurrent infections, lymphadenopathy, and neurologic manifestations	Lymphoma
Albinism	Partial or total absence of pigmentation of skin, hair, eyes ("Pink eye"). Premature aging of skin as noted by actinic chelitis, telangiectasia, keratosis, and cutaneous horns	Several phenotypic varieties, including impairment of vision, hearing, and mental retardation	Basal and squamous cell carcinoma of skin
Fanconi's Aplastic Anemia	Spotty or patchy brown pigmentation	Pancytopenia, bone marrow hypoplasia, congenital abnormalities, including hypoplasia of thumbs, absent radius	Leukemia
Glioma-Polyposis Syndrome* (Turcots' Syndrome)	Café au lait spots	None	Brain tumors, most commonly glioblastoma multiforme (one patient had medulloblastoma) and adenocarcinoma of colon secondary to polyposis coli

*Condition restricted to siblings (male and females) in two unrelated families strongly suggesting autosomal recessive inheritance.

in Celtic people than that which was expected based on distribution of the local population. In addition, the onset of cancer appeared to be about ten years earlier than in the other ethnic populations in that area. It was believed that the susceptibility to skin cancer in the Celtics was related to an inherited inability of the skin to protect them in the usual fashion against the carcinogenic effects of ultraviolet radiation. Racial and ethnic groups used for comparison in this study included Australians born of Mediter-

TABLE 21-III
SEX-LINKED RECESSIVE INHERITANCE

Disorders	Skin Manifestations	Manifestations of Other Systems	Predominant Cancers
Aldrich Syndrome (Wiscott-Aldrich Syndrome)	Chronic eczema, erythroderma, petechiae, purpura, furuncles	Thrombocytopenia, recurrent infections, pyoderma, purulent otitis media; death often due to overwhelming infections	Leukemia, lymphoma
Bruton's Agamma-globulinemia	Pyodermas, furunculosis, cellulitis, conjunctivitis	Multiple recurrent infections; defect in formation of immunoglobulin-producing system	Acute leukemia

TABLE 21-IV
POSSIBLE GENETIC ETIOLOGY—MODE OF INHERITANCE UNKNOWN

Disorders	Skin Manifestations	Manifestations of Other Systems	Predominant Cancers
Scleroderma	"Stiffness of skin" with loss of lines of normal facial expression, history of Raynaud's phenomenon	Esophageal involvement with decreased peristalsis, dilation, dysphagia, alteration of pulmonary function	Bronchiolar carcinoma, malignant carcinoid
Dermatomyositis	Inflammatory changes of skin and muscle, erythema, puffy edematous swelling of eyelids, "heliotrope bloating" minute telangiectasia	Serum enzyme and electromyographic changes, may be preceded by Raynaud's phenomenon	Adenocarcinoma of viscera
Sjögren's Syndrome (Keratoconjunctivitis Sicca)	Dryness of skin and mucous membranes, hyperpigmentation, café au lait spots, purpura and telangiectasia of lips and fingertips	Rheumatoid arthritis	Lymphoma
Systemic Lupus Erythematosus	Malar erythema of "butterfly area," macules: variety of cutaneous and vascular changes	Intermittent fever, arthritis, arthralgia, arteritis, phlebitis, CNS and renal disease (lupus nephritis) biologic false-positive serology, positive LE preps	Thymic tumors, leukemia and lymphoma
Giant Pigmented Nevi* (Bathing Trunk Nevi)	Nevi covering extensive cutaneous surface; variable manifestations ranging from flat to angiomatous, verrucous, and hairy nevi	None	Melanomas in children
Nevus Sebaceous of Jadassohn	Hamartoma often present at birth primarily on scalp, face or neck. Several centimeters or more, circumscribed, round on irregular, slightly raised, waxy, hairless which at puberty, becomes verrucous and nodular and later may be complicated by benign or malignant nevoid tumors	Variable, may find convulsive disorder, focal EEG abnormalities, mental deficiency and brain dysplasia; ocular abnormalities have included colobomas of the irides and choroid, conjunctival lipodermoids, and nystagmus	Basal cell epithelioma (15% to 20%), sebaceous epithelioma, salivary gland adenocarcinoma, syringocystadenoma papilliferum (apocrine duct stage differentiation), and keratoacanthoma

*Hereditary etiology has not yet been established, but the congenital basis and known hereditary factors of certain melanomas raise suspicion about genetic etiology.

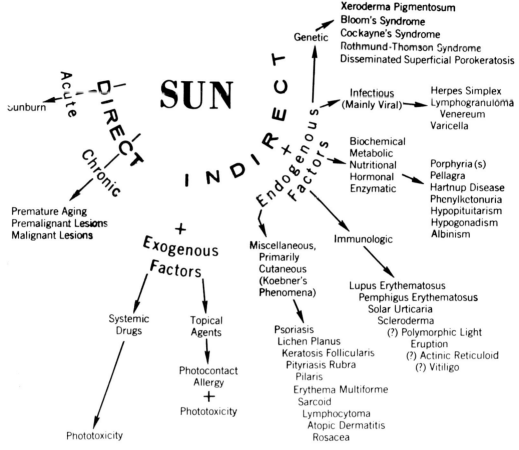

Figure 21–2. Sunlight-related disorders, published by permission of *JAMA* (Isaac Willis, M.D., "Sunlight and the Skin," *Journal of the American Medical Association,* 217:1088–1093, (1971).

ranean or South American ancestry, Asiatics, and Aboriginals of mixed ancestral background. The likelihood of susceptibility to skin cancer increased with the degree of Celtic ancestry.

Willis[10] has surveyed the subject of sunlight-related disorders showing direct effects of solar radiation involving complex interactions of sunlight, genetics, drugs, as well as a variety of endogenous and exogenous factors which are depicted in a rather unique manner in Figure 21–2.

Finally, skin cancer appears to occur with greater frequency in all lightly pigmented individuals who engage in outdoor occupations with much exposure to sunlight such as farming, construction work, and fishing.

Olson[6] has described histologic changes in the skin of Negroes who are protected from solar radiation by their pigmentation and has compared them with persons lacking pigmentary protection and thereby prone to skin cancer. Among the Negroes, he found that the melanocytes of their unexposed skin contained melanosomes which

develop pigment earlier, are larger and are more densely pigmented than those of Caucasians. These melanosomes are transferred to keratinocytes but are predominantly individually distributed throughout the epidermis, including the stratum corneum, since individually disbursed melanosomes are degraded to a lesser degree than melanosomes within melanosome complexes. Thus, the arrangement and distribution of pigment in unexposed Negro skin and tanned Caucasian skin closely resemble one another microscopically. Both are effectively resistant to the effects of ultraviolet light, both acute and chronic.

Finally, in describing the histologic findings in patients prone to skin cancer, Olson[6] states that

fair skinned individuals, with a lifelong history of sunburning and freckling rather than tanning, have characteristic, microscopic alterations in epidermal-melanin units. Hypertrophic melanocytes and dendrites are found focally, but distribution of pigment within melanocytes is uneven. Many keratinocytes contain abundant pigment, while others exhibit none at all. In addition, melanosome complexes tend to be larger than normal. The consequence is uneven pigment distribution and inadequate protection from sunlight since many cells lack pigment umbrella. Individuals with such skin are particularly prone to develop skin cancer.

In addition, Olson found that in a comparable study of the skin of patients with xeroderma pigmentosum the quantity was increased, but melanosome distribution was even more irregular than in fair complexioned individuals with multiple skin cancers. In addition, melanocytes and their dendrites were markedly hypertrophic, but transfer of melanin to keratinocytes was impaired. In addition, keratinocytes were surrounded by numerous hypertrophic dendrites but often they demonstrated little or no melanin. In these patients the quantity of pigment production appears to be adequate but the keratinocytes received inadequate melanin protection from sunlight. Thus, Olson[6] concluded that "color of skin, as well as its capacity to protect against ultra-violet light, depends not only upon the quantity of pigment produced by melanocytes, but also upon melanin transferred to, disbursed within, and degraded by keratinocytes." Therefore, we find repeatedly a set of circumstances involving host factors in interaction with environmental factors linked to the production of the most frequently occurring form of cancer in man, namely, skin cancer.[1]

Genetics and Pigmentation

Most of our information on the genetics of skin color have been derived from the study of mice. These studies have shown conclusively that deviations in skin and coat color are produced by gene mutations. Indeed, practically every phase of the development and function of melanocytes is under the control of specific genes acting alone or in combination with the physiological environment which they inhabit.

The melanocytes appear to be critical cells harboring the pigmentation properties of the skin. No significant sexual or racial differences in their frequency have been established in humans. This observation is in keeping with conclusions derived from the study of mammals which show that variations in skin color are related to differences in melanocyte activity rather than to the sheer numbers of these melanocytes. Szabo[11] reported no regional differences in melanocyte density in the late human fetus but did show a significant increase in their number after birth and these tended to become fewer in old age as shown by Fitzpatrick and associates.[12]

In the case of mice, more than 40 gene loci have been shown to be concerned with pigmentation and Breathnach suggested that even more will be recorded in the future.[13] Breathnach further speculated that melanin pigmentation of the skin in man is under similar precise genetic control.

> Although positive evidence is not easy to obtain because of co-mingling of genes . . . variations in pigmentation are not due to differences in population density of melanocytes per unit area of skin but rather to differences in activity of melanosomes, the degree of melanization of individual granules, possibly the rate of transfer of granules to keratinocytes, and in the final analysis, their concentration and location within the various layers of epidermis.[13]

In summary, the inheritance of skin color (pigmentation) is complex, and involves the functioning capacity of melanosomes, and it appears to be polygenic.[14]

In order to better comprehend the problem of skin, genetics, and cancer, we shall now present several clinical examples showing specific elucidations of these phenomena.

Keratosis

Keratosis (keratoderma) of the palms and soles is a complex disorder which occurs in numerous genetic as well as nongenetic conditions such as arsenical exposure. Reed and Porter[15] constructed a useful genetic classification of the several disorders with a hereditary etiology in which keratosis is manifested (Table 21-V). They have excluded certain entities that were not well-established and they speculate that other conditions will in due time, be added to this classification.

Frequently, the patient is unaware of the presence of keratoderma and when describing the condition, he will state that his hands are slightly rough. Thus, palpation of the palms and soles is important in determining mild keratoderma.

It is important to recognize the several hereditary syndromes in which keratosis is associated with cancer. In these particular rare examples, keratosis could serve as a useful marker indicating an underlying cancer risk to the patient. Contrariwise, one should remember that keratosis also occurs in many genetic and nongenetic disorders which are not associated with cancer and, therefore, the physician should avoid unduly alarming his patients when this condition is recognized. Indeed, knowledge of the clinical characteristics and genetic factors present in the disorders cited in Table 21-V could permit the physician in certain circumstances to provide genetic counseling with emphasis upon the fact that the keratosis is benign and therefore does not denote cancer risk; this is the circumstance for the overwhelming majority of these disorders.

We shall discuss several conditions wherein keratosis is associated with cancer.

Tylosis and Esophageal Cancer (Keratosis Palmaris et Plantaris)

Howel-Evans and associates in 1958[16] found tylosis (hyperkeratosis) of the palms and soles (Figure 21–3) associated with carcinoma of the esophagus in an exceedingly large number of members of two families. The investigators constructed a life table of these families wherein it was predicted that 95 percent of the relatives with tylosis would develop carcinoma of the esophagus by age 65. Interestingly, in 1970, Harper, Harper, and Howel-Evans[17] updated their findings on these families for the twelve-year interval of 1958 to 1970 and found that the predicted

TABLE 21-V
KERATOSIS

	Mode of Inheritance	Type	Other Signs
DISORDER: Localized for Most Part to Keratosis of Palms and Soles			
Tylosis	Autosomal dominant	Diffuse	Hyperhidrosis, friction bullae
Keratosis with carcinoma	Autosomal dominant	Diffuse	**Squamous cell carcinoma of esophagus (4 families known so far)
Keratosis punctata	Autosomal dominant		
Keratosis striata	Autosomal dominant	Localized	
Keratosis mutilans	Autosomal dominant	Diffuse	Ainhum effect on fingers, bony changes
Keratosis mutilans	Autosomal recessive	Diffuse	Ainhum effect on fingers, bony changes, neurosensory deafness
Keratosis with corneal atrophy	Autosomal dominant	Diffuse	Corneal atrophy
Keratosis with multiple changes	Autosomal recessive	Diffuse	Hypotrichosis, nail dystrophy and enamel dysplasia
Papillon-Lefevre syndrome	Autosomal recessive	Diffuse	Other skin involvement seen, loss of teeth in both dentitions (?), calcification of falx cerebri
Mal de Meleda	Autosomal recessive	Diffuse	Other skin areas may be involved
Keratosis with mental changes	Autosomal dominant	Diffuse	Mental deficiency-epilepsy
GENERALIZED DISORDERS: Disorders That May Only at Times be Localized to Palms and Soles Keratosis Palmaris and Plantaris			
Ichthyosiform erythroderma of the bullous type	Autosomal dominant	Diffuse sometimes	
Ichthyosiform erthroderma	Autosomal recessive	Diffuse sometimes	Mental deficiency, variable eccrine function
Darier's disease	Autosomal dominant	Punctate	
Erythrokeratodermia variabilis	Autosomal dominant	Diffuse	Variable configurate ichthyosis
Basal cell nevus syndrome	Autosomal dominant	Punctate	**Basal cell carcinomas, dental cysts, congenital vertebrae and other congenital abnormalities, medulloblastomas of brain
Pityriasis rubra pilaris	Autosomal dominant	Diffuse	Erythroderma, follicular hyperkeratosis
Naegelia and Franceschetti-Jadassohn Syndrome	Autosomal dominant	Diffuse	Pigmentation of skin, defective teeth
Congenital hidrotic ectodermal dysplasia	Autosomal dominant	Diffuse	Nail dystrophy, abnormal dentition
Pachyonychia congenita	Autosomal dominant (May be two types but both dominant)	Diffuse or pressure points	**Premature dentition, friction bullae, nail dystrophy
Dyskeratosis congenita	Sex-linked recessive	Diffuse	**Leukoplakia, defects in other organs, pancytopenia, nail dystrophy
Incontinentia pigmenti	Sex-linked dominant	Localized, fingers and toes mainly	Part of the three stages of development; eye, brain and other organs may be affected
Congenital acanthosis nigricans	? Autosomal	Diffuse	Diffuse skin changes even with involvement of mouth; no cancer, neurosensory deafness
Epidermolysis bullosa dystrophyica	Autosomal dominant	Diffuse	**Bullae with friction with scarring, involvement of gastrointestinal tract
Procupine men (Ichthyosis hystrix)	Autosomal dominant	Diffuse	Mental deficiency

*Permission for publication granted by William B. Reed, M.D., and Editor, *Archives of Dermatology, 104:* 1971.
**Those disorders wherein keratosis is associated with cancer.

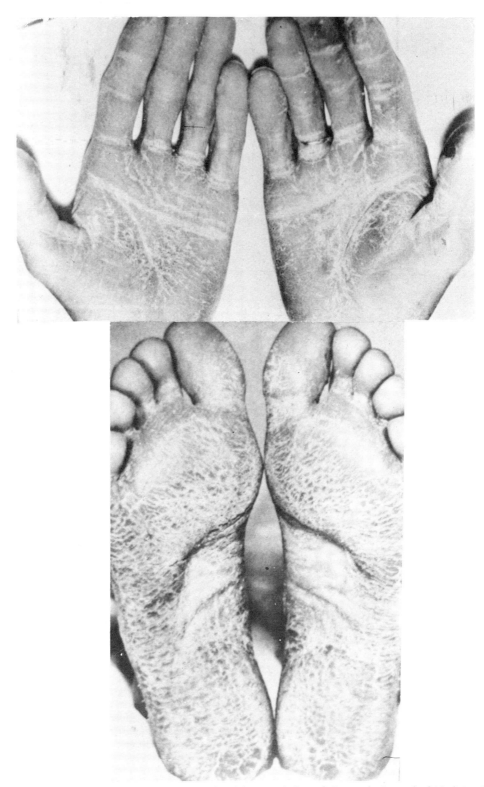

Figure 21–3. Tylosis of palms and soles, reprinted by permission of *Quarterly Journal of Medicine* (W. Howel-Evans, *et al.*, "Carcinoma of the Oesophagus with Keratosis Palmaris et Plantaris (Tylosis), *Quarterly Journal of Medicine,* 27:413–429, (1958).

95 percent occurrence of carcinoma of the esophagus in patients with tylosis was unfortunately occurring in accordance with their earlier predictions. Specifically, six new cases of esophageal carcinoma occurred in this twelve year interval and all in members who had tylosis. In short, no occurrences of esophageal cancer were found in patients without tylosis.

The tylosis in these families is characterized by a later age of onset than that seen in the usual hereditary occurrence of tylosis in the absence of esophageal cancer. Several individuals developed tylosis as late as middle age. In addition, in some members of these esophageal cancer families, tylosis may be confined to the feet as occurred in two women who have died since 1958 of esophageal cancer. Of further interest is the fact that carcinoma of the esophagus occurs in families with tylosis about ten years *earlier* than the usual age at onset of esophageal cancer in the general population.

The management of members of these kindreds who are at risk for carcinoma of the esophagus poses several problems. For example, in 1958 it was not felt justified to undertake regular preventive measures in individuals at risk, since the possibility for successful surgical cure was considered too small when compared to the risk of creating fear of cancer. However, as cancer continued to develop in family members followed by death in every case despite awareness of the condition by family doctors a reappraisal was made. In addition, it was learned that the majority of family members were already aware of and worried about the risk of developing cancer and therefore were more reassured than alarmed by the prospect of having periodic medical evaluation of their problem. As might be expected, many members who did not have tylosis were also worried about the possibility of developing cancer; genetic counseling was able to provide them with some degree of reassurance. The

approaches to preventive care have included barium swallow, esophagoscopy, and more recently, esophageal exfoliative cytology studies. In the case of x-ray evaluation, investigators were concerned about the possibility of excessive x-ray exposure to an esophagus that was already harboring a predisposition to the development of carcinoma; in the case of the performance of esophagoscopy, there was also the consideration of the attendant risks of this procedure, although it is now being performed on individuals who have tylosis and are receiving an anesthetic for any reason. It seems that a practical measure however, would be periodic screening with exfoliative cytology. In addition, members of the family have been advised to abstain from smoking and to minimize their alcohol consumption, since these factors have been clearly shown to be associated with carcinoma of the esophagus. However, practically speaking, the results show that these practices were not being followed by many members of the family. However, one of the youngest individuals to develop esophageal cancer, a 30-year-old patient, neither smoked nor drank. This raised serious question as to the efficacy of stressing the restrictions on smoking and consuming alcohol to these family members. Currently, it is thought that with constant awareness of the problem by both doctors and patients, at the slightest indication of gastrointestinal symptoms an investigation of the esophagus should be undertaken.

In a family described by Shine and Allison[18] tylosis was found in association with a congenital abnormality of the esophagus and esophageal cancer in the proband. This association of tylosis with congenital abnormality of the esophagus was present in two and possibly three generations; an autosomal dominant mode of inheritance was hypothesized.

Cytogenetic studies in patients with tylosis and esophageal cancer have been essentially normal. Esophageal cancer in the absence of tylosis has failed to show any significant familial tendency.[19]

Tylosis and Cancer Other Than Esophageal Cancer

Huriez and associates[20] reported on tylosis of an unusual type known as "Sclerotylosis" which occurred in three families in France. In this particular type of tylosis, hyperkeratosis of the hands and feet is accompanied by atrophic changes of the skin and nails and, interestingly, a frequent occurrence of malignancy in the affected skin. Indeed, 7 of 44 affected individuals developed malignant tumors in the skin, while seven other members died from internal cancers of various anatomic sites including the tongue, tonsil, breast, and uterus. Finally, no cases of esophageal cancer have been found in the families with this unusual form of tylosis, i.e. sclerotylosis. This type of tylosis is probably inherited as an autosomal dominant and appears to be located on a separate chromosomal locus from that of the usual type of tylosis, more particularly that associated with esophageal cancer.

Palmer and Plantar Seed Keratoses

An association has been postulated between palmer and plantar seed keratoses and internal malignancy. For example, Dobson and associates[21] suggested that palmar keratoses occurred four times as frequently in patients with cancer than in those patients who did not manifest cancer. However, a later study by Bean and associates[22] showed that keratoses occurred just as commonly in those with cancer as in those without malignancy. Finally, in a recently reported study, Rhodes[23] surveyed 500 patients over the age of 40 attending a dermatology clinic,

and found that 62 percent had *seed* keratoses on their palms or their soles. However, no statistically significant association was found between the presence of these keratoses and internal malignancy. A slight, but nonsignificant excess association was found between keratoses and basal cell carcinoma.

Several rarely occurring conditions involve the skin and manifest variable histological varieties of cancer with proven or suspected genetic etiology. The following discussion will consider briefly some of these disorders. In each case an attempt has been made to provide sufficient literature for the reader to evaluate when the particular issue might be controversial.

Blue Rubber-Bleb Nevus Syndrome

The Blue Rubber-Bleb Nevus syndrome is characterized by the association of angiomatosis of the skin and of the gut; the cutaneous angiomas may occur anywhere on the skin. They may be nipple- or bladder-like, are soft, bluish and erectile, are easily compressible, and slowly refill with blood when pressure is applied and then released. These angiomas may be pedunculated or they may be sessile. They may be exquisitely painful in certain patients. Angiomas have also been found in the mouth, lungs, spleen, liver, kidneys, adrenals, central nervous system and even the muscles.[24-31] One of the interesting aspects of this disease is the occasional association of spontaneous pain and sweating of the angioma.[26]

Berlyne and Berlyne[25] describe a patient with the syndrome who had an iron deficiency anemia, who complained of bleeding *piles,* and who had undergone surgery for massive hematemesis. He was found to have numerous cavernous hemangiomata in the rectal mucosa which would prolapse on straining. The condition was manifested through five generations of this family; findings were consistent with an autosomal dominant inherited factor. The condition should be distinguished from the Osler-Weber-Rendu syndrome; this differentiation as well as other problems in the differential diagnosis of the Blue Rubber-Bleb Nevus syndrome are clearly delineated in Bean's classic monograph on the subject.[26]

Rice and Fischer[27] reported a 21-year-old Caucasian woman with the syndrome who had hemangiomas of mucous membranes, pleura, lungs, liver, peritoneum, intestines, and skeletal muscles. She also manifested a cerebellar medulloblastoma. This association with cancer has not been previously reported.

The finding of medulloblastoma in a patient with the Blue Rubber-Bleb nevus syndrome could of course be fortuitous. It is of interest here because of the occurrence of medulloblastoma in other hereditary contexts including the multiple nevoid basal cell carcinoma syndrome, another dominantly inherited genodermatosis. Since both of these diseases also have in common multisystem involvement, one wonders about the possibility of a genetic relationship between them. Finally, there is a report of a patient with the Blue Rubber-Bleb Nevus Syndrome and multiple enchondromas in the bones of the fingers and toes, findings consistent with Maffucci's syndrome.[28]

In summary, we have an example of a hereditary disease with distinguishing cutaneous and internal manifestations with a report of cancer in at least one patient. Further studies of this disease will be of interest, in order to determine any other cancer association.

Familial Epidermodysplasia Verruciformis of Lewandowsky and Lutz (EV)

Familial Epidermodysplasia Verruciformis of Lewandowsky and Lutz (EV) was first described by Lewandowsky and Lutz in 1922.[32] This rare disease is characterized by polymorphic verrucose lesions consisting of warty, lichenoid, flat papules which resemble verruca plana. Occasionally, large confluent plaques may occur. These lesions are most often found on the face, neck, trunk, and on the dorsum of the hands and feet. Age of onset is often shortly after birth or during early childhood, and the disease may persist in this form for decades.[33,34] Malignant changes have been recorded with sufficient frequency, i.e. squamous cell carcinoma of the skin in 20 percent[33] so that the condition is referred to by some as a precancerous disorder.[33,35–39] A viral etiology for EV has recently been suggested as of etiological significance in genetically predisposed patients.[40,41]

In the report of Rajagopalan and associates,[33] a Chinese consanguineous family was studied wherein six female members from a sibship of 11 (four brothers and one sister were unaffected) were found to have EV with the suggestion by these authors that it was inherited as an autosomal recessive trait and sex limited in the females. However, in other families reported in the literature, both sexes were equally affected and consanguinity, as mentioned, was a frequent occurrence, thus suggesting autosomal recessive inheritance without sex limitation in these particular kindreds.[33]

Polydysplastic Epidermolysis Bullosa

Polydysplastic epidermolysis bullosa (PEB) usually occurs at birth or shortly thereafter. Its clinical course is characterized by bullous formation, and delayed healing with tissue-paper like scarring. Areas most frequently involved are the extremities, particularly around the joints, acral, and pressure areas. PEB shows a well established association with cancer. According to the review of Wechsler and associates,[42] cancer association was first recognized in 1913 in the report of a 25 year old white lady with PEB who had squamous cell carcinoma of the tongue. Eleven cases of cancer have been described in this condition since that initial report. These carcinomas were primarily squamous cell in type, they appeared between the third and sixth decade, and they almost always occurred in chronic scarred areas. Metastases were occasionally noted, and a common feature of the lesions was a relentless progression of the tumors despite aggressive therapy. Wechsler and associates[42] have now added four additional cases providing additional evidence for the relationship between PEB and squamous cell carcinoma. It was of interest that two of their cases were restricted to a sibship involving two brothers, and another of their patients was a woman whose grandparents were first cousins. These findings are in accord with autosomal recessive inheritance.

Certain similarities are observed between the clinical course of PEB with primary features of bullae, thin scar formation, ulceration, and slow healing, and the carcinogenic process found in thermal-burn scars and in cancer occurrences at the margins of chronic leg ulcers.

Maffucci's Syndrome

The clinical characteristics of Maffucci's syndrome have been described by Bean[43,44] and by Elmore and Cantrell[45] and include the following features: 1) dyschondroplasia in one or more of the long bones which may result in shortening of the bones and fractures; 2) hemangiomas of the skin of any part of the body, including occasional involvement of the lips and palate.

In Maffucci's original report in 1881,[46] he described a 41-year-old woman who in addition to multiple bony-hard masses of the forearm with overlying hemangiomas, also

manifested a malignant scapular tumor which resulted in her death. Subsequent reports have shown that malignant transformation is an important feature in this syndrome. For example, Elmore and Cantrell[45] found that cancer occurred in 14 of 75 (18.6%) patients with Maffucci's syndrome while Strang and Rannie[47] found chondrosarcomatous degeneration of the chondromas in 70 percent of patients with this disease. Johnson and associates[48] report a patient with Maffucci's syndrome who had two sarcomas removed but died from an unrelated adenocarcinoma of the pancreas.

The genetics of Maffucci's syndrome remain unclear. When hemangiomata are associated with osteochrondromatosis, also known as Ollier's disease, we refer to the entity as Maffucci's syndrome. However, neither condition appears to behave genetically in a Mendelian manner. Anderson[49] and Andren, *et al.*[50] discuss a possible familial etiology for this disease.

Porokeratosis

At least three known varieties of porokeratosis have been classified as follows:

1. Mibelli type which is a chronic, progressive disorder of keratinization consisting of annular or gyrate plaques with sharply hyperkeratotic elevated borders. These may occur anywhere on the body with onset at an early age. This type is known as the classic porokeratosis of Mibelli which he described in 1893 and which is discussed by Guss, *et al.*[51]

2. A second type of porokeratosis was described by Chernosky in 1966.[52] This type of porokeratosis occurs in older persons and is a disseminated superficial actinic porokeratosis (DSAP). These lesions differ from the Mibelli type in that they are more superficial and occur on sun-exposed areas of the skin.

3. Finally, Guss, *et al.*[51] have described a third variety of porokeratosis which appears to differ from the first two because of its distinctive distribution: porokeratosis plantaris, palmaris, et disseminata (PPPD).

It is of interest that all three varieties of porokeratosis are inherited as an autosomal dominant. A review of the literature[51] has disclosed two patients with squamous cell carcinomas arising in areas of porokeratosis of Mibelli[53,54] and the propositus in the report by Guss, *et al.*[51] had two squamous cell carcinomas arising from areas of porokeratosis. Guss *et al.*[51] concluded that the occurrence of skin cancer in patients with porokeratosis is probably not coincidental though they believe that more statistical evidence will be necessary to definitely call this a precancerous lesion.

Albinism

Albinism is a genetically determined biochemical defect which results in a partial or a total absence of pigmentation primarily in the skin, hair, and eyes. The skin of patients with albinism has a tendency to age prematurely with such findings as actinic chelitis, telangiectasia, keratosis, and cancer, particularly squamous carcinoma. The skin in this disease has been compared with that found in xeroderma pigmentosum.[55,56]

Albinism was formerly considered as a single clinical entity inherited in an autosomal recessive manner.[56] Several phenotypic varieties of albinism are believed to be the result of different gene mutations. At least two distinct types are: 1) tyrosinase positive albinism which is observed in the San Blas "moon children" and 2) tyrosinase negative albinism.[57,58] Several other rare types of albinism are also associated with a variety of clinical abnormalities.

Patients with albinism are susceptible to skin cancer, including an amelanotic type of malignant melanoma,[59] as well as to basal and squamous cell carcinomas.

Vitiligo and Gastric Carcinoma

Inexplicably, vitiligo has been shown to occur with an increased frequency in patients with pernicious anemia and with gastric carcinoma.[60,61] The implications of this phenomenon are unclear and merit additional study. This finding must be evaluated in the light of existing data showing familial aggregations of gastric carcinoma[62-64] and the occurrence of achlorhydria, gastric carcinoma, and pernicious anemia among relatives of gastric cancer probands.[65]

Xeroderma Pigmentosum*

Xeroderma pigmentosum (XDP) is an exceedingly rare and chronically progressive multisystem disease. It is inherited as an autosomal recessive. The principle target is the skin, and the manifestations are dependent on age and environment. Pathologic changes at this site vary accordingly, but include disturbances of pigmentation and maturation of epidermal cells, leading eventually to the formation of malignant skin tumors, usually basal and squamous cell carcinomas.[66] Malignant melanoma appears to have a frequent association with this disease.[67] Neurologic manifestations may include speech disturbances, mental deficiency, and convulsive disorders.[68] Ocular manifestations may include photophobia, conjunctivitis, keratitis, blepharitis, ectropion, and basal and squamous cell carcinomas.[69] Endocrinologic aberrations have been reported, including aminoaciduria, prolonged erythrocyte glucose-6 phosphate dehydrog-

---

*Portions of this material on xeroderma pigmentosum are reprinted by permission of *Archives of Dermatology* from H.T. Lynch, *et al.*, 96:625–635, (1967).

enase (G-6-PD) activity with suggestion of erythrocyte glutathione deficiency, and possible pituitary adrenal abnormalities.[70] Congenital anomalies, including short stature, microcephaly, and joint abnormalities have been reported also.[71]

Occasionally, two or more hereditary diseases may occur in the same family. Such occurrences provide a unique opportunity to study the interactions of the particular diseases in a common constitutional and environmental milieu. We shall present a detailed clinicogenetic and pathologic study of a family with XDP, congenital ichthyosis, and malignant melanoma.

Family Study

The proband, a 17-year-old white boy, had previous histologically confirmed diagnoses of XDP and malignant melanoma. He was admitted to the University of Texas, M.D. Anderson Hospital and Tumor Institute where detailed medical and genetic studies were performed.[69]

Because of a history of other similarly affected siblings, a *field trip* was made to the patient's home, approximately 1,200 miles away, after his hospital discharge. Participants in the field trip included an internist, a dermatologist, and a geneticist. Complete physical examinations were performed on the six siblings of the patient, his mother, and his father. Skin biopsies were done on each individual except the oldest brother.

Results

The proband was a 17-year-old white boy (Figs. 21–4 and 21–5, II-4) whose birth and gestational history were normal. Lentigines and areas of pigmentation were visible over the entire integument by 4 to 5 months of age. The skin was extremely dry with scaling,

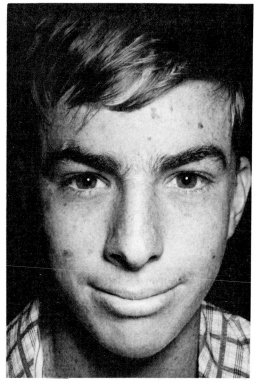

Figure 21–4. Proband with xeroderma pigmentosum. Note increased pigmentation of the face (Fig. 21–5, II-4).

accentuated during the winter months. At 7 years of age, a diagnosis of XDP was made, and at the same time the disease was recognized in an older sister. After this, the patient as well as his other affected siblings were assiduously protected from exposure to solar radiation. At age 13, a dark mole which proved to be malignant melanoma was excised from the right cervical triangle. The following year a basal cell carcinoma was removed from the right supraorbital region. When the patient was 17, a metastatic malignant melanoma was excised from the volar surface of the right arm. The remainder of the medical history was unremarkable. Physical examination revealed an alert well-developed boy. Vital signs were normal.

Results of examination of the head and neck, heart, lungs, abdomen, and neurologic system were within normal limits. The only abnormalities on physical examination were confined to the integument. This showed obvious XDP of moderate severity. The skin of the exposed areas was only slightly more freckled and pigmented than the unexposed areas of skin. The scalp was almost as hyperpigmented and freckled as the face. Freckling of the upper eyelids and dorsum of the feet was noteworthy. Only a few moles (nevus cell nevi) were observed. An unexpected finding was ichthyosis. This was characterized by generalized dryness, scaling of the scalp, face, diffusely hyperkeratotic soles and palms, and horizontally hyperkeratotic folds or ridges of skin over the knees, elbows, and achilles tendon areas. The skin of the legs, especially the pretibial site, was dry, fissured, and resembled fish skin.

Histologically, biopsies from these areas exhibited features of both ichthyosis and XDP. Those of ichthyosis included an absent granular cell layer, keratin layer which was slightly thickened, more dense and homogenous than normal, keratin plugging of hair follicles and eccrine sweat pores. A few scattered parakeratotic foci were encountered. In addition to the features of ichthyosis, the epidermis also exhibited irregular patches of melanin pigmentation, some represented by areas of lentigo, others by increased numbers of melanocytes and melanin pigment in relatively flat epidermis, and others simply by an increase of melanin pigment in cells of the basal and lower malpighian layers without an increase in the number of melanocytes. Focal areas of the nonpigmented epidermis demonstrated abnormal progression of maturation of epidermal cells. In some of these, the cells of the basal and lower malpighian layers were tall, compressed and cylindrical, extending to the upper malpighian layers. In other areas, the cells were arranged more disorderly as in early solar keratoses. These features are consistent with those of XDP.

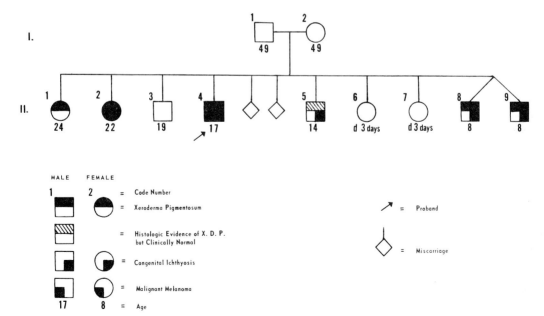

Figure 21–5. Pedigree of family with xeroderma pigmentosum, congenital ichthyosis and malignant melanoma.

The proband's mother was 49 years old (Fig. 21–5, I-2). She admitted she had "dryness of the skin" since age 16, for which she has constantly used lotions and salves. She had symptoms suggestive of tension headache intermittently which began at age 18. She developed a peptic ulcer at age 49 which responded well to medical management. Hypertension of unknown etiology had been controlled medically for several years. Details of the hypertension management were not available. She was put on estrogen therapy at age 49 because of menopausal symptoms. She had had ten pregnancies, two of which terminated in abortion at less than three months' gestation. Two girls died at 3 days (Fig. 21–5, II-6 and II-7). Details on the cause of these deaths were lacking. The remainder of the medical history was unremarkable.

Physical examination revealed a healthy appearing, slightly obese, white woman. Her blood pressure was 160/90 mm mercury (Hg). Examination of the head, neck, breasts, heart, lungs, abdomen, and neurologic system showed normal findings. The skin was universally dry, especially in the pretibial areas and the extensor surfaces of the arms. There was no evidence of XDP. She was not related to her husband.

A skin biopsy from the inner surface of the right upper arm revealed a normal granular cell layer with an overlying normal layer of keratin. There was suggestion of plugging of the eccrine sweat pores and hair follicles, but this was of minimal degree. The epidermis was of uniform thickness. Melanin pigment was evenly distributed through the basal layers of the epidermis, and there was normal progression of maturation of epidermal cells. Diagnostic evidence of either ichthyosis or XDP was lacking, though the slight poral and follicular plugging could possibly be of significance.

The father of the proband is 49 years old (Fig. 21–5, I-1). His growth and development were normal. There was no history of skin disease. He contracted malaria during World War II but had had no recurrence of this disease. He had a perforated duodenal ulcer at age 20 which responded to limited surgical repair. At age 48, he had a venous thrombosis of the right leg and this subsequently was diagnosed as polycythemia. He underwent a splenectomy in 1966, but we have been unable to establish the reasons for splenectomy.

On physical examination, the patient appeared to be healthy though mildly overweight. There were no external manifestations of polycythemia. Examination of the skin showed no evidence of ichthyosis or XDP. Approximately 30 moles were present on his body. Most were intradermal nevi, but two were pigmented macular junctional nevi on the left sole.

A biopsy of the skin of the left arm showed no significant histopathological changes.

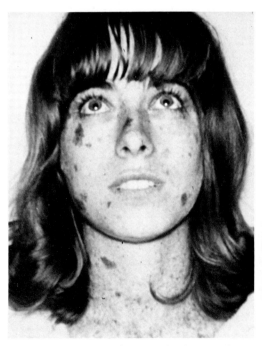

Figure 21–6. Sister of proband with xeroderma pigmentosum (Fig. 21–5, II-1).

There was normal progression of maturation of epidermal cells and normal granular cell and keratin layers. Melanin pigment was evenly distributed through the basal layers.

The oldest sister of the proband is 24 years old (Figs. 21–5 and 21–6, II-1). She was born prematurely at 7 months. Development was normal though her growth rate was slightly retarded. She has had recurrent sinusitis since age 12. Menarche occurred at age 15. She had mild dysmenorrhea through age 22. A diagnosis of XDP was established at age 14. Since then, approximately 20 basal and squamous cell carcinomas have been removed from exposed areas of her body. An active atypical junction nevus was removed in 1957 from an unstated skin site. She has been continually protected from ultraviolet ray exposure since age 14. The remainder of the history was noncontributory.

The physical examination revealed a woman of small stature (5 feet tall) and generally underdeveloped. Vital signs were normal. Complete physical examination results, except for the integument, were normal. Slowly progressive XDP of only a moderate degree of severity was found. There was relatively little difference in the degree of hyperpigmentation and freckling between exposed and unexposed areas of the skin. A striking feature was the presence of giant-sized freckles or lentigines of the face. These were not observed in other affected family members. A careful search was required to detect a slight amount of facial telangiectasia. The surfaces of the extremities were slightly dry without evidence of ichthyosis. Two small nonpigmented papules were detected in the right inner canthus. Clinically these appeared to be keratoses or early basal cell carcinomas. Telangiectasia was present on the lateral portion of the bulbar conjunctivae. A small pigmented macule was observed at the junction of the corea and temporal portion of the left bulbar conjunctiva. The hyperpigmenta-

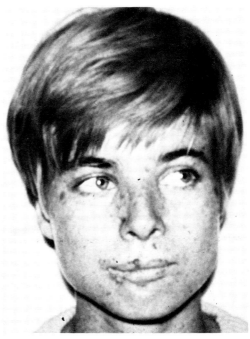

Figure 21–7. Sister of proband showing signs of xeroderma pigmentosum (Fig. 21–5, II-2).

tion in this patient interfered with the detection of moles, but a careful search revealed nevus cell nevi to be scarce.

Biopsy of a small skin lesion on the nose revealed basal cell carcinoma. Of equal interest was the epidermis in the same specimen lateral to this tumor. It demonstrated marked dyskeratosis, accompanied in foci by acantholysis, as observed in some solar keratoses. Melanin pigment was irregularly distributed in areas associated with lentigo. The granular cell layer was present. No changes were present which suggested ichthyosis. A second biopsy from the skin of the leg was also free of ichthyosis, possessing normal granular cell and normal keratin layers. The feature of note was the irregular distribution of melanin pigment in areas associated with a lentigo pattern. Dyskeratosis, while suggested, was not as noticeable as in the exposed skin of the nose. In summary, histologic features consistent with XDP were present, while those of ichthyosis were lacking.

The next oldest sister of the proband is 22 years old (Figs. 21–5, II-2 and 21–7). Gestation, birth, growth, and development were normal. At age 12, this girl was the first member of the family to receive a diagnosis of XDP. However, freckling and areas of pigmentation had been present over her body since infancy. At least 25 basal and squamous cell carcinomas, including a malignant melanoma excised from the integument, since the patient was 12 years old. Melanoma recurred in her thigh several years later and then spontaneously resolved. Menarche occurred at age 13. She has had recent dysmenorrhea. The remainder of the history was unremarkable.

Physical examination of the patient revealed normal vital signs; she was apprehensive and anxious, with emotional lability. Pigmentation was present over the entire body with relatively little difference between exposed and unexposed areas. The upper eyelids were pigmented and freckled. Mild telangiectasia was present over the center of the face. Prominent lentigines were noted over the head and neck, and the lips were freckled. Several small pigmented hyperkeratotic papules were observed over the malar areas and canthi. A scar caused by irradiation of a carcinoma of the right lower lip was noted. The lateral portion of the bulbar conjunctiva had numerous telangiectatic vessels bilaterally. Some atrophy and thinning of the tissues of the nose were present, probably accentuated by prior management of tumors of both alae. The appearance of the facial skin suggested a moderately severe, slowly progressively XDP, but with an increased frequency of cancers and precancerous lesions over the central facial areas. A moderate degree of ichthyosis, characterized by generalized dryness and scaly fishlike skin, was found on the legs and

extensors of the arms. The palms were dry, thickened, and hyperkeratotic.

A representative area of the skin of the leg was biopsied. The granular cell layer proved to be absent and the overlying keratin layer was less flaky and more dense than normal, similar to that observed in the skin of the proband. Keratin plugging of eccrine sweat pores and hair follicles was prominent. The epidermis was irregular, partly as a result of widespread lentigo and cellular nests of junction nevus cells. Melanin pigment distribution was irregular and patchy. Dyskeratotic changes, slight to moderate in degree, were present in the nonpigmented epidermis. These changes illustrate remarkably well the coexisting features of both ichthyosis and XDP.

A 19-year-old brother of the proband (Fig. 21–5, II-3) was delivered at 7 months' gestation without complications. Growth and development were normal. He has never manifested any freckling, increased pigmentation, or dryness of the skin. The remainder of the medical history was unremarkable.

Physical examination revealed a normally developed white boy. Results of the entire physical examination including the skin, were normal, except for the finding of several nevus cell nevi. A skin biopsy was not performed.

A 14-year-old brother of the proband (Fig. 21–8, II-5) was delivered normally, despite the fact that his mother had possible eclampsia at 8½ months' gestation. Growth and development were normal. However, he had a lifelong history of dryness and scaliness of the skin, accentuated in the winter months. The remainder of the medical history was unremarkable.

Physical findings were entirely normal except for the skin. Generalized dryness of the skin was found, including the scalp and face. The palms and soles were slightly thickened and keratosis pilaris of the extensor surfaces

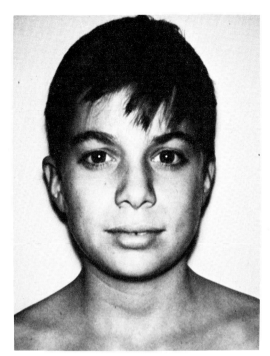

Figure 21–8. Brother of the proband with ichthyosis but no clinical findings consistent with xeroderma pigmentosum (Fig. 21–5, II-5).

of the extremities was present. The skin over the elbows, knees, and Achilles tendons was dry and hyperkeratotic with veruccose folds. Fishskin appearance so characteristic of ichthyosis was prominent over the pretibial sites.

The exposed skin was similar to the unexposed skin and showed no evidence of abnormal sunlight damage. Approximately 12 pigmented nevi were present over the body with a predominance of the junctional type. The only clinical diagnosis in this patient was moderately severe ichthyosis.

Skin biopsies from an arm and a leg presented similar histologic features. In each, the granular cell layer of the epidermis was absent, and the overlying keratin layer, while not noticeably thickened, was more dense and homogeneous than normal. Plugging of eccrine sweat pores and follicles was prominent. Though clinically the patient did not present changes of XDP, slight irregularity and patchiness of melanin pigmentation was noted. This finding, together with the slight focal disorderly arrangement of cells, raises the question of a subclinical degree of XDP.

Eight-year-old brothers of the proband, believed to be identical twins (Figs. 21–5 and 21–9, II-8 and II-9) were born prematurely at 7 months' gestation. Subsequent blood type studies indicated them to be identical for 17 antisera. Deliveries were uncomplicated though the mother had considerable spotting throughout the pregnancy. Growth and development were normal for both children. Both showed freckling and pigmentation of the entire itegument shortly after birth. Both were protected from the sun. To date, no skin cancers have developed. The remainder of the history was noncontributory.

Physical examination showed these boys to be virtually identical in appearance. Both were above average in intelligence. Except for the findings in the skin, physical findings were normal. A mild, slowly progressive XDP was readily recognizable in each child. It was characterized by freckling and hyperpigmentation, particularly on exposed sites. If the pigmentation follows the patterns of the older brother and sisters, the difference between exposed and unexposed sites will probably diminish with time. Slight telangiectasia of the bulbar conjunctiva was present. Both manifested generalized dryness of the skin with a mild ichthyosis of the extensor surfaces of the arms, which was most noticeable on the pretibial areas. One twin had keratosis pilaris of the arms and legs. Relatively few nevus cell nevi were present. The second twin had a hard subcutaneous iceberg-shaped mass of the left malar area which had been present, although asymptomatic, for approximately one year.

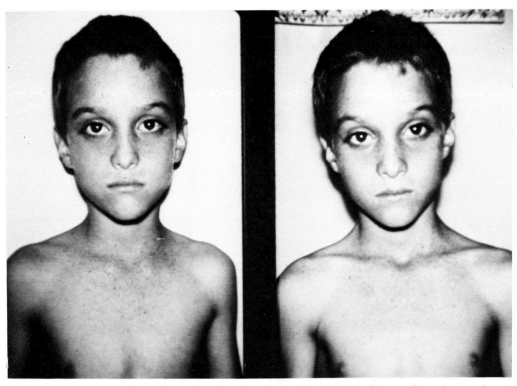

Figure 21–9. Identical twin brothers of proband, each showing clinical evidence of xeroderma pigmentosum (Fig. 21–5, II-8, II-9).

Representative skin from the legs of each of the 8-year-old twins was biopsied. Histologically, the features in each were virtually identical to those of the preceding patients, although they differed with regard to ichthyosis in certain respects. The more pronounced changes were those related to XDP and consisted of irregular melanin pigmentation of the epidermis in areas in the form of lentigo and focal disorderly arrangement of the deeper epidermal cells. These changes coincided with the clinical observations and diagnosis of XDP. The difference histologically from the preceding patients with ichthyosis was the presence of the granular cell layer, though focally diminished, and an overlying essentially normal flaky keratin layer in both twins. However, keratin which plugged hair follicles was relatively promi-

nent. Some plugging of eccrine sweat pores was also present. These findings coincide with the clinical description of each having "mild ichthyosis" and one clinically having keratosis pilaris of the arms and legs. Thus, histologically, features of both diseases were present, though those of ichthyosis were less clear.

Comment

The family presented here is interesting from the standpoint of the occurrence of XDP in five of seven siblings. In addition, four of these five also showed congenital ichthyosis, and two of these had a further and more grave complication, namely, malignant melanoma. One sibling manifested XDP and no ichthyosis and another sibling, while completely free of XDP, clinically presented with a classical and moderately severe form of congenital ichthyosis. This patient histologically, however, presents changes which though minimal were albeit consistent with early changes of XDP. Thus, it appears that in this family we are dealing with two inherited diseases, XDP and congenital ichthyosis. The XDP appears to be behaving as an autosomal recessive factor, while the inheritance of congenital ichthyosis is not clear. A dominant factor with reduced penetrance of the gene cannot be excluded. Note that the mother had dryness of her skin, though histologic evidence for ichthyosis was lacking.

Congenital ichthyosis in association with XDP so far as we can determine, is rare. A literature review has revealed only one authenticated report of this association, namely that of Couillaud[71] in 1898. In addition, a survey of dermatologists from several large institutions revealed that none had ever observed this association. Thus, the association in this family can be most reasonably explained in terms of fortuitous association of two hereditary diseases. It is hoped that other investigators will search carefully for this occurrence in both affected as well as unaffected relatives of probands with XDP.

Congenital ichthyosis has been described previously in association with other genetic disorders. Lynch, *et al.*[72] described congenital ichthyosis in association with secondary male hypogonadism in a family where this combination was present in three members (and two additional members by history) through three generations. A sex-linked mode of inheritance was advanced for this occurrence. Congenital ichthyosis is also an essential component in the syndrome of Rüd.[73] However, etiologic significance of these associations remains unclear.

The occurrence of malignant melanoma in two of the individuals in this family prompted us to make an extensive review of the association of this lesion with XDP. There are a large number of reports documenting this association.[71,74,91] Moore and Iverson[89] summarized 360 cases of XDP which had been reported up to 1959 and estimated that melanoma was an associated finding in 3 percent of these. The present family, with two instances of malignant melanoma among five patients with XDP, provides additional support that these two cutaneous conditions may be associated more frequently than has heretofore been suspected. We emphasize this point because malignant melanoma is rarely considered to be a threat to patients with XDP, with which, generally, basal and squamous cell carcinomas are most frequently associated. From the available data on XDP, malignant melanoma appears to be another manifestation of this severe recessively inherited skin cancer diathesis. When malignant melanoma occurs in families, it usually behaves as an autosomal dominant.[92] The problems of malignant melanoma will be considered below.

Malignant melanoma in XDP may show a peculiarly benign course with frequent spontaneous resolution. Note that the two patients with melanoma and XDP in this family each had metastases from melanoma and each subsequently had a complete remission. I have heard of similar examples of melanoma undergoing spontaneous resolution in XDP patients. These are unpublished accounts from clinical colleagues and are considered by me to be reliable.

Cells from differing tissues of patients with XDP repair ultraviolet-induced deoxyribonucleic acid (DNA) damage slowly (see Dr. Cleaver's discussion in Chapter 8). Cell fusion studies have shown that genetic complementation can occur between fibroblasts from certain pairs of patients and thereby overcome the DNA-repair defect in each member of the pair. This observation suggests heterogeneity of the genetic lesion. Investigations at the NIH on patients with

XDP showing slow DNA repair were found to comprise four distinct complementation groups suggesting that at least four mutations can cause defective DNA repair.[92a]

Finally, there is an additional syndrome involving XDP, with associated neurological complications, known as the de Sanctis-Cacchione syndrome. The cardinal features of the syndrome include xeroderma pigmentosum, microcephaly, mental deficiency, dwarfism, and gonadal hypoplasia. The disorder is inherited as an autosomal recessive.[1]

Cutaneous Malignant Melanoma (CMM)

Malignant melanoma is one of the most poorly understood and perplexing cancers affecting man. The disease shows protean manifestations with frequently erratic behavior which undoubtedly gives rise to the manifold problems in its diagnosis and management.[93] This disease was described by Hippocrates who was the first to recognize its malignant potential. Many writers through the years have referred to the lesion as "fatal black tumor," or "black tumor death," terms describing the discoloration of tissues which may arise from generalized metastasis from this disease.

Approximately 1.3 percent of all cancers are melanomas and about 65 percent of these are believed to arise from pre-existing nevi while congenital moles account for 27 percent of these nevi.[94] Melanomas may arise in multiple sites in any given single nevus, they may arise in multiple areas of the body, or they may occur where no nevi are present. Of those melanomas arising in pre-existing nevi the majority occur at trauma areas such as the palms and the soles of the feet. The tumor has a predilection for fair skinned people, being relatively rare in Negroes; and when it does occur in Negroes, it is often found in nonpigmented areas of their bodies. The most common sites of predilection for melanomas are the head and neck, lower extremities, followed by the trunk.[95] Melanomas have also been described as arising in the gall bladder, esophagus, meninges, vagina, upper respiratory tract, and anorectum.[93] Intraocular melanoma, usually arising in the choroid, is also a frequent site for this disease[96] (See Chap. 23).

There appear to be hormonal associations with melanoma in that the male-female incidence increases with age beyond maturity wherein there is a six-fold increased incidence for men in the third decade of life as opposed to the first decade. There is a secondary peak of incidence in post-menopausal women.[93] Sites of predilection for melanoma also appear to be sex-related in that lesions involving the head and neck occur in men 24 percent of the time as opposed to only 9 percent in women; women show involvement of the extremities 58 percent of the time while in men it is only 25 percent.[97] Survival figures also support hormonal implications in that in pre-menopausal women survival is superior to the survival of men of comparable age groups.

Of all malignant neoplasms affecting the skin of man malignant melanoma is the most serious histologic variety accounting for the greatest number of *dermatologic deaths*. For example, in the United States in 1965, approximately 2,687 individuals died from malignant melanoma. This figure accounted for approximately 27 percent of all patients who died following a dermatologic diagnosis.[98] It is, therefore, no small wonder that heavily pigmented or black lesions of the skin arouse anxiety in physicians and frequently among patients. However, only about 2 percent of all black lesions of the skin are actually malignant melanomas; thus 98 percent, or the overwhelming majority of black lesions of the skin are not malignant melanomas and are, therefore, *not* a threat to the patient's life and well being.[1] However, a difficult problem for patient and physician alike is that of differentiating between those lesions which are benign and those which are either frank melanomas or are destined to become melanomas. Unfortunately, the establishment of a diagnosis of a benign skin lesion versus melanoma by inspection of the skin may be extremely difficult and indeed is often impossible. Competent dermatologists who have had experience and considerable interest in the diagnosis of malignant melanoma may have similar difficulties with the differential diagnosis and may err in 35 to 40 percent of the cases seen clinically. This fact of course dictates the absolute necessity for histopathologic confirmation in order to make a correct diagnosis of black cutaneous growths on the skin.

It is important to realize that many physicians have taken a pessimistic view concerning the prognosis of malignant melanoma. However, with *early* diagnosis and the benefit of skillfully directed therapy, patients with localized disease in the absence of metastatic spread to the lymphnodes, will have a 5 year survival rate of 70 percent and a 10 year survival rate as high as 60 percent. Hence, we should not adopt a hopeless atitude once the diagnosis of malignant melanoma has been established. This not only discourages attempts at successful therapy but also adds to the already severely fatalistic impression about cancer held by many patients.[1]

Family Study†

Four families with malignant melanoma were referred by physicians who were aware of our interest in cancer genetics. In the first two families medical genetic information

†This material is republished by permission of the *Canadian Medical Association Journal* from H.T. Lynch and A.J. Krush, "Heredity and Malignant Melanoma: Implications for Early Cancer Detection, *Canadian Medical Association Journal*, 99:17–21, 1968.

was obtained from probands and their relatives, physicians, hospitals and departments of vital statistics. Verification of the histological diagnosis of malignant neoplasms was obtained whenever possible. The latter two families were referred by an ophthalmologist. Unfortunately, cooperation from these latter two families was restricted to the patients described below.

Results

Family 1

In the first family (Fig. 21–10 and Table 21-VI) CMM was histologically confirmed in the proband (Fig. 21–10, II-4), her sister (Fig. 21–10, II-2) and her son (Fig. 21–10, III-1). Thus, this disease was confirmed in three members of the family in two generations. One patient (Fig. 21–10, III-1) had five primary CMM's histologically verified during a period of six years. Excision of his most recent lesion occurred when the cancer was detected during his visit to us as a result of his concern about the disease in his family

TABLE 21-VI
TUMOR REGISTRY OF FAMILY WITH
CUTANEOUS MALIGNANT MELANOMA
(Family 1)

Pedigree Number (Fig.)	Sex	Age	Malignant Melanoma	Cancer of Other Sites
I-1	F	d67	——	Pancreas
I-2	M	d66		Pancreas
I-3	F	d71		Cervix
I-4	F	d46		Breast, sarcoma fight ilium
II-1	F	42		
II-2	F	54	+	
II-4	↗F	51	+	
II-5	F	50		
III-1	M	26	+ + + + +	
III-3	F	24		
III-4	F	18		
III-5	M	10		

↗ = Proband.
+ = Histologically confirmed.
—— = Medical history only.

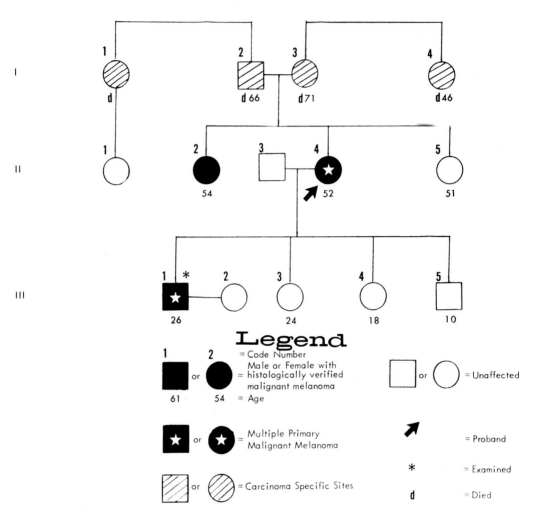

Figure 21–10. Family with malignant melanoma present in two generations. Note occurrence of multiple primary malignant melanoma in a mother and her son.

and his desire to cooperate with us to increase knowledge about its genetic aspects. Of interest is the incidence of other histologic varieties of malignant neoplasms in this family (Table 21-VI), and particularly the occurrence of histologically verified adenocarcinoma of the pancreas in the proband's father and the father's sister (Table 21-VI and Fig. 21–10, I-2 and I-1).

Family 2

In the second family (Fig. 21–11 and Table 21-VII) CMM was histologically confirmed in the proband (Fig. 21–11, II-5), her aunt (Fig. 21–11, II-10) and her first cousin (Fig. 21–11, III-1). It was presented by history in the proband's paternal grandfather (Fig. 21–11, I-6) and two uncles

(Fig. 21–11, II-2 and II-4). Thus CMM was histologically confirmed in three members in two generations and present by history in a third generation. An increased incidence of cancer of the respiratory tract occurred in other relatives. In addition, an aunt of the proband (Fig. 21–11, II-10) had adenocarcinoma of the breast six years before diagnosis of CMM; thus there were two distinct primary cancers.

Family 3

In the third family a 61-year-old woman (Fig. 21–12, II-1) had a diagnosis of intra-ocular melanoma (IMM) (histologically confirmed) while her sister, aged 51 (Fig. 21–12, II-2) had a diagnosis of CMM (histologically confirmed).

Family 4

In the fourth family a 74-year-old man (Fig. 21–12, I-1) had a diagnosis of IMM (histologically confirmed) and his son, aged 44 (Fig. 21–12, II-1), had a diagnosis of CMM (histologically confirmed).

There was no evidence of consanguinity in these four families.

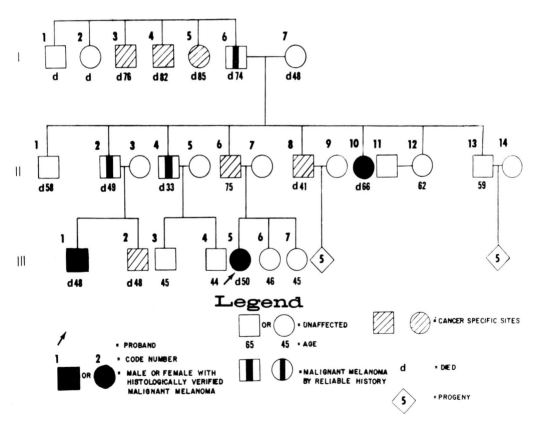

Figure 21–11. Malignant melanoma histologically verified in two generations and present by reliable history in a third generation.

TABLE 21-VII
TUMOR REGISTRY OF FAMILY WITH
CUTANEOUS MALIGNANT MELANOMA
(Family 2)

Pedigree Number (Fig.)	Sex	Age	Malignant Melanoma	Cancer of Other Sites
I-3	M	d76		Unknown site
I-4	M	d82		"Throat Cancer"
I-5	F	d85		Unknown Site
I-6	M	d74	——	
II-2	M	d46	——	
II-4	M	d33	——	
II-6	M	75		Larynx
II-8	M	d41		Lung
II-10	F	d66	+	Breast (age 60)
III-1	M	d48	+	
III-2	M	d48		Lung
III-5	⤢F	d50	+	

⤢ = Proband.
+ = Histologically confirmed.
—— = Medical history only.

Comment

The hereditary aspects of malignant melanoma have only recently received attention in the medical literature. The first familial recording of CMM was that of Cawley,[99] who in 1952 described the disease in a father and two of his three children. Since this report, other investigators have confirmed the existence of a hereditary etiology for this disease in certain families.[92,100-106] Onset at an early age and multiple primary malignant melanomas have characterized the hereditary variety of this disease. The frequency of the hereditary form of malignant melanoma in the general population is unknown. The estimate of approximately 3 percent given by Anderson, Smith and McBride[92] was considered to be an underestimation of the true incidence.[1] In their search of the medical records of approximately 1000 patients with melanoma on file at the M.D. Anderson Hospital and Tumour Institute, they found 28 patients with a family history of malignant melanoma. However, they failed to verify the family histories of the remaining patients since they relied solely upon

statistics supplied by the Department of Epidemiology at that institution.[107] These statistics were based upon family histories from the medical records, which in our experience are often notoriously incomplete. We, therefore, believe that in order to obtain a valid estimate of the frequency of any genetic disease, it is mandatory that hearsay family history be verified.

Possibly a more valid estimate of the frequency of hereditary factors in malignant melanoma is that provided by Wallace and Associates.[108] Specifically, these investigators studied 113 family histories from a total of 125 consecutive cases of malignant melanoma from Brisbane, Australia, and surrounding areas which included the evaluation of 923 first degree relatives. Findings showed a heritability of liability to malignant melanoma of approximately 11 percent. Heritability is a measure of the familial component of liability to a disease and this is readily estimated by a comparison of incidences between first degree relatives of propositi and a control population. Evidence derived from this approach to the problem, suggested that the hereditary factor in malignant melanoma is polygenic in nature. However, the authors freely admit that it may be impossible to distinguish between polygenic inheritance and dominant inheritance with incomplete penetrance because the distinction between the two is a matter of degree rather than of class.[108] However, there were certain features of polygenic inheritance which they considered to be distinctive; these included an increased risk to other relatives if there were more than one in the family with the condition and a tendency for the propositi of the families in which multiple cases occurred to show more extreme forms of the disease. In the case of the severe forms of malignant melanoma, these included early age at onset and the occurrence of more than one primary lesion. Thus, among 68 first degree relatives of the families

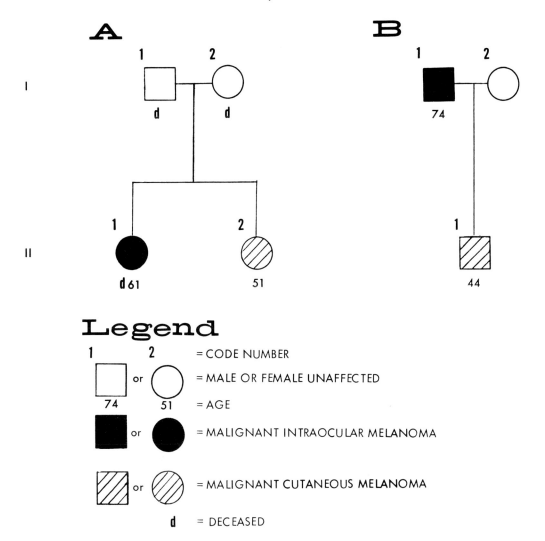

Figure 21–12. Two families showing intra-ocular melanoma and cutaneous malignant melanoma.

with two cases of melanoma, there were three further cases of malignant melanoma, which was four times the expected incidence calculated from the entire data concerning first degree relatives. Similarly, of the 19 cases in that selected group, three had more than one primary lesion, one man having no less than seven histologically proven primary malignant neoplasms. In addition, the affected propositi and their relatives were also younger than would have been expected. Unfortunately, the authors did not report the frequency of associated malignant neoplasms of differing histologic varieties in their sample population.

In analyzing the pedigrees of families with CMM, autosomal dominance is apparent but it is complex, one explanation being reduced penetrance of the gene. It is also possible that more than one gene is involved.[92]

It is of interest that none of the reported genetic studies of CMM included patients with IMM.

Patients with the genetic variety of CMM appear to have a significantly *higher* survival rate than patients manifesting nonfamilial melanoma.[108a] The explanation of this unusual phenomenon is unknown.

IMM has shown a hereditary etiology in some families.[109-112,114,115] Lynch, Anderson and Krush[116] reviewed this work and presented two families in whom the lesion was histologically confirmed in a brother and in the second family it was histologically confirmed in his son and in his granddaughter. The frequency of the hereditary variety of IMM could not be estimated from these studies. However, the rarity of such cases in review of medical reports and the world literature indicates that its familial occurrence is, in fact, infrequent. Overall genetic findings from these families and from those in the literature suggest autosomal dominant inheritance with reduced penetrance of the gene. For further details about intra-ocular melanoma please refer to Chapter 23.

Malignant melanoma may also occur in association with other hereditary diseases, including xeroderma pigmentosum as already mentioned;[117] a review of the world literature showed that malignant melanoma also has a significantly increased association with von Recklinghausen's neurofibromatosis, an autosomal dominantly inherited disorder.[118]

The findings of CMM in Families 1 and 2 reported here are consistent with autosomal dominant inheritance. An interesting observation in both families was the prevalence of malignant neoplasms of differing anatomic sites. Of particular interest was the finding of adenocarcinoma of the pancreas histologically confirmed in siblings (brother and sister) in Family 1 and an increased incidence of carcinoma of the respiratory tract in Family 2. Heretofore, investigations of the familial form of malignant melanoma have failed to record data on the occurrence of other malignant neoplasms in the families. Insight into the inheritance of cancer in man will be increased by meticulous reporting of all varieties of cancer in the particular families under study. In the case of hereditary malignant melanoma, we may ultimately find that there is a specific predilection to this disease, possibly associated with a predisposition to other histologic varieties of cancer. This could be of practical importance in genetic counselling and cancer detection.

A unique finding in the present investigation was the independent occurrence of IMM and CMM in two sisters in Family 3 and in a father and son in Family 4. These families were not related to each other. Additional observations of these types of problems could increase our understanding of inheritance factors in malignant melanoma since CMM and IMM were previously thought to be inherited independently of each other.[119] It is of course possible that the occurrence of both CMM and IMM in these two families was fortuitous.

Implications for Cancer Detection

When malignant melanoma is found in a patient, its possible development in his relatives should be considered. All nevi in relatives at risk should be examined periodically and lesions showing suspicious changes should be biopsied. However, this must be achieved without unduly alarming the family, since provoking apprehension and anxiety could paradoxically cause them to repress the entire issue. This may be one of the most difficult problems encountered in the management of individuals at high genetic risk for cancer.

An unusual opportunity is at hand for cancer control in families with CMM, since this lesion will often be apparent to the patient early in its clinical course. One obvious dilemma, however, concerns how many and which nevi should be biopsied in an individual at high genetic risk for CMM. Unfortunately, no single all-inclusive rule can be stated. At the present time clinical judgement must prevail. An example of such a problem appeared in the first family when the son of the proband advised us that his sister (Fig. 21–10, III-3) had a skin lesion which appeared to be similar to a malignant melanoma which he had recently had excised. She was reticent about seeing her physician and strongly repressed the issue of CMM in her family. When she finally consented to see a physician, biopsy of the lesion revealed a compound pigmented nevus with active junctional activity. Her physician wrote us as follows: "This is certainly a worrisome situation in view of the strong familial tendency for melanoma (in her family) and the fact that she has so many scattered nevi in areas of which we are generally suspicious. I think she should be watched closely and I have instructed her in the usual change to be looked for in moles . . . it is really a problem to determine which lesion to remove." Obviously all nevi on her body could not be removed. However, this physician took the opportunity to establish rapport with his patient and to provide her with a sound educational experience, carefully advising her of characteristic changes in nevi which might indicate malignancy, and urging periodic follow-up.

While some patients in a high cancer-risk category may elect to repress and deny early signs and symptoms of cancer,[120] others may over-react to the increased incidence of cancer in their family. For example, a patient in Family 2 was alarmed about a swift and fulminant course of CMM in his first cousin, a 49-year-old single woman who died from metastatic malignant melanoma three months after excision of a lesion. He explained that many members of the family had moles of varying sizes and shapes. He himself undergoes yearly medical examinations and has been told by his physician that he should see a doctor only if he discovers an alteration in a nevus. He wrote, "In my opinion, however, I suspect that this would already be too late, since the family members who had these spots removed all died within three months." How can such a patient be alerted to the necessity for a wholesome concern about nevi without promoting undue or unrealistic concern or even a hypochondriacal reaction? We do not have the answer to this question, but we believe that such reactions may be avoided through frank and candid discussions between patient and physician. We have been impressed with the intense and crippling fear engendered in patients by their erroneous impressions about cancer. The patient's knowledge of his increased genetic risk for cancer will not necessarily compel him to seek medical attention early for signs and symptoms of cancer. He may react with fear, guilt and anxiety to the point of becoming fatalistic. Such a reaction may be effectively counteracted through the development of a positive philosophy about the cancer problem instilled by the physician early in the patient's life and by emphasizing the cure potential through early diagnosis. On the other hand, a patient who is overly concerned about the cancer risk in his family may also harbor misconceptions and misinterpret signs and symptoms of cancer in his anxiety and fear of its development. This can lead to too frequent visits to the physician for minor symptoms.

In all instances the physician must accept his patient's attitude toward cancer in a sympathetic manner and be willing to take the necessary time not only to explain the significance of early signs and symptoms of malignant disease but also to help the patient gain insight into his feelings and attitudes about the cancer issue.

Porphyria Cutanea Tarda

According to Goldberg[121] the porphyrias can be classified conveniently into two main types, namely, *hepatic* and *erythropoietic*. This division is based upon the principal site of formation of the abnormal porphyrins and their precursors.[122] Hepatic porphyria may present as the acute intermittent variety (autosomal dominant) or as the cutaneous type (porphyria cutanea tarda), (rare examples of autosomal dominant inheritance). Our discussion will be restricted to porphyria cutanea tarda. In this condition an increased fecal excretion of coproporphyrin and protoporphyrin occurs during the course of the disease. During an attack, the urine may be colored orange or red and often contains large amounts of coproporphyrin and zinc-uroporphyrin.[70] Cutaneous manifestations include photosensitivity which is believed to be due to preformed porphyrins in the liver. The cardinal cutaneous features of this syndrome are "bullae, pigmentation, hypertrichosis, and sclerodermoid changes . . . crops of vesicles mixed with bullae up to 2.5 cm in size develop on the exposed part, usually the face, neck, and hands following exposure to sunlight, heat, or other types of local trauma."[70] The skin abrades easily and when healed may leave depigmented scars on exposed surfaces particularly the hands. During acute attacks, abdominal colic, motor paralysis, jaundice, and psychosis may occur similar to that found in acute intermittent porphyria. Barbiturates may precipitate an acute attack and should be avoided assiduously should the diagnosis of porphyria be considered.

Complications of this disease include hemachromatosis, diabetes mellitus, carcinoma of the liver[70] and basal cell carcinoma of the skin.[123]

Porphyria cutanea tarda is inherited as an autosomal dominant with incomplete penetrance.[70] However, more men than women are affected[124] which suggests the possibility of sex-influenced factors.

In a recent report by Waddington[125] a patient with a 10 year history of porphyria was found to have primary liver carcinoma. This case is important because in some cases liver cancer may be responsible for the manifestation of porphyria.

Fanconi's Anemia

Fanconi's anemia (FA)[1] is inherited as an autosomal recessive. Cytogenetic findings from cultured fibroblasts, lymphocytes, and bone marrow have revealed a high incidence of chromosomal structural aberrations including chromatid and isochromatid breaks, exchanges, and endoreduplications.[126,127]

The principal findings in Fanconi's anemia include pancytopenia, bone marrow hypoplasia, and congenital anomalies. The latter may include hypoplasia of the thumbs, absence of the radius, strabismus, microcephaly, microphthalmia, dwarfism, and hypogenitalism. In addition, patients often show a spotty or patchy brown pigmentation of the skin.[1] Indeed, the skin manifestations in some patients may appear similar to those found in patients with dyskeratosis congenita.[128] Some authors consider the conditions identical.[129] Family studies have revealed that relatives in at least one of these families have manifested features of both diseases, suggesting that they are genetically related.[130] The clinical picture is thought to be determined by the extent of mesodermal abnormalities (Franconi's syndrome) versus ectodermal manifestations (dyskeratosis congenita). Cytogenetic studies of patients with dyskeratosis congenita should add clarification to the classification of these disorders.

Cancer shows an increased occurrence in FA though existing data is insufficient for calculating meaningful incidence figures. The most frequently occurring malignant neoplasm in this disease is acute leukemia.[126,127] Interestingly, two of the patients described by Bloom and associates[126] died from acute monocytic leukemia six months and six years respectively after the original diagnosis of pancytopenia. Swift and Hirschhorn,[131] on the other hand, reported a 30-year-old woman with squamous cell carcinoma of the skin of the anus and carcinoma in situ (Bowen's disease) of the vulva.

Cancer, particularly leukemia, shows an increased frequency in presumptive heterozygote relatives of FA probands.[132] This is of particular interest in that cell cultures from obligate FA heterozygotes show an increased susceptibility to malignant transformation by the oncogenic virus SV40.[127] Homozygous (affected) patients show an even greater susceptibility to malignant transformation by SV40 oncogenic virus.

Finally, recent data by Swift and associates[133] have disclosed an apparent increased frequency of diabetes mellitus among relatives of FA probands, wherein some of these relatives would be expected to be heterozygous for the FA gene. These observations were made on the same eight families previously ascertained by Swift[132] for cancer association. There appeared to be a significantly greater risk of diabetes among female relatives in these families, though sampling problems may have accounted for this sex disparity. Thus, the authors suggested that any interpretation based on the association of diabetes and FA must be provisional and should be evaluated in additional FA families.

Dermatoglyphics

One of the objectives of genetic studies is to find biochemical or physical markers which might prove to be helpful in identifying individuals at risk for a specific trait or disease. Dermatoglyphics is an important discipline of which many physicians are unaware, but which is utilized frequently by geneticists in the study of a variety of disorders. Cancer has been no exception in the quest for identifying markers which might be present in the dermal ridges of the hands. This subject has been reviewed recently by Lynch.[1] For example, the simian crease and other dermatoglyphic abnormalities in the hands of children with Down's syndrome has been known for a relatively long period of time. In turn, a significant association with Down's syndrome and leukemia has been confirmed during the past decade.[134]

Studies of dermatoglyphics in leukemia in the absence of Down's syndrome have been controversial though more investigation in this area is obviously necessary.[135,136] For example, Verbov[137] has recently reviewed the subject and has presented findings from 110 patients with leukemia. In this group, he was able to discern dermatoglyphic patterns in males with leukemia which differed from those of a normal control group. Important findings included an increased frequency of finger whorls and a decreased frequency of ulnar loops in patients with acute leukemia. There was also an increased frequency of radial loops and a decreased frequency of arches in chronic leukemia, more particularly in patients with chronic lymphocytic leukemia. These findings are included because of recent interest in the genetics of leukemia,[138-140] and the fact that a variety of dermatologic lesions have been secondarily associated with these diseases.

Hereditary Multiple Benign Cystic Epitheliomas (Brooke-Fordyce Trichoepitheliomas, Epithelioma Adenoides Cysticum of Brooke)

Hereditary multiple benign cystic epithelioma, comprised of multiple tumors derived from hair follicles, is also described in the literature as Brooke's tumor, multiple trichoepithelioma, or epithelioma adenoides cysticum. These lesions are usually multiple and tend to localize predominantly on the skin of the paranasal areas. These lesions develop as small milia-like papules and they lack the significant characteristic changes in the overlying skin which occur in basal cell carcinomas or rodent ulcers. This disorder is inherited as an autosomal dominant.[141]

Malignant transformation to basal cell carcinoma occurs occasionally in this condition. However, the subject of malignant potential remains controversial, particularly because of the problem of determining whether cancer occurrence might be related to previous radiation treatment to the areas affected.[141,142]

Turban Tumors (Ancell-Spiegler Cylindromas)

This disorder is inherited as an autosomal dominant.[141] There are some clinical data suggesting that Turban tumors and hereditary multiple benign cystic epitheliomas may occur concurrently in the same families and result from expression of a common gene.[141] As in trichoepitheliomas discussed above, malignant transformation of Turban tumors to basal cell carcinoma occurs only occasionally. However, again, similar to the trichoepithelioma problem, a prior history of X-ray therapy confuses the issue of a potential for malignant transformation in this disorder.[142]

Multiple Self-Healing Squamous Epithelioma

The disorder now known as multiple self-healing squamous epithelioma was first described by Ferguson-Smith[143] in 1934. This initial report concerned a 23 year old patient who had suffered from the age of 16 with multiple cutaneous tumors of the face, ears, arm, thighs, and legs. These lesions began as red macules and became papular, enlarged, ulcerated and eventually healed, leaving deep pitted scars with irregular, overhanging crenellated borders. The tumors would last for several months and as they would heal, entirely new crops of tumors would appear so that the total number of active lesions would show a continuous increase. Biopsies showed typical appearances of squamous epithelioma, active and malignant in the early stages. As the tumors matured, a progressive cornification would appear and eventually complete involution with scar formation would complete the cycle. This original patient died at age 41 and an autopsy was performed. Numerous tumors and scars were found in the skin of the anus, scrotum, and anterior abdominal wall as well as on the face, legs, ears, and arms. All of the tumors were shown to be well differentiated squamous epitheliomata with lymphatic infiltration of the anal and oral lesions. The anal tumor was found to infiltrate the sphincter and muscle coats of the anal canal.[144] It is this feature of the lesion, as well as other aspects which permits distinguishing it from keratoacanthoma.[145]

Reliable information about multiple self-healing squamous epithelioma have been obtained on 62 cases from the west of Scotland, which accounts for more than twice the number of cases recorded in the World Literature. It is believed that the Scottish cases arose from a single mutation occurring before 1790.[145]

This defect appears to be determined by a rare autosomal dominant gene. Cytogenetic studies have revealed normal findings. No evidence of viral particles have been observed in skin tumors taken from two patients and examined by the electron microscope.[145]

The Multiple Mucosal Neuromata Syndrome

The clinical hallmarks of the multiple mucosal neuromata syndrome are comprised of mucosal neuromas in association with peripheral neurofibromas, medullary thyroid carcinoma, and bilateral pheochromocytomas.[146] Certain features of the syndrome appear to be similar to von Recklinghausen's disease as well as to certain of the endocrine neoplasia syndromes.[147,148] However, in spite of the apparent similarities with these mentioned disorders, the syndrome is considered to be a distinct entity.[146]

Patients with the multiple mucosal neuromata syndrome have phenotypic characteristics which produces a striking similarity in their physical appearance. Specifically, they are tall with arachnodactyly and may show a Marfanoid habitus (Fig. 21–13). They may have skeletal anomalies including scoliosis, pectus excavatum and pes cavus deformity. Neuromuscular components may include a muscular hypotonia. Their facies are characteristic with thickened eyelids, patulous lips, and prognathism which may simulate acromegaly. The most characteristic feature of the syndrome, however, is the presence of multiple mucosal neuromas or neurofibromas which may occur on the tongue (Fig. 21–14 and 21–15), lips, buccal mucosa, and the conjunctiva (Figs. 21–16 and 21–17). Occasionally, peripheral neurofibromas and café-au-lait patches may occur, thus giving rise, as mentioned, to the impression of von Recklinghausen's disease. Other findings may include intestinal neuromas or ganglioneuromas which may present radiographically as a megacolon, and may give rise to clinical signs and symptoms of diarrhea[146] (Fig. 21–18).

The phenotype of this syndrome should suggest to the clinician the possibility of an underlying medullary carcinoma of the thyroid, a potentially curable tumor.[146,148,149]

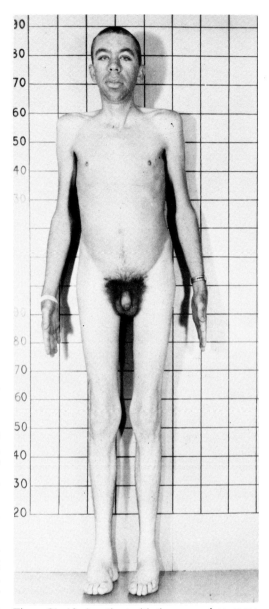

Figure 21–13. A patient with the mucosal neuroma syndrome. Note the heavy facial features and the Marfan-like habitus (Reproduced by courtesy of R. Neil Schimke, M.D.).

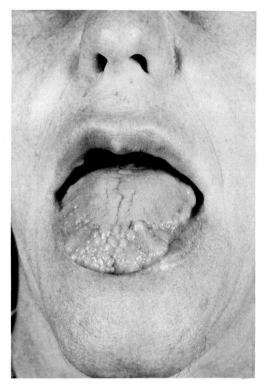

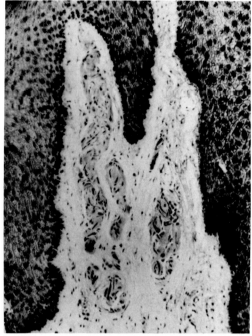

Figure 21–15. Multiple mucosal neuroma syndrome. Histologic section of tongue nodule showing numerous nerve bundles (Reproduced through the courtesy of R. Neil Schimke, M.D.).

Figure 21–14. Multiple mucosal neuroma syndrome. The tongue of this patient is studded with mucosal neuromas (Reproduced through the courtesy of New England Journal of Medicine).

The occurrence of hypertension in such a patient should prompt the exclusion of phenochromocytoma. Measurement of serum calcitonin in relatives at risk at any age will aid significantly in the diagnosis of the underlying medullary thyroid carcinoma.[149] The entire symptom complex in individual patients has been described only on occasion.[150,151]

Most cases have been sporadic. While both sexes are affected, the majority of reports suggest its occurrence more frequently in women. The genetic transmission in the hereditary variety of the syndrome is compatible with autosomal dominant inheritance with variability in the clinical expression of the syndrome.[148]

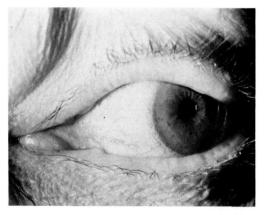

Figure 21–16. Multiple mucosal neuroma syndrome. Typical conjunctival neuromata in an affected patient (Reproduced through the courtesy of R. Neil Schimke, M.D.).

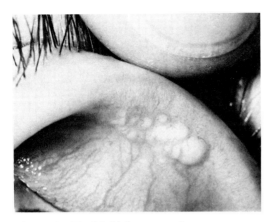

Figure 21–17. Multiple mucosal neuroma syndrome. Note the thickened lid margins and displaced lashes (Reproduced through the courtesy of R. Neil Schimke, M.D.).

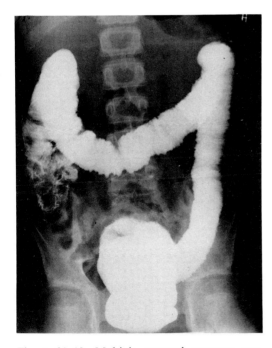

Figure 21–18. Multiple mucosal neuroma syndrome. Barium enema showing the radiographic appearance of intestinal gangliomatosis. The haustral markings are lost and the picture resembles ulcerative colitis (Reproduced through the courtesy of R. Neil Schimke, M.D.).

The Multiple Nevoid Basal Cell Carcinoma Syndrome

The multiple nevoid basal cell carcinoma syndrome was originally characterized by a triad of signs which included multiple nevoid basal cell carcinomas, jaw cysts, and skeletal anomalies. However, with benefit of over 100 publications describing over 250 individuals with this syndrome, the spectrum of anomalies has increased considerably. These now include intracranial calcification, ovarian fibroma, hyporesponsiveness to parathormone, lymphomesenteric cysts, medulloblastoma, and a variety of additional minor associated anomalies.[152]

A characteristic facies which includes frontal and temporoparietal bossing, combined with well-developed supraorbital ridges gives a sunken appearance to the eyes. Exotropia, and a broad nasal root, which may be associated with true ocular hypertelorism may be present. Mild mandibular prognathism may also be observed. Figure 21–19 clearly denotes several of these mentioned anatomic features found in a patient with the disorder and a positive family history of the defect.

For purposes of this discussion, the skin is the primary target organ, with the characteristic lesion consisting of multiple nevoid basal cell carcinomas which usually appear at puberty or during the second or third decade (usually 17–35 years); however, the lesions may occur as early as the second year of life in both exposed and unexposed cutaneous areas. There is a wide range of clinical variation so that in some patients skin lesions may never appear; indeed, in the study of large kindreds, wherein careful examination for all types of stigmata have been conducted, only about half of the affected individuals 20 years or older manifested skin tumors.[153] The lesions are usually numerous and appear as tiny, flesh colored to brownish dome-

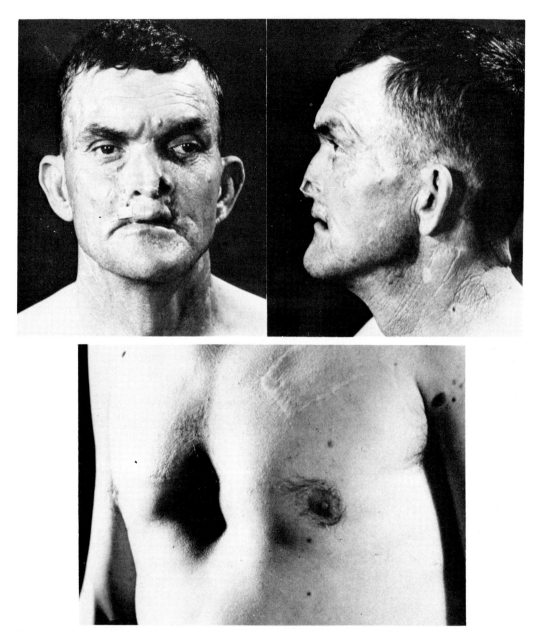

Figure 21–19. Patient showing several striking phenotypic characteristics of the multiple nevoid basal cell carcinoma syndrome. Note ophthalmoplegia, hypertelorism, prognathism, pectus excavatum, and evidence of excision of many basal cell carcinomas.

shaped papules, soft nodules or flat plaques varying in size from one millimeter to one centimeter in diameter. Sites of anatomic location in order of decreasing frequency include the face and neck, back and thorax, abdomen and upper extremities. Occasional patients have manifested more than 1,000 individual lesions.

Other skin lesions have included cysts, comedones, *café-au-lait* pigmentation, hirsutism, and/or multiple pigmented nevi. Palmer-plantar pits have been noted in occasional patients.

Pedigrees of many families manifesting the syndrome clearly demonstrate that it is inherited as an autosomal dominant trait.[154] Penetrance appears to be marked and expressivity is variable. Both sexes are equally affected. No single component of the syndrome will be present in all patients. Thus, in some patients, skeletal anomalies, intracranial calcifications, skin lesions and hyporesponsiveness to parathormone may be prominent while other physical findings may be more subtle and hence often overlooked. Thus, the diagnostician must be fully aware of the complexity of physical signs in the syndrome. The family history should be extremely helpful in indicating patients at risk for the disorder.

Multiple Familial Cutaneous Leiomyomas Associated with Malignant Uterine Leiomyomas

Walker and Reed[155] described a 20-year-old female who at puberty developed multiple small slightly red tumors on the skin of the arms, chest, neck, and legs which were diagnosed as cutaneous leiomyomas. She underwent a hysterectomy where the histologic diagnosis proved to be leiomyosarcoma of the uterus. Approximately one month later she underwent a left nephrectomy. Histologic diagnosis was hypernephroma.

The patient's 25-year-old brother manifested lesions of the skin consistent with cutaneous leiomyomas; these also developed at puberty. An intravenous pyelogram showed normal findings. Two female siblings, ages 16 and 7 were normal. Unfortunately, no mention is given to the remainder of the family history.

There have been previous reports of cutaneous and uterine leiomyomas though only three families showed a genetic disposi-

tion for this disorder;[155] however, one of these families showed the presence of a malignant uterine leiomyoma.[156]

Fisher and Helwig[157] studied 38 patients with cutaneous leiomyomas, and failed to find any association with uterine tumors. They postulated an autosomal dominant mode of inheritance for cutaneous leiomyoma. Rudner and colleagues[156] reported identical twins with both uterine and cutaneous leiomyomas.

Mezzadra[158] reported cutaneous leiomyomata in three generations. Interestingly, uterine myomata were associated in this family.

The association of cutaneous leiomyomas and leiomyosarcoma of the uterus and hypernephroma, as observed by Walker and Reed is presented here because of interest in the association between cutaneous lesions and visceral tumors. However, the limited family history in this single kindred prohibits elucidation of the mode of genetic transmission. However, it will be important to study other families showing similar associations. In such studies it will be helpful if detailed studies of the entire families can be accomplished.

Epidermodysplasia Verruciformis

Epidermodysplasia verruciformis is characterized by numerous circumscribed verrucae which are symmetrically distributed over many sites, most common of which are the dorsum of the hands; and of lesser frequency the wrists, face, trunk and penis. (Spared are the palms, soles, axillae, nails and mucous membranes). The lesions often occur early in life, even at birth and during early childhood. These lesions grossly resemble verruca vulgaris or verucca plana.[159] There is a strong proclivity for malignant degeneration, the most frequent type being basal cell carcinoma.[160] A papova virus has been considered strongly in the etiology of this disorder.[161,162] However, parental consanguinity and familial aggregations have suggested autosomal recessive inheritance.[162,163] Thus, this condition may provide another clinical example supporting an hypothesis invoking the interaction of genetic and viral factors in its etiology.

Discussion

Many medical diseases have a hereditary etiology in which the skin involved has shown a slight statistical association with cancer but wherein the overall cancer risk in the particular patient may nevertheless be rather minimal. Because of space limitations, many of these conditions have not been discussed in this chapter. For example, patients with Down's syndrome harbor a definite risk for development of acute leukemia when they are compared with the risk for leukemia in patients from the general population. Down's syndrome would also qualify for inclusion in this chapter since there are definite cutaneous manifestations in this particular disease. However, the cytogenetic aspects of this disease have been one of its major interests; therefore, this condition as well as several others with cytogenetic aberrations, occasionally dermatologic abnormalities and cancer association are discussed in Chapter 9 by Sandberg and Sakurai.

In addition, many other diseases with varying cancer predisposition are discussed in other chapters throughout this book though they are also included in the tables in this chapter. Their discussion in other chapters may be under a variety of categories such as collagen vascular diseases, in the chapter on miscellaneous disorders (Chapter 22) which includes such diseases as scleroderma and lupus erythematosis, or they may be discussed in context with neurology implications in Chapter 17, treating these subjects; this includes such disorders as tuberous sclerosis and von Recklinghausen's neurofibromatosis. However, in the interest of brevity, they have not been given any additional discussion in this chapter.

REFERENCES

1. Lynch, H.T.: *Skin, Heredity, and Malignant Neoplasms.* New York, Med Exam, 1972, pp. 300.
2. Lynch, H.T.: Skin, heredity, and cancer. *Cancer, 24*:277–288, 1969.
3. Newbold, P.C.H.: Skin markers of malignancy. *Arch Dermatol, 102*:680–692, 1970.
4. Wiener, K.: *Skin Manifestations of Internal Disorders (Dermadromes).* St. Louis, Mosby, 1947, pp. 690.
5. Freeman, R.G.: Carcinogenic effects of solar radiation and prevention measures. *Cancer, 21*:1114–1120, 1968.
6. Olson, R.L.: Skin colon, pigment distribution, and skin cancer. *Cutis, 8*:225–239, 1971.
7. Blum, H.F.: *Carcinogenesis by Ultraviolet Light.* Princeton, Princeton U Pr, 1959.
8. Silverston, H.: Sited as a personal communication by Urback, F., *et al.*: Ultraviolet radiation and skin cancer in man. In Montagna, W., and Dobson, R.L. (Eds.): *Advances in Biology of Skin Carcinogenesis,* Oxford, Pargamon Pr, 1965, Vol. 7, Ch. 12, pp. 195–214.
9. Silverston, H., and Searle, J.H.A.: The epidemiology of skin cancer in Queensland: the influence of phenotype and environment. *Br J Cancer, 24*:235–252, 1970.
10. Willis, I.: Sunlight and the skin. *JAMA, 217*: 1088–1093, 1971.
11. Szabó, G.: Quantitative histological investi-

gations on the melanocyte system of the human epidermis. In Gordon, M., (Ed.): *Pigment Cell Biology.* New York, Acad Pr, 1959, pp. 99–125.

12. Fitzpatrick, T.B., Szabó, G., and Mitchell, R.E.: Age changes in the human melanocyte system. *Advan Biol Skin, 6:*36–50, 1964.

13. Breathnach, A.S.: Normal and abnormal melanin pigmentation of the skin. In M. Wolman, (Ed.): *Pigments in Pathology.* New York, Acad Pr, 1969, pp. 551.

14. Wolman, M.: *Pigments in Pathology.* New York, Acad Pr, 1969, pp. 551.

15. Reed, W.B., and Porter, P.S.: Keratosis, *Arch Dermatol, 104:*99–100, 1971.

16. Howel-Evans, McConnell, R.B., Clarke, C.A., and Sheppard, P.M.: Carcinoma of the oesophugus with keratosis palmaris et plantaris (Tylosis): a study of two families. *Quart J Med, 27:*413–429, 1958.

17. Harper, P.S., Harper, R.M.J., and Howel-Evans, A.W.: Carcinoma of the oesophagus with tylosis. *Quart J Med, 39:*317–333, 1970.

18. Shine, I., and Allison, P.R.: Carcinoma of the oesophagus with tylosis (keratosis palmaris et plantaris). *Lancet, 1:*951–953, 1966.

19. Mosbech, J., and Videbaek, A.: On the etiology of esophageal carcinoma. *J Natl Cancer Inst, 15:*1665–1673, 1955.

20. Huriez, C., Deminatti, M., and Agache, P., et al.: Une Gёnodysplasie non Encore Individualisёe: La Genodermatose Sclero-Atrophiante et Keratodermigue des Ex-

20. Huriez, C., Deminatti, M., and Agache, P., et al.: Une Gёnodysplasie non Encore Individualisёe: La Genodermatose Sclero-Atrophiante et Kёratodermigue des Extrёmitёs Frequemment Dёgёnёrative. *Sem Hop Paris, 44:*481–488, 1968.

21. Dobson, R.L., Young, M.R., and Pinto, J.S.: Palmar keratoses and cancer. *Arch Dermatol* (Chicago), *92:*553–556, 1965.

22. Bean, S.F., Foxley, E.G., and Fusaro, R.M.: Palmar keratoses and internal malignancy: a negative study. *Arch Dermatol* (Chicago), *97:*528–532, 1968.

23. Rhodes, E.L.: Palmar and plantar seed keratoses and internal malignancy. *Br J Dermatol, 82:*361–363, 1970.

24. Braverman, I.M.: *Skin Signs of Systemic Disease.* Philadelphia, Saunders, 1970, pp. 302–303.

25. Berlyne, G.M., and Berlyne, N.: Anaemia due to the "Blue Rubber-Bleb" naevus disease. *Lancet, 2:*1275–1277, 1960.

26. Bean, W.B.: *Vascular Spiders and Related Lesions of the Skin.* Springfield, Thomas, 1958.

27. Rice, J.S., and Fischer, D.S.: Blue rubber-bleb nevus syndrome: generalized cavernous hemangiomatosis or venous hamartoma with medulloblastoma of the cerebellum: case report and review of the literature. *Arch Dermatol, 86:*503–511, 1962.

28. Sakurane, H.F., Sugai, T., and Saito, T.: The association of blue rubber-bled nevus and Maffucci's syndrome. *Arch Dermatol, 95:*28–36, 1967.

29. Fine, R.M., Derbes, V.J., and Clark, W.H.: Blue rubber-bled nevus. *Arch Dermatol, 84:*802–805, 1961.

30. Fretzin, D.F., and Potter, B.: Blue rubber-bleb nevus. *Arch Intern Med, 116:*924–929, 1965.

31. Talbot, S., and Wyatt, E.H.: Blue rubber-bleb naevi. *Br J Dermatol, 82:*37–39, 1970.

32. Lewandowsky, F., and Lutz, W.: Ein Fall einer bisher nicht beschriebenen Häwterkrankung (Epidermodysplasia vercuiformis). *Arch Dermatol Syph,* (Berlin), *141:*193–203, 1922.

33. Rajagoplan, K., Bahru, J., Loo, D.S.C., Tay, C.H., Chin, K.N., and Tan, K.K.: Familial epidermodysplasia verruciformis of Lewandowsky and Luts. *Arch. Dermatol, 105:*73–78, 1972.

34. Oehlschlaegel, G., Röckl, H., and Muller, E.: Die Epidermodysplasia Verruciformis, eine sog. Praecancerose. *Hautarzt, 17:*450–458, 1966.

35. Mashkilleison, L.N.: Ist die Epidermodysplasia Verruciformis (Lewandowsky-Lutz) eine selbständige Dermatose? Ihr Beziehungen zur Verrucositas. *Dermat Wochenschr, 92:*569–578, 1931.

36. Ormea, F.: Epidermodysplasia verruciformis und hautcarcinoma. *Arch Dermatol Syph* (Berlin), *188*:278–296, 1949.

37. Lutz, W.: Zur Epidermodysplasia Verruciformis. *Dermatologica, 115*:309–314, 1957.

38. Sullivan, M., and Ellis, F.A.: Epidermodysplasia verruciformis (Lewandowsky-Lutz). *Arch Dermat Syph* (Chicago), *40*:422–432, 1939.

39. Costa, O.G., and Junqueira, M.A.: Epidermodysplasia Verruciformis (Lewandowsky and Lutz). *Arch Dermatol Syph, 46*: 469–479, 1942.

40. Kraus, Z., and Vortel, V.: (Epidermodysplasia verruciformis). *Cesk Dermatol, 35*: 95–99, 1960.

41. Jablonska, S., Biczysko, W., and Jakubowicz, K., *et al.*: On the viral etiology of epidermodysplasia verruciformis lewandowsky-Lutz: Electron microscope studies. *Dermatologica, 137*:113–125, 1968.

42. Wechsler, H.L., Krugh, F.J., Domonkos, A.N., Scheen, S.R., and Davidson, C.L.: Polydysplastic Epidermolysis Bullosa and development of epidermal neoplasms. *Arch Dermatol, 102*:374–380, 1970.

43. Bean, W.B.: Dyschondroplasia and hemangiomata (Maffucci's syndrome). *Arch Intern Med, 95*:767–781, 1955.

44. Bean, W.B.: Dyschondroplasia and hemangiomata (Maffucci's syndrome), II. *Arch Intern Med, 102*:544–550, 1958.

45. Elmore, S.M., and Cantrell, W.C.: Maffucci's syndrome: case report with a normal karyotype. *J Bone Joint Surg Am, 48*:1607–1613, 1966.

46. Maffucci, A.: Di un caso di encondroma ed angioma multiplo: Contribuzione alla genesi embrionale dei tumori, *Movimento Napoli, 3*:399–412, 1881.

47. Strang, C., and Rannie, I.: Dyschondroplasia with hemangiomata (Maffucci's syndrome); report of case complicated by intracranial chondrosarcoma. *J Bone Joint Surg, 32*:376–383, 1950.

48. Johnson, J.L., Webster, J.R., Jr., and Sippy, H.I.: Maffucci's syndrome (dyschondroplasia with hemangioma). *Am J Med, 28*: 864–866, 1960.

49. Anderson, I.F.: Maffucci's syndrome: report of a case with a review of the literature. *S Afr Med J, 39*:1066–1070, 1965.

50. Andren, L., Dymling, J.F., Elner, A., *et al.*: Maffucci's syndrome: report of four cases. *Acta Chir Scand, 126*:397–405, 1963.

51. Guss, S.B., Osbourn, R.A., and Lutzner, M.A.: Porokeratosis plantaris, palmaris, et disseminata: a third type of porokeratosis. *Arch Dermatol, 104*:366–373, 1971.

52. Chernosky, M.E.: Porokeratosis: report of 12 patients with multiple superficial lesions. *South Med J, 59*:289–294, 1966.

53. Johnston, E.N.M.: Porokeratosis of Mibelli with squamous cell carcinoma. *Br J Dermatol, 70*:381, 1958.

54. Savage, J.: Porokeratosis (Mibelli) and carcinoma. *Br J Dermatol, 76*:489, 1964.

55. Tietz, W.: A syndrome of deaf-mutism associated with albinism, showing dominant autosomal inheritance. *Am J Hum Genet, 15*:259–264, 1963.

56. Keeler, C.E.: Albinism, xeroderma pigmentosum, and skin cancer. *Nat Cancer Inst* (Monograph 10): International conference on the biology of cutaneous cancer. U.S. Department of Health, Education, and Welfare, Public Health Service, 1963, pp. 349–359.

57. Witkop, C.J., Van Scott, E.J., and Jacoby, G.A.: Evidence for two forms of autosomal recessive albinism in man. *Proc Second Int Conf Hum Genet*, Rome, 1961, pp. 1064–1065.

58. Witkop, C.J., Nance, W.E., Rawls, R.F., and White, J.G.: Autosomal recessive oculacutaneous albinism in man: evidence for genetic heterogeneity. *Am J Hum Genet, 22*:55–74, 1970.

59. Keeler, C.E., and MacKinnon, J.H.: The albino-moon child research project. *MSH Bull Curr Res, 2*:3–27, 1963.

60. Wright, P.D., Venables, C.W., and Dawber, R.P.R.: Vitiligo and gastric carcinoma. *Br Med J, 3*:148, 1970.

61. Allison, J.R., Jr., and Curtis, A.C.: Vitiligo and pernicious anemia. *AMA Arch Dermatol, 72*:407–408, 1955.

62. Vidabaek, A., and Mosbech, J.: The aetriology of gastric carcinoma elucidates by a study of 302 pedigrees. *Acta Med Scand, 149*:137–159, 1954.

63. Woolf, C.M.: Further study on the familial aspects of carcinoma of the stomach. *Am J Hum Genet, 8*:102–109, 1956.

64. Gorer, P.A.: Genetic interpretation of studies on cancer in twins. *Ann Eugen, 8*:219–232, 1938.

65. Mosbech, J.: *Heredity in Pernicious Anemia: A Proband Study of the Heredity and the Relationship to Cancer of the Stomach.* Copenhagen: E. Munksgaard, 1953, p. 107.

66. Lynch, H.T.: Hereditary factors in carcinoma. In *Recent Results in Cancer Research.* Monograph series, New York: Springer-Verlag, Vol. 12, 1967, pp. 1–186.

67. Attie, J.L., and Khafif, R.A.: *Melanotic Tumors: Biology, Pathology, and Clinical Features.* Springfield, Thomas, 1964, pp. 160–183.

68. Reed, W.B.: Mary, S.B., and Nickel, W.R.: Xeroderma pigmentosum with neurological complications: the de Santis-Cacchione syndrome. *Arch Dermatol* (Chicago), *91*:224–226, 1965.

69. Moss, H.V., Jr.: Xeroderma pigmentosum: report of two cases with metabolic studies. *Arch Dermatol, 92*:638–642, 1965.

70. Butterworth, T., and Strean, L.P.: *Clinical Genodermatology.* Baltimore, Williams & Wilkins, 1962.

71. Couillaud, P.: Xeroderma pigmentosum de Kaposi. *Ann Dermatol Syphiligr, 9*:443–448, 1898.

72. Lynch, H.T., Ozer, F., McNutt, C.W., Johnson, J.E., and Jampolsky, N.A.: Secondary male hypogonadism and congenital ichthyosis: association of two rare genetic diseases. *Am J Hum Genet, 12*:440–447, 1960.

73. MacGillivary, R.C.: Syndrome of Rüd. *Am J Ment Defic, 59*:62–72, 1954.

74. Pick, F.J.: Ueber melanosis lenticularis progressiva. *Wochenschr Dermatol Syph, 11*:3–32, 1884.

75. Mendes da Costa, S.: Xeroderma Pigmentosun. *Nederl T Geneesk, 1*:1117–1118, 1900.

76. Elsenberg, A.: Xeroderma pigmentosum (Kaposi): progressive lenticular melanosis. *Arch Dermatol Syph, 22*:49–70, 1890.

77. Benziger, K., and Heuss: *Paracelsus,* Zurich, 1897.

78. Wesolowski, W.: Beitrag zur Pathologischen Anatomie dex Xeroderma Pigmentosum. *Centralbl Allg Path, 10*:990–997, 1899.

79. Havas, cited by Nicolas, J., Favre, M., and Dupasquier, D.: Du Cancer Melanique Dans Le Xeroderma Pigmentosum. *Ann Dermatol Syph, 8*:457–572, 1927.

80. Stout: A case of xeroderma pigmentosum. *J Cutan Dis, 26*:380–381, 1908.

81. Rouvière, G.: Deux Nouvesux Cas de Xeroderma Pigmentosum. *Ann Dermatol Syph, 1*:34–37, 1910.

82. Nakagawa, cited by Nicolas, J., Favre, M., and Dupasquier, D.: Du Cancer Mélanique Dans Le Xeroderma Pigmentosum. *Ann Dermatol Syph, 8*:457–472, 1927.

83. Nicolas, J., Favre, M., and Dupasquier, D.: Du Cancer Mélanique Dans Le Xeroderma Pigmentosum. *Ann Dermatol Syph, 8*:457–472, 1927.

84. Foldvàri, F.: Métastase Sarcomteuse Hépatique de Xeroderma Pigmentosum. *Acta Dermatol Syph, 15*:253–262, 1934.

85. Flarer, F.: Discheratosi: Epiteliomi Multipli E Melanosarcoma in Bambino di Tre Anni Con Xeroderma Pigmentoso. *Riforma Med, 53*:635–638, 1937.

86. Merelender, I.J., and Ginzburgowa, B.: Xeroderma Pigmentosum (Melanoneurinoma Consecutivum). *Acta Dermatovener, 19*:75–87, 1938.

87. Ronchese, F.: Spontaneous bleaching of melanotic freckles. *Arch Dermatol, 94*:739–741, 1966.

88. Van Patter, H.T., and Drummond, J.A.: Malignant melanoma occurring in xeroderma pigmentosum: report of a case. *Cancer, 6*:942–947, 1953.

89. Moore, C., and Iverson, P.C.: Xeroderma pigmentosum; showing common skin cancers plus melanocarcinoma controlled by surgery. *Cancer, 7*:377–382, 1954.

90. Iijima, S., Watanabe, S., and Shimoda, C.: A case of xeroderma pigmentosum with melanoma: report of a case with review of literature. *Acta Dermatol, 52:*163–167, 1957.

91. Lemaire, M., and Gaumond, E.: Xeroderma pigmentosum, Huit Cas D'évolution Différente Dans Deux Familles. *Can Med Asso J, 92:*406–412, 1965.

92. Anderson, D.E., Smith, J.L., Jr., and McBride, C.M.: Hereditary aspects of malignant melanoma. *JAMA, 200:*741–746, (May 29) 1967.

92a. Robbins, J.H., Kraemer, K.H., Lutzner, M.A., Festoff, B.W., and Coon, H.G.: Xeroderma Pigmentosum: An inherited disease with sun sensitivity, multiple cutaneous neoplasm, and abnormal DNA repair. *Ann Int Med, 80:*221–248, 1974.

93. Wilkinson, T.S., and Paletta, G.X.: Malignant melanoma: current concepts. *Am Surg, 35:*301–309, 1969.

94. McNeer, G., and Das Bupta, T.: Life history of melanoma. *Am J Roentgen, 93:*686–694, 1965.

95. Pack, G.T., Lenson, N., and Gerber, D.M.: Regional distribution of moles and melanomas, *AMA Arch Surg, 65:*862–870, 1952.

96. Lynch, H.T., Anderson, D.E., and Krush, A.J.: Heredity and intraocular malignant melanoma: study of two families and review of forty-five cases. *Cancer, 21:*119–125, 1968.

97. Nathanson, L., Hall, T.C., and Farber, S.: Biological aspects of human malignant melanoma. *Cancer, 20:*650–655, 1967.

98. Joint Committee on Planning for Dermatology: National Program for Dermatology. The Academy of Dermatology, 1964, p. 69.

99. Cawley, E.P.: Genetic aspects of malignant melanoma. *AMA Arch Dermatol Syph, 65:*440–450, 1942.

100. Katzenellenbogen, I., and Sandbank, M.: Malignant melanoma in twins. *Arch Dermatol, 94:*331–332, 1966.

101. Moschella, S.L.: A report of malignant melanoma of the skin in sisters. *Arch Dermatol, 84:*1024–1025, 1961.

102. Salamon, T., Schnyder, U.W., and Storck, H.: A contribution to the question of heredity and malignant melanoma. *Dermatologica* (Basel), *126:* 66–75, 1963.

103. Schoch, E.P., Jr.: Familial malignant melanoma: a pedigree and cytogenetic study. *Arch Dermatol, 88:*445–456, 1963.

104. Smith, F.E., Henly, W.S., Knox, J.M., and Lane, M.: Familial melanoma. *Arch Intern Med, 117:*820–823, 1966.

105. Greifelt, A.: Malignes Melanom: Beziehungen zu Schwangerschaft, Pubertat, Kindheit: Familiare Maligne Malanoma. *Arztl Wochenschr, 7:*676–679, July 18, 1952.

106. Miller, T.R., and Pack, G.T.: The familial aspect of malignant melanoma. *Arch Dermatol* (Chicago), *86:*35–39, 1962.

107. Anderson, D.E.: Personal Communication, 1967.

108. Wallace, D.C., Exton, L.A., and McLeod, G.R.: Genetic factor in malignant melanoma. *Cancer, 27:*1262–1266, 1971.

108a. Anderson, D.E.: Clinical characteristics of the genetic variety of cutaneous melanoma in man. *Cancer, 28:*721–725, 1971.

109. Bowen, S.F., Brady, H., and Jones, V.L.: Malignant melanoma of eye occurring in two successive generations. *Arch Ophthalmol* (Chicago), *71:*805–806, 1964.

110. Davenport, R.C.: Family history of choroidal sarcoma. *Br J Ophthalmol, 11:*443–445, 1927.

111. Gutmann, G.: Casuisticher Beitrag zur Lehre von den Geschwülsten des Augapfels. *Arch Augenh, 31:*158–180, 1895.

112. Parsons, J.H.: *The Pathology of the Eye.* Vol. II, Histology, Part II, New York, Putnam's, 1905, pp. 496–497, Vol. II.

113. Pfingst, A.O., and Graves, S.: Melanosarcoma of choroid occurring in brothers. *Arch Ophthalmol* (Chicago), *50:*431–439, 1921.

114. Silcock, A.Q.: Hereditary sarcoma of the eyeball in three generations. *Br Med J, 1:* 1079, 1892.

115. Tucker, D.P., Steinberg, A.G., and Cogan, D.G.: Frequency of genetic transmission of sporadic retinoblastoma. *Arch Ophthalmol* (Chicago), *57:*532–535, 1957.

116. Lynch, H.T., Anderson, D.E., and Krush,

A.J.: Heredity and intraocular malignant melanoma: study of two families and review of 45 cases. *Cancer, 21:*119–125, 1968.

117. Lynch, H.T., Anderson, D.E., Smith, J.L., Jr., Howell, J.B., and Krush, A.J.: Xeroderma pigmentosum, malignant melanoma, and congenital icthyosis: a family study. *Arch Dermatol, 96:*625–635, 1967.

118. Gartner, S.: Malignant melanoma of the choroid and von Recklinghausen's disease. *Am J Ophthalmol, 23:*73–78, 1940.

119. Turkington, R.W.: Familial factor in Malignant melanoma. *JAMA, 192:*77–82, 1965.

120. Krush, A.J., Lynch, H.T., and Magnuson, C.: Attitudes toward cancer in a "Cancer Family." Implications from cancer detection. *Am J Med Sci, 249:*432–438, 1965.

121. Goldberg, A.: Diagnosis and treatment of the porphtrias. *Proc R Soc Med, 61:*193–196, 1968.

122. Stanbury, J.B., Wyngaarden, J.B., and Fredrickson, D.S.: *The Metabolic Basis of Inherited Disease.* New York, McGraw, 1960.

123. Falls, H.F.: The Eye and Hand as an Aid to Diagnosis of Hereditary Constitutional Syndromes, paper presented by Third International Congress of Human Genetics, Chicago, Illinois, September 9, 1966.

124. Waldenstrom, J.: The porphyrias as inborn errors of metabolism. *Am J Med, 22:*758–773, 1957.

125. Waddington, R.T.: A case of primary liver tumor associated with porphyria. *Br J Surg, 59:*653–654, 1972.

126. Bloom, G.E., Warner, S., Gerald, P.S., and Diamond, L.K.: Chromosome abnormalities in constitutional aplastic anemia. *New Engl J Med, 274:*8–14, 1966.

127. Todaro, G.J., Green, H., and Swift, M.R.: Susceptibility of human diploid fibroblast strains to transformation by SV40 virus. *Science, 153:*1252–1254, 1966.

128. Hitch, J.M.: Dyskeratosis congenita. *Cutis, 4:*1229–1232, 1968.

129. Cole, H.N., Rauschklob, J.E., and Toomey, J.: Dyskeratosis congenita with pigmentation, dystrophia unguis and leukokera-

tosis oris. *Arch Dermatol Syph, 21:*71–95, 1930.

130. Bryan, H.G., and Nixon, R.J.: Dyskeratosis congenita and familial pancytopenia. *JAMA, 192:*203–208, 1965.

131. Swift, M.R., and Hirschhorn, K.: Fanconi's anemia: inherited susceptibility to chromosome breakage in various tissues. *Ann Intern Med, 65:*496–503, 1966.

132. Swift, M.: Fanconi's anaemia in the genetics of neoplasia. *Nature, 230:*370–372, 1971.

133. Swift, M., Scholman, L., and Gilmour, D.: Diabetes mellitus and the gene for Fanconi's anemia. *Science, 178:*308–310, 1972.

134. Milyer, R.W.: Down's syndrome (Mongolism), other congenital malformations and cancers among the sibs of leukemic children. *New Engl J Med, 268:*393–401, 1963.

135. Rosner, F.: Dermatoglyphics of leukemic children. *Lancet, 2:*272–273, 1969.

136. Wertelecki, W., Plato, C.C., and Fraumeni, J.F., Jr.: Dermatoglyphics in leukemia. *Lancet, 2:*806–807, 1969.

137. Verbov, J.L.: Dermatoglyphics in leukemia. *J Med Genet, 7:*125–131, 1970.

138. Heath, C.W., Jr., and Moloney, W.C.: Familial leukemia. Five cases of acute leukemia in three generations. *New Engl J Med, 272:*882–887, 1965.

139. Steinberg, A.G.: The genetics of acute leukemia in children. *Cancer, 13:*985–999, 1960.

140. Fraumeni, J.F., Jr., Vogel, C.L., and Devita, V.T.: Familial chronic lymphocytic leukemia. *Ann Intern Med, 71:*279–284, 1969.

141. Welch, J.P., Wells, R.S., and Kerr, C.B.: Ancell-spiegler cylindromas (Turban-Tumours) and Brooke-Fordyce trichoepitheliomas: evidence for a single genetic entity. *J Med Genet, 5:*29–35, 1968.

142. Ziprokowski, I., and Schewach-Millet, M.: Multiple trichoepithelioma in a mother and two children. *Dermatologics* (Basal), *132:*248–256, 1966.

143. Smith, J. Ferguson: A case of multiple primary squamous-celled carcinomata of the skin in a young man, with spontaneous healing. *Br J Dermatol, 46:*267–272, 1934.

144. Currie, A.R., and Smith, J. Ferguson: Multiple primary spontaneous-healing squa-

mous-cell carcinomata of the skin. *J Pathol Bacteriol, 64:*827–839, 1952.

145. Ferguson-Smith, M.A., Wallace, D.C., James, Z.H., and Renwick, J.H.: Multiple self-healing squamous epithelioma. *Birth Defects: Original Article Series, 7:*157–163, 1971.

146. Schimke, R.N.: Multiple mucosal neuromata syndrome. In Lynch, H.T., (Ed.). *Skin, Heredity and Malignant Neoplasms.* New York, Med Exam, 1972, Chapt. 13, p. 200.

147. Rimoin, D.L., and Schimke, R.N.: *Genetic Disorders of the Endocrine Glands,* St. Louis, Mosby, 1971, p. 383.

148. Schimke, R.N.: Phenotype of malignancy: the mucosal neuroma syndrome. *Pediatrics, 52:*283–287, 1973.

149. Melvin, K.E.W., Tashjian, A.J., Jr., and Miller, H.H.: Studies in familial (Medullary) thyroid carcinoma. *Recent Progr Horm Res, 28:*399–470, 1972.

150. Forsman, P.J., and Jenkins, M.E.: Medullary carcinoma of the thyroid with marfan-like body habitus. *Pediatrics, 52:*188–196, 1973.

151. Levin, D.L., Perlia, C., and Tashjian, A.H., Jr.: Medullary carcinoma of the thyroid gland: the complete syndrome in a child. *Pediatrics, 52:*192–196, 1973.

152. Gorlin, R.J., and Sedano, H.O.: The multiple nevoid basal cell carcinoma syndrome revisited. In Lynch (Ed.): *Skin, Heredity, and Malignant Neoplasms.* New York, Med Exam, 1972.

153. Gilhuus-Moe, O., Haugen, L.K., and Dee, P.M.: The syndrome of multiple cysts of the jaws, basal cell carcinomata and skeletal anomalies. *Br J Oral Surg, 6:*211–222, 1968.

154. Gorlin, R.J., Vickers, R.A., Kelln, E., and Williamson, J.J.: The multiple basal-cell nevi syndrome. An analysis of a syndrome consisting of multiple nevoid basal-cell carcinoma, jaw cysts, skeletal anomalies, medulloblastoma and hyporesponsiveness to parathormone. *Cancer, 18:*89–104, 1967.

155. Walker, R.H., and Reed, W.B.: Genetic cutaneous disorders with gynecologic tumors. *Am J Obstet Gynecol, 116:*485–492, 1973.

156. Rudner, R.J., Schwartz, O.D., and Grekin, J.N.: Multiple cutaneous leiomyoma in identical twins. *Arch Dermatol, 90:*81–82, 1964.

157. Fisher, W.L., and Helwig, E.B.: Leiomyomas of the skin. *Arch Dermatol, 88:*510–520, 1963.

158. Mezzadra, G.: Leiomioma Cutaneo Multiplo Eredittario, Studio Di Un Caso Sistematizzato In Soggetto Maschile Appartenente A Famiglia Portatrice Di Leiomiomatosi Cutaneo E Fibromiomatosi Uterina. *Minerva Derm, 40:*388–393, 1965.

159. Sullivan, M., and Ellis, F.A.: Epidermodysplasia verruciformis (Lewandowsky and Leitz). *Arch Derm Syph, 40:*422–432, 1939.

160. Aaronson, C.M., and Lutzner, M.A.: Epidermodysplasia verruciformis and epidermoid carcinoma. Electron microscopic observations. *JAMA, 201:*775–777, 1967.

161. Baker, H.: Epidermodysplasia verruciformis with electron microscopic demonstration of virus. *Proc R Soc Med, 61:*589–590, 1968.

162. Jablonska, S., Fabjanska, L., and Formas, I.: On the viral etiology of epidermodysplasia verruciformis. *Dermatologica, 132:*369–385, 1966.

163. Midana, A.: Sulla Questione Dei Rapporti Tra Epidermodysplasia Verruciformis E Verrucosi Generalizzata. *Dermatologica, 99:*1–23, 1949.

CHAPTER 22

CANCER RESISTANCE

HENRY T. LYNCH AND HODA GUIRGIS

Introduction

CANCER IS NOT uniformly distributed in the population. There are marked variations in cancer incidence at different anatomic sites, in different populations and in different areas of the world. Numerous etiologic differences account for such variations in cancer incidence, including differences in genotypes, environmental exposures, habit patterns, occupations, socioeconomic status, and educational factors.[1,2] A comprehensive exploration of cancer etiology involves integrated consideration of all potentially mitigating factors, not only individually, but also collectively as they interact with each other.[1,3-5]

As we studied families with significantly increased incidences of cancer, compared to the general population, we observed a significant paucity of occurrences of cancer in certain branches of these families and in a number of other families, some of which included the kin of spouses of patients in high-incidence families. We concluded that some kindreds may be characterized by unusual resistance or decreased susceptibility to cancer, just as other kindreds may be characterized by unusual cancer-proneness. This observation is not surprising because significant differences in cancer resistance have been well established in inbred strains of a variety of animals.[6-8] Recent studies in tumor immunology have revealed a crucial relationship between an animal's immune defense system and its response to carcinogens as well as to transplanted cancer cells.[9,10] Stephenson, et al.[11] have discussed spontaneous regression of tumors in humans in relation to tolerance and/or resistance to malignancy.

Several examples of possible cancer resistance will be discussed. They will include: 1) two families noteworthy for a paucity of carcinoma wherein no other known associated genetic trait or disorder has been identified; 2) data on an autosomal dominantly inherited disorder, namely, osteogenesis imperfecta which seemingly shows a paucity of cancer in affected individuals; 3) a discussion of cancer variations in diabetes mellitus, a condition known to be familial but for which the genetic mechanism has not yet been determined; 4) cancer frequencies in patients manifesting a deficiency of the enzyme glucose-6-phosphate dehydrogenase (G-6-PD); finally, 5) we shall present data showing cancer frequency variations in a normal population.

Cancer-Resistant Family (Family A)

The schematic pedigree shown in Figure 22-1 is noteworthy for a paucity of malignant neoplasms. Interestingly, longevity was rather advanced in many of its members. The average age at death of all members was 57.4 years. When deaths below age 30 were excluded, the average age at death was 70.3 years. Cardiovascular disease was responsible for 12 of the 32 recorded causes of death at ages which ranged from 53 to 86. Two family members are living in their eighties and seven in their seventies. The histologic varieties

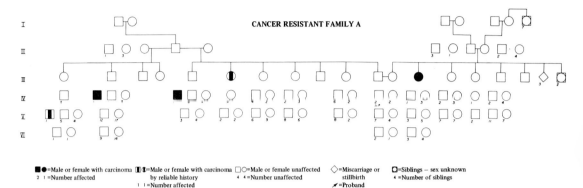

Figure 22–1. A schematic pedigree of a cancer-resistant family (Family A) depicting the occurrence of cancer by generation (and not by sibships in a generation).

of cancer in several patients, significantly, were usually associated with nongenetic factors, i.e. bronchogenic carcinoma in a heavy smoker; "youth cancer," which we believe may have been leukemia, occurred in a 13-year-old child (Table 22-I). Thus, in this family we see that among 266 relatives at risk for cancer, only five have developed malignant neoplasms. In considering those who reached the age of 40, 3.5 percent developed cancer (Table 22-I).

Cancer-Resistant Family (*Family B*)

Among 589 members of Family B, 16 have developed cancer (2.7%, Fig. 22–2, and Table 22-II).

When each of the 13 branches of this family is considered separately (considering those who reached the age of 40) one notes that branch 7 has an incidence rate for cancer of 18 percent which is the approximate rate expected in the general population. Branches

TABLE 22-I
CANCER INCIDENCE BY FAMILY BRANCH IN A CANCER-RESISTANT FAMILY
FAMILY A

Branch of Family	Total No. (all ages)	No. with Cancer (all ages)	Percent	No. Members Over Age 40	No. with Cancer After Age 40	Percent	Multiple Primary Lesions
1	17	1	8%	5	—	—	—
2	62	1	2%	18	1	6%	—
3	19	1	5%	10	—	—	—
4	8	1	12%	8	1	12%	—
5	22	—	—	22	—	—	—
6	20	—	—	6	—	—	—
7	19	—	—	7	—	—	—
8	30	—	—	14	—	—	—
9	20	1	5%	11	1	9%	—
10	20	—	—	5	—	—	—
11	4	—	—	2	—	—	—
12	25	—	—	6	—	—	—

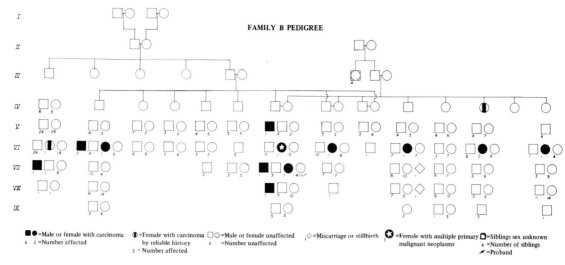

Figure 22–2. A schematic pedigree of a cancer-resistant family (Family B) depicting the occurrence of cancer by generation (and not by sibships in a generation).

2 and 12 have rates of 11 and 10 percent respectively, while all of the remaining branches have rates of 5 percent or less which gives the overall rate of 4.2 percent.

Breast cancer occurred in four individuals (among whom one survived two primary breast lesions and died at age 76 of a CVA). Basal cell carcinoma occurred in two patients as did bladder cancer. Bladder cancer oc-

curred in persons who were known to be cigar smokers. Cancer of the esophagus occurred in a 56-year-old man who was known to have been a heavy drinker. The late age of cancer onset is noteworthy in four individuals (i.e. 77, 79, 71, and 84). One child developed a brain tumor at the age of six years and died at the age of nine years. The average age at death of 197

TABLE 22-II
CANCER INCIDENCE BY FAMILY BRANCH IN A CANCER-RESISTANT FAMILY
FAMILY B

Branch of Family	Total No. (all ages)	No. with Cancer (all ages)	Percent	No. Members Over Age 40	No. with Cancer After Age 40	Percent	Multiple Primary Lesions
1	116	2	—	105	2	2%	—
2	68	3	4%	28	3	11%	—
3	25	—	—	22	—	—	—
4	12	—	—	10	—	—	—
5	17	—	—	12	—	—	—
6	18	—	—	14	—	—	—
7	53	5	9%	22	4	18%	1
8	42	1	2%	30	1	3%	—
9	10	—	—	6	—	—	—
10	57	1	2%	35	1	3%	—
11	56	—	—	23	—	—	—
12	64	3	5%	29	3	10%	—
13	51	1	2%	19	1	5%	—

family members who died at any age was 52.2, but when only the 150 members who reached the age of 30 were considered, the average age at death was 65.1. Seven individuals are alive in their seventies and 14 in their eighties.

Osteogenesis Imperfecta

Osteogenesis imperfecta (OI) is a multisystem collagen disease most noteworthy for bone involvement wherein fractures occur with only minimal trauma. The condition is inherited as an autosomal dominant with marked variable expressivity of the gene.[12]

We have reviewed the world literature on the subject through 1965 and found that cancer was reported infrequently in this disease (Table 22-III). These reports concern osteogenesis imperfecta tarda which in most instances does not impair normal expectations of longevity. Furthermore, the validity of the reports of malignancy in several of these studies is in question. The one instance reported by Bell[13] was based on a vague statement by Greenish[14] "... he is said to have died from cancer." The two cases suspected to be sarcoma found in families studied by Seedorff[12] were later proven to be normal on biopsy. The study by Werner[15]

showing three cases of sarcoma associated with OI in members of a family did not contain histologic verifications. This point is exceedingly important in that the hyperplastic callous formation during healing at the fracture site in OI may simulate sarcoma in every detail only to be proven normal when a biopsy is obtained.[16-18] Finally, our review of the subject has shown only one additional malignancy, namely that of Roschlau[17] showing sarcoma (histologically verified) in a patient with OI. However, this case must be evaluated from the standpoint of another disease which this patient had, namely the Rothmund syndrome, in addition to OI.

Diabetes Mellitus

Diabetes and cancer have many interesting features in common, the most prominent of which is the fact that both are chronic diseases with a relatively late age of onset. Thus, their prevalence significantly outnumbers incidence. In many cases hereditary factors have been strongly invoked for these diseases although in each there are also many examples wherein environmental factors appear to be of critical importance in their etiology. In turn, each disease may be

TABLE 22-III
TABLE OF REPORTED MALIGNANCIES FOUND IN WORLD LITERATURE
ASSOCIATED IN OSTEOGENESIS IMPERFECTA

	Date Reviewed	Number of Families Studied	Total Number Afflicted With OI	Number With Malignancy
Bell	to 1928	102	605	—
Greenish				1*
Seedorff	to 1948	55	180	2**
Jewell and Lofstrom				1
Werner				3*
Blatt				1
Caniggia et al.	to 1958	4	20	0
Lynch	to 1965	—	—	—
Roschlau		1	2	1
Total		162	807	9

* Unconfirmed.
** Biopsy normal.

associated with a wide range of endocrino-logic abnormalities including the well established aberrations in carbohydrate tolerance. Thus, with such common ground as this, it is not surprising that intense interest has been expressed in the possibility of meaningful associations between these two diseases.[19]

Limitations to the interpretation of data linking cancer to diabetes are: 1) the problem of whether diabetes in a cancer patient results from a diabetogenic action of the tumor and/or some type of hormonal imbalance related to the tumor; 2) whether diabetes mellitus per se is a disease either predisposing to cancer in certain patients or whether the presence of this disease protects or spares the patient from the development of cancer. To help resolve these issues scientifically so that meaningful data might be obtained would obviously be a major undertaking. Unfortunately, at the present time no data exists which can materially elucidate the problem. Practically all of the available information is retrospective.[19] The majority of studies fail to take into consideration the family history of cancer and/or of diabetes mellitus and in many cases the data fail to clearly illuminate the chronological relationship of these diseases. A prospective study of a large series of patients with diabetes mellitus is needed with careful medical evaluation of the diabetes history and laboratory findings with a well documented family history of diabetes, cancer, and other disorders. Finally, a matched control population, selected for the absence of diabetes mellitus, should be available. A study of this magnitude would obviously be expensive and would require a prolonged period of time; nevertheless it would undoubtedly be of merit in helping to settle the controversy about the association of diabetes mellitus and cancer.

An extensive review of the current literature has been provided by Kessler[19] covering several categories of the problem as follows: 1) clinical studies of carbohydrate metabolism in cancer patients; 2) laboratory studies of carbohydrate metabolism of tumors; 3) studies of cancer and diabetes in autopsy populations; 4) studies of cancer risk among diabetics; and 5) miscellaneous studies.

This extensive review uncovered a serious problem which influenced the majority of these works, namely, the fact that methods utilized in the study of patients and controls as well as the criteria for assessing diabetes differed widely. However, in spite of these shortcomings, when all studies were considered collectively, clinical evidence supported a positive association between cancer and a concomitant dysfunction in sugar metabolism. These studies were retrospective and a temporal relationship in this association could not be elucidated; nor could information be obtained concerning metabolic derangement, particularly with respect to whether it was characteristic of cancer or whether it was consistent with the presence of a chronic disease in general.

On the other hand, in contrast to the positive association between diabetes and cancer in the clinical studies, a negative association between cancer and diabetes was observed in the majority of the autopsy-based studies. However, methodologic problems in these studies, as in the clinical studies, impose limitations and warrant caution in their interpretation. For example, a bias may have been present in that cancer patients may have been preferentially selected for autopsy when compared with patients dying from diabetes mellitus. Also, the number of autopsies may differ among certain ethnic, racial and socioeconomic groups, and as a result a particular group may be more prone to diabetes, but less likely to have autopsies performed. While the autopsy data in general tended to show a decreased association with cancer, one noteworthy exception was found in pancreatic carcinoma, the prevalence of which was significantly increased among descendants of diabetic patients.

Kessler[20] evaluated cancer mortality among 21,447 diabetic patients who were seen at the Joslyn Clinic in Boston during a 26 year period ending in 1956. This analysis was made through the calculation of standardized mortality ratios wherein the observed numbers of deaths due to cancer were compared with those expected for age and sex specific ratios from the general Massachusetts population during the same period of time. Results showed that cancer mortality among the female diabetic patients was approximately that which was found in the general population of Massachusetts. However, in contrast to the females, the male diabetics showed a significantly reduced risk for death from cancer. This reduced cancer risk was even present when deaths from lung cancer were included. Kessler suggested that this reduced cancer risk among the diabetics was attributable to two factors, namely an excessive risk of deaths from other causes among the diabetics (excluding cancer), and an over representation of Jews among the diabetic patients. This study confirmed previous studies which indicated an increased risk of death from carcinoma of the pancreas among patients with diabetes mellitus. However, the explanation for this association is exceedingly complex and may involve possible carcinogenic potentialities of exogenous animal insulin influence. Finally, Kessler's data[20] provided evidence that diabetic females did not show an increased mortality from endometrial carcinoma. This observation is in contradistinction to several large retrospective studies of endometrial carcinoma patients.[21-23] Interestingly, diabetes mellitus has been shown to be negatively correlated with intracranial neoplasms.[24]

Glucose-6-Phosphate Dehydrogenase (G-6-PD)

Glucose-6-phosphate dehydrogenase deficiency is inherited as a sex-linked factor. Beaconsfield, *et al.*[25] noted an inverse association between G-6-PD deficiency and cancer mortality. These observations were based primarily on comparisons between occidental and oriental Jews. Thus, these findings suggested that individuals with G-6-PD deficiency have a relatively decreased cancer risk when they are compared with nondeficient individuals.

Naik and Anderson[26] found a lower frequency of G-6-PD deficiency in both male and female American Negroes when compared with controls.

Kessler[27] suggested a similar inverse association between diabetes and cancer, based in part, upon the positive association between diabetes mellitus and G-6-PD deficiency.

The associations between G-6-PD deficiency, cancer, and diabetes mellitus merit further study. It also suggests the importance of searching for additional biochemical factors in studies of cancer prone as well as cancer resistant genotypes.

It has been suggested that a hereditary deficiency of G-6-PD may inhibit the hexosemonophosphate (HMP) glycolytic pathway and thus diminish the risk of developing cancer.[25] The relatively high incidence of G-6-PD deficiency among Oriental Israeli males[28] and the low cancer death rates reported for this group[29] may be correlated through this mechanism. And, in view of the heightened proclivity of Jews to the development of diabetes,[30] it may be of some significance that the HMP shunt is stimulated by insulin and depressed in diabetes mellitus.

Cancer Variations in Families in a Normal Population*

Despite world-wide interest in the epidemiology of cancer, the literature includes very little reliable data on the distribution of cancer in families derived from large numbers of consecutively ascertained normal subjects in the general population.

We studied cancer occurrences in the families of more than 4,000 consecutively ascertained normal subjects (constituting more than 5,000 families) who were under evaluation at two geographically separate medical centers. Special attention was given to carcinoma of the breast. (See Chapter 20).

Family histories of cancer of all anatomic sites were evaluated in more than 4,000 consecutive persons who underwent either routine cancer screening examination in a mobile multiphasic cancer detection unit (group I /Omaha/, all ages considered, 3,261 patients) or were seen as part of a breast milk study (group II /Detroit/, women 45 years or younger, 1,058 patients), from which 2,044 maternal and paternal lineages were studied. These investigations were conducted independently at the two medical centers.

Approximately one half of all families studied did not manifest any evidence of cancer. In 33.2 percent of group I families and 29.3 percent of group II families, cancer occurred in one first degree relative; two or more first degree relatives had cancer in 20.2 percent of families in group I and 24.1 percent in group II. Comparison of the results of the cancer histories of group I and group II show great similarity, though ascertained independently at the two medical centers. This same observation was present for practically all statistical categories in this study, regardless of the specific histologic variety of cancer or the specific age category analyzed.

Differential Cancer Expression in Families of Variable Cancer Probands

In any cancer prone population certain histologic varieties of cancer may occur in excess; therefore, it is logical that other varieties of cancer would occur less frequently in these particular individuals. For example, childhood leukemia with its high death rate would obviously restrict the occurrence of many of the adenocarcinomas and other forms of cancer which more typically occur in adulthood. Similarly, patients with autosomal dominantly inherited familial polyposis coli harbor a high risk for adenocarcinoma of the colon (assuming that prophylactic colectomies have not been performed); this will then restrict the occurrence of other malignant neoplasms in affected patients due primarily to their high death rate from colon cancer.

Our studies have shown that specific patterns of malignant neoplasms may occur in excess in certain cancer prone families. For example, this might involve a wide assortment of differing histologic varieties of cancer, i.e., the familial complex of brain tumors, sarcoma, leukemia, and breast cancer, as discussed in Chapters 17 and 20. In certain families showing differing histologic varieties of cancer, certain specific malignant neoplasms occur infrequently. Again, death from the predominant cancers comprising the particular familial cancer syndrome may be a significant factor. An example of this is demonstrated in the cancer family syndrome which is characterized by a variety of adenocarcinomas, particularly adenocarcinoma of the colon and endometrium. In this particular situation carcinoma of the uterine cervix occurs only rarely in the face of a marked excess of endometrial carcinoma. It might be argued that factors which predispose these patients

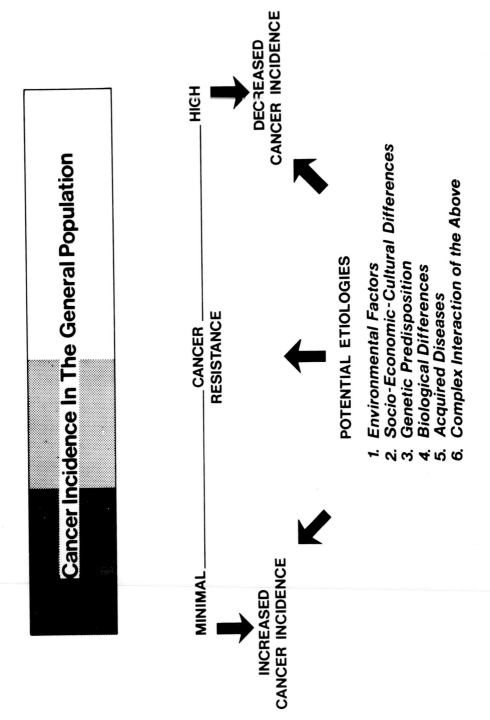

Figure 22–3. Diagrammatic scheme depicting variation in cancer resistance in the general population.

to endometrial carcinoma, possibly certain endocrine aberrations, might also counteract the development of cervical cancer.

It is conceivable that we are dealing with a complex problem of cancer predisposition as well as cancer resistance for specific histologic varieties of cancer in the general population and in certain families. For example, Kaposi's sarcoma predisposition occurs frequently in the Bantu of South Africa while squamous and basal cell carcinomas of the skin occur rarely (probably due to resistance from pigmentation) in these individuals. (See Chapter 19).

We have assembled data from three of our ongoing cancer genetic studies. The first study deals with 154 probands with verified adenocarcinoma of the colon, seen in the greater Omaha area during 1964. This represented the total incidence of colon cancer in this community during the single year. The second study involved breast cancer probands seen at the University of Nebraska College of Medicine. This involved 89 pathologically verified breast cancer cases. The third study involved lung cancer probands seen at the Omaha Veterans Administration Hospital (91 verified cases) and the University of Nebraska College of Medicine (39 verified cases), (for a total of 130 lung cancer cases). The present discussion will focus upon the distribution of cancer of all anatomic sites in the families of these probands from these three studies.

Figure 22–3 provides a diagramatic model indicating our theoretical concept which designates cancer resistance as a continuum with extremes of marked resistance versus minimal resistance. Using this model we speculate that in the case of the occurrence of cancer of all anatomic sites in families in the general population we might find families with a specific histologic type and/or multiple anatomic sites manifesting an increased incidence while other families have significantly less cancer prevalence. Factors that determine cancer resistance or susceptibility may be primarily environmental, genetic, and/or result from an interaction of these factors. The interaction of genetic and environmental factors much more likely will explain the overwhelming majority of these cases.

Table 22-IV and Figure 22–4 present the cancer distribution of the families in the three studies taking all anatomic sites of cancer into consideration. Note that the familial distribution of cancer of all anatomic sites in the three studies is remarkably similar with respect to the total number of cancers per family. For example, families in the colon cancer study showed approximately 49 percent absence of cancer in first degree relatives; those in the lung cancer studies showed 45 percent absence of cancer in first degree relatives; and finally, those in the breast cancer study showed 40 percent absence of cancer in first degree relatives. In the other extreme, namely cancer proneness (or decreased cancer resistance), we find that 6 percent of the colon cancer families had three or more first degree

TABLE 22-IV
FAMILY HISTORY OF ALL CANCER SITES IN FIRST-DEGREE RELATIVES

No. of Relatives	Colon Study (154) No.	Colon Study (154) %	Lung Study (130) No.	Lung Study (130) %	Breast (89) No.	Breast (89) %
Proband only	76	49	58	45	36	40
Proband + one relative	40	26	34	26	18	20
Proband + two relatives	18	12	27	21	17	19
Proband + three or more relatives	9	6	11	8	7	8
No information Colon (11)						
Breast (11)						

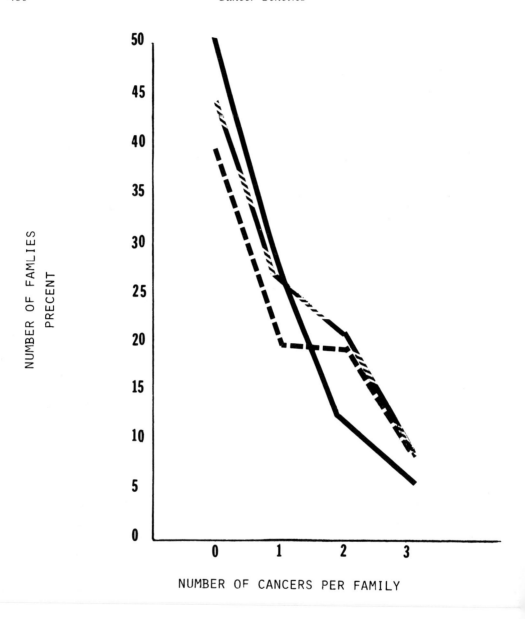

NUMBER OF CANCERS PER FAMILY

COLON
BREAST
LUNG

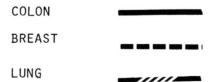

Figure 22–4. Family history of cancer of all sites in the three studies involving colon, breast and ovary.

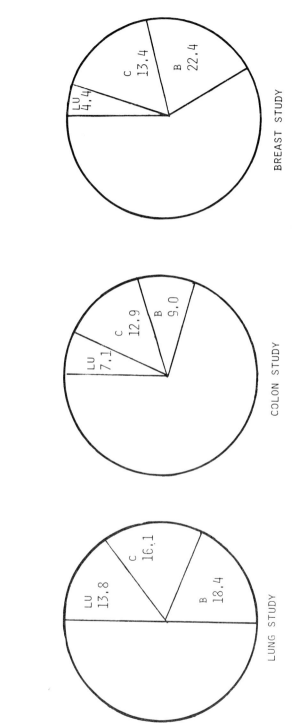

Figure 22–5. Common cancer associations (percent) in the three studies.

relatives with cancer; while 8 percent of the families from the lung cancer study had three or more first degree relatives with cancer; and finally, 8 percent of the families with breast cancer had three or more relatives with cancer of all anatomic sites. Thus, of the three most commonly occurring cancers affecting man, we find a remarkably similar pattern of relative cancer resistance versus relative cancer proneness when considering all anatomic varieties of cancer.

Common cancer associations in the three studies, such as (a) colon cancer in association with colon, lung and breast cancer; (b) lung cancer in association with lung, colon, and breast cancer; (c) and breast cancer in association with colon, lung and breast cancer are shown in Table 22-V and Figure 22–5. Interestingly, carcinoma of the colon was relatively uniformly distributed in the families from these three studies.

Note that carcinoma of the lung (Figure 22–5) as opposed to colon cancer, shows a nonuniform distribution. Specifically we find 13.8% association with lung, 4.4% association with breast, and 7.1% association with colon. A similar nonuniform pattern is found with respect to the breast cancer. The associations being 9.0% with colon cancer, 18.4% with lung cancer and 22.4% with breast cancer. The distribution of these cancer associations in families suggests that certain factors influence resistance or susceptibility to site specific cancers which differ according to the cancer site. For example, in the case of lung cancer the nonuniform distribution could be due to a stronger component of environmental forces while in breast cancer it could be due to endogenous (hormonal) and genetic influences. Therefore, the basis for cancer resistance cannot be made solely on the association of specific cancer sites but must also take into consideration certain biological, environmental and genetic factors. These data while novel must be evaluated cautiously. They are presented primarily to stimulate further investigations.

Comment

In spite of intensive studies in cancer epidemiology during the past several decades, the role of heredity in cancer remains enigmatic. Moreover, surprisingly little is known about the frequency of low and high risk cancer families in the general population. The majority of studies in cancer genetics have been concerned with relatively large numbers of cancer probands and their families showing a specific anatomic variety of cancer compared with families of matched controls selected for the absence of that particular type of cancer.[31,32,33] Other studies have involved various cancer predisposing syndromes such as familial polyposis coli, Gardner's syndrome, von Recklinghausen's neurofibromatosis, hereditary exostoses, multiple nevoid basal cell carcinoma syndrome, and others,[34] as well as selected cancer prone families lacking associated

TABLE 22-V
COMMON CANCER ASSOCIATIONS IN THE THREE STUDIES

| | Colon Study (154) | | Lung Study (130) | | Breast Study (89) | |
	No.	%	No.	%	No.	%
Colon	20	12.9	21	16.1	12	13.4
Lung	11	7.1	18	13.8	4	4.4
Breast	14	9.0	24	18.4	20	22.4

physical stigmata, such as Family G of Warthin.[35]

An interesting observation from these data is that approximately one half of all the families studied showed an absence of cancer (all sites) in first degree relatives of the screened individuals. On the other hand, only approximately 7 percent of all families studied show a marked predominance (three or more cancers among first degree relatives) of cancer (all sites). These observations reveal a lack of uniformity in cancer distribution in families, and suggest that some of the families may be relatively cancer resistant while others may be relatively cancer prone. Nonuniformity of cancer distribution is observed repeatedly when specific histologic varieties of cancer are studied in different areas of the world. While the overall frequency of cancer of specific anatomic sites varies from country to country and continent to continent, the overall frequency of cancer of all anatomic sites in the total population remains remarkably similar. However, the worldwide cancer statistics do not reflect cancer incidence in individual families, although this situation prevails at the infrahuman level.[1] While specific strains of mice are cancer resistant, other strains are remarkably cancer prone.[6,7] Preliminary investigations by Lynch and Krush[36] based upon detailed studies of a limited number of families showed that certain kindreds have a marked paucity of cancer (frequency of 1% or less) while other families were classified as cancer prone with rates of cancer exceeding 40 percent. Moreover, when individual branches of these cancer prone families were carefully analyzed, it was found that cancer rates in some branches were as high as 50 percent, demonstrating that cancer frequency may vary considerably even within families due possibly to the segregation of the gene(s) predisposing to

cancer. Furthermore, while individuals were members of different branches of the family, their environment exposures, occupations, habit patterns and general socio-economic and educational backgrounds did not differ significantly. Therefore, we suggest that cancer prone genotypes as well as cancer resistant genotypes may exist in the population. Findings in this study are consistent with this hypothesis.

Our data indicates that multiple breast cancer prone families occur infrequently in the population with approximately 12 sporadic or nonfamilial occurrences to every multiple case family. This undoutedly is an underestimate of multiple breast cancer prone families since breast cancer occurs relatively late in adulthood; thus, patients at risk for this disease may die from other causes before developing breast cancer. Also, other histologic varieties of cancer may be occurring in so-called breast cancer prone families. Thus, if certain potentially breast cancer prone families had an excess of males, these individuals might manifest other varieties of tumors such as carcinoma of the gastrointestinal tract and, lacking females at risk for breast cancer, the families might go unrecognized as breast cancer families. In addition, ascertainment for breast cancer may not be complete in every family studied.

We found breast cancer associated with carcinoma of the breast, stomach and colon most frequently in both groups. There is epidemiologic precedence for these observations. For example, Hill and associates[37] were impressed with striking similarities between the epidemiology of breast and colon cancer, i.e. both tumors show similar geographic variations and both occur more frequently in higher socio-economic groups. They suggested that the incidence of these tumors may be correlated with variation in the fat content of the diet. Lynch and associates[38,39] have confirmed familial associations between cancer of the stomach and colon in the study of a large number of breast cancer prone families as well as from retrospective and prospective studies of the families of a relatively large number of colon cancer probands. In addition, in a review of a large series of multiple primary malignant neoplasms, Schoenburg and associates[40] found that colon cancer was the most frequently occurring extra primary malignant neoplasm associated with breast cancer.

Carcinoma of the breast may also be associated with carcinoma of the ovary and endometrium. Familial associations of these lesions were reported previously by Lynch and associates,[41,42] and the literature includes similar documented observations by others. In addition, Schottenfeld and Berg[43] reported a positive association of multiple primary carcinomas of the breast, ovary, and endometrium, suggesting demographic characteristics and etiologic factors common to these diseases. Geographic and racial variations in these lesions are also consistent with these associations. For example, Smith[44] showed that death rates from cancer of the breast, uterine corpus and ovary were lower among Japanese-Americans than in the general United States population, while death rates from cancer of the breast and ovary tended to be higher in Japanese-Americans than in native Japanese. Thus, certain unknown factors appear to influence the association of carcinoma of the breast and ovary causing an increase in rates of both of these lesions in migrant Japanese and their descendants.

While genetic implications have been discussed throughout, it should be understood that the type of associations we have mentioned do not restrict the etiologic issue to genetic or host factors. Rather, they suggest the importance of *familial* factors, which could be either primary genetic factors or common environmental exposures and/or interactions of both of these phenomena. Thus, it should be realized that the family history is just one of many epidemiologic variables in the cancer problem; and, in the case of breast cancer, additional risk factors must be carefully appraised, including geographic variations, age at first pregnancy, age at menarche, natural or surgical menopause, the presence or absence of benign breast cancer, exposures to certain medications including hormones and tranquilizers, diet, particularly fat content, height and weight and, finally, we must consider the intricate problems involving interactions by multiples of these factors.[45,46] Thus, the ideal cancer genetic study should be designed with careful consideration of genealogy, confirmation of cancer, search for genetic markers in order to aid in the eventual understanding of genetic mechanisms and, finally, it should evaluate these phenomena in context with the myriad environmental interactions of the patient.[36,39,42,47] While Mac-Mahon and associates[47] have correctly called attention to risk events (pregnancy) early in the life of the patient, we would like to extend the concept back to conception. Thus, in certain circumstances, genetic factors may predispose the patient to breast cancer, particularly when other initiating events, i.e. possibly oncogenic viruses, are present and thereby acting in concert with cancer-predisposing genomes.

Conclusions

Variation is a ubiquitous biological phenomenon, complex in its origin, involving interactions of genetic determinants, environmental determinants, and the individual's activities. The familial clustering of disease may result from genetic or environmental factors or from interactions of both intrinsic and extrinsic factors. Different points of view and varied lines of attack are entirely justified and natural products of the vast amount of data already published.

The medical literature includes many references to so-called host factors, testifying to ancient as well as contemporary observations that causes are to be found in the characteristics of individual members of the population affected, as well as in the environments in which both host and 'causative agent' are found. In order to recognize the role of the 'host' in the etiology of a disease, the nature of genetic-environment interaction must be understood: an individual's genotype determines an indefinite but limited assortment of different phenotypes associated with differences in environment. When there is a manifest difference between members of two extended kinships in their cancer risks, then two or more different genotypes are involved with different constitutional effects associated with different cancer diatheses, and/or environmental circumstances are involved which increase the nongenetic differences of the liability. Both types of relevant variables are extremely difficult to discern in a heterogeneous population of affected individuals, especially if multiple etiologies are involved. Therefore, we have endeavored to determine and characterize familial clusters of high-cancer-risk individuals as well as familial clusters with remarkably low cancer risks. These studies indicate that factors relevant to cancer diatheses and cancer resistance show familial associations. Future studies on such families will endeavor to identify familial variables associated with the differences in cancer predisposition and resistance.

Discussion

Cancer resistance may be determined on a multifactorial basis. Therefore, it is reasonable to ask the question, "Are families which show a remarkable freedom from cancer receiving this protection on the basis of multiple-gene-transmitted constitutional characters?" Falconer[48] suggests that, when considering diseases which may fall into the category of multifactorial inheritance, one should consider together both genetic and environmental factors which make a particular individual more or less likely to develop a disease such as cancer or diabetes mellitus, and that these should be combined into a single measure which he refers to as the individual's "liability." He reasons that the "liabilities" (susceptibility) of individuals in a population form continuous variables and that the apparent discontinuities between "affected" and "normal" arise from "threshold" differences at some levels of the liabilities. Thus, individuals with liabilities above the threshold are affected, and individuals with liabilities below the threshold are not. The liability of any one individual cannot be measured with precision. On the other hand, however, mean liability may be evaluated for a population or group from the incidence of the disease in that population or group. Thus, liability can in principle be expressed in units on a scale that renders its distribution normal (i.e. fitting a Gaussian or normal curve), and measurements of the mean liability are the standard deviations on the scale.

According to Falconer[48]

The analysis provides an estimate of the correlation between relatives in respect to liability, and this leads, with certain assumptions, to an estimate of the heritability of liability in the population. The heritability is the proportion of the variance of liability that is ascribable to additive genetic variance. This is the nearest to which one may approach, with human data, the degree of genetic determination of liability. The data required for the analysis are the incidence of the disease in the population and the incidence in relatives of affected propositi drawn from the population.

The liability or proneness to a disorder is a function of interacting environmental and genetic factors. These factors operate in differing orders of magnitude depending upon the individual's specific genetic and environmental circumstances. Thus, when environmental factors are more significant, the relative effects of hereditary factors will be less significant. Families like A and B (cancer-resistant) and certain cancer-prone families discussed elsewhere in this book may be associated with environments which are not strikingly different from each other. These families, however, show different heritabilities of cancer predisposition and resistance.

A heritability determination is an estimate of the proportion of the total phenotypic variation (i.e. individual differences) that can be attributed to genetic variation in a single generation of some particular population under one set of environmental conditions. The heritability of cancer may be defined as the extent to which variation in individual risk of acquiring cancer is due to genetic differences. A disease will show a greater-than-zero heritability if two or more segregating genetic alleles, which manifest different effects upon predisposition and resistance to the disease, occur on at least one chromosomal locus. Such a trait may show different heritabilities in different populations which are characterized by genotypic and/or environmental differences, because the manifestations of any particular gene depend upon interactions between that gene and the overall genotype as well as with nongenetic or environmental variables. An individual's predisposition or resistance to a particular disease process depends upon that individual's genetic norm or range of reaction and the environmental factors interacting with his genotype. A genetic factor may be manifested only be appropriate genotype-environment combinations. A gene's harmfulness or usefulness is determined by the bearer's environment. Thus, the genetic epidemiologist functions as an ecologist seeking significant correlations between a disorder and one or another variable from the great array of environmental influences. One's success in such research is related to the uniqueness of the variable and the directness of its effect, to the frequency of the disorder, and to the ease of diagnosing the disorder.

In families with the cancer family syndrome discussed in Chapter 19 an autosomal dominant genetic factor has been postulated; but in Families A and B, it is not possible to delineate a simple Mendelian pattern of genetic transmission for an alleged cancer resistance. Of the few cancers that have developed in kindreds A and B, most can be accounted for on an environmental basis. On the other hand, tumors in the cancer-prone branches of the families with the cancer family syndrome indicate a meaningful pattern or association.

The available vital statistics in all of these families range from the early part of the nineteenth century to the present time. During the period before World War II, more persons died from infectious diseases, childbirth, etc., than at the present time. It is also relevant to consider the number who died or were killed during or after the major U.S. and foreign wars of the nineteenth and twentieth centuries. These conditions have all affected the longevity figures in the studied families.

For further testing of the above hypothesis, an analysis of cancer occurrences from the standpoint of families prone to the disease as well as families showing a paucity of malignant neoplasms is needed. Furthermore, additional analyses must be made of the particular varieties of cancer, given the known epidemiological factors relating to the specific malignant neoplasms. For example, smoking is associated with bronchogenic carcinoma; promiscuity, multiple matings, and poor female hygiene, are associated with carcinoma of the uterine cervix, etc.[49]

The cancer epidemiologist must constantly scrutinize all possible hereditary and environmental factors which could be of etiologic importance in the development of cancer. Unfortunately, many studies have concerned themselves only with single carcinogenic factors. Very few attempts have been made to relate nongenetic factors to host factors, e.g. cigarette smoking and family history[50] (Chapter 13) solar radiation and cancer induction in patients with xeroderma pigmentosum (Chapter 21). Few studies have been specifically concerned with cancer resistance in humans.[9,10]

The observations brought forth in this chapter show a wide variation in tumor incidence among four extended families. They also demonstrate marked variability in cancer distribution in families of *normal* individuals from the general population. Biological variations structure the expectation that such distributions might occur in many families. Marked variations in life span exist between different species and between individuals within a given species. Goldstein[51] stated that this phenomenon implicates genetic factors and suggested that an explanation for variations in the aging process resides "in genomes with either different genetic programs or specific rates of mutability." Since cancer is generally an age-related disease, it is consistent with Goldstein's hypothesis that certain genetic programs "turn on" in different individuals in our population and thus elicit different diseases which partly account for variations in life expectancy of those individuals. Untreated patients with such classically inherited disorders as familial polyposis coli (Mendelian autosomal dominant) show a marked reduction in longevity due to the development of adenocarcinoma of the colon at a relatively early age as the result of an inherited cancer diathesis associated with disease. Xeroderma pigmentosum is another example of a hereditary disease (Mendelian autosomal recessive) which imposes a serious compromise on a patient's longevity. Other families are prone to coronary artery disease, either through inheritance of lipid or other metabolic abnormalities and/or gene-transmitted differences for factors yet undetermined but which predispose to coronary artery disease. Such individuals are additional examples of persons whose longevity may be seriously compromised by gene-transmitted constitutional characteristics. It is reasonable to postulate that genetic differences play prominent roles in a family's cancer proneness as well as its cancer resistance. This observation does not exclude the role of nongenetic factors such as the interaction of an oncogenic virus in a genetically and immunologically susceptible host whose constitution favors the development of malignant neoplasms.

The genetic basis of a disease is a reflection of the genetic basis of health and that due to the interaction of the large number of relevant hereditary factors or genes and the large number of environmental factors which influence the liability of persons of any given constitution to the particular disease.[51] The first step in understanding the etiologic role of biological heredity is to realize that the genotype (i.e. total genetic material) of an individual, the chromosomal material derived from his parents, is a set of potentialities and not a set of already-formed or predetermined characteristics. The relative contributions of heredity and environment for a particular disease differ with different overall heredities (i.e. total genotypes) and with different environments.

The only unequivocally reliable approach to a nonexperimental system is deferment of any final determination of the relevant modes of genetic transmission until each responsible gene can be recognized. An alternative investigative approach involves comparative studies in members of high-risk versus those in low-risk or sporadic families.[52] Even if predisposition to a given disease in an individual may be associated with a simple Mendelian mode of genetic transmission, some cases would be sporadic due to occurrence of phenocopies (i.e. the apparently same disease, characteristically associated with a particular gene or group of genes, brought about as a manifestation of other etiologies), diagnostic errors, etc.

The demonstration of both the occurrence of sporadic cancer occurrences (as in Families A and B) and of familial cases (as in the cancer family syndrome) shows heterogeneity in data which were previously considered as if they were homogeneous. Such data even show that the risk in selected families is great enough to suggest a simple genetic hypothesis[53] for transmission of major differences in the predisposition to cancer. The data have not established that any particular genotype is either necessary or sufficient for development of cancer. They do show, however, that certain types of cancer are particularly liable to develop in genetically predisposed individuals. Whether or not the disease actually develops in a genetically predisposed individual, or at

what age it develops, and details of its symptomatology and severity, are determined by interactions with environmental variables and other genes. The happenings of nature are characterized by probability laws, rather than by simple causality.[54] The cancer epidemiologist can define his best posits, but he never knows beforehand whether or not they will come true in any specific case.

Summary

We have attempted to show that certain families in the general population show a profound paucity of cancer as demonstrated in families A and B. Certain genetic disorders such as diabetes mellitus and G-6-PD may show a negative correlation with cancer. Furthermore, we have demonstrated that a sizeable proportion of the normal population (approximately 46%) show an absence of cancer amongst first degree relatives, while a minority of the population (approximately 7%) are cancer prone, as evidenced by three or more occurrences of cancer in first degree relatives.

These findings have implications for research in carcinogenesis, in that it may be as important to know why certain members of the population are at *reduced* risk for cancer as it is to know why those in the population are remarkably *cancer prone*. Cancer control implications also exist in that an important risk factor to be considered in any cancer control program is family history. This even applies to other obvious risk factors such as cigarette smoking, wherein it is well known that family history of lung cancer significantly increases the likelihood of the cigarette smoker developing lung cancer.

Finally, these studies indicate a wide range of cancer susceptibility in humans, a phenomenon that is a function of both genetic and nongenetic factors, and which is very similar to findings observed at the infra-human level.

REFERENCES

1. Lynch, H.T.: Hereditary factors in carcinoma. In *Recent Results in Cancer Research.* New York, Springer-Verlag, 1967.

2. Steward, G.T.: Limitations of the germ theory. *Lancet, 1*:1077–1081, 1968.

3. Gianferrari, L., and Morganti, G.: Ricerche sulla familiaritá neoplastica. *Acta Genet Med Gemellol, 6*:217–224, 1957.

4. Beolchini, P.E., Cresseri, A., Gianferrari, L., Malcovati, P., and Morganti, G.: Ricerche genetiche sulle neoplasia dell' utero I. *Acta Genet Med Gemellol (Roma), 5*:462–468, 1956.

5. Serra, A., and Soini, A.: Ricerche sulla familiaritá del carcinoma ovarico. *Acta Genet Med Gemellol, 8*:1–22, 1959.

6. Jacobs, B.B.: Growth of tumors in allogenic hosts after organ culture explanation, II tumor-host interactions. *J Natl Cancer Inst, 42*:537–543, 1969.

7. Stern, K., and Goldfeder, A.: Radiation studies on mice of an inbred tumor-resistant strain, VI., immune responses to heterologous red cells of nonirradiated and radiated mice. *Int Arch Allergy, 35*:504 513, 1969.

8. Water, N.F., and Burmester, B.R.: Mode of inheritance of resistance of rous sarcoma virus in chickens. *J Natl Cancer Inst, 27*: 655–661, 1961.

9. Moore, G.E.: Cancer immunity: fact or fiction? *Tex Med, 64*:54–59, 1969.

10. Hellström, I., Hellström, K.E., Pierce, G.E., and Yang, J.P.S.: Cellular and humoral immunity to different types of human neoplasms. *Nsture, 220*:1352–1354, 1968.

11. Stephenson, H.E., Delmex, J.A., Renden, D.E., Kimpton, R.S., Todd, P.C., Charron, T.L., and Lindberg, D.A.B.: Host immunity and spontaneous regression of cancer evaluated by computerized data reduction study. *Surg Gynecol Obstet, 133*:649–655, 1971.

12. Seedorff, K.S.: *Osteogenesis Imperfecta; a Study of Clinical Features and Heredity Based on 55 Danish Families Comprising 180 Affected Members.* Arhus, Uneversitetsforlaget, 1949.

13. Bell, J.: *Blue Sclerotics and Fragility of Bone.*

New York, Cambridge U Pr, 1925, pp. 269–324.

14. Greenish, R.W.: A case of hereditary tendency to fragilitas ossium. *Br Med J, 2*:966–967, 1880.

15. Werner, R.: Mehrfaches Vorkommen Einer Neigung Zu Knochenbruchen und Sarkomentwicklung in Einer Familie. *Z fur Krebsforsch, 32*:40–42, 1930.

16. Koskinen, E.V.S.: Massive hyperplastic callus formation stimulating osteogenic sarcoma in osteogenesis imperfecta; report of a severe case. *Ann Chir Gynaecol Fenn, 47*: 257 271, 1958.

17. Roschlau, G.: Rothmund-Syndrome, Kombiniert Mit Osteogenesis Imperfecta Tarda und Sarkom des Oberschenkels. *Z Kinderheilk, 86*:289–298, 1962.

18. Caniggia, A., Stuart, C., and Guideri, R.: Fragilitas ossium hereditaria tarda; Ekman-Lobstein disease. *Acta Med Scand* [Suppl], *340*:1–172, 1958.

19. Kessler, I.I.: Cancer and diabetes mellitus: a review of the literature. *J Chronic Dis, 23*:579–600, 1971.

20. Kessler, I.I.: Cancer mortality among diabetics. *J Natl Cancer Inst, 44*:673–686, 1970.

21. Moss, W.T.: Common peculiarities of patients with adenocarcinoma of the endometrium; with special reference to obesity, body build, diabetes and hypertension. *Am J Roentgenol, 58*:203–210, 1947.

22. Benjamin, F.: Glucose tolerance in dysfunctional uterine bleeding and in carcinoma of the endometrium. *Br Med J, 1*:1243–1246, 1960.

23. Lynch, H.T., Krush, A.J., and Larsen, A.L.: Endometrial carcinoma: multiple primary malignancies, constitutional factors, and heredity. *J Med Sci, 252*:381–390, 1966.

24. Aronson, S.M., and Aronson, B.E.: Central nervous system in diabetes mellitus: lowered frequency of certain intracranial neoplasms. *Arch Neurol, 12*:390–398, 1965.

25. Beaconsfield, P., Rainsbury, R., and Kalton, G.: Glucose-6-phosphate dehydrogenase deficiency and the incidence of cancer. *Oncologia* (Basel), *19*:11–19, 1965.

26. Naik, S.N., and Anderson, D.E.: The association between glucose-6-phosphate dehydrogenase deficiency and cancer in American Negroes. *Oncology, 25:*356–364, 1971.

27. Kessler, I.: A genetic relationship between diabetes and cancer. *Lancet, 1:*218–220, 1970.

28. Szeinberg, A., Sheba, C., and Adam, A.: Selective occurrence of glutathione instability in red blood corpuscles of various Jewish tribes. *Blood, 13:*1043–1053, 1958.

29. Kallner, G.: Mortality statistics in Israel; a survey of the years 1950–1960. *Israel Med J, 21:*1–11, 1962.

30. Entmacher, P.S., and Marks, H.H.: Diabetes in 1964, a world survey. *Diabetes, 14:*212–223, 1965.

31. Macklin, M.T.: Comparison of the number of breast cancer deaths observed in relatives of breast-cancer patients and the number expected on the basis of mortality rates. *J Natl Cancer Inst, 22:*927–951, 1959.

32. Oliver, C.P.: Studies on human cancer families. *Ann NY Acad Sci, 71:*1198–1212, 1958.

33. Penrose, L.S., MacKenzie, H.T., and Karn, M.N.: A genetical study of human mammary cancer. *Br J Cancer, 2:*168–176, 1948.

34. Lynch, H.T.: *Skin, Heredity, and Cancer.* Flushing, Med Exam, 1972.

35. Lynch, H.T., and Krush, A.J.: Cancer family "G" revisited: 1895–1970. *Cancer, 27:*1505–1511, 1971.

36. Lynch, H.T., Krush, A.J., and Kaplan, A.R.: Cancer frequency variations among and within families. *Acta Genet Med Gemellol, 21:*53–65, 1972.

37. Hill, M.J., Goddard, P., and Williams, R.E.O.: Gut bacteria and aetiology of cancer of the breast. *Lancet, 2:*472–473, 1971.

38. Lynch, H.T., Guirgis, H., Swartz, M., Lynch, J., Krush, A.J., and Kaplan, A.R.: Genetics and colon cancer. *Arch Surg, 106:*669–675, 1973.

39. Lynch, H.T., Krush, A.J., and Guirgis, H.: Genetic factors in families with combined gastrointestinal and breast cancer. *Am J Gastroenterol, 59,*31–40, 1973.

40. Schoenburg, B.S., Greenberg, R.A., and Eisenberg, H.: Occurrence of certain multiple primary cancers in females. *J Natl Cancer Inst, 43:*15–32, 1969.

41. Lynch, H.T., and Krush, A.J.: Carcinoma of the breast and ovary. *Surg Gynecol Obstet, 133:*644–648, 1971.

42. Lynch, H.T., Krush, A.J., Lemon, H.M., Kaplan, A.R., Condit, P.T., and Bottomley, R.H.: Tumor variation in families with breast cancer. *JAMA, 222:*1631–1635, 1972.

43. Schottenfeld, D., and Berg, J.: Incidence of multiple primary cancers. IV. Cancers of the female breast and genital organs. *J Natl Cancer Inst, 46:*161–170, 1971.

44. Smith, R.L.: Recorded and expected mortality among Japanese of the United States and Hawaii with special reference to cancer. *J Natl Cancer Inst, 17:*359–473, 1956.

45. Vakil, D.V., and Morgan, R.W.: Etiology of breast cancer. I. Genetic aspects. *Can Med Assoc J, 109:*29–32, 1973.

46. Vakil, D.V., and Morgan, R.W.: Etiology of breast cancer. II. Epidemiologic aspects. *Can Med Assoc J, 109:*201–206, 1973.

47. MacMahon, B., Cole, P., and Brown, J.: Etiology of human breast cancer: a review. *J Natl Cancer Inst, 50:*21–42, 1973.

48. Falconer, D.S.: The inheritance of liability to diseases with variable age of onset, with particular reference to diabetes mellitus. *Ann Hum Genet, 31:*1–20, 1967.

49. Beolchini, P.E., Cresseri, A., Gianferrari, L., Malcovati, P., and Morganti, G.: Ricerche Genetiche Sulle Neoplasie Dell' Utero III. *Acta Genet Med Gemellol (Roma), 7:*47–90, 1958.

50. Tokuhata, G.K.: Familial factors in human lung cancer and smoking. *Am J Public Health, 54:*24–32, 1964.

51. Goldstein, S.: The biology of aging. *New Engl J Med, 285:*1120–1129, 1971.

52. Morton, N.E.: *Computer Applications in Genetics,* Honolulu, U of Hawaii Pr, 1969.

53. Morton, N.E.: In Burdette, W.J., (Ed.): *Methodology in Human Genetics,* San Francisco, Holden-Day, 1962.

54. Reichenbach, H.: In Jarrett, J.L., and McMurrin, S.M., (Eds.): *Contemporary Philosophy.* New York, HRW, 1954.

CHAPTER 23

MISCELLANEOUS PROBLEMS, CANCER,

AND GENETICS

Henry T. Lynch

As knowledge accumulates about the importance of host factors and/or genetics in cancer, the complexity of these relationships becomes more apparent. For example, we know that a specific histologic type of cancer may in the majority of circumstances appear to be "nongenetic"; yet in certain circumstances simple inheritance patterns might prevail. This is seen in the case of carotid body tumors wherein only 3 percent appear to be inherited (autosomal dominant). It is also apparent in esophageal cancer in which environmental factors such as cigarette smoking, alcoholism, and poor socioeconomic background appear to be of etiologic importance. Yet we find esophageal cancer occurring in exceedingly rare circumstances in association with keratosis palmaris et plantaris where it behaves as a classical autosomal dominant.[1] Of course, intriguing questions pertain to those as yet uknown genetic and/or environmental factors which may exist in certain families which predispose certain relatives to carotid body tumors on the one hand and to esophageal cancer on the other. We believe that a search for constitutional or host factors in context with nongenetic factors, utilizing a broad epidemiologic approach to the problem in families prone to these as well as many other varieties of cancer, might in due time provide vital information about carcinogenesis.

The purpose of this chapter is to discuss a variety of cancer problems which have not previously been described in detail in this book; these will include certain diseases or traits which appear to have a cancer association, which show either a simple genetic inheritance pattern or which appear to be "familial" in that they occur in excess in certain families, though precise etiologic factors have yet to be determined. Finally, new and developing areas of research in cancer genetics will be discussed briefly.

Cancer and Collagen Diseases

Inter-relationships between autoimmune phenomena, collagen disease, and cancer have received considerable attention in the quest for cancer etiology particularly in the study of such diseases as lupus erythematosus, dermatomyositis, and scleroderma.[1-4] An experimental animal model, namely New Zealand Black (NZB) in-bred strains of mice, is now available in which spontaneous lymphoma and autoimmune hemolytic anemia arise.[5] It is also established that normal immune mechanisms are dependent upon the normal functioning of lymphocytes and plasmacytes; however, these laboratory animals provide a model in which to study mechanisms involved when abnormal lymphocytes proliferate and in turn produce abnormal globulins which may react with normal tissues of the host and lead to the production of an "autoimmune state."[6,7]

Investigations during the past 20 years have indicated that patients afflicted with the several varieties of rheumatic diseases including rheumatoid arthritis, systemic lupus erythematosus, progressive systemic sclerosis, dermatomyositis, Sjögren's syndrome, and rheumatic fever may also manifest immunological abnormalities. Indeed, studies of lesions from patients with these diseases have revealed lymphoid hyperplasia, vasculitis, and fibrinoid necrosis which resemble closely the lesions produced experimentally through induced allergic reactions in animals. In spite of these observations, the pathogenesis of the immunological abnormalities in these disorders remains enigmatic. One hypothesis under consideration is that of "cryptoinfection" by some type of viable agent which might initiate the phenomenon of hypersensitivity or autoimmunity as part of the disease process. Virus particles have been found in cell-free extracts of organs of the mentioned NZB strain of mice, at birth, suggesting the possibility of transplacental transmission.[5]

Circulating DNA may be found in the serum of patients with lupus erythematosus. This has been found to coincide with a decrease or disappearance of anti-DNA antibodies and serum complement. One hypothesis is that this process is related to virus-like particles which have been found in renal and other biopsy specimens from laboratory animals as well as from man.[5]

It is believed that some of the above mechanisms in certain human patients may be responsible for the development of collagen diseases. Indeed, similar events may occur in certain cancers in man including multiple myeloma and chronic lymphocytic leukemia wherein abnormal globulins or lymphocytes react aberrantly to certain antigenic stimulations. Finally, when viewing these events collectively in their experimental and clinical contexts, one might postulate a relationship between certain autoimmune states associated with cancer and immunoproliferative disorders, wherein a breakdown in the host defense against cancer is heralded by the production of abnormal lymphocytes and plasmacytes, fol-

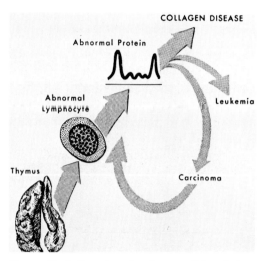

Figure 23–1. Drawing showing possible relationship between "collagen" disease, leukemia, and carcinoma which might be mediated through abnormal Lymphocytes producing abnormal globulines. Reproduced by permission of Robert P. Barden, M.D. and Editor of *Radiology,* 92:972–974, 1969.

lowed by the elaboration of defective globulin antibodies which in turn, leads to a decrease in resistance to cancer. These events have been depicted schematically by Barden[8] to show a possible "bridge" between collagen disease and cancer (Fig. 23–1).

Lupus Erythematosus

Lupus erythematosus is a multi-system disease with frequent occurrences of any combination of intermittent fever, arthritis, arthralgia, arteritis, phlebitis in the central nervous system, renal disease (lupus nephritis), and a wide variety of cutaneous manifestations most noteworthy of which is the malar erythema of the so-called "butterfly area" of the face.[9–10] Smith and associates[11] have recently proposed a theoretically possible relationship between immunological deficiency, lymphoma, and connective tissue disease in a patient with systemic lupus erythematosus, dysgamma-globulinemia and lymphoma; in addition, these investigators included a review of eight additional patients with SLE and lymphoma. They suggest that a spectrum of immune abnormalities exists in patients with SLE, and they further postulate the existence of a selective immunoglobulin deficiency in connective tissue diseases in general with an association with cancer or lymphoma and other connective tissue diseases including dermatomyositis and Sjögren's syndrome.[11] Their patient was of interest because of manifestations of a high titer of IgM, antinuclear antibodies, profuse development of extracellular hematoxylin material and cryoglobulinemia which may have been related predominantly to the presence of IgM. Histopathological findings in this patient showed the concurrent presence of connective tissue disease, dysgamma-globulinemia, and lymphoma, implying the likelihood of an immunopathogenic relationship among these disorders.

This entire problem has been elucidated further by studies of Dr. Eric R. Hurd, of the University of Texas Southwestern Medical School. He and his associates have demonstrated viral antibody levels as well as the existence of cytoplasmic myxovirus-like tubular structures in patients with SLE. These studies may in time prove that there is a link between viruses and cancer in certain circumstances in humans. Of further importance is that it is related to a known precancerous autoimmune disease which appears to aggregate in certain families.

The mode of inheritance of SLE has not been clearly delineated at this time though several studies have suggested the likelihood of an autosomal dominant gene in some families.[12-14] With respect to the cancer relationships, increased occurrences of lymphomas have been mentioned and we must also consider the known increased frequency of thymic tumors in this disease.[15,16]

Dermatomyositis

Dermatomyositis is a rarely occurring collagen disease considered by some to be a nonsuppurative form of polymyositis which may present as an acute, subacute, or chronic disease process. Intermittent fever may occur in some patients. This systemic disease is characterized by inflammatory and degenerative changes involving skin and muscle primarily; the disease process may lead to associated muscular atrophy, weakness, and tenderness. Muscle weakness occurs in the primary musculature of the shoulder girdle, arms, and the gluteal and femoral areas; this involvement may give rise to a characteristic posture which includes drooping of the head and difficulty in sitting up or assuming an erect position. Skin changes include a form of erythema and puffy edematous swellings of the eyelids, i.e. *heliotrope bloating;* other cutaneous manifestations may include minute telangiectasia, erythematous patches on the face and extremities, and a brown pigmentation which may mimic the appearance and anatomic distribution of the cutaneous manifestations of lupus erythematosus. Vasomotor disturbances may occur similar to those found in Raynaud's disease. In spite of their prominence and unusual characteristics, the skin changes in dermatomyositis are not diagnostic and may often resemble those of a nonspecific or toxic dermatitis.[17]

Dermatomyositis can be distinguished from generalized scleroderma during certain phases of its clinical course. However, differentiation may prove difficult in the acute edematous phases of each disease and multiple histologic sections from characteristic areas of skin and muscle may be required in order to make this differentiation.

Variable associations of cancer in patients with dermatomyositis have been reported. For example, in 1959, Williams[18] found that cancer occurred in 15 percent of 92 patients with dermatomyositis. Other series have reported a cancer association as high as 50 percent in patients with the adult variety of dermatomyositis, the most common malignant lesions being those of the gastrointestinal tract, sarcoma of soft tissues, lymphoma, multiple myeloma, and malignant melanoma.[19-21] When assessing the cancer risk in dermatomyositis, it is important to differentiate carefully between the *adult* and the so-called *juvenile* variety of this disease.[22,23] The juvenile variety (onset before age 20), does not show an increased association with cancer. The mechanism involved in carcinogenesis in dermatomyositis remains unknown at this time.

The genetics of dermatomyositis are exceedingly complex and to date no precise mode of inheritance has been delineated.[24,25] In one kindred, two female first cousins manifested the disease and interestingly there was an increased occurrence of rheumatoid arthritis and certain protein abnormalities suggesting a relationship between dermatomyositis and connective tissue disorders.[25]

Scleroderma

Scleroderma is a systemic disease with skin as the primary target organ. The average age of onset of this disorder is between the third and fifth decades. Females are affected more often than males. Interestingly, the name scleroderma, referred to by its German name "Hautscleren," means hide-bound skin which provides an excellent clinical description of the disorder. This disease may not always be present as a clear-cut entity and some authors have suggested an interrelationship or transition between scleroderma, lupus erythematosus and dermatomyositis;[26] others consider scleroderma and Raynaud's phenomenon to be integral parts of systemic scleroderma.[27] Scleroderma may be divided into a generalized form showing predominance of systemic manifestations and a localized variety which lacks systemic manifestations and has a more favorable prognosis. In the generalized form, the abnormalities in internal organs are believed to result primarily from vascular changes which include thickening of the walls of vessels with subsequent ischemia. Shortening of the esophagus, probably due to atrophy of its musculature, is frequently manifested in the generalized systemic form of the disease.

An increased frequency of cancer is associated with scleroderma; possibly a premorbid cancerous state may be promulgated by the sclerodermatic process. This is seemingly most evident in patients with scleroderma and bronchogenic carcinoma. In this case, the malignancy appears to be secondary to dense pulmonary fibrosis caused by scleroderma.[28] On the other hand, certain reports suggest that malignant neoplasms, per se, may produce systemic manifestations, which give rise to a syndrome mimicking dermatomyositis, polyarthritis, and scleroderma.[29]

The inheritance of scleroderma, like that of dermatomyositis, is not clear at this time. Familial occurrences have been reported and in one family the disorder was confirmed in two brothers while their sister was probably "affected."[30] In a review of the genetic literature, Burge and associates[31] found four incidences of familial scleroderma and eight cases in which the documentation was less complete. These authors also investigated a family in which two sisters manifested scleroderma and other close relatives showed a variety of connective tissue disorders including lupus erythematosus, Sjögren-Larson syndrome, and other diseases in the autoimmune category including chronic glomerulonephritis. In addition, biochemical studies revealed abnormalities of the serum immune globulins which also may be associated with autoimmune disease.

A rapidly accumulating body of data supports the hypothesis that autoimmune diseases may be under genetic influence.[32-36] Familial scleroderma has been reported in association with other connective tissue disorders[37,38] including the report by Tuffanelli.[32] Finally, Camus *et al.* report a family which includes a mother and her four daughters, all of whom manifested varying degrees of scleroderma associated with Sjögren's syndrome.[39]

Burch and Rowell[39a] studied the genetic aspects of scleroderma in a large population survey. They speculated that the sex patterns and age of onset rates in lupus erythematosus, scleroderma, and other autoimmune diseases were quite similar. They speculated further that these diseases which predominantly affect females were caused by dominantly inherited mutations on the X chromosome but they also believed that a certain number of somatic mutations occurred with these problems.

Tuffanelli[32] emphasized that familial clustering of connective tissue disorders and the presence of auto-antibodies among asymptomatic relatives in these families does not necessarily imply a genetic etiology. He stressed that such familial concentrations could also be caused by environmental agents such as a virus.

Sjogren's Syndrome

The associated findings of keratoconjunctivitis sicca, disorders of lacrimal and salivary glands, xerostomia, and rheumatoid arthritis were described in a series of patients by Sjögren, a Swedish ophthalmologist, in 1933. Subsequent observations of additional patients have shown that these findings constitute a syndrome which is now known as Sjögren's syndrome. The spectrum of physical findings in this condition has increased and now includes additional collagen-vascular disorders including progressive systemic sclerosis, Raynaud's phenomenon, polyarteritis, polymyositis, and systemic lupus erythematosus. Symptoms and signs include dryness and keratosis of mucous membranes, particularly in the mouth, conjunctiva, nose, throat, and occasionally in the urinary bladder and vagina. The eye symptoms may be severe and occasionally include corneal ulceration and loss of visual acuity. The salivary glands may be palpably enlarged, inflamed, and exquisitely tender. Anemia and achlorhydria may also occur and there have been rare cases of granuloma annulare. Dental hygiene may be poor with many carious teeth. The fingernails may be brittle, the scalp may be dry, and alopecia is often found. Osteoporosis is also a frequent finding.[40]

Hypergammaglobulinemia occurs frequently in patients with this condition. They may also show the rheumatoid factor, antinuclear factors, precipitating antibodies, and anti-IgM. Because of these associations, this syndrome is considered by many to be an autoimmune disease.[41] Increased incidences of cancer occur in association with this disease. For example, in one series of 58 patients with Sjögren's syndrome, three developed reticulum cell sarcoma.[42] Another report showed malignant lymphoma of the salivary glands[43] while another patient had adenocarcinoma of the parotid gland.[44]

There is a paucity of available information concerning the role of heredity in Sjögren's syndrome.[40] It is suggested that a hereditary predisposition to this condition might exist because it is frequently associated with other collagen diseases in which hereditary factors are known to be implicated.

Childhood Malignancies: Epidemiologic Surveys

The retrospective approach to childhood malignancies has been a favorite and generally acceptable epidemiologic method to determine cancer susceptibility in children. Attempts have also been made to elucidate cancer risks in order to augment our knowledge of cancer etiology. Although retrospective surveys have several serious handicaps, they provide insight into some of the perplexing areas of cancer epidemiology; hopefully they will also provide leads or clues which can then be studied by long-range prospective investigations. In cancer research, events, however unlikely on a priori grounds, may nevertheless prove to be highly significant.

Stewart and Barber[45] discussed data based on the *Oxford Survey of Childhood Cancers* —a study based primarily on retrospective surveys.[46] While differences between patients and controls were not striking, initial results revealed that the sibship position, maternal age, findings of mongolism and recent attacks of pneumonia were likely to be associated in children with leukemia. It was also suspected that children who had been x-rayed before birth, children whose mothers had had several abortions, and children who had brothers and sisters with cancer were more likely to develop cancer than were children in whose families none of these events occurred.[45]

The influence of carcinogenic factors on the host is difficult to appraise through retrospective surveys. Thus, while radiation effects are known to be carcinogenic it would be important to know whether their effects are differentially influenced by host factors such as an inherited susceptibility or resistance to cancer. It would be difficult to determine the influence of such host factors but conceivably, through a painstaking appraisal of the family history of all patients whose mothers had received diagnostic radiation during pregnancy, and determining dose-response relationships between radiation exposure and certain genotypic factors

in the host, meaningful information might be obtained. However, the amount of roentgen dose used in diagnostic radiology is exceedingly difficult to quantify since it may vary considerably in different radiology departments; finally most radiology departments do not consider it necessary to keep records of the dose of irradiation associated with each film exposure. Indeed, in many cases the records may not even reveal the number of films which have been taken during an examination. Finally, machine designs have been changed periodically so that within any particular department, the irradiation dosage may vary, depending upon the time of exposure.

Surveys of childhood cancer, particularly that of the *Oxford Survey of Childhood Cancers,* have revealed a need to develop new theories about carcinogenesis from the standpoint of age. Specifically, existing theories are primarily oriented to adult cancer and their assumptions cannot be transferred to cover infantile and juvenile cancers. For example, the fact that children are more susceptible to specific histological varieties of cancer than young adults is at marked variance with hypotheses which propose that cancer susceptibility invariably increases with age from birth. In addition, present theories of carcinogenesis attach more importance to extrinsic factors than to intrinsic or host factors, probably because an overwhelming majority of epidemiologic surveys have been concerned with the appraisal of known carcinogenic factors such as smoking, radiation, and certain occupational exposures. They have been far less often concerned with intrinsic factors in the host which could be significant determinants for cancer development in concert with above-mentioned exogenous carcinogenic factors.

Specific examples of childhood cancer, i.e. retinoblastoma, are mentioned in other chapters in this book.

Wilms' Tumor

Wilms' tumor accounts for approximately 6 percent of all renal malignant neoplasms, and about three fourths of these tumors occur in children under the age of 4 years.[47] This malignant neoplasm has an insidious clinical course and unfortunately may reach a massive size before the first symptoms are recognized.

Wilms' tumor is associated with a number of congenital anomalies. The most frequent association is with aniridia.[48-50] Other congenital anomalies include hemihypertrophy, pigmented nevi, hemangiomas, horseshoe kidney, duplication of the upper urinary tract, aplastic or hypoplastic kidneys, cryptorchidism, hypospadias, undescended testes, bilateral small fibrous ovaries, recurved pinna, microcephaly, mental retardation, and multiple neurofibromatosis. Associated cardiac anomalies include tetralogy of Fallot with patent foramen ovale (one case), aortic stenosis (one case), patent ductus arteriosus (two cases), and patent foramen ovale in two patients at ages 4 and 6 years.[51]

Lynch and Green[52] presented a patient with bilateral Wilms' tumor and congenital abnormalities of the heart (transposition of the great vessels and Ebstein's anomaly) confirmed at autopsy. This patient was of additional interest because of his family

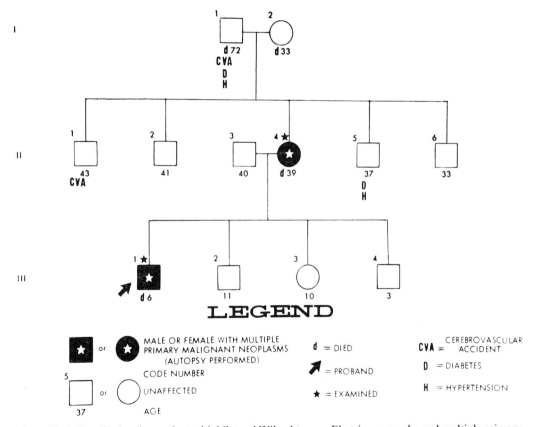

Figure 23–2. Family showing patient with bilateral Wilms' tumor, Ebsteins anomaly, and multiple primary cancer in his mother. From Lynch and Green, *Am J Dis Child, 115:*723, 1968.

history. Specifically, his mother had had four primary malignant neoplasms, which included bilateral pheochromocytomas (age 39) solid thyroid carcinoma with amyloid stroma (age 22), and a mucin-producing breast carcinoma (age 33) (Fig. 23 2). All of these tumors were histologically confirmed. Findings in the mother were consistent with a pluriglandular syndrome with carcinoma. Of further interest was the finding that the proband's maternal uncle had suffered a cerebral vascular accident at age 21 with residual hemiplegia of the left side. He had hypertension and diabetes mellitus by history. Similar findings of hypertension and diabetes mellitus were observed in other members of the family; and subsequent studies by other investigators showed that certain relatives in the maternal line manifested medullary thyroid carcinoma with amyloid and pheochromocytoma, with a mode of transmission in the family consistent with an autosomal dominant factor.[53]

Another remarkable family (Fig. 23–3) has been studied by Kontras and Newton[54] wherein three patients in two generations had histologically verified Wilm's tumor. A fourth member died in early childhood from "kidney tumor" which was not verified but was suspected of being a Wilms' tumor.

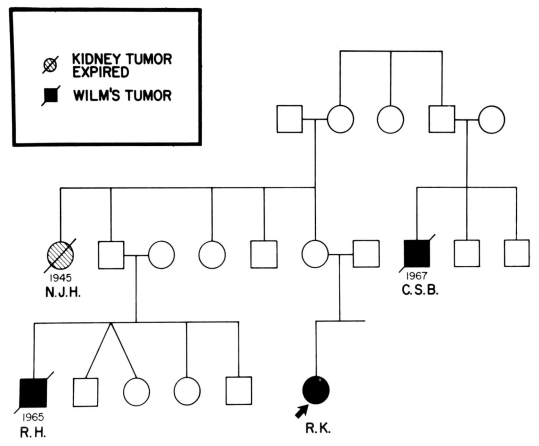

KIDNEY TUMOR
EXPIRED

WILM'S TUMOR

Figure 23–3. Pedigree of family with Wilms' tumor, courtesy of Stella B. Kontras, M.D., Genetics Division, Department of Pediatrics, Ohio State University, Columbus, Ohio.

Dominant inheritance with reduced penetrance was postulated to explain the genetics in this family. Similarly, Wilms' tumor was recently verified in three generations in a family.[55]

In spite of reports of several remarkable families prone to Wilms' tumor, hereditary factors in this problem have not been systematically studied. Lynch and Green[52] reviewed the literature and were able to find several additional reports of families with two or more affected relatives. For example, MacKay[56] reported a family which included seven siblings, five with congenital kidney lesions, of whom two had congenital Wilms' tumors. Wilms' tumor has also been described in identical twins.[50,51] In a family reported by Miller, *et al.*[50] two brothers and a first cousin were reported to have Wilms' tumor. Findings from their series also included a child with Wilms' tumor with a sib who had a brain cyst; another proband had a sib with hemangioendothelioma of the external ear and congenital adrenal hypoplasia, while the sib of another proband was reported to have died of liver cancer at 15 years of age.

Wilm's tumor has been described in context with pseudohermaphroditism and chronic glomerulonephritis in a five-year-old boy with a suggestion that this might constitute a clinical syndrome.[57] This patient was said to have had the first histologically documented case of infantile glomerulonephritis associated with pseudohermaphroditism, though several instances of the combination of glomerulonephritis and pseudohermaphroditism discerned later in childhood are reported in the literature. Interestingly, in two reports of glomerulonephritis with pseudohermaphroditism,[58,59] the tumors were derivatives of the urogenital ridge. Specifically, Drash, *et al.*[58] reported Wilms' tumors involving the right kidney in each patient and Frasier, *et al.*[59] reported on gonadoblastomas and teratoma. The review by

Spear, *et al.*[57] contains other reports of Wilms' tumor occurring in association with pseudohermaphroditism and in the nephrotic syndrome. These authors also called attention to the frequent occurrence of gonadal tumors in hermaphrodites. Before these combinations can be considered in terms of a syndrome, serious thought should be given to their etiology with special attention to hereditary factors as well as to the action of teratogenic agents during pregnancy.

A recent report by Meadows and associates[59a] described a family wherein a mother had congenital hemihypertrophy, and three of her children had verified Wilms' tumor.

Knudson and Strong[59b] have proposed a two-mutation model for Wilms' tumor. This theory assumes that cancer is caused by two mutational events, and that the malignant neoplasm arises from a single cell. When the first mutation occurs in a germ cell the mutation will then be present in all cells of the particular individual, and will of course be hereditary. Possibilities for cancer in the gene carrier will include no cancer, a single tumor, or multiple tumors. Where the first mutation is somatic, it will then be restricted to a single cell and the particular malignant neoplasm will be non-hereditary. The second mutation is always somatic in both the hereditary and non-hereditary types. All tumors require two mutational events. Thus, in the hereditary variety the first event has already transpired, and will be present in all of the cells. Therefore, only a single second mutational event is necessary for tumor development.

Hereditary cancers occur on the average at an earlier age than non-hereditary cancers, and they are more likely to be multiple. The non-hereditary variety will be late and more frequently single, since two infrequent mutational events for tumor development in a single or derivative cell is a requirement. Further discussion of this theory is found in Chapter 1.

Thus, from this review of Wilms' tumor, we find a challenging field of investigation for cancer epidemiologists as well as embryologists, pediatricians, and geneticists.

Rhabdomyosarcoma

Li and Fraumeni[60] studied the death certificates of 418 children in the United States who died of rhabdomyosarcoma between 1964 and 1969, and reviewed 280 medical records from 17 hospitals. It is of interest that these authors were able to identify five families in this series in which a second child showed soft tissue sarcoma; three siblings (vs. 0.06 expected by chance), and two cousins. In addition, they also noted a high frequency of carcinoma of the breast and a variety of other malignant neoplasms including acute leukemia, carcinoma of the lung, pancreas, and skin occurring at relatively young ages among the parents, grandparents, and other relatives of these affected children. Of additional interest was the occurrence of adrenal cortical carcinoma and brain tumor in first degree relatives of two other children with rhabdomyosarcoma. The authors found no increased frequency of congenital abnormalities associated with rhabdomyosarcoma in their series of patients.

These authors suggested that the etiology of this problem is complex and may result from the interaction of genetic and environmental factors, including the possibility of an oncogenic virus.[60]

Neuroblastoma

Neuroblastoma, a relatively common malignant neoplasm occurring in childhood, (approximately one case per 10,000 live born children) has been reported on rare occasions to effect more than one member of a family. One of the earliest reports of familial neuroblastoma was that of Dodge and Benner[61] who in 1945 treated a brother and sister for neuroblastoma of the adrenal medulla. Chatten and Voorhess[62] reported a family in which an asymptomatic mother showed an abnormally high urinary excretion of dopamine, norepinephrine, and V.M.A., during pregnancy, which persisted for 23 months. Four of her five children had neuroblastomas (three overt and one *in situ*). Cytogenetic evaluations of both parents and one of the affected children were normal. One of the affected children also manifested aganglionosis; another showed patent ductus arteriosus. Miller[63] could not find any unusual incidences of congenital abnormalities in patients manifesting neuroblastoma. However, he did comment upon the theoretical probability of such an association.

In their review of the literature, Chatten and Voorhess[62] were able to find only four reports in which a second sibling was either suspected or known to have neuroblastoma. This review included the mentioned report by Dodge and Benner.[61] They also collaborated in the study of another family which included two affected siblings with neuroblastoma whose mother had normal urinary catecholamine excretion.

Griffin and Bolande[64] reported a family in which two sisters had disseminated neuroblastoma. Interestingly, regression of the retroperitoneal neoplasm to fibrocalcific residues and maturation to ganglioneuroma occurred; and in one a metastatic nodule in the skin matured to a ganglioneuroma and through progressive loss of ganglion cells eventually showed a close resemblance to neurofibroma.

Wong, Hanenson, and Lampkin[65] reported neuroblastomas in two siblings whose father had increased levels of V.M.A. in his urine but no clinical evidence of tumor. Results in this particular family suggest that neuroblastoma may be inherited in an autosomal dominant pattern resulting from mutation of the gene(s) governing the neural crest formation. The above authors support the hypothesis of an autosomal dominant factor involving the neural creast; this mechanism is similar to that which includes the inheritance of multiple neurofibromatosis and pheochromocytoma and is enforced by the fact that neurofibromas, ganglioneuromas, pheochromocytomas and neuroblastomas, all of which are of neural crest origin, have been shown to coexist in various combinations within the same individual.

Finally, Hardy and Nesbitt[66] presented a kindred in which neuroblastoma occurred in two siblings, namely, a six-month old boy (proband) and his four-year-old sister. Neuroblastoma was also diagnosed in a two-year-old male, first cousin of these children. It was of further interest that other childhood neoplasms occurred in several members of the family. Specifically, a paternal aunt of the proband died of a tumor "on the head and scalp" (no histologic diagnosis) at the age of four years and another cousin died of "renal tumor" at the age of four months, histologic diagnosis not established, though a note on the chart indicated the lesion as being "Wilms' tumor." Another cousin died at the age of six months of "renal tumor." The diagnosis on the medical record stated "hypernephroma with pulmonary metastases" though a search of the record did not reveal any more specific pathologic material.

To summarize, we find in the literature nine kindreds in which neuroblastoma has occurred in more than one member of a family. In the family of Chatten and Voorhess[62] the mother had abnormally high urinary catecholamine excretion, and in the report of Wong and associates[65] the father had elevated levels of V.M.A. This is of interest in that the report by Zimmermann[67] showed that the common father of affected half siblings had an apparently benign mass of the posterior mediastinum. Collectively these studies support the contention of dominant inheritance. Of further interest in this context is the observation of Beckwith and Perrin[68] that *in situ* neuroblastoma occurs 40 times more frequently than its clinical appearance. Therefore, it is possible that the incidence of clinically undetectable neuroblastoma in siblings of children with overt neuroblastoma is more common than recognized, and it may possibly be present in one of the parents. Finally, Helson and co-workers[69] found increased catecholamines in five asymptomatic siblings in four families each of which had one child affected with neuroblastoma, supporting the possibility of greater frequency of "silent" affected relatives.

The etiology of neuroblastoma remains enigmatic though further light might be shed on this problem through specific studies (such as biochemical analysis of catecholamines) on the relatives of children with neuroblastoma and on the children of survivors of neuroblastoma.

Hepatoblastoma

Hepatoblastoma has been shown to be related to congenital defects in children, particularly hemihypertrophy, a congenital anomaly which is also associated with neoplasms of the adrenal cortex and kidney in children.[70–72]

Fraumeni, *et al.*[73] described two infant sisters from a sibship of four with hepatoblastoma. No other members of the family showed evidence of cancer nor congenital abnormalities of the type associated with childhood neoplasms save for the presence of congenital hip dislocation in one of the girls with hepatoblastoma. In addition, alpha$_1$-fetoprotein persisted in the serum of one of the affected infants. This fetal alpha$_1$-globulin normally disappears from the serum during the neonatal period though it may reappear with non-neoplastic liver disease, hepatic cellular carcinoma, or embryonal gonadal tumors.[74,75]

This is the first known report of familial hepatoblastoma. The authors were unable to provide specific etiologic clues; however, the rarity of the condition in the United States suggests that the involvement was more than coincidental.[73] Further study of this disease in the population, including careful scrutiny of the families of probands with this condition, in due time might provide additional etiological information.

Hepatocellular Carcinoma*

The etiology of hepatocellular carcinoma is exceedingly complex. This lesion is known to occur in patients with coarse or macronodular cirrhosis which in many cases has been found to be a consequence of viral hepatitis. It has an unusual geographic distribution, occurring frequently in inhabitants of East Africa, in Africa south of the Sahara, and in Southeast Asia.[76,77] Half of all cancers among male Bantus under age 45, arise in the liver.[78] Etiologic considerations include the possible role of hemochromatosis, thorotrast (for diagnostic purposes), parasitic infections (liver flukes), mycotic infections, including aflatoxins and foods contaminated with *penicillium islandicum,* and kwashiorkor.[79] Finally, it is of interest that populations with a high frequency of hepatocellular carcinoma as well as hemochromatosis, parasitic infections, and kwashiorkor, also have a relatively high frequency of persistence of Australia antigen.[80-82]

*While not a tumor of childhood, hepatocellular carcinoma is described here for continuity purposes in context with hepatoblastoma.

There has been considerable interest in the Australia antigen problem though its specific relationship to hepatocellular carcinoma remains inconclusive. Smith and Blumberg performed a retrospective study of the occurrence of Australia antigen in 65 patients with hepatocellular carcinoma but found that Australia antigen in the sera from these patients did not occur more frequently than in a similar population of patients who did not have hepatic cancer.[83] However, data from other investigators documented high incidence of Australia antigen in patients with hepatocellular carcinoma from Greece and Africa where this disease occurs with greater frequency.[84-87]

Finally, there is evidence for the occurrence of the Australia antigen in patients with familial hepatoma. For example, Denison and associates[88] described a family with concurrent Australia antigen and familial hepatoma, and finally, Sutnick and associates[89] quoted data from two Japanese kindreds showing an excess of hepatoma, post-necrotic cirrhosis, and chronic hepatitis, as well as persistent Australia antigen.[90]

In 1915 Hedinger[91] reported familial occurrences of primary hepatic carcinoma in two sisters who died within a week of each other. Kaplan and Cole[92] described primary hepatocellular carcinoma in three siblings of Jewish extraction, ages 64, 64, and 49. No consanguinity was reported.[93,94] Hepatoma has also been described in three of fourteen patients with homozygous alpha$_1$ antitrypsin deficiency.[95] All fourteen showed an accumulation of periodic-acid-Schiff-positive globules in the hepatocytes. Pulmonary emphysema was found in 12 of these patients. With the limited number of familial reports of this lesion, it is not possible to delineate the genetic mechanism. Certainly any hypothesis would have to include interaction with genetic and environmental factors.

Sacrococcygeal Teratomas in Children

Sacrococcygeal teratomas may be found in newborn infants and where the tumor is massive it may pose an obstetrical problem during delivery. The tumor contains cells from all three germ layers. Currently accepted theory suggests that the sacrococcygeal teratoma is derived from the totipotent cells of the primitive knot (Hensen's node).[96]

This lesion is seen predominantly in female children where a ratio of four females to one male has been observed in several clinical series.[97-99] The incidence of cancer rises significantly as the child grows older. For example, Hickey reported that 95 percent of the teratomas removed prior to four months of age were benign while 61 percent of teratomas removed after four months were malignant.[97]

Interestingly, the incidence of twins in the immediate family of a child affected with sacrococcygeal teratoma is increased significantly over that for twinning in families of normal children.[97] Congenital abnormalities are also increased in children with sacrococcygeal teratomas. For example, Hickey[97] found a frequency of 11 percent in 112 patients with this lesion. The congenital abnormalities involved primarily the long axis of the child such as spina bifida, cleft palate, meningocele, undescended testicles, and patent urachus.[97]

There is marked variation in the gross appearance of these tumors. They range in size from a few centimeters in diameter to massive proportions. The tumor may be solid, cystic, or it may show a combination of the two. The surface may be grossly irregular or it may be smooth. The cystic spaces may contain fluid which may be clear, cloudy, or it may be composed of sebaceous material. It is generally believed that the more cystic the tumor the greater the likelihood that it is benign.[96] Microscopically one sees a large variety of tissues involving all germ layers though one particular germ layer may predominate. Thus, one may find muscle, bone, cartilage, nerve tissues, skin, and other structures in the benign tumors while the malignant tumors present largely as embryonal adenocarcinoma.[96]

The differential diagnosis of sacrococcygeal teratoma should include problems consistent with a mass occurring in a child in the region of the buttocks, sacrococcygeal, or presacral area. These include meningocele, hemangioma, lipoma, rectal duplication, infected pilonidal cyst or ischiorectal abscess.

It is extremely important to recognize sacrococcygeal teratoma as early in the life of the child as possible since the prognosis is often excellent when the lesion is excised at a very early stage. Significant delay may result in an extremely grave prognosis.

The role of heredity in the etiology of sacrococcygeal teratoma is unknown. However, the occurrence of an excess of twinning in families of affected children, the high female to male ratio and the association with congenital abnormalities suggest that hereditary factors should be studied.

Beckwith-Wiedemann Syndrome

In 1963, Beckwith[100] described three patients with a newly-recognized syndrome now referred to as the Beckwith-Wiedemann syndrome. Features of this syndrome include macroglossia, omphalocele, cytomegaly of the adrenal cortex, renal medullary dysplasia, hyperplastic visceromegaly, and hyperplasia of the gonadal interstitial cells. Later Cohen and associates[101] added other patients with the syndrome and described additional features including postnatal somatic gigantism, mild microcephaly, and severe hypoglycemia. Wiedemann[102] reported affected sibs and added an additional feature to the syndrome, namely, a dome-shaped defect of the diaphragm. However, it is important to realize that all of the mentioned features may not necessarily occur in each patient with this syndrome. For example, though gigantism may not be present at birth and growth may be normal during the first few months, somatic gigantism eventually occurs in the majority of patients; height and weight above the 90th percentile is a frequent occurrence.

Cancer appears to occur in excess in this syndrome. For example, Sherman and associates[103] and Necman[104] described patients with adrenal cortical carcinoma, while Wilson and Orlin[105] and Tower and Beck[16] described patients with nephroblastoma. It is of interest that some of these patients manifesting cancer also had associated hemihypertrophy. The latter has been shown by Fraumeni, et al.[70-72] to be associated with neuroblastoma, adrenocortical carcinoma, and embryonal tumors of the liver.

Differential diagnosis of the Beckwith-Wiedemann syndrome poses a problem because of its similarities to other disorders. For example, patients with the Beckwith-Wiedemann syndrome may show findings suggesting hypothyroidism or mucopolysaccharidosis, while other patients may have features of the syndrome which overlap those of the hemihypertrophy syndrome. Down's syndrome, cerebral gigantism, and gangliosidosis also should be considered in the differential diagnosis of the Beckwith-Wiedemann syndrome.

The outlook for survival in patients with this syndrome is guarded. Of the 33 patients described by Thorburn and associates,[107] 13 died. The cause of death in several cases was believed to be due to associated malformations while 5 of these patients had intra-abdominal neoplasms.

The clinician is provided an opportunity to practice preventive medicine in this condition in that the association of an umbilical defect, macroglossia, and macrosomia in a neonate should alert him to the possibility of this syndrome; investigation for hypoglycemia with prompt treatment, should it be present, would be of prime importance in the prevention of neurologic sequellae. In addition, the doctor should be constantly on the alert for the possibility of intra-abdominal malignancy in the long-term follow-up of the patient.[108]

The genetics of this syndrome are not clear. This disease has been reported several times in siblings and indeed, Wiedemann[102] reported three affected sibs in a family; consanguinity was established in one of the cases reported by Cohen and associates[101] thus indicating an autosomal recessive mode of transmission. However, Cohen and associates[101] report a personal communication with Opitz and associates concerning a large kindred with at least five affected males in several generations. These authors postulated that the Beckwith-Wiedemann syndrome was inherited in an autosomal dominant manner with incomplete penetrance and variable expressivity. They further noted that some affected individuals had only minor anomalies, such as ear lobe grooves. Irving[109] described the Beckwith-Wiedemann syndrome in two siblings and one first cousin; a second cousin was noted to have nephroblastoma.

Cohen and associates[101] reviewing the cytogenetics in this syndrome found them to be essentially normal. They reported one example from the literature of a C/D translocation and excessive material on the short arm of a Group G chromosome though they admitted that the case was poorly documented.

Renal Hamartomas, Nephroblastomatosis and Fetal Gigantism

Perlman, *et al.*[109a] described a family of Jewish Yemenite origin wherein a marriage between second cousins resulted in six children, five of whom died in infancy. All five of the children who expired are believed to have manifested the same disorder, which will be described below as it occurred in the proband. Pathology material was said to have been available for three of these five children. This condition was considered by the authors to represent a new familial cancer predisposing syndrome. It was believed to have certain similarities with the Beckwith syndrome, though clinical and pathologic features differentiating it from this syndrome will be described.

The proband died at 27 days of age. He had an unusual facies. The following features were noted: endophthalmos, small nose with depressed ridge, everted upper lip, serrated alveolar margins, and low set ears. The xiphisternum was broad, bifid, and prominent. Physical examination revealed enlarged and irregular kidneys. Intravenous urography performed at two hours of age revealed bilateral enlarged renal shadows with prompt excretion of the medium. The findings were interpreted as consistent with bilateral diffuse Wilms' tumor; the possibility of adult-type polycystic disease of the kidneys could not be excluded. The child experienced marked weight loss, peripheral edema and developed clinical and laboratory evidence of hyperosmolar dehydration; he developed urinary tract infection and died at 27 days of age, presumably of overwhelming infection.

Autopsy revealed generalized visceromegaly including cardiomegaly, hepatomegaly, splenomegaly, and enlargement of the pancreas. The kidneys were enlarged and showed exaggerated lobulation. The pelvis and ureters were dilated. Microscopic examination of the kidneys showed severe acute pelonephritis. The unaffected areas of the renal cortex, especially the subcapsular zone showed immature glomeruli, hamartomas, and foci of nephroblastomatosis. Microscopic examination of the pancreas showed an increase in the number of islet cells wherein approximately five percent of them were giant in size; there was ductal and acinar dilitation. The adrenals, testes, and liver were histologically normal. The pituitary gland was not examined. The final pathological diagnoses were as follows: 1) visceromegaly, 2) renal immaturity, hamartomas, and nephroblastomatosis, 3) acute severe pelonephritis, 4) pancreatic islet hyperplasia, and 5) ductular and acinar dilitation in the pancreas.[109a]

Family history revealed the father to be age 27 and the mother to be 25. Both were normal. As mentioned, four of the proband's siblings died in the perinatal period, and each of these individuals was assumed to have been affected. The sixth child was considered to be normal and lacked any of the stigmata of this disorder.

Points of overlap with Beckwith's syndrome included fetal gigantism, visceromegaly, islet cell hypertrophy, and the association with nephroblastoma. The conditions differ, however, in that macroglossia and umbilical anomalies, the most constant clinical features of Beckwith's syndrome, were lacking in this particular sibship. Differences in renal morphology were also noted. Cortical hamartomas and nephroblastomatosis were characteristic findings in this family, while in Beckwith's syndrome medullary dysplasia is a typical finding. The syndrome described here was lethal in the perinatal period, whereas most patients with Beckwith's syndrome survive infancy. And finally, the facies of the proband was distinct from that of infants with Beckwith's syndrome.

Because of parental consanguinity, affliction of both sexes, and a negative family history apart from the disorders present in the sibship, autosomal recessive inheritance was suggested.

Cowden's Disease (Multiple Hamartoma Syndrome)

Cowden's disease is the eponym assigned to honor the single patient in whom the disorder was originally described by Lloyd and Dennis.[110] Weary and associates[111] add five additional cases of the syndrome which is composed of a complex assortment of ectodermal, mesodermal, and endodermal hamartomatous lesions. The distinctive features of the syndrome involve mucocutaneous lesions consisting of lickenoid and papillomatous anomalies of the face and ears, gingival hypertrophy, massive "virginal" bilateral fibroadenomatous enlargement of breasts, acrokeratotic lesions of the hands, papillomatous and papular oral lesions, multiple lipomas and angiomas. Other associated aberrations have included carcinoma of the breast, lesions of the gastrointestinal system which included polyposis of the colon, and thyroid lesions (goiters, adenomas and carcinomas).[111]

A dominant inheritance pattern has been tentatively assigned to the multiple hamartoma syndrome. No cytogenetic abnormalities have as yet been identified in this condition (a name which Weary and associates[111] prefer to Cowden's disease).

Down's Syndrome

Miller,[112] in a review of the subject of cancer in Down's syndrome, traced the history of its association with leukemia

stating that the first etiologic relationship was suggested in 1954 when three cases were described in France; and two years later, reports appeared showing similarly affected children in North Carolina and four others in Minnesota. Systematic studies soon followed showing that the risk for leukemia in children with Down's syndrome was significantly greater than that in the general population.[46,113,114,115,116]

An extra autosome in the G group is found in Down's syndrome. It is not certain whether this chromosomal abnormality predisposes to leukemia per se or is a concomitant of this disease. However, the leukemogenic influence appears to occur at the time that the chromosomal abnormality arises, namely, before conception.

The peak for leukemia mortality among individuals with Down's syndrome occurs significantly earlier than that for the general population. One study showed the peak to be at the age of one year in Down's syndrome patients.[112] The relative risk of leukemia in patients with Down's syndrome under 10 years of age is more than 18 times normal; and this risk is even higher when children under the age of 5 years are considered.

It was commonly believed that the type of leukemia associated with Down's syndrome was usually of the myelogenous variety. However, Miller[112] found no documentation for this assumption in the literature. On the contrary, Miller cited then unpublished data by Fraumeni and associates[117] which indicate that the percentage of patients with Down's syndrome having the myelogenous variety of leukemia is similar to that found among children with leukemia in the general population.

Since mosaicism and translocations involving the G chromosomes are rare, the evaluation of the frequency of these chromosome aberrations and the association of leukemia and Down's syndrome is unavailable. However, Miller cited several case reports suggesting that there is, in fact, such a relationship. One report concerned two sibs with G/G translocation Down's syndrome with a leukemoid reaction at birth. One of the siblings recovered and the other died at 10 days of age. Autopsy disclosed the presence of chronic myelocytic leukemia. Other case reports showed acute lymphocytic leukemia in a D/G translocation carrier and in a child whose three siblings had Down's syndrome and whose mother was a D/G translocation carrier.[118]

Siblings of children with Down's syndrome appear to have an increased risk for leukemia.[112] For example, Zsako and Kaplan[119] reviewed the maternal histories of children with Down's syndrome and reported that two or more relatives were affected by cancer to a degree more significant than that found amongst the relatives of staff members and patients at the same clinic. Miller[112] suggests that the overall epidemiologic data with respect to the risk of leukemia amongst the sibs of children with Down's syndrome, are equivocal but nevertheless they are less than 5 times greater than the normal expectation.[120]

The data is scarce concerning the association of tumors other than leukemia with Down's syndrome. In reviewing these data, Miller suggests that the results cast suspicion on only two malignant neoplasms, namely, retinoblastoma and cancer of the testis.[112] However, in order to establish a real association, more investigation will be required. Miller urges that physicians record Down's syndrome on death certificates with specific mention of the existence of cancer even though the particular tumor may not have been the direct cause of death.

Renal Carcinoma (Hypernephroma)

Carcinoma of the kidney has been infrequently reported as hereditary in families.

Brinton[121] reported three cases of "hypernephroma" occurring in siblings based on autopsy or biopsy reports. The father was also allegedly treated for a kidney tumor and the mother died of "cancer," though a pathology report was not available. Riches[122] studied a series of 130 cases of renal cancer and found only one familial occurrence, in this case in siblings. Specifically, a brother had a renal tumor composed of a mixture of clear and granular cells while his sister had a renal tumor consisting entirely of clear cells. Rusche[123] reported two brothers with renal carcinoma who presented clinically with metastases. Klinger[124] reported a brother and sister with renal cell carcinoma.

Steinberg and associates[125] reported the occurrence of carcinoma of the kidney in a mother and her daughter. Consanguinity was absent in this family. Karyotypes from peripheral blood were normal in both patients. No unusual environmental exposures were found which could be responsible for renal neoplasms. Cancer was not present in any other members of this family.

A remarkable family was reported by Franksson and associates[126] in which all five siblings in the sibship developed renal carcinoma (hypernephroma). In four of these siblings renal carcinoma was bilateral. Symptoms appeared in the patients between the ages of 37 and 53; they were typical of renal carcinoma. Interestingly, one of the siblings had polycystic kidneys in addition to renal carcinomas, while another sibling had fibrosarcoma in the region of the scapula. Another sibling with renal carcinoma had optic atrophy, and finally another sibling had mental retardation. The father of these patients died of a cerebral vascular accident. However, an autopsy was not performed. Their mother had schizophrenia.

It was of interest that the hypernephromas in each of these siblings were remarkably similar. Specifically, the tumors consisted of tubular or papillary structures with poorly developed connective tissue matrix. The epithelial cells were regularly cylindrical, with granular cytoplasm and small monomorphic chromatin-rich nuclei. The frequency of mitosis was low. No invasion was apparent in the growth of the large veins in the hilum. In limited areas of some tumors, cells of a clear cell type were seen in apparently tubular or completely irregular grouping in a fine fibrillary matrix.[126]

The authors were impressed with the possibility that the findings in this family were consistent with autosomal dominantly inherited Lindau-von Hippel's disease[127-130] wherein bilateral multiple renal carcinoma has been described previously.[127,130] In addition, renal carcinoma has been described previously in polycystic kidneys.[131] Hamartomas of the kidney have been found in patients with autosomal dominantly inherited tuberous sclerosis.[132-135]

Therefore, we find that the overwhelming majority of cases of renal carcinoma are apparently nongenetic and due to differing etiologies. However, the occasional reports of carcinoma of the kidney in siblings and in more than one generation of the family suggest the possibility of hereditary etiologic factors in certain circumstances but they are insufficient to delineate the precise genetic mechanism. On the other hand, the occurrence of renal carcinoma in a known hereditary disorder, i.e. Lindau-von Hippel's disease, is intriguing since this autosomal dominantly inherited disorder harbors a propensity for the production of cerebellar hemangioblastoma and apparently also predisposes through unknown mechanisms to the production of renal carcinoma.

Testicular Tumors

The genetic literature on testicular tumors reveals a paucity of familial occurrences of these lesions.[136-142] To date, five sets of twins and four sets of nontwin brothers with primary testicular tumors have been reported according to a review by Young and Bohne.[141] In addition, these authors reported the first example of nontwin siblings with histologically documented tumors of the same cell type, and in this case, seminoma. It was also of interest that two of the five pairs of twins reported in the literature have been afflicted with seminoma alone.[141]

We are aware of a family wherein a father and son both had testicular tumors. The son had a histologically verified seminoma and had undergone treatment for an undescended testicle several years prior to the occurrence of the malignant neoplasm. His father allegedly had seminoma, though histological verification of this lesion was lacking.[142]

Finally, we have recently studied a large segment of an inbred Dutch kindred containing more than 2000 members. Noteworthy were occurrences of several hereditary precancerous diseases among the family members. These included two siblings with xeroderma pigmentosum and two siblings from another sibship who manifested a syndrome which may possibly be a variant of Fanconi's aplastic anemia. Four patients had histologically verified testicular malignant neoplasms. Other generally rarely occurring cancers included Wilms' tumor, thymic carcinoma, and astrocytoma. At present there is no satisfactory etiologic explanation for these events in this family. Environmental factors common to the family cannot be excluded. Hereditary factors conditioned strongly by consanguinity may be operating in concert with as yet unknown non-genetic factors such as an oncogenic virus.[142a]

Ovarian Carcinoma

Ovarian carcinoma accounted for 6.7 percent of cancer deaths in white and 5 percent among non-Caucasian women in the United States in 1965.[143] Statistics for this lesion were compared with age-adjusted death rates in 1962 to 1963 in Japan (1.69) and in Denmark (11.02) revealing a marked variation in occurrence. While small differences in rate may be attributable to differences in diagnostic facilities, nevertheless, Wynder, *et al.* concluded that major differences such as those between Japan and the western countries are real and therefore, require an epidemiologic explanation.[143]

The first study to deal specifically with the epidemiology of ovarian cancer was that of West, in 1966.[144] He evaluated 97 patients with ovarian cancer and 97 patients with benign disease of the ovary. Of the several variables under investigation, only one showed significant findings and this was related to a history of mumps in one woman. Specifically, the control group had more histories of mumps parotitis than had the patients with ovarian cancer. West concluded that mumps in childhood may produce protection against development of ovarian malignancy in later years. He speculated that some unknown factor that provides a woman with resistance to the development of clinically recognizable mumps may at the same time decrease her resistance to the development of ovarian cancer. Two other variables examined in West's study included previous exposure to diagnostic and therapeutic x-radiation and the therapeutic use of hormones. With respect to x-ray exposure, the results did not warrant the conclusion that this was important in influencing the production of ovarian malignancies. Hormones in therapeutic doses did not appear to pose a significant risk for ovarian carcinoma.

Wynder, *et al.*[143] studied 150 ovarian cancer patients and compared these with 300 age-matched control patients. They found no difference in marital status between the groups, and pregnancy factors were not noteworthy. However, the study did suggest that dysmenorrhea occurred more frequently among the ovarian cancer patients, who also more often had a history of early menstrual bleeding and earlier menopause than in the control group. They studied mortality rates among Americans and Japanese-Americans and found possible differences in the etiologic background of pre- and post-menopausal ovarian cancer patients. Their accumulated data suggested that the increase in ovarian cancer among Japanese immigrants in the United States could provide a primary clue to the etiology of ovarian cancer. They suggested that in both immigrant groups and native Americans studies be made of such factors as diet and steroids and their possible role in the production of cancer. Another suggestive finding from Wynder's study is the possibility that cancer of the ovary may be somewhat more common among upper as opposed to lower income groups in the western world. Ovarian cancer was also found to be more common among Jewish women in New York City than among other religious groups, particularly in postmenopausal women. However, in interpreting these data, one must realize that ovarian cancer is likely to be diagnosed more often among individuals in higher socioeconomic groups who are receiving better medical care than in women in lower socioeconomic groups.

One must also realize that among native Japanese, breast cancer occurs infrequently, though its incidence rises slowly among Japanese immigrants in the United States.[145] Wynder suggested that future studies of the epidemiology of ovarian cancer should be concerned with the collection of chemical data on steroid excretion. Again, it would appear that clues might be obtained by comparing native Japanese, Japanese immigrants to the United States, and native American women, with respect to these biochemical parameters.

Other epidemiologic evidence from the literature has shown that patients with ovarian cancer more frequently have blood group A.[146] In their work on multiple primary malignant neoplasms, Moertel[147] and Cook[148] suggested a possible relationship between ovarian and endometrial carcinoma.

The first large-scale study of the genetics of ovarian cancer was reported by Lynch in 1936.[149] This involved a review of 110 patients with ovarian carcinoma. Findings showed that 40 percent of these patients had a history of cancer in other members of the family; 12 percent had never been pregnant.

Serra and Soini[150] made a genealogical study of 138 ovarian cancer families and compared these with 138 control families. They observed a significant excess of cancer among relatives in the ovarian cancer families as opposed to the control group. Predominant cancers were of the gastrointestinal and reproductive systems and breast. There was also an excess of ovarian cancer in their relatives. Liber[151] reported site specific ovarian carcinoma in a mother and five of her daughters.

More recently, Li, et al.[152] studied a family in which seven women, four of whom were sisters, had ovarian carcinoma. The lesion was also suspected in three other relatives in this family. In their review of the world literature they found that their family represented the third familial aggregation of ovarian carcinoma wherein a pattern consistent with a dominant gene or a possible polygenic mechanism was found.

The relationship between ovarian carcinoma and carcinoma of the breast is discussed by Lynch and associates in Chapter 20.

Ovarian Dysgerminoma

Ovarian Dysgerminoma is a rare disease accounting for only 1 percent of malignant ovarian neoplasms. This neoplasm appears to arise from an early germ cell and is similar to seminoma of the testes in the male. The tumor has no hormonal effect. Grossly it may be quite large though small tumors have also been observed. The tumor has a smooth, rather dense capsule and may be rubbery in consistency.

According to Jackson,[153] of approximately 650 cases reported in the world literature, none have shown a family history of the disease. Jackson described what appears to be the first family wherein ovarian dysgerminoma was present in two (mother and daughter) and possibly three generations (maternal grandmother) of a Jamaican family. The grandmother was known to have had an ovarian cancer but unfortunately no pathology was available.

Jackson[153] has made some interesting calculations from the Liverpool Cancer Registry concerning the probability of dysgerminoma of the ovary occurring in three generations of the same family. According to this Cancer Registry, "the probability of developing cancer of the ovary is 1.506×10^{-4}, and assuming the incidence of dysgerminoma to be 1 percent of ovarian cancer, the probability of a female developing dysgerminoma is 1.506×10^{-6}. The probability of a female and her daughter both having dysgerminoma is 2.3×10^{-12}, and of a female, her daughter, and granddaughter all having the disease is 3.4×10^{-18}. If it is assumed that the grandmother had ovarian cancer, but not dysgerminoma, then the probability of her daughter and granddaughter having dysgerminoma of the ovary would be 3.4×10^{-16}. If the female population of the world is taken as 10^{-9}, then using the probability figures, the association of a grandmother, daughter, and granddaughter all having dysgerminoma of the ovary may be expected to occur by chance once every 300 million years. Even the chance of a mother and daughter both having dysgerminoma is rare and might occur only once in every 450 years.[153]

Endometrial Carcinoma *

Carcinoma of the endometrium differs strikingly from carcinoma of the uterine cervix. Differentiating characteristics include the age at onset, clinical course, relationship to ethnic and socioeconomic groups, associated constitutional factors which have included diabetes mellitus, obesity, and hypertension, incidence, and apparent association of multiple primary malignant diseases. All too frequently clear-cut histologic differentiation is not reported in the literature; in many cases the material is classified merely as "uterine" carcinoma. This has posed serious problems in the interpretation of genetic factors in these two conditions.[154,155]

We reviewed all medical records of patients with histologically confirmed carcinoma of the endometrium treated at the University of Nebraska Hospital during a 20-year period (1946–1965). Pathological reports as well as available tissue specimens were reappraised. An attempt was made in every case to obtain tissue confirmation for malignancy. When any question arose concerning the status of multiple primary malignancies, opinions from additional pathologists were sought. A detailed genetic inquiry for the presence of carcinoma and other medical disorders in the families of the respective propositi was made through personal interviews with the available surviving probands and their relatives. Table 23-I summarizes the findings of associated constitutional features.

*Portions of this material are reprinted by permission of the publishers of Southern Medical Journal. Lynch, *et al.*, "Heredity and Endometrial Carcinoma," *Southern Medical Journal, 60*:231–235, 1967.

TABLE 23-I
CLINICAL AND CONSTITUTIONAL
ASSOCIATIONS FOUND IN 154 CONSECUTIVE
PATIENTS WITH HISTOLOGICALLY
CONFIRMED ENDOMETRIAL CARCINOMA

	Number of Patients	%
Endometrial carcinoma	154	100
Obesity	123	80
Hypertension	100	65
Diabetes mellitus	66	42
Triad of obesity, hypertension and diabetes	46	30
Arthritis	58	38
Arteriosclerotic heart disease	58	38
Cholecystitis	36	23
Cholelithiasis	25	16
Gallbladder disease	45	29
Leiomyomata uteri	33	21
Endometrial hyperplasia	13	8
Endometrial polyps	10	6

Obesity was the most frequently occurring constitutional factor. It was present in 123 (80%) of the 154 patients. Obesity was extreme in many of these patients; several weighed more than 300 pounds and two weighed more than 400 pounds. Hypertension was present in 100 patients (65%) and diabetes mellitus was present in 66 patients (43%). Multiple primary malignant neoplasms were found in 17 patients (11%). Five of the 17 patients had three primary malignant neoplasms.

Abbreviated pedigrees of 26 patients (16%) who had first degree relatives with endometrial carcinoma are shown in Figure 4. In family No. 17, three sisters had endometrial carcinoma with histologic confirmation. In families No. 5 and No. 7 each proband had a mother and a daughter with histologically confirmed endometrial carcinoma. In families No. 4 and No. 6, two sisters had histologically confirmed endometrial carcinoma.

Previous investigations of carcinoma of the endometrium have been concerned primarily with selective evaluation of patients for the related incidences of obesity, diabetes mellitus, endometrial hyperplasia, hypertension, cardiovascular disease, parity, and

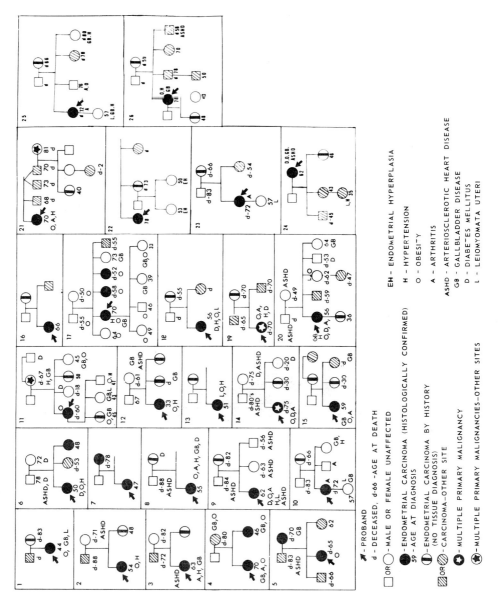

Figure 23–4. Abbreviated pedigrees of 26 patients (16%) of the 154 probands with histologically verified endometrial carcinoma. These pedigrees reflect those probands who had first degree relatives with endometrial carcinoma.

other constitutional associations, as well as with a study of hereditary factors. Much confusion has arisen from some of these studies partly because of the lack of clarity of histologic diagnosis of the malignancy, as well as from variations in the criteria used in evaluating associated diseases and constitutional findings.[154,155]

Several rather consistent observations from past investigations pertaining to differences between carcinoma of the uterine corpus and carcinoma of the uterine cervix are as follows: 1) Jewish people have a relatively increased incidence of endometrial carcinoma over carcinoma of the uterine cervix; 2) Negroes and Puerto Ricans have a greatly increased incidence of carcinoma of the uterine cervix; 3) carcinoma of the endometrium occurs in higher socioeconomic groups and appears to have distinct constitutional associations, most frequent of which are obesity, diabetes mellitus, and hypertension, which are not associated with carcinoma of the uterine cervix; 4) early sexual intercourse, multiparity, and lack of circumcision of the spouse appear to show a positive correlation with uterine cervical carcinoma and do not appear to have a relationship to carcinoma of the uterine corpus. Whereas uterine cervical carcinoma was formerly 5 to 10 times as frequent in incidence as endometrial cancer, at the present time the ratio is approximately 2 to 1.[154]

The most frequent associated constitutional factor in our series of patients was obesity (80%) which was extreme in many cases. Indeed, this was also a frequent finding in first degree relatives of probands including affected as well as unaffected individuals. While this observation appears to be significant, caution must be drawn in interpreting this finding in the absence of a control population. Obesity, in spite of its frequency in our civilization, is poorly understood.

The finding of 43 percent of probands with endometrial carcinoma showing diabetes mellitus is also high when compared with the incidence in the general population. However, the age factor must be considered since the incidence of diabetes mellitus is positively correlated with advancing age; the average age of probands with endometrial carcinoma in our series was 63 years.

Similar reasoning must be applied to the incidence of hypertension (65%), arterio-

sclerotic heart disease (38%), and gall bladder disease (29%), which are also positively correlated with advanced age.

The 11 percent incidence of multiple primary malignancies in this study is not significantly different from that of Moertel and associates[156] who found an incidence of 9.9 percent of multiple primary malignancies in the study of 807 patients with endometrial cancer. These investigators found carcinoma of the breast and endometrium to be the most frequently associated primary sites. They found carcinoma of the colon as a separate primary site in 14 percent of their endometrial carcinoma patients. It is interesting that none of the probands in our endometrial carcinoma series showed carcinoma of the colon as a second primary site, yet this is the most frequent site for a second primary in patients with endometrial cancer in the cancer family syndrome (See Chapt. 19). The occurrence of a second primary malignancy in the endometrial cancer probands and in the cancer family syndrome appears to be increased over that expected for most malignancies in the general population and is also higher than that found in studies of uterine cervical cancer. We should, therefore, follow such patients carefully, realizing that they have an increased risk for the development of additional primary malignancies. The second primary cancer may well be of more clinical importance than the original one.[156]

The finding of 16 percent of the probands whose first degree relatives had endometrial carcinoma is conservative. Rigorous documentation either through personal examination of tissue, evaluation of pathologic reports, or highly reliable information from physicians formed the basis for our statistics. In all cases, the search for tissue verification continues. Factors impeding the search among relatives include: 1) daughters or younger sisters of the proband may be clinically normal at the time of the investigation, but have a risk for developing the lesion at a later age; 2) mother and aunts of the proband may have had endometrial carcinoma but tissue confirmation is lacking because of death of a family physician, destruction of the old hospital records, or migration of the family to distant areas; 3) in many cases, women in the direct genetic line have had hysterectomy for dysfunctional uterine bleeding, leiomyoma uteri, or endometrial hyperplasia at an age preceding that of the risk age of endometrial carcinoma; and 4) death at earlier ages from other major causes of mortality. This could be a critical factor in the mentioned frequent association of obesity, diabetes mellitus, and hypertension, since these factors also mitigate against longevity.

The inherited gene defect leading to endometrial carcinoma may have a direct effect upon the endocrine system, possibly involving the pituitary-adrenal axis. This is shown by the associated endocrinologic and constitutional findings including dysfunctional uterine bleeding and endometrial hyperplasia in the patients. These findings suggest that estrogenic hyperactivity could predispose to the development of endometrial carcinoma.[157] The endocrine aberration may be more complex and may, in addition to hyperestrinism, also include pituitary hyperplasia. Other evidence in favor of estrogenic involvement in the etiology of endometrial carcinoma is seen in its frequent association with functional estrogenic ovarian tumors and with the Stein-Leventhal syndrome.[158] It has also been suggested that prolonged treatment with estrogens may have a causal effect. For instance, a patient with Turner's syndrome received 1 to 5 mg of stilbesterol daily for 6 years and developed endometrial carcinoma at the age of 22 years.[159]

More than one genotype may be implicated in endometrial carcinoma. Specifically, there could be a separate genotype responsible for the occurrence of this lesion in the cancer family syndrome in which cancer of all sites is involved, but in which endometrial carcinoma is the most frequent malignancy in females; it also occurs at a significantly younger age than in the general population. A second genotype may account for the lesion in many of the probands and their relatives in this series, wherein the lesion appears to be site-specific.

Chondrosarcoma

Chondrosarcomas differ from osteosarcomas because of their distinctive pathology, clinical behavior, response to therapy and prognosis. These lesions occur about half as frequently as osteosarcomas, but they occur twice as frequently as Ewing's sarcomas. Chondrosarcomas occur more frequently in males than in females.

Schajowicz and Bessone[160] described chondrosarcoma (histologically verified) in three males in a sibship of seven children (six males and one female). One of the brothers died at eighteen years of age from chondrosarcoma of the pelvis; another brother had chondrosarcoma of the fibula when he was sixteen years old (treated by resection); he later developed a second tumor of the femur 2½ years following the resection of the initial chondrosarcoma; this was not believed to be a metastasis. The third brother had chondrosarcoma of the femur at the age of 14. The authors emphasized the almost identical macroscopic and microscopic appearance of the three tumors which were located in the fibula and femur. No other cases of cancer were found among the siblings of the three affected children.

Cytogenetic studies were performed on two of the brothers with chondrosarcoma and on the twin brother (zygosity not determined) of the third affected brother. The findings were within normal limits.

Unfortunately, no details were given regarding the health status of the parents or of their other close relatives.

The authors speculated about the possibility of a dominant mutation existing only in the germinative cells of one of the parents. While this possibility cannot be excluded, it will be necessary to evaluate additional families in order to delineate a genetic and/or environmental factor responsible for the familial occurrences of chondrosarcoma. In addition, in this particular study, it would have been helpful to know whether hereditary exostosis had occurred prior to the appearance of chondrosarcoma.

Osteogenic Sarcoma

Osteogenic sarcoma usually occurs sporadically. However, occasional families may have more than one member affected with this disease, suggesting that in certain contexts, familial factors may be important. The only pedigree we have been able to find in which osteogenic sarcoma was found in two generations, occurred in the family recorded by Epstein, *et al.*[161] In this family osteogenic sarcoma occurred in a father and his daughter. However, the family was also noteworthy because of an excess of cancer of other histologic varieties. Other family reports of sarcoma show the lesion to be restricted to siblings. In one such report by Roberts and Roberts,[162] osteogenic sarcoma was diagnosed in three siblings over a 4-month span, thus suggesting the possibility that etiologic factors were related to a particular time period in the life of these individuals. Pohle and associates[163] reported two affected siblings; Harmon and Morton[164] reported four siblings with osteogenic sarcoma; and Robbins[165] reported another family. A common antigen has recently been found in patients with osteogenic sarcoma and their close contacts, thereby suggesting the possibility of an infectious agent in the etiology of this cancer.[166]

Esophageal Cancer

The incidence of esophageal carcinoma varies widely geographically. This permits epidemiologists to analyze critically environmental factors which may be important in the etiology of this lesion and which appear to be particularly prevalent in the specific area where the tumor occurs most frequently. For instance, the incidence of esophageal cancer is high in India while it is fairly uncommon in most western countries. Paymaster, *et al.*[167] also noted the occurrence of second primaries in several patients with esophageal cancer and it was of further interest that these were invariably in the mouth and pharynx, suggesting a possible common cause. Habit patterns which were common among these people were the smoking of bidi and the chewing of pan. Bidi is a type of cigarette in which the tobacco is rolled in dried leaves; pan on the other hand, may be almost anything that is chewable including betel leaf, betel nut, and slaked lime. Finally, patients with either or both of these habits were found to have increased incidences of cancer of the upper and middle thirds of the esophagus. Cancer of the lower third of the esophagus did not show this association.

Esophageal cancer also occurs frequently in such varied climatic areas as the Alaskan tundra[168] and equatorial Africa.[170,171] In addition to the mentioned habit patterns noted among the inhabitants of India, in other parts of the world esophageal cancer has been associated with cultural habits such as increased consumption of alcohol, dietary customs, smoking habits, and a general association with lower socioeconomic groups.[168-177] In addition, certain structural aberrations resulting from congenital stenosis of the esophagus, and esophageal webs, and acquired lesions of the esophagus including inflammatory stenosis, peptic stenosis and lye stricture, have all been associated with esophageal cancer.[171] It is of further interest that when these lesions are present, esophageal cancer occurs at an earlier age than in the general population.[173-175]

Lynch, *et al.*[176] studied the incidence and prevalence of esophageal cancer in Omaha-Douglas County, Nebraska, a community of 350,000 (1960 census) during 1964 and identified 16 patients with histologically verified carcinoma of the esophagus (14 cases were squamous cell carcinoma and 2 were anaplastic carcinoma of the esophagus). The incidence rate was 4.6 per 100,000 population; the prevalence of the condition approximated the incidence since few patients survived in this particular series longer than one year (2 were alive after one year, though both succumbed within one and one-half years after their diagnoses). The United States mortality rate for esophageal cancer based on 1957 statistics was 2.7 per 100,000 population. Therefore, the incidence rate in the community under study exceeded that of the United States mortality rate with statistical significance at the 5 percent level. It was of extreme interest in this study that the economic level of all of the patients with esophageal cancer was distinctly lower than that of the median family income for the community, and furthermore, the distribution of esophageal cancer in the community was restricted to the lowest socioeconomic census tracts. This area was characterized by the greatest unemployment and lowest income per family in the city. *All* of the cases occurred in this area of the community, which represented a total population of 89,000 in the census tracts in which the lesion was found, and when compared with the United States mortality rates of

2.7 per 100,000, the difference was highly significant at the 1 percent level.

Esophageal cancer occurred more frequently among Negroes than whites in this community (after due correction was made for the overall population of Negroes and whites) though this difference was significant only at the 10 percent level.

No familial occurrences of esophageal cancer were found in this particular study. In addition to racial and socioeconomic factors, other aspects of potential epidemiologic importance included the occurrence of alcoholism among approximately 75 percent of the 16 patients with esophageal cancer. It should be noted that alcoholism has been a constant source of interest in the etiology of esophageal cancer, though its etiological role cannot be fully determined until additional factors are studied such as the specific types of alcoholic beverages consumed and the level of contaminants such as nitrosamines, zinc, lead, and other possible carcinogenic agents.[177,178]

Some of the highest incidences of esophageal cancer in the world are found in Iran. Pour and Ghadirian[178a] report a remarkable family from Iran wherein thirteen descendants of the same parents manifested esophageal cancer. The authors postulate that the intense aggregation of esophageal cancer in this family may have resulted from environmental influence on genetically susceptible individuals.

The only association of esophageal cancer with hereditary factors of which we are aware, is that with autosomal dominantly inherited tylosis palmaris et plantaris[179] (see Chapter 21).

Gastric Cancer

The marked decline in mortality from stomach cancer among Caucasians in the United States during the past 40 to 50 years has been dramatic. For example, the age adjusted mortality rates for males has declined from 28 per 100,000 in 1930 to 9.7 per 100,000 in 1967. On the other hand, the incidence of this disease is exceedingly high in Japan, Finland, and Chile. While the decline in incidence in the United States has been noted in both sexes, it affects males twice as often as females. Noteworthy, also, has been a relationship between the incidence of gastric cancer and the patient's socioeconomic status; specifically, an inverse relationship exists between the lowest and highest socioeconomic groups, the lowest having an incidence of gastric cancer approximately 3 times higher than the upper socioeconomic populations. Foreign-born groups in the United States also have higher mortality rates from stomach cancer than the native-born. In reviewing these data, Lilienfeld[180] suggested that the data are consistent with environmental etiological factors for gastric carcinoma. Environmental factors which have been under consideration have included dietary habits with a suggestion that the lesion is increased in areas where people eat fewer green vegetables and citrus fruits but consume more starchy foods. Soil in areas where gastric cancer occurs excessively has been analyzed particularly with respect to trace metals; air pollution has also been under scrutiny including occupational exposures, particularly with respect to the textile industry and mining. However, epidemiologic factors to date have not been consistent enough to pinpoint any distinct etiology.[181] Familial factors have been recorded in investigations of gastric cancer though these studies have not delineated specific genetic mechanisms nor their specific interaction with common environmental exposures in specific families.[182]

Pastore, *et al.*[183] have demonstrated a relationship between low serum pepsinogen levels and gastric carcinoma in Japanese males. It is suggested that possibly dietary habits may influence pepsinogen levels and these might provide clues to the etiology of gastric carcinoma. Thus, using a measurable parameter such as pepsinogen we might be provided with a profitable epidemiologic approach to the problem of gastric cancer in other population studies.

One of the enigmas of gastric cancer is an unexplained and consistent statistical relationship between this lesion and pancreatic carcinoma. Specifically, in the United States, pancreatic carcinoma has increased in the face of the mentioned decrease in gastric cancer. For example, Krain[184] cites a 383 percent increase in the age adjusted mortality rate from pancreatic cancer between 1920 and 1965 in the United States. Soberingly, approximately one in every 16 cancer deaths in patients of all ages is pancreatic cancer.[185] Statistics from the American Cancer Society have revealed that pancreatic cancer is the most lethal malignancy among men from age 35 to 54 and accounts for the most frequent site of cancer in men from age 55 to 74; pancreatic cancer accounted for more deaths in males in 1971 than that from any other malignant neoplasm except cancer of the lung, colon, and rectum.[185]

Thus, we find remarkable changes in incidence in these two malignant neoplasms in that 40 years ago stomach cancer resulted in more male deaths than from any other cancer and occurred approximately 12 times more frequently than pancreatic cancer; today, we see almost an inverse relationship between these two malignancies.[185,186] We also find world wide implications for this inverse relationship between gastric and pancreatic cancer. Specifically, in countries where a high incidence of gastric cancer exists, we find a low incidence of pancreatic carcinoma, and vice versa. For example, as mentioned, the Japanese have one of the highest rates of gastric cancer and yet, they have one of the lowest rates in the world for pancreatic cancer.[187] Other contrasts have been less well documented but merit further study. For example, there appears to be a significant urban preponderance of pancreatic cancer while gastric cancer appears to occur more frequently in rural populations.[185] The average age at onset of gastric cancer appears to be increasing while that for pancreatic cancer appears to be decreasing. While familial factors have been mentioned for gastric cancer, there is less evidence that familial factors are involved in pancreatic cancer.[185]

Possibly the most renowned family with a history of stomach cancer is that of Napoleon Bonaparte. Specifically, Napoleon died in 1821 from carcinoma of the stomach. It is alleged that his grandfather, his father, his brother, and his three sisters all died from carcinoma of the stomach.[188]

Genetic studies of stomach cancer probands and their families have failed to disclose simple inheritance patterns for this disease. Males are affected twice as frequently as females. Pernicious anemia appears to be associated frequently with carcinoma of the stomach.[189] Gastric cancer is also frequently associated with blood group A.[190-193]

The general concensus of opinion from studies of families with gastric cancer is that there is a three-fold increased risk for gastric cancer among relatives of gastric cancer probands over that in the general population.[194] [195] In addition, Mosbech[196] reported increased occurrences of achlorhydria, gastric carcinoma, and pernicious anemia among the relatives of patients with stomach cancer. Thus, Videbaek has reasoned that possibly it is the tendency to achlorhydria which is inherited and which in turn predisposes the patients to both gastric cancer and pernicious anemia.

Studies of identical twins have revealed only a weak tendency for concordance of gastric cancer in monozygous as opposed to dizygous twins.[197,198] Finally, stomach cancer may be found in association with another genetic disease. Specifically, Haerer, *et al.*[199]

report two sibs with ataxia telangiectasia, each of whom developed mucinous adenocarcinoma of the stomach in the second decade of life. Their mother also developed gastric cancer.

Gallbladder Cancer

The etiology of carcinoma of the gallbladder is unknown although an association with gallstones has been documented repeatedly in the medical literature.[200] Another interesting facet of this disease is its apparent prevalence among American Indians in southwestern United States.[201-205] Indeed it has been verified that American Indians in the Southwest have an unusually high incidence of gallbladder disease of all types.[202] Cholecystectomy is the most frequent surgical procedure performed at the Phoenix Indian Hospital; this operation outnumbered appendectomies by a ratio of 2.7:1.[204] Autopsies from various Indian tribes showed a 40 percent incidence of gallbladder disease indicating an incidence more than double that found in American non-Indian populations. In one epidemiologic study of the Pima Indians a prevalence of 48.6 percent of gallbladder disease was observed.

Nelson and associates[202] reviewing medical records from the Fort Defiance Hospital located on the Navajo Indian Reservation in Northern Arizona found that about 95 percent of its patients are full-blooded Navajo Indians while about 5 percent are Hopi Indians. This record review revealed an inordinantly high incidence of gallbladder disease of all varieties, a high rate of common duct stones, and a high incidence of gallbladder cancer (6% of patients undergoing laparotomy for gallbladder disease). Rates for gallbladder cancer from other reports of various southwest Indian tribes ranged from 3 percent to 3.8 percent.[203] These figures are higher than the generally accepted 1 to 2 percent incidence for the non-Indian population.[206-208]

In a similar study at the Phoenix Hospital, Reichenbach[209] noted that the rate of gallbladder and biliary tract cancer in Indians was six times that of the non-Indian population. This observation was based upon a review of autopsy studies in this population.

An important observation in the study by Nelson and associates[202] was the likelihood of the presence of cancer in females over 50 years of age who underwent laparotomy for suspected gallbladder or biliary tract disease.

An interesting observation among the Indians in the Southwest is a marked paucity of duodenal ulcer disease. This fact facilitates the differential diagnosis of cholecystitis in these Indians. Thus, signs or symptoms of right upper quandrant peritonitis are almost uniformly due to cholecystitis in Indians.

In summary, Nelson and associates[202] concluded that gallbladder disease is a frequent and virulent public health problem in southwestern American Indians. It appears particularly to affect young women with production of a high incidence of common duct stones and cancer.

Of epidemiologic interest is the fact that these American Indians are relatively homogeneous by virtue of fairly uniform dietary habits; they are centrally located on reservations with obviously similar environmental exposures.

Intraocular Malignant Melanoma *

Although primary intraocular malignant melanoma comprises a relatively small proportion of all malignant melanomas, it is, nevertheless, the most common malignant

*Portions of this material are reprinted by permission of the publishers of *Cancer*, from Lynch, H.T., *et al.* Heredity and Intraocular Malignant Melanoma, *Cancer* 21:119–125, 1968.

neoplasm of the eye. The lesion occurs most frequently after the fifth and sixth decades of life and is extremely rare in children. It seems to have a definite racial predilection, being most frequently found in Caucasians and rarely in Negroes. This racial difference is reflected by the Registry of Ophthalmic Pathology of the Armed Forces Institute of Pathology, where the ratio of ocular melanoma in Caucasians to non-Caucasians is 250:1.[210] There is no significant difference in frequency in men and women. The clinical behavior of metastases of this lesion is highly unpredictable. In some patients the disease may have a fulminant course; in others, as many as 20 or more years may elapse after enucleation of the affected eye before widespread dissemination occurs.[211] The principal site of metastasis is the liver. In some cases the liver may be the only site of metastasis and, indeed, may seemingly represent a new primary tumor; however, in other patients, virtually every organ and tissue of the body ultimately may be involved with metastatic disease.

The etiology of ocular malignant melanoma is unknown.[210 220] Several studies[212,213,215,217-219] have suggested a hereditary basis for this lesion in particular families.

We have studied two families in each of whom this lesion has appeared in two or more relatives.[221] In addition, we have analyzed medical records from 45 consecutive patients with histologic confirmation of ocular melanoma. Finally, we also surveyed practicing ophthalmologists and dermatologists in Texas, with respect to their experience with this lesion from the standpoint of its familial occurrence in their practice.

Genetic Studies

Our survey was made of the medical records of 45 patients with histologic diagnosis of intraocular melanoma who were seen at the University of Texas M.D. Anderson Hospital and Tumor Institute between March, 1944 and September, 1966. Search was made for information on the presence of this same lesion in relatives of these patients. Only one patient (Family 1) had a similarly affected relative; in this case, a sister of the patient had a histologically verified intraocular malignant melanoma. A second family (Family 2), completely unrelated to Family 1, was referred to us because of our interest in cancer genetics. Study of both families included correspondence with relatives, physicians, hospitals and bureaus of vital statistics to substantiate genealogic, general medical, and pathologic information. Histologic confirmation for intraocular melanoma was sought in every case and, when possible, slides from the tissue specimens were obtained for review.

Further information concerning the possible familial occurrence of intraocular melanoma was sought through a survey of all ophthalmologists and dermatologists in Texas listed in the 1965 AMA Membership Directory. This listing included 213 ophthalmologists and 103 dermatologists. Our reason for attempting to ascertain cases known to dermatologists was to determine if there were any familial occurrences of concurrent cutaneous and intraocular melanomas.

Results

Review of 45 records of patients with histologically confirmed intraocular melanoma revealed only one example of the lesion occurring in a relative (Family 1). There were 26 males and 19 females in this series. The average age at diagnosis of ocular melanoma was approximately 58 years. There were 43 Caucasian and two Negro patients. The left eye was affected in 23 patients and the right eye in 22 patients. Blood group data were available on only 22 of these individuals; of these, 12 had blood group "A" and 10 had

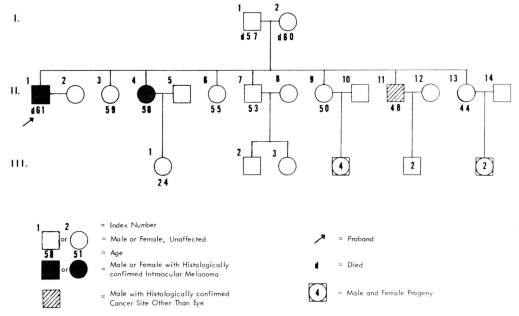

Figure 23–5. Pedigree of Family 1 with intraocular melanoma histologically confirmed in two siblings, published by permission of *Cancer* (Lynch and Krush, *Cancer*, 21:119–125, 1968).

blood group "O"; 19 were Rh positive and 3 were Rh negative.

Family 1

The proband (Fig. 23–5, II-1) was a 61-year-old Caucasian man whose past medical history up to age 59 was noncontributory; however, at age 59, he underwent enucleation of the right eye (January 1964). Histologic diagnosis was malignant melanoma. He did

well until January, 1966, at which time he lost weight and had generalized malaise. Biopsy of liver revealed metastatic malignant melanoma. The clinical course was progressively downhill and the patient died in July, 1966. Autopsy revealed that the cause of death was pulmonary embolism. There was evidence of widespread dissemination of malignant melanoma.

The family history revealed that the patient's mother had "cancer of the womb" and

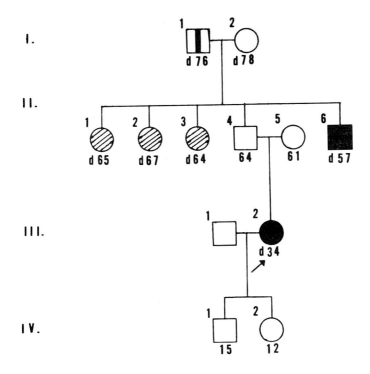

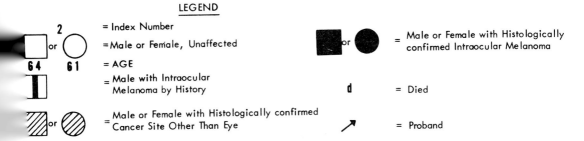

LEGEND

Figure 23–6. Intraocular Melanoma. Family 2.

died at age 60; the father died because of a traumatic injury at age 57. A sister of the proband (Fig. 23–5, II-4) is a 58-year-old Caucasian woman who had a history of "tearing of the right eye" since 1957. An elevated pigmented mass was seen temporal to the macular area of the right eye in 1963, and she was examined periodically until May, 1965, at which time the lesion extended towards the macular area. The right eye was enucleated and the histologic diagnosis was malignant melanoma. The remainder of the medical history is noncontributory. This sister has one child (Fig. 23–5, III-1), a girl, age 24, whose medical history is unremarkable. A brother of the proband (Fig. 23–5, II-11), age 48, had a histologically confirmed diagnosis of papillary adenocarcinoma of the rectum in 1965. The remainder of the family history is noncontributory. There is no evidence of consanguinity in this family.

Family 2

The proband (Fig. 23–6, III-2) was a 34-year-old Caucasian woman. She had a diagnosis of episcleritis of the left eye at age 31 in August, 1959. Dilation of the eyes at that time revealed no abnormal findings. In January, 1962, she complained of "blurring of vision." Dilation at that time showed a "large black mass at 12 o'clock" in the left eye. Immediate enucleation of the left eye was performed. The histologic diagnosis was malignant melanoma of the choroid and ciliary body.

In August, 1962, a large nodule, palpable in the region of the left lobe of the liver, was presumed to be metastatic malignant melanoma. Chlorambucil was prescribed; there was no significant improvement in her condition and she died two months later. Autopsy permission was refused. The remainder of her medical history was not remarkable.

The patient had two children, a son, age 15, and a daughter, age 12 (Fig. 23–6, IV-1

and IV-2), both in good health. Her father (Fig. 23–6, II-4), age 64, except for recurrent renal lithiasis since 1951, was in good health. A paternal aunt (Fig. 23–6, II-1) died at age 65 because of histologically confirmed cholangiocarcinoma of the liver; another paternal aunt (Fig. 23–6, II-2) died at age 67 because of histologically confirmed adenocarcinoma of the stomach; a third paternal aunt (Fig. 23–6, II-3) died at age 64 of histologically confirmed adenocarcinoma of the rectum; a paternal uncle (Fig. 23–6, II-6) died at age 57 from histologically confirmed malignant melanoma of the choroid of the right eye; and, finally, her paternal grandfather (Fig. 23–6, I-1) allegedly had intraocular melanoma and died at age 76. This patient died in a foreign country, and thus far, we have been unsuccessful in obtaining histologic confirmation of this lesion. There was no evidence of consanguinity in this family.

Questionnaires were answered by 113 ophthalmologists and 72 dermatologists practicing in Texas. Of these physicians, only three (all ophthalmologists) stated that they had observed intraocular melanoma in more than one relative of a family; however, details of these familial occurrences are insufficient for genetic analysis.

Comment

Intraocular melanoma has received little systematic epidemiologic study and minor attention has been directed toward the possible role of hereditary factors.[221] A review of the world literature revealed several reports of intraocular melanoma occurring in more than one relative. Highlights from these reports are as follows:

1. Gutmann[215] in 1895 reported five patients with intraocular melanoma, one of whom had a positive family history of this lesion. This patient was a Caucasian woman

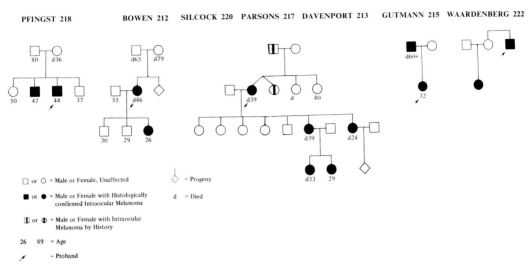

Figure 23–7. Series of patients with intraocular melanoma from world literature.

who underwent enucleation of her right eye at age 32 for spindle cell sarcoma of the choroid. Her father died of melanotic sarcoma of the choroid two years before the diagnosis in his daughter. His age at death was not recorded (Fig. 23–7).

2. Silcock[220] (1892), Parsons[217] (1905) and Davenport[213] (1927) reported familial occurrences of intraocular melanosarcoma. Silcock and Parsons described the tumor in two generations and Davenport described it in three generations; however, these reports refer to the same family. We have taken the liberty of consolidating the information in the three reports to construct the pedigree shown in Figure 23–7, and the following summary: The proband was a 38-year-old woman whose left eye was enucleated for a spindle cell pigmented melanoma. Her father had an eye removed but the reason for enucleation was not given; however, it was stated that it was not from an injury. Her twin sister also had an eye removed, again for reasons other than an injury. Another sister had a tumor removed from the breast at age 40. The proband had seven children, two of whom were affected. The youngest

child had her left eye enucleated at age 19 for a pigmented mixed round spindle cell sarcoma of the choroid. She died 5 years later from metastatic melanoma. An older daughter had her left eye removed at about age 30 and her right eye was removed at about age 38 because of melanotic sarcoma of the ciliary body and choroid. She apparently had disseminated melanoma at her last operation and died the following year. She had two daughters, each of whom had had the right eye removed for sarcoma of the choroid. The elder daughter had her eye removed at age 29 and died of metastatic melanoma 4 years later; the younger daughter had her eye removed at age 19 and, though having freely movable, sharply defined, painless, subcutaneous "lumps," she was still alive 10 years after her enucleation. The average age of the five authenticated cases in this family was 28.6 years, according to Davenport, and all died from metastatic melanoma except one, who is known to have survived at least 10 years.

3. A familial occurrence of ocular melanoma in two brothers was reported by Pfingst and Graves[218] in 1921 (Fig. 23–7). The older

brother had his left eye enucleated at age 47 for an intraocular spindle cell melanoblastoma (melanosarcoma). The tumor was located close to the optic nerve on its temporal side. The younger brother had his left eye enucleated at age 44. The tumor in his eye appeared to arise from the choroid anteriorly and extended to the ciliary body. Its general cellular structure was similar to that seen in his older brother. An older sister and younger brother apparently were unaffected.

4. Waardenberg[222] (1940) described melanosarcoma of the eye in an uncle and niece (Fig. 23–7).

5. A 1964 report by Bowen, *et al.*[212] (Fig. 23–7) described a Caucasian woman who had her right eye enucleated in 1953, at age 45. Histologic diagnosis was malignant melanoma of mixed cell type-spindle A and spindle B cells. She died 12 months later in 1954. Autopsy revealed metastatic malignant melanoma of the spindle cell type. In 1963, her 26-year-old daughter had her left eye enucleated. Histologic examination revealed a mixed tumor composed mainly of spindle A but with some spindle B cells.

Findings in our series of 45 patients with intraocular melanoma showed no significant statistical difference with respect to sex, the occurrence of the tumor in the right or left eye, or expected frequencies of the ABO and RH blood types. The ratio of 43 Caucasian and two Negro patients was not significantly different from the total ratio of Caucasian to Negro patients who have been admitted to this hospital since 1941. Only one familial occurrence of this lesion was encountered in this series, that of an affected brother and sister (Fig. 23–5, II-1 and II-4).

In most cases, the recorded family history was less than desirable for genetic study. Unfortunately, this is often the case in medicine and probably reflects lack of interest by the examiner in this aspect of the medical work-up; however, the advanced age of these patients (average age 58) and the overall

morbidity in some precluded obtaining accurate genealogic information. A further factor that could seriously compromise genetic expectations for intraocular melanoma is the advanced age of the patients at onset. Therefore, many patients could be genotypically predestined to develop this neoplasm (phenotypic expression) but because of mortality from other causes at advanced years, it does not appear. In addition, it is almost impossible to obtain reliable medical documentation on parents of elderly patients, many of whom may have come from foreign lands or whose records are not available because of deaths of their physicians, etc. Furthermore, the progeny of these patients are currently younger than the expected age for the development of intraocular melanoma though they may be at risk. Follow-up of such individuals on a longitudinal basis could be rewarding.

The findings of three families with intraocular melanoma from the survey of ophthalmologists and dermatologists is of genetic interest in the light of the over-all rarity of this disease; however, we are unable to speculate further on these families at this time because of the limited data.

The inheritance of ocular melanoma appears to be independent of cutaneous melanoma. Study of patients with familial intraocular melanoma reported in the literature and the two families reported here did not show cutaneous melanoma occurring in relatives. Moreover, of 28 families with cutaneous melanoma,[211] not a single example of intraocular melanoma was found. Exceptions to this problem are discussed in Chapter 23.

The age of occurrence of ocular melanoma in the familial cases, i.e. in our own two families, and those found in the literature averaged 20 years younger than those in the hospital series. This is in keeping with an earlier age of occurrence for hereditary malignant neoplasms as opposed to the same histologic variety occurring on a sporadic basis.[221]

The findings in Family 2 (Fig. 23–6) and those reported by Gutmann,[215] Silcock,[220] Parsons,[217] Davenport,[213] Waardenberg,[222] and Bowen and associates[212] (Fig. 23–7) are compatible with autosomal dominant inheritance. The fact that the father of the proband in Family 2 is as yet unaffected does not in any way negate autosomal dominant inheritance. Possible explanations for this are that of reduced penetrance of the gene and/or that the subject may ultimately manifest this disease should he survive long enough.

Autosomal recessive inheritance or autosomal dominant inheritance with reduced penetrance of the gene provides a possible explanation for the remaining families; however, the absence of consanguinity, while not excluding a recessive factor, tends to mitigate against this mode of inheritance.

Intraocular melanoma also has shown an increased association with von Recklinghausen's neurofibromatosis, an autosomally dominant inherited disorder.[214] Thus we have further evidence suggesting the importance of hereditary or constitutional factors.

The overwhelming majority of cases of intraocular melanoma appear sporadically, seemingly caused by factors other than heredity. This in no way weakens the argument favoring the role of heredity for some families with this disease. Other rarely occurring tumors, including retinoblastoma[223] may behave similarly to intraocular melanoma; i.e. most cases are sporadic but, when occurring in families, the mode of inheritance may be clear-cut, namely, autosomal dominant.

Carotid Body Tumors

The carotid body is composed of a network of chemoreceptor tissue located on both sides of the upper cervical region in the area of the bifurcation of the common carotid artery. Variations in oxygen, carbon dioxide tension and pH all stimulate this organ causing reflex changes in respiration and vasomotor activities.

Malignant transformation of carotid body tumors is a relatively infrequent event. For example, of approximately 500 cases of carotid body tumors described by Staats and associates,[224] 8.4 percent showed definite changes of malignancy. Metastasizing carotid body tumors are rare. Reese and associates[225] reported a case and reviewed 14 examples from the literature. Whimster and Masson[226] reported a case of metastasizing carotid body tumor and in reviewing the subject they found two other cases in addition to the 14 reviewed by Reese and associates.[225]

The first carotid body tumor was described in 1891 by Marchand[227] while the first description of a familial occurrence of carotid body tumors was reported by Chase[228] in 1944. He described bilateral occurrences of carotid body tumors in the proband with histologic confirmation of carotid body tumor occurring unilaterally in the proband's sister. In reviewing the subject, Rush,[229] found several kindreds with the lesion occurring in two or more family members. Again, bilateral occurrence of the lesion was found in at least one affected member in each family. Rush concluded that bilateral occurrence is a more likely event in the familial variety of carotid body tumors than in the sporadic variety. Kroll and associates[230] reported carotid body tumors in 12 individuals in two generations of a family and interestingly, five of the twelve showed bilateral occurrence of the lesion. A review of familial carotid body tumors by Resler and associates[231] also showed a significant occurrence of bilateral lesions. These studies show clearly that bilateral tumors are significantly frequent in individuals having the familial variety and furthermore bilateral tumors may appear simultaneously or at intervals of

months or years in these patients. The
hereditary variety of carotid body tumors
occurs in about 3 percent of the cases and
the mode of transmission is consistent with
an autosomal dominant inheritance pattern.
Thus, the overwhelming majority of occurrences of carotid body tumors are sporadic
and of unknown etiology.[231] Examination of
all members of a family is therefore advo-
cated with removal of the tumors while they
are small. Angiography is a useful procedure
in the diagnosis of carotid body tumors.

Werner's Syndrome

In 1940, Werner[232] reported the combination of short stature and cataracts, skin
changes, which included atrophy, hyperkeratosis, tautness, and ulceration of the
feet and hands, muscle and joint changes,
early menopause, early graying of the hair
and a premature and progressive senility in
four siblings. These are characteristic of the
condition now known as Werner's syndrome.

For many years Rothmund's syndrome[233]
was considered essentially the same disorder
as Werner's syndrome, though recently a
clear delineation between these two disorders has been established, primarily as a
result of the work of Thannhauser.[234] Epstein, *et al.*[235] have reviewed the subject of
Werner's syndrome, and have described this
disease in 3 members of a sibship. Their review of the world literature included 122
additional cases of Werner's syndrome and
have characterized the primary features of
the syndrome as follows:

> ... symmetrical retardation of growth
> with absence of the adolescent growth
> spurt, graying of the hair, atrophy and
> hyperkeratosis of the skin, generalized
> loss of hair, alteration of the voice,
> cataracts (subcapsular and cortical,
> usually posterior), ulcerations of the

feet, and mild diabetes in about half of
the cases ... (other features included):
> ... atrophy of the muscle, fat, and
> bones of the extremities, vascular
> calcification, soft tissue (usually peri-
> articular) calcification, and general-
> ized osteoporosis , . . 'Hypogonad-
> ism' ... (in both sexes) was frequently
> present.

It is significant that approximately 10 percent of the patients described in this series
manifested malignant neoplasms, the predominant form being sarcomas as opposed
to carcinomas. Meningiomas were also found
to occur frequently.

A difficulty in the diagnosis of Werner's
syndrome is that the diagnosis cannot usually
be made until the patient is over age 30,
since the cardinal features of the syndrome,
i.e. cataracts and skin ulcerations, do not
usually present until this age. However, the
index of suspicion for any particular patient
might be increased through knowledge of
the presence of the disease in the family in
which case an earlier diagnosis might be
possible.

The basic metabolic derangement in Werner's syndrome is unclear despite about 65
years of accumulated clinical experience with
the disease. Possible etiologies have included
defects in ectoderm as well as primary endocrinopathies implicating the parathyroid or
pituitary glands.[236] Recently, investigators
have considered the role of enzymatic defects in this disease.[236-238] However, in
spite of frequent allusions to endocrinologic
etiologic factors, particularly the gonads and
diabetes mellitus, the role of these phenomena in Werner's syndrome is not yet clearly
understood. As a matter of fact, Riley and
associates[239] have recently discounted an
endocrinologic basis for this disease (Fig.
23–8).

Werner's syndrome is inherited in an autosomal recessive manner. The association of

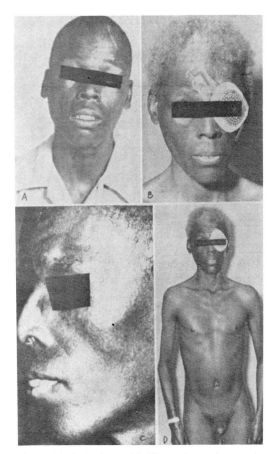

Figure 23–8. Patient with Werner's syndrome. A. The patient at age 24; B. The same patient at age 34 showing the marked aging; C. Demonstrates the characteristic beaking of the nose; D. Shows the slender tapering of the extremities, tight skin, and normal external genitalia. Reproduced by permission of Thomas R. Riley, M.D., and the Editor, *Annals of Internal Medicine*, 63:285–294, 1965.

malignant neoplasms in Werner's syndrome has been well documented[237,240–247] and as mentioned above, there is an unusually high incidence of sarcomas. However, in evaluating these cancer associations, we must realize that this is a relatively rare disease and it is possible that some of the cases were reported primarily because of the rarity of the condition and interest generated by the associated cancer.

Celiac Disease (Nontropical Sprue; Gluten-Induced Enteropathy)

The triad of intestinal malabsorption, abnormal small-bowel structure, and gluten intolerance comprises the main clinical characteristics of celiac disease. This disease has also been referred to in the literature as gluten-induced enteropathy. It should also be noted that celiac disease in children and so-called nontropical sprue are the same disorder with apparently the same pathogenesis.[248] The statistical incidence of this disease in the general population is not known, primarily because its incidence may vary significantly from one population to the next, and the disease itself may also vary in each individual. For example, an individual may have typical mucosal changes and yet have no overt manifestations of the disease, thus making the diagnosis virtually impossible unless a mucosal biopsy were obtained for other reasons. However, in the usual case, patients with celiac disease manifest typical features of the malabsorption syndrome, including weight loss, abdominal distention and bloating, diarrhea, steatorrhea, and abnormal absorptive function. Patients also may present with iron deficiency anemia, hypoprothrombinemia, or puzzling metabolic bone disease with demineralization, compression deformities, kyphoscoliosis, or Milkman's fractures, all in the absence of significant diarrhea or steatorrhea. In addition, for reasons unknown at the present time, emotional disturbances appear to be common in patients with celiac disease.

In the absence of specific diagnostic tests for nontropical sprue, the following three factors should be evaluated in order to arrive at a definitive diagnosis: evidence of malabsorption; an abnormal jejunal biopsy showing subtotal villous atrophy; and clinical, biochemical, and histological improvement following a gluten-free diet.

Occasionally, the diagnosis might be made more clear through challenging the patient with 30 to 50 Gms of gluten taken orally. If this causes increased diarrhea and steatorrhea immediately, the diagnosis of gluten-induced enteropathy will be confirmed.

Mounting evidence indicates that celiac sprue is an inherited disease resulting from an autosomal dominant gene with incomplete penetrance.[249] A sex-influenced factor is likely in that women are affected twice as frequently as men. However, the specific pathogenetic mechanism accounting for the difference in sex ratio is not known.

In 1962, Gough and associates identified the association of celiac sprue with cancer, and described intestinal reticulosis complicating idiopathic steatorrhea.[250] This association was confirmed by other investigators, including Harris and associates[251] in their study of 202 patients with adult celiac disease and idiopathic steatorrhea; 6.9 percent of these patients developed either lymphoma or carcinoma of the gastrointestinal tract (predominantly carcinoma of the esophagus). The mean duration of symptoms of celiac disease prior to the diagnosis of lymphoma in these patients was 21.2 years and for carcinoma of the gastrointestinal tract, 38.5 years. Interestingly, a gluten-free diet appeared to diminish the risk of malignant transofrmations in these patients.

In reviewing the subject, Harris and associates[251] noted that an association between adult celiac disease and malignant lymphoma had been identified more than thirty years earlier and more recently the association of this disease with carcinoma has been observed. Austad and associates[252] reviewed this problem and described 7 patients with histologically confirmed idiopathic steatorrhea in whom lymphoma developed. They called attention to 17 additional patients in whom this association was probable and suggested further that possibly in as many as 50 percent of reported cases, the patients had idiopathic steatorrhea prior to the development of lymphoma. These authors believed that the most frequent mode of presentation of reticulosis in this disease is the result of failure of response to treatment for steatorrhea or recurrence of symptoms in patients who had improved as a result of treatment. They found that abdominal pain, skin rashes, fever, and an abdominal mass occurred frequently in these patients and that laparotomy with biopsy offered the best chance for diagnosis. When steatorrhea occurs with malignant lymphoma, the tumor is most often found in the proximal small intestine. Finally, these authors also suggested that the incidence of Hodgkin's disease is increased in these patients and that the onset of lymphoma is often later than that expected in the general population, and the prognosis is generally poorer.

Additional reports,[253] including one describing acute myeloid leukemia in a patient with celiac disease[254] tend to support the assumption that cancer is closely associated with this disorder.

Harris and associates[251] summarize the problem by stating that the celiac patient in whom lymphoma is most likely to develop is most often a male, over age 40, with a history of celiac disease for more than ten years and who is *not* on a gluten-free diet.

Autoimmune factors[253-255] may be the underlying mechanism in this disease which leads to irreversible malignant change. Observations of disturbance of immunoglobulins[256,257] in patients with celiac disease support this possibility.

Familial Fibrocystic Pulmonary Dysplasia

In 1944 Hamman and Rich[258] described 4 patients with a fatal form of acute diffuse interstitial pulmonary fibrosis (all died a few months after the diagnosis was made). Since that time, others have noted patients with similar pathological findings but manifesting a less acute clinical course of this disease; in general these patients have been considered to have the same disease. In 1959 Donohue and associates[259] reported three families with this condition suggesting a hereditary form of the disease and they suggested the term, "familial fibrocystic pulmonary dysplasia." Additional families have now been documented and these have been reviewed briefly by Young[260] who reported an additional affected patient in a previously reported family. The review by Koch[261] revealed 31 cases of familial fibrocystic pulmonary dysplasia within 10 families described in the world literature through 1965. He added a new family in which three unequivocal and 5 probable cases of familial fibrocystic pulmonary dysplasia occurred among 56 relatives. The findings were consistent with an autosomal dominant mode of inheritance.

Diagnostic criteria for familial fibrocystic pulmonary dysplasia include digital clubbing which may precede clinical onset by several years, progressive dyspnea and cyanosis, plumonary hypertension, polycythemia, arterial hypoxia and hypocapnia, negative sweat tests, and x-ray findings of diffuse bilateral pulmonary fibrosis. Diffuse fibrocystic pulmonary dysplasia may be confirmed postmortem.[262] These patients have a significantly increased risk for bronchogenic carcinoma. McKusick and Fisher[263] discussed the role of carcinoma as a complication of cystic disease of the lung in terms of a situation comparable to malignant degeneration in hereditary polyposis of the colon and in hereditary neurofibromatosis. They gave a second analogy, namely, the possible occurrence of malignancy in this disease in terms of its superimposition upon chronically infected and scarred areas such as occurs in the esophagus in achalasia, in the skin in lupus vulgaris, in burn scars, and in chronic vari-

cose ulcers, in the colon in ulcerative colitis, and in the lung in bronchiectasis.

Nasopharyngeal Carcinoma (NPC)

Nasopharyngeal carcinoma occurs infrequently in most parts of the world. However, in Asia this particular cancer is the most frequently occurring malignant neoplasm in male Chinese who originate from the Southern Province of Kwangtung.[264] Historically, during the past 10 centuries, the Southern Chinese have migrated often and interestingly, an increased frequency of NPC (nasopharyngeal carcinoma) has been found in those individuals who have migrated to Singapore,[265] Java,[266] Australia,[267] and more recently, California.[268] For example, the minimal age-adjusted incidence rate of NPC in the Hong Kong population was 25.2 per 100,000 males and 10.6 for females in 1965[269] while it was only 0.7 in the Swedish population.[270]

Whenever cancer epidemiologists note such striking relationships between a particular racial or ethnic group and an extreme susceptibility to develop a particular malignant neoplasm, they wonder immediately about the role of genetic factors, environmental factors, and/or their interaction. Thus, de-The and associates began detailed studies of this problem[271] and they directed their efforts toward both genetic and environmental factors; in the latter they have paid particular attention to the possibility of a virological factor interacting with host factors.[272] Biopsies of NPC tissue were cultured and permanent lymphoblastoid lines were established in which a Herpes-type virus was discovered. Indirect immunofluorescence test showed that this virus shared structural antigens with Epstein-Barr virus, of the type associated with Burkitt's lymphoma. de-The and associates consider this association exceedingly complex; more work will be necessary to discern its true meaning.[271] de-The has also noted occasional aggregations of NPC in families. In one remarkable family, NPC was found in the propositus who was one of 10 children. Analysis of the family revealed that no fewer than 6 of the 10 children had died of NPC. The father of the propositus had been married twice. Interestingly, none of the three children from one wife had the disease but 6 of the 7 children from his second wife were affected with NPC. There was a definite case of NPC in the parental generation, one in the grandparental generation and a possible case even in one generation further back.[273] de-The postulates a genetically determined susceptibility to viral tumorigenesis comparable to the situation in certain inbred mice where oncogenic viruses are common but wherein tumors arose only in genetically susceptible animals.[274]

Hereditary Multiple Exostosis

Hereditary multiple exostosis is characterized clinically by numerous cartilage-capped exostoses which are located primarily in areas of actively growing bone of the endochondral skeleton. These lesions appear to be juxtaepiphysial in origin and therefore are found typically at the ends of the tubular bones, vertebral borders of the scapula, the iliac crest, and the ribs. Areas which are usually unaffected are the vertebral bodies, the patella, and the carpal and tarsal bones.[275] Bone growth is also involved giving rise to readily recognizable deformities in approximately 3 out of every 4 affected patients. The most common deformities include shortness of stature, bowing of the radius with ulnar deviation of the wrist, subluxation of the humoral radial joint, valgus deformity of the knee and ankle, tibiofibular synostosis, and asymmetry of the pectoral and pelvic girdles. These abnormal-

ities frequently occur in a haphazard manner with the exception of the ankle deformity which is usually bilateral and symmetrical.[275]

The disorder may be diagnosed at birth in certain patients through radiologic studies. Approximately 30 percent of patients will show manifestations of the defect during the first decade of life.

The most ominous complication of this disorder is the potential for malignant transformation of exostoses to chondrosarcoma. The frequency of this complication has varied considerably in the several reported series. For example, Dahlin[276] found an incidence of chondrosarcoma in approximately 10 percent of patients with the disorder while Jaffe[277] suggested that the frequency of chondrosarcoma was 25 percent. Solomon[275] on the other hand, allowing that cancer is a frequent occurrence, believed that these figures were higher than the observations of most clinicians.

The most common sites for this malignancy are the ilium and the proximal end of the femur. The tumor is slow-growing and metastases occur late. These lesions are radiation-resistant, making surgical extirpation the treatment of choice. Any increase in the size of an exostoses after normal maturation should be considered to be a sign of malignancy, until proven otherwise.

Exostoses may compress nerves and tendons, interfere with movement, and cause pain and other neurological sequelae. Thus, surgical resection for these reasons as well as for cosmetic purposes may be necessary. The prognosis for normal life expectancy is generally good unless chondrosarcomas develop.

Hereditary multiple exostosis is inherited by a single autosomal dominant gene with high penetrance. The mutation rate for this defect is believed to be high. In a study of 46 probands, Solomon[275] found that approximately 63 percent had affected relatives.

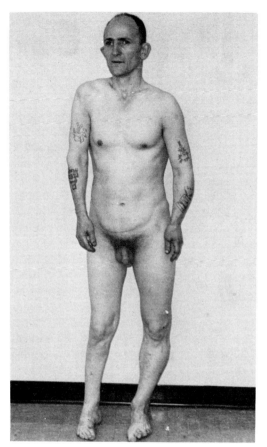

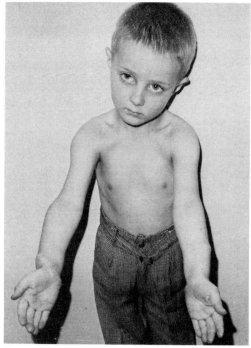

Figure 23–10. This is the son of the patient shown in Figure 23–9. Note the presence of exostoses of the upper extremities with minimal but albeit significant deformities.

Figure 23–9. Patient with hereditary multiple exostoses showing deformities of all four extremities which are more prominent in left arm and left leg, all of which are secondary to multiple exostoses.

There was no sex predilection and there is variable expressivity for this trait. These genetic observations have been confirmed by others.[278–280]

We have studied a family wherein a father and his son were both affected with hereditary multiple exostosis (Fig. 23–9 and 23–10). Note the numerous exostoses of the long bones with marked deformities of the left arm and both legs in the father (Fig. 23–9). Lesser but albeit significant exostoses and deformities are noted in the upper extremities of his son (Fig. 23–10).

Thymoma

Thymoma occurs only rarely in childhood. For example, of the 107 cases of thymomas reported by Lattes[281] only one example was in a child, and in this case the child was two years old; and of 51 cases of thymoma reported by Legg and Brady[282] only one was in a patient under 10 years of age.

Recently Matani and Dritsas[283] reported thymoma in a 27-month-old girl, which histologically was predominantly of the lymphocytic type. Two years prior to this diagnosis her older brother, age 9 months, died with symptoms of respiratory insufficiency, and at autopsy a thymoma was found which histologically was comprised solely of mature lymphocytes with scattered Hassall's corpuscles.

This example of familial thymoma documented in a brother and sister during infancy and early childhood are apparently the only examples of this problem reported in the literature.[283]

Metastasizing Carcinoid Tumors

Moertel and Dockerty[284] have documented multicentric and metastasizing carcinoid tumors of the ileum occurring in three patients through two generations of a family. It was of interest that one of the patients had two primary carcinomas, one being a metastasizing carcinoid tumor and the second primary was breast cancer. Her mother was related to the family by marriage. She also had had breast cancer.

In the review of the literature there are only two additional reports of the familial occurrence of carcinoid tumors. In one[285] a brother and sister had metastasizing carcinoid tumors of the ileum, and in the second a father and daughter had nonmetastasizing carcinoids of the appendix discovered as incidental findings at appendectomy.[286]

Alpha₁ Antitrypsin Deficiency and Hepatoma

Alpha$_1$ antitrypsin deficiency is inherited as an autosomal recessive and has been shown to be associated with chronic obstructive pulmonary disease when the genetic defect is present in the homozygous state.[287-289] While the clinical picture may differ among individuals, early onset of emphysema is the rule. Although the issue of pulmonary disease had previously captured the attention of clinical investigators, Sharp, et al.[290] were the first investigators to document an association between liver disease and alpha$_1$ antitrypsin deficiency. Specifically, they reported 10 children with cirrhosis in six families manifesting alpha$_1$ antitrypsin deficiency. These observations have now been confirmed by several other investigators and are recorded in a recent review by Berg and Eriksson.[291] In addition, these authors examined liver tissue from autopsy specimens in 13 patients and a biopsy specimen in another patient all showing homozygous alpha$_1$ antitrypsin deficiency. They found that the hepatocytes contained periodic-acid-Schiff-positive globular material similar to that found in infantile cirrhosis with alpha$_1$ antitrypsin deficiency. Five of these patients died of cirrhosis and three had fibrosis of the liver. Of these 8 patients, all of whom were over 50 years of age, 3 also had hepatomas. Of the 13 autopsy cases, 12 had either bullous or panacinar emphysema.

This study suggests that in the genetic disorders, alpha$_1$ antitrypsin deficiency, pulmonary emphysema and liver disease are linked. While the association of hepatoma with this problem is limited, based upon three verified cases, nevertheless, it indicates a greater need to study the cancer association in this metabolic defect. Models of this type could provide invaluable clues to carcinogenesis.

Poland's Syndrome

Poland's syndrome shows the following clinical manifestations: usual absence of the pectoralis major; less frequent features include syndactyly, bony abnormalities of the thorax and hypoplasia of the hand or arm.

In a review of the subject, Mace and associates[292] reported a patient with both Poland's syndrome and acute lymphocytic leukemia. Hoefnagel and associates[293] described another patient with both Poland's syndrome and acute myelocytic leukemia. Finally, Walters and associates[294] have reported an additional patient with both Poland's syndrome and acute leukemia.

All reports of this syndrome to date have described it as sporadic and of unknown etiology. However, the association of multiple congenital abnormalities of the muscular and skeletal systems suggest the possibility of a genetically determined defect. David,[295] on the other hand, suggested that poland's syndrome may result from exposure to a teratogenic agent in utero.

Hereditary Bone Dysplasia with Sarcomatous Degeneration: Study of a Family

A previously undescribed problem of bone dysplasia manifested as multiple areas of necrosis in the diaphyses of the large tubular bones has been described in a family.[296] It is of interest that an alarming frequency of medullary fibrosarcoma has occurred in affected members of this family. The cancers appear to arise primarily in the actively proliferating fibrous tissue that borders the islands of dead bone.

The family study involved 60 to 65 living members of the kindred of Irish extraction who had resided in midwestern Vermont and adjacent New York State for six generations. Bone dysplasia was present on historical evidence in father to son passage, thereby excluding X-linked inheritance. The trait (bone dysplasia) was expressed in four generations. The age of onset was 14 years or older. Symptoms included aching, tenderness over affected areas and occasional weakness of the involved extremity. Sarcoma was verified in four individuals in two generations; three affected individuals were members of a sibship of six. The inheritance pattern appears to be consistent with that of an autosomal dominant factor.[296]

Genetic counseling is difficult since phenotypic evidence of the disorder as shown by radiographic findings occur usually past puberty. The investigators plan a program of periodic radiographs of the legs in younger patients at risk. Scintiscans may aid in distinguishing sarcoma from underlying dysplasia and will be performed annually. Immediate biopsy of any suspicious area will hopefully improve cancer control.

Myxoma of the Heart

Myxomas are being diagnosed more frequently today, the result of increased interest in the problem combined with clinical evaluation and cineangiography. The first familial report of this problem was by Krause, *et al.*[297] in a report involving a 34-year-old man with myxoma of the pulmonic valve whose brother was said to have died of a myxoma involving the left atrium, at age 25. Kleid, *et al.*[298] report two brothers, one 14 years old with left atrial myxoma, and the other 16 years old with right atrial myxoma. Both of these individuals manifested the tumor at the same time. These two reports suggest a familial tendency to cardiac myxoma. The evidence, however, is insufficient to ascribe a mode of inheritance. Unfortunately no mention is made of consanguinity in these reports.

Tumors of the heart are exceedingly rare, with statistics showing that only 0.0017 percent of autopsies reveal this lesion. Interestingly, more than 50 percent of primary heart tumors are myxomas, and they may occur in any chamber of the heart.[299] These statistics attest to the possible role of familial factors in myxoma when multiple occurrences in any one particular family are found. Since myxoma is a treatable lesion, but one that may present great diagnostic difficulties unless it is given primary consideration, it may behoove us to be on the alert for other familial occurrences of this disease. Finally, rhabdomyomas of the heart have been a frequent finding in autosomal dominantly inherited tuberous sclerosis.[1]

X-linked Recessive Reticuloendothelial Syndrome with Hyperglobulinemia

Lymphoreticular malignancies[300] and certain reticuloendothelial syndromes may occur in families;[301] while generally rare, they have with few exceptions involved both males and females in single sibships in a single generation.[302] Efforts at determining specific modes of inheritance have for the most part been unsuccessful. However, Omenn[303] reported an inbred family with a fatal reticuloendothelial syndrome which suggested an autosomal recessive inheritance pattern.

Recently Falletta and associates[302] described a fatal reticuloendothelial disorder which appears to have been inherited as an X-linked recessive trait. This condition occurred in a Latin American family wherein consanguinity was not present. Only males of less than six years of age who were related through their mothers were affected. All of these affected boys had an affected maternal uncle. This comprised 17 affected boys from eight sibships in two generations. The disorder was characterized by fever, hepatosplenomegaly, lymph node enlargement, purpura, jaundice, and in some patients terminal convulsions occurred. The illness was brief with a clinical course lasting less than two months, and then followed by death. At onset of the illness, the youngest patient was four months of age and the oldest was five and one-half years of age. All of the children were phenotypically normal at birth with the exception of one, who manifested cataracts, deafness, and heart disease during the first month of life. All 17 of the children had fever and 12 out of 12 who had been carefully examined had lymphadenopathy and splenomegaly. Of these 12, eleven had hepatomegaly, nine had purpura, eight had pallor and jaundice, seven had rales and five had terminal convulsions.

Tissue was available from 13 patients including 12 from post-mortem material. Findings from these evaluations showed the following:

A mononuclear cell infiltrate was present in the liver (portal areas), lymph nodes, spleen, bone marrow, lungs, thymus, kidneys, meninges, brain, adrenals, heart, intestines, and testes, and, in one case, parathyroids. Mature plasma cells were also seen in most of the involved tissues, most prominently in the bone marrow.

The mononuclear cells were heterogeneous, many with large nuclei of different shapes—oval, round, fusiform, or indented. The nuclear chromatin was finely granular in some cells and coarsely granular in others. Prominent nucleoli (sometimes two) were found in many of the larger cells. The cytoplasm varied from a scanty pink rim around the larger nuclei to a plentiful maroon concentric or eccentric zone in smaller cells. The cytoplasm in most of the cells, large and small, stained with pyroninmethyl green stain. Occasional mitotic figures were seen.[302]

Hyperglobulinemia was a frequent finding; interestingly, approximately one half of the unaffected first degree relatives showed elevated immunoglobulin levels. The authors concluded that the patients' fatal disorder might have been due to a clonal proliferation of malignant cells which resemble T cells in their phytohemagglutinin responsiveness, as described previously by Davies, et al.[304]

This fascinating syndrome will merit careful longitudinal study, which fortunately is in the planning. Thus, of great concern will be the significance of the issue of elevated immunoglobulin levels amongst unaffected members of the family in order to determine if this finding is related to the occurrence of the fatal disorder or to any other types of malignant neoplasms.

Urinary Bladder Cancer

Fraumeni and Thomas[305] reported the occurrence of carcinoma of the urinary bladder in a man and his three sons. This was a white family of Russian-Jewish origin who had emigrated to the United States in 1910 and had settled in the Washington, D.C. area. There were no consanguinous marriages in the family. None of the family members had been exposed to dyes, chemicals, or occupational agents which have been either incriminated or suspected in bladder carcinogenesis. Each affected patient, however, had smoked approximately one package of cigarettes daily since adolescence, though the proband had discontinued his smoking habit 17 years prior to the diagnosis of bladder cancer.

In a single family report of this type it is not possible to define clearly the mechanism involved in the familial aggregation of cancer. The possibility of a chance event cannot be excluded, though the frequency of this site-specific malignant neoplasm in the family suggests either a common environmental exposure or a genetic effect and/or the interaction of both. With the exception of cigarette smoking, no common carcinogeneic exposure was observed. However, we should note that it has been estimated that cigarette smokers have a two- to three-fold greater risk of developing carcinoma of the urinary bladder than do nonsmokers.[306]

The only large genetic study on the subject is that of Morganti and associates;[307] this involved a comparison of 160 patients with urinary bladder cancer with 160 age-matched healthy controls. The authors found a history of bladder cancer in four relatives of the probands in the experimental group and in two relatives of the control group, a difference which was not statistically significant.

It will be important that evidence of bladder cancer in families be meticulously documented. Such studies should include a critical evaluation of potentially significant carcinogenic exposures including habit patterns such as cigarette smoking, which may be operating in concert with host factors.

Carcinoma of the Ureter

Carcinoma of the ureter has been histologically verified in a 68-year-old white woman and in her 53-year-old son.[308] There was no evidence of tumors of the genito-urinary system in any other relatives. However, details of the search for and documentation of cancer genealogy were not presented in this study.

This is the only report of familial occurrences of carcinoma of the ureter that we have been able to locate. It is possible that this familial association is due to chance, and therefore it may not harbor any epidemiologic significance. However, carcinoma of the ureter occurs relatively infrequently in the population, and the occurrence in a mother and her son merits further careful inquiry.

Carcinoma of Larynx

Laryngeal carcinoma comprises approximately 2.5 percent of all human cancers. However, in spite of the frequency of this lesion in the population very few references to its occurrence in families have been reported. In one such investigation Wynder and associates[309] studied 347 cases of laryngeal cancer, and from this group found only two examples of this lesion in siblings. This involved the occurrence of carcinoma of the epiglottis in sisters at ages 36 and 39 respectively. Interestingly, both of these ladies smoked more than one and one-half packages of cigarettes per day. Recently, Marlowe[310] has reported the occurrence of cancer of the larynx, histologically verified, in sisters ages 52 and 48 years respectively. Both sisters had similar smoking histories, with each smoking one package of cigarettes per day for approximately 15 years. The tumors were diagnosed within two weeks of each other, were similar histologically, and involved similar anatomic locations (base of the epiglottis). Remainder of the family history was reportedly unremarkable.

Genetics and Virilizing Adrenal Carcinoma

Hyperplasia of the adrenal cortex with virilization has been shown to occur in families. However, the occurrence of two or more patients with virilizing adrenal carcinoma in families is an exceedingly rare occurrence; specifically, there are only three reports of familial occurrence of this lesion available in the literature.[311-313] In the case of virilization due to adrenal hyperplasia (adrenal genital syndrome) the mode of inheritance of the several varieties of this condition is autosomal recessive.

A report by Mahloudji and associates[313] presented an example of virilizing adrenal carcinoma in two siblings wherein parental consanguinity was documented. Because of histologic documentation of the adrenal lesion in two siblings, parental consanguinity, absence of abnormality in the parents, and the mixed sexes of the affected sibs, the authors suggested an autosomal recessive mode of inheritance.

Associated congenital abnormalities in patients and in their relatives, including hemihypertrophy and brain tumors have been reported. It was, therefore, of interest that in the family reported by Mahloudji and associates one of the siblings had hydrocephalus and another died of myelogenous leukemia.

Leucocytic Mucopolysaccharides in Cancer Patients

Riesco and Leyton[314] described the presence of mucopolysaccharides (MPS) in leucocytes of peripheral blood of cancer patients which differed significantly from controls. Specifically, MPS appeared only in approximately 3 percent of leucocytes of normal controls, while in the cancer patients 56 percent of polynuclear and 90 percent of mononuclear cells contained this material, the differences being highly significant. In a subsequent study, Riesco and Coke[2] studied MPS in cancer patients, their first degree relatives, and in controls. They found that a first degree relative of a cancer patient had a three times greater probability of having MPS in their lymphocytes than that observed in individuals from the general population. Furthermore, they found that through genetic segregation analysis, a high leucocytic MPS trait segregated in the families of cancer patients according to expectations for an autosomal dominantly inherited trait. They postulated that the disturbance of the lymphocytic MPS represented a subclinical variant of the clinical mucopolysaccharidoses. This assumption will merit critical testing in differing cancer prone and cancer free populations.

Burkitt's Lymphoma

Burkitt's tumor is an unusual multicentric lymphoma which involves primarily the mandible and maxilla of children between the ages of two and fourteen.[316] This disease was initially described in Africa where considerable epidemiological interest developed because of patterns involved in its occurrence including geography, climate, arthropod vectors, age, and migratory patterns of the population. Time-space clustering of the disease has been observed repeatedly in Africa.[317,318] Collectively these observations have suggested an infectious etiology.[316] Elevated serum antibody titers of Epstein-Barr virus have lent credence to this theory.

Burkitt's lymphoma has occurred in siblings in Africa.[318,319,320] Thus, one wonders about a genetic oncogenic susceptibility to an infectious agent such as the Epstein-Barr virus.[321]

Stevens and associates[322] reported an eight-year-old white male who succumbed to malignant lymphoma, undifferentiated, Burkitt's type. This boy's 17-year-old sister simultaneously developed acute leukemia with cells identical to those seen in Burkitt's lymphoma. This latter phenomenon had not been previously described and the authors referred to this phenomenon as acute leukemia, undifferentiated, Burkitt's type.

The family was of English-German-Dutch descent and they resided in the Los Angeles area. Consanguinity was absent. There was a history of skin cancer in the patient's father and the maternal grandmother. However, there was no other documented history of cancer in the preceding four generations. There was no known chemical, industrial, or other potential carcinogenic exposure to the affected children. The parents and children had never been outside the continental United States, nor had they been outside of California for more than five years preceding the illness.

The simultaneous occurrence of these tumors, particularly the histological identity of cell types, was considered to be more consistent with an environmental component. However, serological studies for the presence of Epstein-Barr viral antibodies in the two siblings were unremarkable.[322]

Additional studies of this problem in more patients will hopefully elucidate the contributory role of host and/or environmental factors in its etiology.

Arrhenoblastoma

Arrhenoblastomas are rarely occurring tumors which are believed to arise from embryonic remnants of the presumptive seminiferous tubules in an area in proximity to the hilus of the ovary. These lesions are almost always unilateral, solid, and are usually hemorrhagic.[323] These neoplasms have masculinizing or femininizing effects, and rarely, tumors producing *both* femininizing and virilizing signs may occur; these latter type have been designated as gynandroblastomas. Arrhenoblastomas, while rare, nevertheless are the most common of the masculinizing ovarian tumors. These lesions characteristically occur in young women, and they will recur or metastasize in approximately 25 percent of the patients.[324]

Since this tumor is so exceedingly rare, its familial occurrence raises considerable interest about its etiology. The lesion has been reported in three separate families. In one family, a mother and daughter were affected,[325] in another family two sisters were affected,[326] and more recently the lesion was described in two first cousins.[324]

Infantile Genetic Agranulocytosis (Kostmann's Syndrome)

In 1956 Kostmann[327] described a new disease which he referred to as Infantile Genetic Agranulocytosis, and which has now become more popularly known as Kostmann's syndrome. The onset of this anomaly occurs during early infancy, and is manifested by fever and skin infections which include multiple furuncles. There are a paucity, and in some patients a complete lack of granulocytes in the peripheral blood. Bone marrow biopsy and autopsy specimens show a marked retardation or arrest in the maturation of myelopoietic cells. If treatment is not given promptly the disease progresses rapidly and the patient may die from overwhelming infection. The first report of this disorder involved 14 children of both sexes from nine families.[327] It was of interest that most of the affected children were found to come from a common pedigree, once detailed genealogic studies were completed. Close consantuinity between the parents was found in five of the nine families. Genetic analysis was consistent with a single autosomal recessive genetic mode of transmission.

Recently, Schroeder and Kurth[328] have demonstrated spontaneous chromosomal breakage in Kostmann's agranulocytosis. They infer an increased association between Kostmann's agranulocytosis and leukemia, and support this hypothesis on the strength of the reported correlation between spontaneous chromosomal breakage and leukemia in other disorders including Bloom's syndrome, Fanconi's aplastic anemia, and ataxia telangiectasia. However, they do not present concrete evidence which would confirm the association with cancer.

It will be important to document cancer associations with Kostmann's agranulocytosis in order to determine statistical significance so that we can ascertain with greater certainty whether or not this disease harbors an increased proclivity for development of cancer.

Hereditary Pancreatitis

Hereditary pancreatitis was first described in 1952 by Comfort and Steinberg.[329] It is transmitted by an autosomal dominant gene.[330] This form of pancreatitis has an age of onset usually in the 10 to 15 year range, and the condition may vary considerably in severity. Of the 18 kindreds reported in the literature, members in about half of the families were found to excrete a cystine-like amino acid in their urine. Excretion of this amino acid does not appear to have any significance so far as the clinical course of the disease is concerned.[331] The clinical picture of pancreatitis may be variable, consisting of episodes of mild abdominal pain with elevation of serum amylase levels in some of the patients, while in others severe hemorrhagic pancreatitis may occur. Pseudocysts of pancreas have been found in some patients with this disease. It is of interest that biliary calculi have been a rare occurrence in this disease. About 20 percent of patients with clinical forms of pancreatitis have required surgery, though this has been generally unsatisfactory.[331]

The occurrence of pancreatic cancer in association with this disease has been invetigated.[332] Eight cases of pancreatic cancer have been described in patients with hereditary pancreatitis, the youngest of whom was a 39-year-old male. Seven of the tumors have been adenocarcinomas of the pancreas, and one was a cystadenocarcinoma. Further study is necessary in order to help elucidate the significance of these observations.

Cancer of the Prostate

Cancer of the prostate is the second most common cause of death from cancer in males in the United States. Despite its frequency its epidemiology has not been investigated extensively. Wynder and associates[333] have recently studied a large number of patients with prostate cancer and compared them with a control group; they have also reviewed recent epidemiologic findings for this disease. In their comparison of prostate cancer patients with controls they found no differences with respect to educational level, tobacco and alcohol habits, past surgical or medical histories, circumcision, weight, height, or blood groups. Their literature review showed clinical prostatic cancer to be exceedingly rare in Japan, with an increase in its frequency among Japanese immigrants in the United States. No major environmental factors were found which could explain the possibility that prostatic cancer is hormone related. However, it was agreed that factors that might influence endocrine etiology are difficult to determine through interview methods.

Breast cancer also shows an epidemiologic pattern somewhat similar to prostate cancer, in that breast cancer occurs relatively infrequently in Japan, but increases in frequency among Japanese immigrants in the United States. Another possible link to the epidemiology of cancer of the prostate and breast stem from recent observations[334] which showed a significant familial association between carcinoma of the breast and prostate. Thus, common epidemiologic factors that influence both these lesions may be manifested through interactions with certain as yet unclear familial factors.

Cancer of the prostate has a low incidence rate among Jewish men in the United States. This may be related to the relatively low rate of prostatic cancer observed generally among immigrants from eastern Europe. However, native-born Jews appear to have rates for prostatic cancer which are similar to those of other Caucasians born in the United States.[333] Wynder believes that further elucidation of etiology for prostatic cancer may be expedited through multidisciplinary studies concentrating on the apparent differences in the incidence of prostatic cancer among native Japanese and Japanese immigrants to the United States, and among Caucasians and Negroes native to the United States.

Lynch, *et al.*[335] previously studied family histories of 109 consecutive patients with prostatic cancer. Only 4.5 percent of these patients had first degree relatives who manifested this disease. Due to the advanced age of the propositi, however, their family histories were often incomplete. One noteworthy feature of this survey was the observation that 20 percent of the patients showed multiple primary malignant neoplasms, with two of them each showing five separate primary malignant neoplasms.

There has been relatively very little investigation of the hereditary aspects of prostate cancer. Two studies on the subject[336,337] indicated approximately a three-fold increase of this lesion among fathers and brothers of affected propositi compared to controls. A major limitation of these studies, however, has been their dependency upon data derived from death certificates, which are therefore characterized by the lack of critical clinicopathologic correlation.

Multiple Myeloma

Multiple myeloma is a neoplastic process in which a clone of plasma cells autonomously proliferates. This leads to the production of a large amount of antigenically homogeneous globulin, which gives rise to a monoclonal protein that is often referred to as M-protein. The incidence of multiple myeloma in persons over age 20 is approximately five per 100,000 per year.[338] Although the cause of this disease is unknown, radiation has been implicated, because radiologists show a higher incidence of multiple myeloma than other physicians.[339]

Viral-like particles in inclusion bodies within myeloma cells have been identified in human beings.[340] There is no substantial evidence, at this time, that chemical agents are of etiologic importance, although mineral oil has been implicated in the induction of plasma-cell neoplasms in mice.[341] Myeloma has recently been reported in four sets of spouses who had been married from six to 41 years before myeloma was diagnosed in one of the spouses. In these cases, the interval between the onset of myeloma in one spouse and the diagnosis in the mate ranged from one month to 15 years.[342]

There have been at least 12 familial reports of multiple myeloma.[343,344] Kyle and associates[342] state that they know of three additional families with myeloma which have not been reported.

McKusick has listed multiple myeloma in his catalogue of genetic diseases[345] as being associated with autosomal recessive mode of genetic transmission. There is at least one study of monozygotic twins in which one member of the pair had multiple myeloma and the co-twin was allegedly free of this disease.[343] An interesting feature of this investigation, however, was that a cytogenetic study of both of these twins, in addition to showing cytogenetically normal cells, each showed aneuploid cells with numerous inconsistent abnormalities. One consistent abnormality was the occurrence of an extra chromosome the size of which corresponded with the F or G group. These abnormalities occurred in a small percentage of the cells. The cytogenetic findings were more pronounced in the twin who was afflicted with multiple myeloma. The authors speculate about the possibility that the normal twin might eventually develop a form of paraproteinemic malignancy.

Myeloma and asymptomatic paraproteinemia has been described recently in first and second degree relatives in two generations of a Dutch family without consanguinity.[346]

We, of course, must fully appreciate the fact that discordance for any disorder may occur in monozygotic twins and not necessarily discount the role of genetic factors. In diseases as complicated as cancer and, in particular, those cancerous diseases which have an unusually late onset in life, there are undoubtedly a multitude of environmental factors that might be necessary for complete expression of the full predisposition for the particular tumor in the host. Thus, in any given set of circumstances, one co-twin of a pair of monozygotic twins might be spared specific environmental insults and, even though genetically "susceptible," might not develop the disease.

C-Monosomy Myeloproliferative Syndrome

Three patients with a myeloproliferative disorder and a missing C-group chromosome in bone marrow cells were reported in 1964 by Freireich and associates.[347] Transformation to acute myelomonocytic leukemia occurred as a terminal event in two of these patients.

Macdougall and associates[348] reviewed the literature on this disorder and found six additional patients, all children. They report the salient clinical and hematologic features of the disorder to include hepatosplenomegaly, anemia, thrombocytopenia, peripheral blood leukocytosis, bone marrow erythroid, and myeloid hyperplasia with myeloid metaplasia, normal or increased leukocyte alkaline phosphatase, and C-group chromosome monosomy in bone marrow cells with a normal chromosome pattern in peripheral blood leukocytes. The disease has a chronic course, extending from one to six years. Acute myeloblastic leukemia has developed as a terminal event in three of the six reported children, erythroleukemia in one of them, and myelofibrosis in another. One child, still alive 44 months after onset, had early evidence of myeloblastic leukemic transformation. They have also described a four-year-old child with C-group monosomy and a myeloproliferative disorder with a terminal myelomonocytic leukemia. Autoradiography was performed on bone marrow cultures, and the investigators concluded that the missing chromosome was a No. 7 autosome. The child had developed erythroleukemic and myelomonoblastic phases of the disease, factors which support the theory of an abnormal precursor stem cell, and the speculation that one or more of the C-group chromosomes may have a regulatory role in hemopoiesis.[348]

Summary

In summary I have discussed several malignant neoplasms and precancerous disorders wherein variable evidence in support of genetic etiology has been given. In many circumstances the conditions are currently receiving intense interest from a variety of medical disciplines; for example work is currently in progress on nasopharyngeal carcinoma where geneticists, epidemiologists, and virologists are working either independently or as teams in quest for new information regarding the complex issues of etiology and pathogenesis in this lesion. New methodologies in the study of cancer genetics show great promise for elucidation of some of the mysteries in this perplexing field. Selected topics discussed in this area emphasize the importance of multi-disciplined approach to cancer etiology and show clearly the need to study host factors in context with the myriad environmental inter-actions.

REFERENCES

1. Lynch, H.T.: *Skin, Heredity and Malignant Neoplasms.* New York, Med Exam, 1972, pp. 300.
2. Damashek, W.: Chronic lymphocytic leukemia. An accumulative disease of immunological incompetent lymphocytes. *Blood, 29:*556–584, 1967.
3. Deaston, J.G., and Levin, W.C.: Systemic lupus erythematosus and acute myeloblastic leukemia: report of their coexistence and a survey of possible associating features. *Arch Intern Med* (Chicago), *120:* 345–348, 1967.
4. Thompson, J.S.: Immunity and systemic lupus erythematosus. *Postgrad Med, 37:*619–627, 1965.
5. Mellors, R.C.: Autoimmune disease in NZB-B1 Mice: II. Autoimmunity and malignant lymphoma. *Blood, 27:*435–448, 1966.
6. Burnet, F.M.: The concept of immunological surveillance. *Prog Exp Tumor Res, 13:*1–27, 1970.
7. Sophocles, A.M., and Nadler, S.H.: Immunologic aspects of cancer. *Surg Gynecol Obstet, 133:*321–331, 1971.
8. Barden, R.P.: Collagen disease and cancer. *Radiology, 92:*972 974, 1969.
9. Tuffanelli, V.L., and Debois, E.L.: Cutaneous manifestations of systemic lupus erythematosus. *Arch Dermatol* (Chicago), *90:* 337–386, 1964.
10. Tay, C.H.: Cutaneous manifestations of systemic lupus erythematosus: a clinical study from Singapore. *Aust J Dermatol, 11:*30–41, 1970.
11. Smith, C.K., Cassidy, J.T., and Bole, G.G.: Type I dysgammaglobulinemia, system lupus erythematosus and lymphoma. *Am J Med, 48:*113–119, 1970.
12. Brunjes, S., Zike, K., and Julian, R.: Familial systemic lupus erythematosis; a review of the literature with a report of ten additional cases in four families. *Am J Med, 30:*529–536, 1961.
13. Leonhard, T.: Family studies in systemic lupus erythematosis. *Acta Med Scand* (Suppl), *416:*1–156, 1964.
14. Pollack, V.E.: Antinuclear antibodies in families of patients with systemic lupus erythematosis. *New Engl J Med, 271:*165–171, 1964.
15. Barnes, R.D.: Thymic neoplasms associated with refractory anaemia. *Guy Hosp Rep, 114:*73–82, 1965.

16. Beickert, A.: Lupus-erythematosus—syndrom bei lymphogranulomatose. *Schweiz Med Wochenschr, 88:*668–669, 1958.

17. Andrews, G.E., and Domonkos, A.N.: *Diseases of the Skin,* 5th ed. Philadelphia, Saunders, 1964, p. 749.

18. Williams, R.C.: Dermatomyositis and malignancy: a review of the literature. *Ann Intern Med, 50:*1174, 1959.

19. Christianson, H.B., Brunsting, L.A., and Perry, H.O.: Dermatomyositis: unusual features, complications, and treatment. *Arch Dermatol, 74:*581–589, 1956.

20. Grace, J.T., and Dao, T.L.: Dermatomyositis in cancer: a possible etiological mechanism. *Cancer, 12:*648–650, 1959.

21. Katz, A., and Digby, J.W.: Malignant melanoma and dermatomyositis. *Can Med Assoc J, 93:*1367–1369, 1965.

22. Arundell, F.D., Wilkinson, R.D., and Haserick, J.R.: Dermatomyositis and malignant neoplasms in adults: a survey of 20 years' experience. *Arch Dermatol, 82:*772–775, 1960.

23. Curtis, A.C., Heckaman, J.H., and Wheeler, A.H.: Study of the autoimmune reaction in dermatomyositis. *JAMA, 178:*571–573, 1961.

24. Lambie, J.A., and Duff, I.F.: Report of familial occurrence of dermatomyositis and a family survey. *J Lab Clin Med, 58:*935–936, 1961.

25. Lambie, J.A., and Duff, I.F.: Familial occurrence of dermatomyositis: case reports and a family survey. *Ann Intern Med, 59:*839–847, 1963.

26. Kierland, R.R.: The collagenoses: transitional forms of lupus erythematosus, dermatomyositis, and scleroderma. *Mayo Clinic Proc, 39:*53, 1964.

27. Farmer, R.G., Gifford, R.W., Jr., and Hines, E.A., Jr.: Prognostic significance of Raynaud's phenomenon and other clinical characteristics of systemic scleroderma: a study of 271 cases. *Circulation, 21:*1088–1095, 1960.

28. Montgomer, R.D., Stirling, G.A., and Hamer, N.A.: Bronchiolar carcinoma in progressive systemic sclerosis. *Lancet, 1:*586–587, 1964.

29. Basten, A., and Bonnin, M.: Scleroderma in carcinoma. *Med J Aust, 1:*452, 1966.

30. McAndrew, G.M., and Barnes, E.G.: Familial scleroderma. *Ann Phys Med, 8:*128–131, 1965.

31. Burge, K.M., Perry, H.O., and Stickler, G.B.: "Families" Scleroderma. *Arch Dermatol* (Chicago), *99:*681–687, 1969.

32. Tuffanelli, D.L.: Scleroderma, immunological and genetic disease in three families. *Dermatologica, 138:*93–104, 1969.

33. Holly, H.: Evidence for a predisposition of rheumatic disease in families of patients developing drug-induced systemic lupus erythematosus. *Arth Rheum, 7:*684–686, 1964.

34. Joseph, R.R., and Zarafonetis, C.J.D.: Fatal systemic lupus erythematosus in identical twins: case report and review of the literature. *Am J Med Sci, 249:*190–199, 1965.

35. Leonhardt, T.: Familial hypergammaglobulinemia in systemic lupus erythematosus. *Lancet, 11:*1200–1203, 1957.

36. Orabona, M.L., and Albano, O.: Progressive systemic sclerosis (or visceral scleroderma), *Acta Med Scand* (Suppl), *333:*1–170, 1958.

37. Leonhardt, T.: Familial occurrence of collagen diseases, II. Progressive systemic sclerosis and dermatomyositis. *Acta Med Scand, 169:*735–742, 1961.

38. Rodnan, G.P., Maclachlin, M.J., Fisher, E.R., Zlotnick, A., and Creighton, A.: Serum proteins and serological reactions in patients with progressive systemic sclerosis (diffuse scleroderma) and their relatives. *Clin Res, 9:*149, 1961.

39. Camus, J.P., Emerit, I., Reinert, Ph., Guillien, P., Crouzet, J., and Fourot, J.: Sclerodermie Familiale avee Syndrome de Sjögren et Anomalies Lymphocytes et Chromosomes. *Ann Med Interne Fevrier, 121:*149–161.

39a. Burch, P.R.J., and Rowell, N.R.: Autoimmunity, etiological aspects of chronic discoid and systemic lupus erythematosus, systemic sclerosis, and hashimoto's thyroiditis. *Lancet, 11:*507–513, 1963.

40. Sinkovics, J.G., Trujillo, J.M., Pienta, R.J., and Ahearn, M.J.: Leukemogenesis stemming from autoimmune disease. In *Genetic*

Concepts of Neoplasia, A Collection of Papers Presented at the Twenty-third annual Symposium on Fundamental Cancer Research. Baltimore, Williams and Wilkins, 1970, p. 619.

41. Denko, C.W., and Bergenstal, D.M.: The sicca syndrome (Sjögren's Syndrome): a study of sixteen cases. *Arch Intern Med, 105:*849–858, 1960.

42. Talal, N., and Bunim, J.J.: The development of malignant lymphoma in the course of Sjögren's Syndrome. *Am J Med, 35:*529–540, 1964.

43. Rothman, S., Block, M., and Hauser, F.V.: Sjögren's Syndrome associated with lymphoblastoma and hypersplenism. *Arch Derm Syph, 63:*642–643, 1951.

44. Delaney, W.E., and Balogh, K., Jr.: Carcinoma of the parotid gland associated with benign lymphoepithelial lesion (Mikulicz's disease) in Sjögren's Syndrome. *Cancer, 19:*853–860, 1966.

45. Stewart, A., and Barber, R.: The epidermiological importance of childhood cancers. *Br Med Bull, 27:*64–70, 1971.

46. Stewart, A., Webb, J., and Hewitt, D.: A survey of childhood malignancies. *Br Med J, 1:*1495–1508, 1958.

47. Scott, L.S.: Wilms' tumor: its treatment and prognosis. *Br Med J, 1:*200–203, 1956.

48. Lynch, H.T.: Hereditary factors in carcinoma. In Rentchnick, P., *et al.* (Eds.): *Recent Results in Cancer Research.* Berlin, Springer-Verlag, 1967, Vol. 12, p. 186.

49. Fontana, V.J., Ferrara, A., and Perciaccante, R.: Wilms' tumor and associated anomalies. *Am J Dis Child, 109:*459–461, 1965.

50. Miller, R.W., Fraumeni, J.F., Jr., and Manning, M.D.: Association of Wilms' tumor with aniridia, hemihypertrophy, and other malformations. *New Engl J Med, 270:*922–927, 1964.

51. Gaulin, E.: Simultaneous Wilms' tumors in identical twins. *J Urol, 66:*547–550, 1951.

52. Lynch, H.T., and Green, G.S.: Wilms' tumor and congenital heart disease. *Am J Dis Child, 115:*723–727, 1968.

53. Hill, S.: Personal Communication, 1970.

54. Kontras, S.B., and Newton, W.A.: Familial Wilms' tumor, in press.

55. Brown, W.T., Puranik, S.R., Altman, D.H., and Hardin, H.C., Jr.: Wilms' tumor in three successive generations. *Surgery, 72:*756–761, 1972.

56. Mackay, H.: Congenital bilateral megaloureters with hydronephrosis: remarkable family history. *Proc Roy Soc Med, 38:*567–568, 1945.

57. Spear, G.S., Hyde, T.P., Gruppo, R.A., and Sluser, R.: Pseudohermaphroditism, glomerulonephritis with the nephrotic syndrome, and Wilms' tumor in infancy. *J Pediatr, 79:*677–681, 1971.

58. Drash, A., Sherman, F., Hartmann, W.H., and Blizzard, R.M.: A syndrome of pseudohermaphroditism, Wilms' tumor, hypertension, and degenerative renal disease. *J Pediatr, 76:*585, 1970.

59. Frasier, S.D., Bashore, R.A., and Mosier, H.D.: Gonadoblastoma associated with pure gonadal dysgenesis in monozygous twins. *J Pediatr, 64:*740, 1964.

59a. Meadows, A.T., Lichtenfeld, J.L., and Koop, C.E.: Wilms's tumor in three children of a woman with congenital hemihypertrophy. *New Eng J Med, 291:*23–24, 1974.

59b. Knudson, A.G., Jr., and Strong, L.C.: Mutation and Cancer: A model for Wilms' tumor of the kidney. *J Nat Cancer Inst, 48:*313–324, 1972.

60. Li, F.P., and Fraumeni, J.F., Jr.: Rhabdomyosarcoma in children: epidemiologic study and identification of a familial cancer syndrome. *J Natl Cancer Inst, 43:*1365–1373, 1969.

61. Dodge, H.J., and Benner, M.C.: Neuroblastoma of the adrenal medulla in siblings. *Rocky Mt Med J, 42:*35–38, 1945.

62. Chatten, J., and Voorhess, M.L.: Familial neuroblastoma: report of a kindred with multiple disorders, including neuroblastomas in four siblings. *New Engl J Med, 277:*1230–1236, 1967.

63. Miller, R.W.: Relation between cancer and congenital defects in man. *New Engl J Med, 275:*87–93, 1966.

64. Griffin, M.E., and Bolande, R.P.: Familial neuroblastoma with regression and maturation to ganglioneurofibroma. *Pediatrics, 43:*377–382, 1969.

65. Wong, K.Y., Hanenson, I.B., and Lampkin, B.C.: familial neuroblastoma. *Am J Dis Child, 121:*415–416, 1971.

66. Hardy, P.C., and Nesbitt, M.E.: Familial neuroblastoma, report of a kindred with a high incidence of infantile tumors. *J Pediatr, 80:*74–77, 1972.

67. Zimmermann, N.J.: Ganglioneuroblastome als erbliche System-erkrankung des Sympathicus. *Beitr z path Anat u z Allg Path, 111:*355–372, 1951.

68. Beckwith, J.B., and Perrin, E.V.: *In situ* neuroblastomas: a contribution to the natural history of neural crest tumors. *Am J Pathol, 43:*1089–1104, 1963.

69. Helson, L., Blasco, P., and Murpht, M.L.: Familial neuroblastoma. *Clin Res, 17:*614, 1969.

70. Fraumeni, J.F., Jr., Geiser, C.F., and Manning, M.D.: Wilms' tumor and congenital hemihypertrophy: report of 5 new cases and review of literature. *Pediatrics, 40:* 886–899, 1967.

71. Fraumeni, J.F., Jr., and Miller, R.W.: Adrenocortical neoplasms with hemihypertrophy, brain tumors, and other disorders. *J Pediatr, 70:*129–138, 1967.

72. Fraumeni, J.F., Jr., Miller, R.W., and Hill, J.A.: Primary carcinoma of the liver in childhood: an epidemilogic study. *J Natl Cancer Inst, 40:*1087–1099, 1968.

73. Fraumeni, J.F., Rosen, P.J., Hull, E.W., Barth, R.F., Shapiro, S.R., and O'Connor, J.F.: Hepatoblastoma in infant sisters. *Cancer, 24:*1086–1090, 1969.

74. Houstek, J., Masopust, J., Kithier, K., and Radl, J.: Hepatocellular carcinoma in association with a specific fetal alpha$_1$-globulin, fetoprotein. *J Pediatr, 72:*186–193, 1968.

75. Mawas, C., Kohen, M., Lemerle, J., Buffe, D., Schweisguth, O., and Burtin, P.: Serum alpha$_1$ foeto-protein (fetuin) in children with malignant ovarian or testicular teratoma. Preliminary Results. *Int J Cancer, 4:*76–79, 1969.

76. Higginson, J.: The geographical pathology of primary liver cancer. *Cancer Res, 23:* 1624–1633, 1963.

77. Stewart, H.L.: In Burdette, W.J. (Ed.): *Geographic Distribution of Hepatic Cancer, Primary Hepatoma.* Salt Lake City, U of Utah Pr, 1965, pp. 31–36.

78. Oettlé, A.G.: The incidence of primary carcinoma of the liver in the southern vantu, 1., critical review of the literature. *J Natl Cancer Inst, 17:*249–280, 1956.

79. Miyake, M., Saito, M., and Enomoto, M., *et al.*: Toxic liver injuries and liver cirrhosis induced in mice and rats through long term feeding with penicillium islandicum sopp-growing rice. *Acta Path Jap, 10:*75–123, 1966.

80. Blumberg, B.S., Alter, H.T., and Visnich, S.: A "new" antigen in leukemia sera. *JAMA, 191:*541–546, 1965.

81. Blumberg, B.S., Melartin, L., and Guinto, R.A., *et al.*: Family studies of a human serum isoantigen system (Australia antigen). *Am J Hum Genet, 18:*594–608, 1966.

82. Myerson, R.M., Soroush, A., and Skerrett, P.V.: Hepatocellular carcinoma, positive Australia (hepatitis-associated) antigen and sarcoidosis. *Am J Dig Dis, 16:*857–862, 1971.

83. Smith, J.B., and Blumberg, B.S.: Viral hepatitis, postnecrotic cirrhosis, and hepatocellular carcinoma, *Lancet, 2:*953, 1969.

84. Sherlock, S., Niazi, S.P., and Fos, R.A., *et al.*: Chronic liver disease and primary liver cell cancer with hepatitis-associated (Australia) antigen in serum. *Lancet, 1:*1243–1247, 1970.

85. Hadziyannia, S.J., Merikas, G.E., and Afroudakis, A.P.: Hepatitis-associated antigen in chronic liver disease. *Lancet, 1:*100, 1970.

86. Vogel, C.L., Anthony, P.P., and Mody, H., *et al.*: Hepatitis-associated antigen in Ugandan patients with hepatocellular carcinoma. *Lancet, 2:* 621–624, 1970.

87. Prince, A.M., Leblanc, L., and Kron, K., *et al.*: S.H. antigen and chronic liver disease. *Lancet, 2:*717–718, 1970.

88. Denison, E.K., Peters, R.L., and Reynolds, T.B.: Familial hepatoma with hepatitis-associated antigen. *Ann Intern Med, 74:* 391–394, 1971.

89. Sutnick, A.I., London, W.T., and Blumberg, B.S.: Australia antigen: a genetic basis for chronic liver disease and hepatoma? *Ann Intern Med, 74:*442–444, 1971.

90. Ohbayashi, A., Mayumi, M., and Okochi, K.: Australia antigen in two families with multiple recurrences of cryptogenic cirrhosis of liver. In press.

91. Hedinger, E.: Primary hepatic cancer in two sisters. *Centralbl Allg Path, 15:*385–387, 1915.

92. Kaplan, L., and Cole, S.L.: Fraternal primary hepatocellular carcinoma in three male, adult siblings. *Amer J Med, 39:*305–311, 1965.

93. Hagstrom, R.M., and Baker, T.D.: Primary hepatocellular carcinoma in three male siblings. *Cancer, 22:*142–150, 1968.

94. Miller, M.C.: Familial cirrhosis with hepatoma. *Amer J Dig Dis, 12:*633–638, 1967.

95. Berg, N.O., and Eriksson, S.: Liver disease in adults with alpha$_1$ antitrypsin deficiency. *New Engl J Med, 287:*1264–1267, 1972.

96. Exelby, P.R.: Sacrococcygeal teratomas in children. *Ca-A Cancer J Clinicians, 22:*202–208, 1972.

97. Hickey, R.C., and Layton, J.M.: Sacrococcygeal teratoma. Emphasis on the biological history and early therapy. *Cancer, 7:*1031–1043, 1954.

98. Waldhausen, J.A., Kolman, J.W., Vellios, F., and Battersby, J.S.: Sacrococcygeal teratoma. *Surgery, 54:*933–949, 1963.

99. Chretien, P.B., Milam, J.D., Foote, F.W., and Miller, T.R.: Embryonal adenocarcinomas (a type of malignant teratoma) of the sacroccygeal region. 01 clinical and pathologic aspects of 21 cases. *Surg Gynecol Obstet, 92:*341–354, 1951.

100. Beckwith, J.B.: Extreme Cytomegaly of the Adrenal Fetal Cortex, Omphalocele, Hyperplasia of Kidneys and Pancreas, and Leydig-cell Hyperplasia: Another Syndrome? Read before the Western Society for Pediatric Research, Los Angeles, 1963.

101. Cohen, M.M., Gorlin, R.J., Feingold, M., and ten Bensel, R.W.: The Beckwith-Wiedemann syndrome. *Amer J Dis Child, 122:* 515–519, 1971.

102. Wiedemann, H.R.: Complexe Malformatif Familial Avec Hernie Obilicale et Macroglossie: Un Syndrome Nouveau? *J Genet Hum, 13:*223–232, 1964.

103. Sherman, F.E., Bass, L.W., and Fetterman, G.H.: Congenital metastasizing adrenal cortical carcinoma associated with cytomegaly of the fetal adrenal cortex. *Amer J Clin Pathol, 30:*439–446, 1958.

104. Neeman, cited by Beckwith, J.B.: Macroglossia, omphalocele, adrenal cytomegaly, gigantism, and hyperplastic visceromegaly. In Bergsma, D. (Ed.): *Birth Defects: Original Article Series.* New York, National Foundation, *5:*188–196, 1969.

105. Wilson, F.C., and Orlin, H.: Crossed congenital hemihypertrophy associated with Wilms' tumor. *J Bone Joint Surg, 47:*1609–1614, 1965.

106. Tower, J., and Beck, P.C., cited by Beckwith, J.B.: Macroglossia omphalocele, adrenal cytomegaly, gigantism, and hyperplastic visceromegaly. In Bergsma, D. (Ed.): *Birth Defects: Original Article Series.* New York, National Foundation, *5:*188–196, 1969.

107. Thorburn, M.J., Miller, C.G., and McNeil Smith-Read, E.H.: Exomphalosmacroglossia-gigantism syndrome in Jamaican infants. *Amer J Dis Child, 119:*316–321, 1970.

108. Eaton, A.P., and Maurer, W.F.: The Beckwith-Wiedemann syndrome. *Amer J Dis Child, 122:*520–525, 1971.

109. Irving, I.: Exomphalos with macroglossia: a study of 11 cases. *J Pediat Surg, 2:*499–507, 1967.

109a. Perlman, M., Goldberg, G.M., and Danovitch, G.: Renal hamartomas and nephroblastomatosis with fetal gigantism: a familial syndrome. *J Pediatr, 83:*414–418, 1973.

110. Lloyd, K.M., and Dennis, M.: Cowden's Disease: a possible new symptom complex with multiple system involvement. *Ann Intern Med, 48:*136–142, 1963.

111. Weary, P.E., Gorlin, R.J., Gentry, W.C., Comer, J.E., and Greer, K.E.: Multiple

hamartoma syndrome (Cowden's Disease). *Arch Dermatol, 106:*682–690, 1972.

112. Miller, R.W.: Neoplasia and Down's syndrome. *Ann NY Acad Sci, 171:*637–644, 1970.

113. Wald, N., Borges, W.H., Li, C.C., Turner, J.H., and Harnois, M.D.: Leukemia associated with mongolism, *Lancet, 1:*1228, 1961.

114. Holland, W.W., Doll, R., and Carter, C.O.: The mortality from leukemia and other cancers among patients with Down's syndrome (Mongols) and among their parents. *Br J Cancer, 16:*178–186, 1962.

115. Jackson, E.W., Turner, J.H., Klauber, M.R., and Norris, F.D.: Down's Syndrome: variatiln of leukemia occurrence in institutionalized populations. *J Chronic Dis, 21:*247–253, 1968.

116. Lashof, J.C., and Stewart, A.: Oxford survey of childhood cancers. Progress report III: leukaemia and down's syndrome. *Monthly Bull Minist Health* (London), *24:*136–143, 1965.

117. Fraumeni, J.F., Jr., Manning, M.D., and Mitus, W.J.: Acute childhood leukemia: epidemiologic study by cell type of 1,263 cases at the children's cancer research foundation in Boston, 1947–65. *J Natl Cancer Inst, 46:*461–470, 1971.

118. Buckton, K.E., Harnden, D.G., Baikie, A.G., and Woods, G.E.: Mongolism and leukemia in the same sibship. *Lancet, 1:*171–172, 1961.

119. Zsako, S., and Kaplan, A.R.: G_1-Trisomy and familial mental retardation, congenital anomalies and malignancy. *Am J Ment Defic, 72:*809–814, 1968.

120. Miller, R.W.: Radiation, chromosomes and viruses in the etiology of leukemia. Evidence from epidemiologic research. *New Engl J Med, 271:*30–36, 1964.

121. Brinton, L.F.: Hypernephroma: familial occurrence in one family. *JAMA, 173:*888–890, 1960.

122. Riches, E.: On carcinoma of the kidney. *Ann Roy Coll Surg* (Eng), *32:*201–208, 1963.

123. Rusche, C.F.: Silent adenocarcinoma of the kidney with solitary metastases occurring in brothers. *J Urol, 70:*146–151, 1953.

124. Klinger, M.: Renal-cell carcinoma in siblings: a case report. *J Am Geriatr Soc, 16:*1047–1052, 1968.

125. Steinberg, S.M., Brodovsky, H.S., and Goepp, C.E.: Renal carcinoma in mother and daughter. *Cancer, 29:*222–225, 1972.

126. Franksson, C., Bergstrand, A., Ljungdahl, I., Magnusson, G., and Nordenstam, H.: Renal carcinoma (hypernephroma) occurring in 5 siblings. *J Urol, 108:*58–61, 1972.

127. Kaplan, C., Sayre, G.P., and Greene, L.F.: Nephrogenic carcinomas in Lindau-von Hippel disease. *J Urol, 86:*36–42, 1961.

128. Kernohan, J.W., Woltman, H.W., and Adson, A.W.: Intramedullary tumors of the spinal cord: a review of 51 cases with attempt at histologic classification. *Arch Neurol Psychiat, 25:*679–701, 1931.

129. Levine, S.R., Witten, D.M., and Greene, L.F.: Nephrotomography in Lindau-von Hippel disease. *J Urol, 93:*660–662, 1965.

130. Greene, L.F., and Rosenthal, M.H.: Multiple hypernephromas of the kidney in association with Lindau's disease. *New Engl J Med, 244:*633, 1951.

131. Johnson, W.F.: Carcinoma in a polycystic kidney. *J Urol, 69:*10–12, 1953.

132. Hulse, C.P., and Palik, E.E.: Renal hamartoma. *J Urol, 66:*506–515, 1951.

133. Moolten, S.E.: Hamartial nature of tuberous sclerosis complex and its bearing on tumor problem. *Arch Intern Med, 69:*586–623, 1942.

134. Perou, M.L., and Gray, P.T.: Mesenchymal hamartomas of the kidney. *J Urol, 83:*240–261, 1960.

135. Viamonte, M., Jr., Ravel, R., Poltano, V., and Bridges, B.: Angiographic findings in a patient with tuberous sclerosis. *Am J Roentgen, 98:*723–733, 1866.

136. Blandy, J.P., Hope-Stone, H.F., and Dayan, A.D.: *Tumors of the Testicle.* New York, Grune & Stratton, 1970, 0. 26.

137. Raven, R.W.: Tumors of the testis in two brothers. *Lancet, 2:*870–871, 1934.

138. Lownes, J.B., and Leberman, P.: Tumors of testes in brothers. *Urol Cutan Rev, 43:*205–206, 1939.

139. Willis, R.A.: *Pathology of Tumours,* 3rd ed.

London, Butterworth & Co., Ltd., 1960, p. 561

140. Hutter, A.M., Jr., Lynch, J.J., and Shnider, B.I.: Malignant testicular tumors in brothers. *JAMA, 199*:155–156, 1967.

141. Young, J.A., and Bohne, A.W.: Seminoma in nontwin brothers: a case report. *J Urol, 107*:1000–1101, 1972.

142. Moorhead, E.L.: Personal Communications, 1972.

142a. Lynch, H.T., Krush, A.J., Mulcahy, G.M., and Reed, W.B.: Familial occurrences of a variety of premalignant diseases and uncommon malignant neoplasms. *Cancer, 33*:1474–1479, 1974.

143. Wynder, E.L., Dodo, H., and Barber, H.R.K.: Epidemiology of cancer of the ovary. *Cancer, 23*:352–370, 1969.

144. West, R.O.: Epidemiologic study of malignancies of the ovaries. *Cancer, 19*:1001–1007, 1966.

145. Haenszel, W., and Kurihara, M.: Studies of Japanese migrants—I. mortality from cancer and other disease among Japanese in the United States. *J Natl Cancer Inst, 40: 40*:43–68, 1968.

146. Osborne, R.H., and De George, F.V.: The ABO blood groups in neoplastic disease of the ovary. *Amer J Hum Genet, 15*:380–388, 1963.

147. Moertel, C.G., Dockerty, M.B., and Baggenstoss, A.H.: Multiple primary malignant neoplasms. *Cancer, 14*:221–248, 1961.

148. Cook, G.B.: A comparison of single and multiple primary cancers. *Cancer, 19*:959–966, 1966.

149. Lynch, G.W.: Clinical review of 100 cases of ovarian carcinoma. *Am J Obstet Gynecol, 32*:753–777, 1936.

150. Serra, A., and Soini, A.: Ricerche Sulla Familiarità del Carcinoma Ovarico. *Acta Genet Med Gemellol* (Roma), *8*:409–430, 1959.

151. Liber, A.F.: Ovarian cancer in mother and five daughters. *Arch Pathol, 49*:280–290, 1950.

152. Li, F.P., Rapoport, A.H., Fraumeni, J.F., and Jensen, R.D.: Familial ovarian carcinoma. *JAMA, 214*:1559–1561, 1970.

153. Jackson, S.M.: Ovarian dysgerminoma in three generations? *J Med Genet, 4*:112–113, 1967.

154. Lynch, H.T., Krush, A.J., Larsen, A.L., and Magnuson, C.W.: Endometrial Carcinoma: multiple primary malignancies, constitutional factors, and heredity. *Am J Med Sci, 252*:381–390, 1966.

155. Lynch, H.T., Krush, A.J., and Larsen, A.L.: Heredity and endometrial carcinoma. *South Med J., 60*:231–235, 1967.

156. Moertel, C.G., Dockerty, M.B., and Baggenstoss, A.H.: Multiple primary malignant neoplasms. II. Tumors of different tissues or organs. *Cancer, 14*:231–237, 1961.

157. Way, S.: Aetriology of carcinoma of the body of uterus. *J Obstet Gynecol Br Emp, 61:* 46–58, 1954.

158. Jackson, R.L., and Dockerty, M.B.: The Stein-Leventhal syndrome: analysis of 43 cases with special reference to association with endometrial carcinoma. *Am J Obstet Gynecol, 73*:161–173, 1957.

159. Dowsett, J.W.: Corpus carcinoma developing in a patient with Turner's syndrome treated with estrogen. *Am J Gynecol, 86:* 622–625, 1963.

160. Schajowicz, F., and Bessone, J.E.: Chondrosarcoma in three brothers. *J Bone Joint Surg, 49-A*:129–141, 1967.

161. Epstein, L.I., Bixler, D., and Bennett, J.E.: An incident of familial cancer: including three cases of osteogenic sarcoma. *Cancer, 25*:889–891, 1970.

162. Roberts, C.W., and Roberts, C.P.: Concurrent osteogenic sarcoma in brothers and sisters. *JAMA, 105*:181–185, 1935.

163. Pohle, E.A., Stovall, W.D., and Boyer, H.N.: Concurrence of osteogenic sarcoma in two sisters. *Radiology, 27*:545–548, 1936.

164. Harmon, T.P., and Morton, K.S.: Osteogenic sarcoma in four siblings. *J Bone Joint Surg, 48*:493–498, 1966.

165. Robbins, R.: Familial osteosarcoma, fifth reported occurrence. *JAMA, 202*:1055, 1967.

166. Morton, D.L., and Malmgren, R.A.: Human osteosarcomas: immunologic evidence suggesting an associated infectious agent. *Science, 162*:1279–1281, 1968.

167. Paymaster, J.C., Sanghvi, L.D., and Gangad-

haran, P.: Cancer in the gastrointestinal tract in Western India. *Cancer, 21:*279–288, 1968.

168. Fortuine, R.: Characteristics of cancer in the Eskimos of Southwestern Alaska. *Cancer, 23:*468–474, 1969.

169. Burrell, R.J.W.: Distribution maps of esoph ageal cancer among Bantu in the Transkei. *J Nat Cancer Inst, 43:*877–888, 1969.

170. Higginson, J., and Oettle, A.G.: Cancer incidence in the Bantu and "Cape Colored" races of South Africa: report of a cancer survey in the Transvaal (1953–1955). *J Natl Cancer Inst, 24:*558–671, 1960.

171. Wynder, E.L., and Brass, I.J.: A study of etiologic factors in cancer of the esophagus, *Cancer, 14:*398–412, 1961.

172. Cliffton, E.E.: Surgery and irradiation in the treatment of esophageal cancer. *Hosp Pract, 4:*88–98, 1969.

173. Mosbech, J., and Videbaek, A.: On the etiology of esophageal carcinoma. *J Natl Cancer Inst, 15:*1655–1673, 1955.

174. Just-Viera, J.O., and Haight, C.: Achalasia and carcinoma of the esophagus. *Surg Gynecol Obstet, 128:*1081–1095, 1969.

175. Lortat-Jacob, J.L., Richard, C.A., and Fekete, F., *et al.:* Cardiospasm and esophageal carcinoma: report of 24 cases. *Clin Surg, 66:*969–975, 1969.

176. Lynch, H.T., Ewers, D.D., Krush, A.J., Sharp, E.A., and Swartz, M.J.: Esophageal cancer in a Midwestern community. *Am J Gastroent, 55:*437–442, 1971.

177. Reilly, C., and McGlashan, N.D.: Zinc and copper contamination in Zambian alcoholic drinks. *S. Afr. J Med Sci, 34:*43–48, 1969.

178. McGlashan, N.D.: Oesophageal cancer and alcoholic spirits in Central Africa. *Gut, 10:*643–650, 1969.

178a. Pour, P., and Ghadirian, P.: Familial cancer of the esophagus in Iran. *Cancer, 33:*1649–1652, 1974.

179. Shine, I., and Allison, P.R.: Carcinoma of the oesophagus with tylosis (Keratosis Palmaris et Plantaris). *Lancet, 1::*51–953, 1966.

180. Lilienfeld, A.: Epidemiology of gastric cancer. *New Engl J Med, 286:*316–317, 1972.

181. Wynder, E.L., Kmet, J., and Dungal, N., *et al.:* An epidemiological investigation of gastric cancer. *Cancer, 16:*1461–1496, 1963.

182. Graham, S., and Lilienfeld, A.M.: Genetic studies of gastric cancer in humans: an appraisal, *Cancer, 11:*945–958, 1958.

183. Pastore, J.O., Kato, H., and Belsky, J.L.: Serum pepsin and tubeless gastric analysis as predictors of stomach cancer: a 10-year follow-up study, Hiroshima. *New Engl J Med, 286:*279–284, 1972.

184. Krain, L.S.: The rising incidence of carcinoma of the pancreas—real or apparent. *J Surg Oncol, 2:*115, 1970.

185. Stephenson, H.E.: Cancer of the pancreas and stomach: a study in contrasts. *Surgery, 71:*307–308, 1972.

186. Silverberg, E., and Holleb, A.I.: Cancer Statistics, 1971. *Cancer, 21:*13–31, 1971.

187. Segi, M., Kurihara, M., and Matsuyama, T.: Cancer mortality for selected sites in 24 countries (No. 5 [1964–1965]), Sendai, Japan, Tohoku University School of Medicine, 1969, pp. 66–67.

188. Sokoloff, B.: Predisposition to cancer in the Bonaparte family. *Am J Surg, 40:*673–678, 1938.

189. Mosbech, J., and Bidebaek, A.: Mortality from and risk of gastric carcinoma among patients with pernicious anemia. *Brit Med J, 2:*390–394, 1950.

190. Shearman, D.J.C., and Finlayson, N.D.C.: Familial aspects of gastric carcinoma. *Am J Dig Dis, 12(5):*529–534, 1967.

191. Hoskins, L.C., Loux, H.A., Britten, A., and Zamcheck, N.: Distribution of ABO blood groups in patients with pernicious anemia, gastric carcinoma, and gastric carcinoma associated with pernicious anemia. *New Engl J Med, 273:*633–637, 1965.

192. Buckwalter, J.A., Wohlwend, C.B., Colter, D.C., Tidrick, R.T., and Knowler, L.A.: The association of the ABO blood groups to gastric carcinoma. *Surg Gynecol Obstet, 104:*176–179, 1957.

193. Mosbech, J.: ABO blood groups in stomach cancer. *Acta Genet Stat Med, 8:*219–227, 1958.

194. Videbaek, A., and Mosbech, J.: The aetiology

of gastric carcinoma elucidated by a study of 302 pedigrees. *Acta Med Scand, 149:* 173–148, 1954.

195. Woolf, C.M.: A further study on the familial aspects of carcinoma of the stomach. *Am J Hum Genet, 8:*102–109, 1956.

196. Mosbech, J.: *Heredity in Pernicious Anemia: A Proband Study of the Heredity and the Relationship to Cancer of the Stomach.* Copenhagen, Muskgard, 1953, pp. 107.

197. Goren, P.A.: Genetic interpretation of studies on cancer in twins. *Ann Eugen, 8:*219–232, 1937–1938.

198. Lee, F.I.: Carcinoma of the gastric antrum in identical twins. *Postgrad Med J, 47:*622–632, 1971.

199. Haerer, A.F., Jackson, J.F., and Evers, C.G.: Atasia-telangiectasia with gastric adeno-carcinoma. *JAMA, 210:*1884, 1969.

200. Lieber, M.M.: The incidence of gall stones and their correlation with other diseases. *Ann Surg, 135:*394–405, 1952.

201. Brown, J.E., and Christensen, C.: Biliary tract disease among the Navajos. *JAMA, 202:*1050–1052, 1967.

202. Nelson, B.D., Porvaznik, J., and Benfield, J.R.: Gallbladder disease in Southwestern American Indians. *Arch Surg, 103:*41–43, 1971.

203. Kravetz, R.E.: Etiology of biliary tract disease in Southwestern American Indians. *Gastroenterology, 46:*392–398, 1964.

204. Sievers, M., and Marquis, J.: The Southwestern American Indian's burden: biliary disease. *JAMA, 182:*570–572, 1962.

205. Sampliner, J.E., and O'Connell, D.J.: Biliary surgery in the Southwestern American Indian. *Arch Surg, 96:*1–3, 1968.

206. Briele, H.A., Long, W.B., and Parks, L.C.: Gallbladder disease and cholecystectomy: experience with 1500 patients managed in a community hospital. *Am Surg, 35:*218–222, 1969.

207. Derman, H., Gerbarg, D., and Kelly, J., *et al.:* Are gall stones and gallbladder cancer related? *JAMA, 176:*450–451, 1961.

208. Newman, H.F., and Northup, J.D.: Gallbladder carcinoma in cholelithiasis. *Geriatrics, 19:*453–456, 1964.

209. Reichenbach, D.D.: Autopsy incidence of diseases among Southwestern American Indians. *Arch Pathol, 84:*81–85, 1967.

210. Allen, J.C., and Jaeschke, W.H.: Recurrence of malignant melanoma in an orbit after 28 years. *Arch Ophthalmol* (Chicago), *76:* 79–81, 1966.

211. Anderson, D.E., Smither, J.L., Jr., and Mc-Bride, C.M.: Hereditary aspects of malignant melanoma. *JAMA, 200:*741–746, 1967.

212. Bowen, S.F., Brady, H., and Jones, V.L.: Malignant melanoma of the eye occurring in two successive generations. *Arch Ophthalmol* (Chicago), *71:*805–806, 1964.

213. Davenport, R.C.: Family history of choroidal sarcoma. *Br J Ophthalmol, 11:*443–445, 1927.

214. Gartner, S.: Malignant melanoma of the choroid and von Recklinghausen's disease. *Am J Ophthalmol, 23:*73–78, 1940.

215. Gutmann, G.: Casuisticher Beitrag zur Lehre von den Geschwülsten des Augapfels. Augapfels. *Arch Augenheikunde, 31:*158–180, 1895.

216. Hogan, M.J., and Zimmerman, L.E.: *Ophthalmic Pathology, An Atlas and Textbook,* 2nd ed. Philadelphia, Saunders, 1962, p. 413.

217. Parsons, J.H.: *The Pathology of the Eye.* New York, Putman, 1905, pp. 496–497.

218. Pfingst, A.O., and Graves, S.: Melanosarcoma of choroid occurring in brothers. *Arch Ophthalmol* (Chicago), *50:*431–439, 1921.

219. Resler, D.R., Snow, J.B., and Williams, G.R.: Multiplicity and familial incidence of carotid body and glomus jugulare tumors. *Ann Otol, 75:*114–122, 1966.

220. Silcock, A.Q.: Hereditary sarcoma of eyeball in three generations. *Br Med J, 1:*1079, 1892.

221. Lynch, H.T., Anderson, D.E., and Krush, A.J.: Heredity and intraocular malignant melanoma: study of two families and review of forty-five cases. *Cancer, 21:*119–125, 1968.

222. Waardenberg, P.J.: Melanosarcoma of the eye in more than one member of a family. *Nederl T Geneesk, 84:*4718, 1940.

223. Tucker, D.P., Steinberg, A.G., and Cogan,

D.G.: Frequency of genetic transmission of sporadic retinoblastoma. *Arch Ophthalmol, 57*:532–535, 1957.

224. Staats, E.F., Brown, R.L., and Smith, R.R.: Carotid body tumors, benign and malignant. *Laryngoscope, 76*:907–916, 1966.

225. Reese, H.E., Lucas, R.N., and Bergman, P.A.: Malignant carotid body tumors. *Ann Surg, 157*:232–243, 1963.

226. Whimster, W.F., and Masson, A.F.: Malignant carotid body tumor with extradural metasteses. *Cancer, 26*:239–244, 1970.

227. Marchand, F.: Beiträge zur Kenntniss der normalen und Pathologischer Anatomie der Glandula Carotica und der Nebennieren. *Int Beitr Wiss Med* (Berlin), *1*:535–581, 1891.

228. Chase, W.H.: Familial and bilateral tumors of the carotid body. *J Pathol Bact, 36*:1–12, 1933.

229. Rush, B.F.: Familial bilateral carotid body tumors. *Ann Surg, 157*:633–636, 1963.

230. Kroll, A.J., Alexander, B., Cochios, F., and Pechet, L.: Hereditary deficiencies of clotting factors VII and X associated with carotid body tumors. *New Engl J Med, 270*:6–13, 1964.

231. Resler, D.R., Snow, J.B., and Williams, G.R.: Multiplicity and familial incidence of carotid body and Glomus tumors. *Ann Otol, 75*:114–122, 1966.

232. Werner, O.: *Ueber Kataract in Verbindung mit Sklerodermie.* Doctoral Dissertation, Kiel University, Schmidt & Klaunig, Kiel, 1904.

233. Rothmund, A.: Ueber Katarakt in Verbindung mit einer Eigentümlichen Hautdegeneration. *Arch Ophthalmol, 14*:158–182, 1868.

234. Thannhauser, S.J.: Werner's syndrome (progeria of the adult) and Rothmund's syndrome: two types of closely related heredofamilial atrophic dermatosis with juvenile cataracts and endocrine features: a critical study with five new cases. *Ann Intern Med, 23*:559–626, 1945.

235. Epstein, C.J., Martin, G.M., Schultz, A.L., and Motulsky, A.G.: Werner's syndrome: a review of its symptomatology, natural history, pathologic features, genetics, and

relationship to the natural aging process. *Medicine* (Balt), *45*:177–221, 1966.

236. Oppenheimer, B.S., and Kugel, V.H.: Werner's Syndrome: heredo-familial disorder with scleroderma, bilateral juvenile cataract, precocious graying of hair and endocrine stigmatization. *Trans Assoc Am Physicians, 49*:358–370, 1934.

237. Boyd, M.W., and Grant, A.P.: Werner's syndrome (progeria of the adult), further pathological and biochemical observations. *Br Med J, 2*:920–925, 1959.

238. Petrohelos, M.A.: Werner's syndrome: a survey of three cases, with review of the literature. *Am J Ophthalmol, 56*:941, 1963.

239. Riley, T.R., Wieland, R.G., Markin, J., and Thamwi, G.J.: Werner's syndrome. *Ann Intern Med, 63*:285–294, 1965.

240. Epstein, C.J.: Werner's syndrome. *Ann Intern Med, 63*:343–345, 1965.

241. Ellison, D.J., and Pugh, D.W.: Werner's Syndrome. *Br Med J, 2*:237, 1955.

242. Muller, L., and Andersson, B.: Werner's Syndrome: survey based on two cases. *Acta Med Scand* (Suppl), *283, 146*:3–17, 1953.

243. Agatston, S.A., and Gartner, S.: Precocious cataract and scleroderma (Rothmund's syndrome; Werner's syndrome). *Arch Ophthalmol* (Chicago), *21*:492–496, 1939.

244. Oppenheimer, B.S., and Kugel, V.H.: Werner's syndrome: report of the first necropsy and of findings in a new case. *Am J Med Sci, 202*:629–642, 1941.

245. Jacobson, H.G., Rifkin, H., and Zucker-Frankling, D.: Werner's Syndrome: A clinical roentgenological entity. *Radiology, 74*:373–385, 1960.

246. Boatwright, H., Wheeler, C.E., and Cawley, E.P.: Werner's syndrome. *AMA Arch Intern Med* (Chicago), *90*:243–249, 1952.

247. McKusick, V.A.: Medical genetics 1962. *J Chronic Dis, 16*:457–634, 1963.

248. Rubin, C.E., and Dobbins, W.O., III: Peroral biopsy of the small intestine: a review of its diagnostic usefulness. *Gastroenterology, 49*:676–697, 1965.

249. McDonald, W.C., Dobbins, W.O., III, and Rubin, C.E.: Studies of the familial nature

of celiac sprue using biopsy of the small intestine. *New Engl J Med, 272:*448–456, 1965.

250. Gough, K.R., Read, A.E., and Naish, J.M.: Intestinal reticulosis as a complication of idiopathic steatorrhea. *Gut, 3:*232–239, 1962.

251. Harris, O.D., Cooke, W.T., Thompson, H., and Waterhouse, J.A.H.: Malignancy in adult coeliac disease and idiopathic steatorrhea. *Am J Med, 42:*899–912, 1967.

252. Austad, W.I., Cornes, J.S., Gough, K.R., McCarthy, C.F., and Read, A.E.: steatorrhea and malignant lymphoma: the relationship of malignant tumors of lymphoid tissue and celiac disease. *Am J Dig Dis, 12:*475–490, 1967.

253. Tonkin, R.D.: Reticulosis of small bowel as a late complication of idiopathic steatorrhea. *Proc R Soc Med, 56:*167–168, 1963.

254. Whitehead, R.: Primary lymphadenopathy complicating idiopathic steatorrhea. *Gut, 9:*569–575, 1968.

255. Gupte, S.P., Perkash, A., Mahajan, C.M., Aggarwal, P.K., and Gupta, P.R.: Acute myeloid leukemia in a girl with celiac disease. *Am J Dig Dis, 16:*939–941, 1971.

256. Hobbs, J.R., and Hepner, G.W.: Deficiency of m-globulin in celiac disease. *Lancet, 1:*217–220, 1968.

257. Asquith, P., Thompson, R.A., and Cooke, W.T.: Serum-immunoglobulins in adult celiac disease. *Lancet, 2:*129–131, 1969.

258. Hamman, L., and Rich, A.R.: Acute diffuse interstitial fibrosis of the lungs. *Bull Hopkin's Hosp, 74:*177–212, 1944.

259. Donohue, W.L., and Laski, B., Uchida, I., and Munn, J.D.: Familial fibrocystic pulmonary dysplasia and its relation to the Hamman-Rich syndrome. *Pediatrics, 24:*786–813, 1959.

260. Young, W.A.: Familial fibrocystic pulmonary dysplasia: a new case in a known affected family. *Can Med Ass J, 94:*1059–1061, 1966.

262. Womack, N.A., and Graham, E.A.: Epithelial metaplasia in congenital cystic disease of the lung: its possible relation to carcinoma of the bronchus. *Am J Pathol, 17:*645–653, 1941.

263. McKusick, V.A., and Fisher, A.M.: Congenital cystic disease of the lung with progressive pulmonary fibrosis and carcinomatosis. *Ann Intern Med, 48:*774–690, 1958.

264. Ho, H.C.: Nasopharyngeal carcinoma in Hong Kong. In Muir, C.S., and Shanmugaratnam, K., (Eds.): *Cancer of the Nasopharynx*, UICC Monograph Series, Vol. 1, pp. 58–63, Copenhagen, Munksgaard, 1967.

265. Muir, C.S., and Shanmugaratnam, K.: The incidence of nasopharyngeal carcinoma in Singapore. In Muir, C.S., and Shanmugaratnam, K., (Ed.): *Cancer of the Nasopharynx*, UICC Monograph Series, Vol. 1, pp. 47–53, Copenhagen, Munksgaard, 1967.

266. Djojopranoto, M.: *Beberapa Segi Patologi Tumour Ganas Nasopharynx di-Diawa-Timu.* Thesis. Gita Karya, Surabaja, Indonesia, 1960.

267. Scott, G.C., and Atkinson, L.: Demographic features of the Chinese population in Australia and the relative prevalence of nasopharyngeal cancer among Caucasians and Chinese. In Muir, C.S., and Shanmugaratnam, K., (Eds.): *Cancer of the Nasopharynx*, UICC Monograph Series, Vol. 1, pp. 64–72, Munksgaard, Copenhagen, 1967.

268. Zippin, C., Tekawa, I.S., Bragg, K.U., Watson, D., and Linden, G.: Studies on heredity and environment in cancer of the nasopharynx, *J Natl Cancer Inst, 29:*483–490, 1962.

269. Ho, H.C.: Nasopharyngeal carcinoma in Hong Kong. *Proceedings of the 9th International Cancer Congress Tokyo, 1966.* Panel 11. UICC Monograph Series, Vol. 10, pp. 110–116, 1967.

270. Shanmugaratnam, K.: Cancer of the nasopharyngeal carcinoma: origin and structure. In Muir, C.S., and Shanmugaratnam, K., (Eds.): *Cancer of the Nasopharynx*, UICC Monograph Series, Vol. 1, pp. 153–162. Copenhagen, Munksgaard, 1967.

271. de-The, G., Ho, H.C., Kwan, H.C., Desgranges, C., and Favre, M.D.: Nasopharyngeal carcinoma (NPC). I. Types of cultures derived from tumour biopsies and nontumorous tissues of Chinese patients with special reference to lymphoblastoid transformation. *Intl J Cancer, 6:*189–206, 1970.

272. de-The, G., Ambrosioni, J.C., Ho, H.C., and Kwan, H.C.: Lymphoblastoid transformation and presence of herpes-type viral particles in a Chinese nasopharyngeal tumour cultured *in vitro. Nature, 221:* 770–771, 1969.

273. de-The, G.: Personal Communication, 1962.

274. Lilly, F.: The histocompatibility 2-locus and susceptibility to tumour induction. *Natl Cancer Inst Monograph, 22:*631–642, 1966.

275. Solomon, L.: Hereditary multiple exostosis. *J Bone Joint Surg* (Brit), *45:*292–304, 1963.

276. Dahlin, D.C.: *Bone Tumors.* Springfield, Thomas, 1957.

277. Jaffe, H.L.: *Tumors and Tumorous Conditions of the Bones and Joints.* London, Henry Kimpton, 1958.

278. Lynch, H.T., unpublished data, 1972.

279. Fejer, R., and Revay, S.: Exostosis cartilaginea multiplex familiaris. *Am J Med, 39:* 296–297, 1965.

280. Vial, K.J.: Hereditary multiple exostosis: a genetic analysis. *Med J Aust, 1:*213–215, 1966.

281. Lattes, R.: Thymoma and other tumors of the thymus: an analysis of 107 cases. *Cancer, 15:*1224–1260, 1962.

282. Legg, M.A., and Brady, W.J.: Pathology and clinical behaviour of thymomas: a survey of 51 cases. *Cancer, 18:*1131–1144, 1965.

283. Matani, A., and Dritsas, C.: Familial occurrence of metastasizing carcinoid tumors. *Ann Intern Med, 78:*389–390, 1973.

284. Moertel, C.G., and Dockerty, M.B.: Familial occurrence of metastasizing carcinoid tumors. *Ann Intern Med, 78:*389–390, 1973.

285. Eschbach, J.W., and Rinaldo, J.A., Jr.: Metastatic carcinoid. A familial occurrence. *Ann Intern Med, 57:*647–650, 1962.

286. Anderson, R.E.: A familial instance of appendiceal carcinoid. *Am J Surg, 111:*738–740, 1966.

287. Fagerhol, M.K., and Laurell, C.B.: The pi system-inherited variants of serum alpha$_1$ antitrypsin. *Prog Med Genet, 7:*96–111, 1970.

288. Eriksson, S.: Studies in alpha$_1$ antitrypsin deficiency. *Acta Med Scand* (Suppl), *432:* 1–85, 1965.

289. Talamo, R.C., Blennerhassett, J.B., and Austen, K.F.: Familial emphysema and alpha$_1$ antitrypsin deficiency. *New Engl J Med, 275:*1301–1304, 1966.

290. Sharp, H.L., Bridges, R.A., Krivit, W., and Freier, E.F.: Cirrhosis associated with alpha$_1$ antitrypsin deficiency: a previously unrecognized inherited disorder. *J Lab Clin Med, 73:*934–939, 1969.

291. Berg, N.O., and Eriksson, S.: Liver disease in adults with alpha$_1$ antitrypsin deficiency. *New Engl J Med, 287:*1264–1267, 1972.

292. Mace, J.W., Kaplan, J.M., Schanberger, J.E., and Gotlin, R.W.: Poland's syndrome: report of seven cases and review of the literature. *Clin Pediatr, 11:*98, 1972.

293. Hoefnagel, D., Rozycki, A., Wurster-Hill, D., Stern, P., and Gregory, D.: Leukaemia and Poland's Syndrome. *Lancet, 2:*1038, 1972.

294. Walters, T.R., Reddy, B.N., Bailon, A., and Vitale, L.F.: Poland's Syndrome Associated with Leukemia. *J Pediatr, 82:*889, 1973.

295. David, T.J.: Nature and etiology of the Poland anomaly. *N Engl J Med, 287:*487, 1972.

296. Arnold, W.H.: Hereditary bone dysplasia with sarcomatous degeneration. *Ann Intern Med, 78:*902–906, 1973.

297. Krause, S., Adler, L.N., and Reddy, P.S. *et al.*: Intracardiac myxoma in siblings. *Chest, 60:*404–406, 1971.

298. Kleid, J.J., Klugman, J., Haas, J., and Battock, D.: Familial atrial myxoma. *Am J Cardiol, 32:*361–364, 1973.

299. Straus, R., and Merliss, R.: Primary tumor of the heart. *Arch Pathol* (Chicago), *39:*74–78, 1945.

300. Ferguson, S.W., and Lynn, T.N.: Familial leukemia. A report of four cases of acute leukemia in four consecutive generations. *South Med J, 63:*1337–1340, 1970.

301. Weinberg, A.G., and Rogers, L.E.: Hepato-

splenomegaly, pancytopenia, and fever. *J Pediatr, 82:*879–884, 1973.

302. Falletta, J.M., Fernbach, D.J., Singer, D.B., South, M.A., Landing, B.H., Heath, C.W., Jr., Shore, N.A., and Barrett, F.F.: A fatal X-linked recessive reticuloendothelial syndrome with hyperglobulinemia. *J Pediatr, 83:*549–556, 1973.

303. Omenn, G.S.: Familial reticuloendotheliosis with eosinophilia. *N Engl J Med, 273:* 427–432, 1965.

304. Davies, A.J.S., Festenstein, H., Leuchars, E., Wallis, V.J., and Doenhoff, M.J.: A thymic origin for some peripheral-blood lymphocytes. *Lancet, 1:*183–184, 1968.

305. Fraumeni, J.F., Jr., and Thomas, L.B.: Malignant bladder tumors in a man and his three sons. *JAMA, 201:*97–99, 1967.

306. Lilienfeld, A.M.: The relationship of bladder cancer to smoking. *Am J Public Health, 54:* 1864–1875, 1964.

307. Morganti, G., et al.: Recherches Clinico-Statistiques et Génétiques sur les Neoplasies de la Vessie. *Acta Genet, 6:*306–307, 1956.

308. Burkland, C.E., and Juzek, R.H.: Familial occurrence of carcinoma of the ureter. *J Urol, 96:*602–701, 1966.

309. Wynder, E.L., Bross, I.J., and Day, E.: Epidemiological approach to etiology of cancer of the larynx. *JAMA, 160:*1384–1391, 1956.

310. Marlowe, F.I.: Simultaneous laryngeal tumors in sisters. *Arch Otolaryngol, 92:* 195–197, 1970.

311. Fraumeni, J.F., Jr., and Miller, R.W.: Adrenocortical neoplasms with hemihypertrophy, brain tumors, and other disorders. *J Pediatr, 70:*129–138, 1967.

312. Kenny, F.M., Hashida, Y., Askari, H.A., Sieber, W.H., and Fetterman, G.H.: Virilizing tumors of the adrenal cortex. *Am J Dis Child, 115:*445–458, 1968.

313. Mahloudji, M., Ronaghy, H., and Dutz, W.: Virilizing adrenal carcinoma in two sibs. *J Med Genet, 8:*160–163, 1971.

314. Riesco, A., and Leyton, C.: Mucopolysaccharides in peripheral leucocytes of cancer patients. *Br J Cancer, 25:*284–290, 1971.

315. Riesco, A., and Coke, C.: The genetic origin of leucocytic mucopolysaccharides in cancer patients. *Br J Cancer, 28:*269–274, 1973.

316. Burkitt, D.P., and Wright, D.H.: *Burkitt's Lymphoma.* Edinburgh, E. & S. Livingstone, Ltd., 1970.

317. Pike, M., Williams, E.H., and Wright, B.: Burkitt's Tumour in the West Nile District of Uganda, 1961–1965. *Br Med J, 2:* 395–399, 1967.

318. Wright, D.H.: The epidemiology of Burkitt's Tumor. *Cancer Res, 27:*2424–2438, 1967.

319. Dalldorf, G., Linsell, C.A., and Barnhart, F.E.: An epidemiological approach to the lymphomas of African children and Burkitt's sarcoma of the jaws. *Perspect Biol Med, 7:*435–449, 1964.

320. Morrow, R.H., Pike, M.C., and Smith, P.G., et al.: Burkitt's Lymphoma: A time-space cluster of cases in Bwamba county of Uganda. *Br Med J, 1:*491–492, 1971.

321. Hirshaut, Y., Cohen, M., and Stevens, D.: Serological differences between American and African Burkitt's lymphoma. *Fed Proc, 30:*301, 1971.

322. Stevens, D.A., O'Conor, G.T., Levine, P.H., and Rosen, R.B.: Acute leukemia with "Burkitt's Lymphoma Cells" and Burkitt's lymphoma. *Ann Intern Med, 76:*967–973, 1972.

323. Novak, E.: Endocrine effects of certain dysontogenetic tumors of the ovary. *Endocrinology, 30:*953–958, 1942.

324. Goldstein, D.P., and Lamb, E.J.: Arrhenoblastoma in first cousins: report of 2 cases. *Obstet Gynecol, 35:*444–450, 1970.

325. Javert, C.T., and Finn, W.F.: Arrhenoblastoma. The incidence of malignancy and the relationship to pregnancy, to sterility, and to treatment. *Cancer, 4:*60, 1951.

326. Accardo, M., and Condorelli, B.: Arrhenoblastoma in due sorelle. *Riv Pat Clin Sper, 7,*171, 1966.

327. Kostmann, R.: Infantile genetic agranulocytosis (agranulocytosis infantilis hereditaria). *Acta Paediatr* (Scand), *45:*1–78, 1956.

328. Schroeder, T.M., and Kurth, R.: Spontaneous chromosomal breakage and high incidence of leukemia in inherited disease. *Blood, 37:* 96–112, 1971.

329. Comfort, M.W., and Steinberg, A.G.: Pedigree of a family with hereditary chronic relapsing pancreatitis. *Gastroenterology, 21:*54–63, 1952.

330. Davidson, P., *et al.*: Hereditary pancreatitis: a kindred without gross aminoaciduria. *Ann Intern Med, 68:*88–96, 1968.

331. Appel, M.F.: Hereditary pancreatitis: review and presentation of an additional kindred. *Arch Surg, 108:*63–65, 1974.

332. Castleman, B.: Case records of the Massachusetts general hospital. *N Engl J Med, 286:*1353–1359, 1972.

333. Wynder, E.L., Mabuchi, K., and Whitmore, W.F., Jr.: Epidemiology of cancer of the prostate. *Cancer, 28:*344–360, 1971.

334. Lynch, H.T., Guirgis, H.A., Albert, S., Brennan, M., Lynch, J., Kraft, C., Pocekay, D., Vaughns, C., and Kaplan, A.R.: Familial association of carcinoma of the breast and ovary. *Surg Gynecol Obstet,* in press.

335. Lynch, H.T., Larsen, A.L., Magnuson, C.W., and Krush, A.J.: Prostate carcinoma and multiple primary malignancies. *Cancer, 19:*1891–1987, 1966.

336. Woolf, C.M.: An investigation of the familial aspects of carcinoma of the prostate. *Cancer, 13:*739–744, 1960.

337. Morganti, G., Gianferrari, L., Cresseri, A., Arrigoni, G., and Lovati, G.: Recherches Clinico-Statistiques et Génétiques sur les Néoplasies de la Prostate. *Acta Genet, 6:* 304–305, 1956.

338. Kyle, R.A., Nobrega, F.T., and Kurland, L.T.: Multiple myeloma in Olmsted County, Minnesota, 1945–1964. *Blood, 33:* 739–745, 1969.

339. Lewis, E.B.: Leukemia, multiple myeloma, and aplastic anemia in American radiologists. *Science, 142:*1492–1494, 1963.

340. Sorenson, G.D.: Virus-like particles in Myeloma cells of man. *Proc Soc Exp Biol Med, 118:*250–252, 1965.

341. Potter, M., and Boyce, C.R.: Induction of plasma-cell neoplasms in strain BALB/c mice with mineral oil and mineral oil adjuvants. *Nature, 193:*1086–1087, 1962.

342. Kyle, R.A., Heath, C.W., Jr., and Carbone, P.: Multiple myeloma in spouses. *Arch Intern Med, 127:*944–946, 1971.

343. Ogawa, M., Wurster, D.H., and McIntyre, O.R.: Multiple myeloma in one of a pair of monozygotic twins. *Acta Haematol, 44:* 295–304, 1970.

344. Robbins, R.: Familial multiple myeloma: the tenth reported occurrence. *Am J Med Sci, 254:*848–850, 1967.

345. McKusick, V.A.: *Mendelian Inheritance in Man: Catalogs of Autosomal Dominant, Autosomal Recessive, and X-Linked Phenotypes,* 3rd ed. Baltimore, Johns Hopkins, 1971, p. 465.

346. Meijers, K.A.E., DeLeeuw, B., and Voormolen-Kalova, M.: The multiple occurrence of myeloma and asymptomatic paraproteinaemia within one family. *Clin Exp Immunol, 12:*185–193, 1972.

347. Freireich, E.J., Whang, J., Tjio, J.H., Levin, R.H., Brittin, G.M., and Frei, E. III: Refractory anemia, granulocytic hyperplasia of bone marrow and a missing chromosome in marrow cells. A new clinical syndrome? *Clin Res, 12:*284, 1964.

348. Macdougall, L.G., Brown, J.A., Cohen, M.M., and Judisch, J.M.: C-Monosomy myeloproliferative syndrome: a case of 7-monosomy. *J Pediatr, 84:*256–259, 1974.

CHAPTER 24

GENETIC COUNSELING AND CANCER

HENRY T. LYNCH AND JANE LYNCH

G ENETIC COUNSELING INVOLVES communication of genetic risk information in context with diagnosis, prognosis, and disposition of the medical genetic disorder to individual patients and their concerned relatives. This subject continues to receive major attention in the medical literature as well as in the lay press. The improved control of infectious and other controllable diseases has undoubtedly influenced the trends in medicine with increasing interest now being given to birth defects, metabolic disorders, and chronic diseases, many of which have a hereditary etiology.

In spite of the increased number of studies concerning genetic counseling, one still encounters considerable lack of knowledge among physicians concerning its role in medicine. It will, therefore, be the purpose of this chapter to attempt to clarify this issue and to relate it to the cancer problem.

Scope of Genetic Counseling Problems

Any patient or relative of a patient who manifests a disorder which has either a presumptive or proven hereditary etiology should be advised concerning the possible role of genetic factors. However, in order to provide accurate and satisfying advice about a medical-genetic problem which, incidentally, will frequently involve diagnosis, therapy, and prognosis, we believe that it is mandatory for a physician to offer genetic counseling. Unfortunately, to some individuals "genetic counseling" implies the quotation of simple stereotyped mathematical risks. However, we consider medical genetic problems in the same context as any other medical problem, requiring the establishment of a patient-physician relationship.[1]

Genetic problems are unique in that they often affect the entire family directly or indirectly; occasionally even the patient's peer group as well as members of the community in which the family resides may be concerned with the "family disorder." Certain hereditary disorders present in a family may arouse misdirected guilt, fear, anxiety, apprehension, fatalism, denial, and accusation directed toward the spouse, parents, or other members of the family. In some cases, guilt and even an expressed need for punishment, resulting from misdirected feelings of "blame" may also occur. Therefore, in order to proceed with positive goal-directed genetic counseling, the physician must evaluate the problem in context with all of these emotional components. Thus, hereditary disorders, including those forms of cancer which are considered to be genetic or "familial" must be considered within the frame of reference of the patient, his family, and his community; the complex interaction of these problems with their frequent emotional overtones provides the material for genetic counseling. Accepting this premise, one realizes that genetic counseling limited solely to any single facet of the problem, such as mere recitation of genetic risk is completely inadequate and leads only to frustration and failure of the process. Thus, genetic counseling must involve a sensitive appraisal and reflection of family interactions, financial problems which a chronic hereditary disease might engender, disability with possible loss of employment, occasional depersonalization and even family disruption as sequelae of emotional stress.

Genetic Counseling in Specific Genetic-Oncologic Problems

Clinically oriented genetic counseling can only be accomplished satisfactorily when detailed epidemiologic information is available pertaining to the specific cancer problem of concern; this should include its distribution in the family, its probable risk to living relatives, and its predicted risk to future progeny of family members. In addition, preventive measures should be discussed whenever possible. Such examples would include colectomy for patients with familial multiple adenomatous polyposis coli, and possible gonadectomy for patients with the testicular feminization syndrome. On the other hand, watchful expectation with periodic diagnostic examinations, are indicated for persons who are thought to be at increased risk for some of the common malignant neoplasms such as carcinoma of the breast and colon, whose modes of inheritance either are not established or specific markers are not present so that the cancer risk must be judged empirically.

Clinical examples of cancer-genetic problems are listed in Tables 1-I–1-V in the introductory chapter of this book. These tables provide a cursory presentation of cancerous and precancerous disorders, aggregations of which in families have led to various hereditary etiological hypotheses. They should be used cautiously, with full knowledge of the fact that multiple etiologic factors may be involved in any one particular condition.

For example, in the case of carotid body tumors, depicted in Table 1-I, it should be realized that while autosomal dominant inheritance has been shown in families with this tumor, the overwhelming majority of occurrences apparently do not involve primary genetic factors; specifically, about 97 percent of the occurrences are sporadic, i.e. nonfamilial with unknown etiology. Similarly, retinoblastoma (Table 1-I) has a classical genetic etiology in between 20 and 40 percent of the cases; however, certain undefined nongenetic factors (fresh gene mutations cannot be excluded) may also be of etiologic importance. On the other hand, though heredity appears to play a significant role in lupus erythematosis (Table 1-IV) no genetic mechanism has yet been proven. In addition, the significance of malignant transformation in this disease must be critically scrutinized so that its full relationship to this immune disorder may be appreciated. Table 1-V lists those conditions wherein the risk to a first degree relative of an affected patient is increased, often about two to three fold. This is referred to as an empiric risk and by itself does not provide knowledge as to etiology, i.e. genetic or familial factors and/or both may be important. Thus, in the case of lung cancer it is clear that cigarette smoking is of crucial importance, but nevertheless familial factors also must be considered.[2]

These tables reflect the fact that considerable knowledge about cancer genetics has been accrued during the past several decades as evidenced by the number of listings in the several categories presented. However, the incompleteness of this listing attests to the need for continued diligent genetic investigations concerning carcinogenesis.

Breast Cancer

An example of the above problem is found in breast cancer for which no reliable marker has been determined to date. It is estimated that breast cancer will occur in about 6 percent of all women in the United States when appropriate age correction is made. However, given a first degree relative with breast cancer, the empirical risk becomes approximately three times as great (18%) as that occurring in the general population. The familial risk is greater in patients from families with bilateral breast cancer and/or onset at premenopausal age. The risk for breast cancer is also increased in women with early menarche, late natural or surgical menopause, in those who are nulliparous or have their first pregnancy after age 30. It may also be accentuated in obese women and those from higher socio-economic strata. In certain families, the risk may approach 50 percent, as is expected for a dominantly inherited factor.[3] In addition, risk factor estimates may be required for other histologic varieties of cancer in certain breast cancer prone families, i.e. breast cancer in association with carcinoma of ovary or endometrium (see Chapter 20). When breast cancer prone families are identified, genetic risk information should be given in context with cancer control techniques such as instruction in self-breast examination, and the patients should be encouraged to visit their physicians annually for careful breast examinations; additional diagnostic measures such as mammography and thermography should be instituted after age 35 or 40, or even at a younger age for members of families in which an unusually early onset of breast cancer may prevail.

Testicular Feminization Syndrome

The testicular feminization syndrome (TFS) is a relatively rare disorder which assumes importance in genetic counseling because of the increased risk for testicular cancer in certain members of affected families.[4-7] Typical patients have a female habitus with absence of or scanty axillary and pubic hair, female external genitalia, with variable stages of underdevelopment of the labia with a blind-ending vagina (which is usually adequate for sexual relations). Patients with TFS appear outwardly as females and they manifest the psycho-sexual orientation of a female. They frequently marry and often enjoy a normal sex life.[6,8] There is an absence of development of internal genitalia except for a rudimentary uterus and for gonads (testes) which may be intraabdominal or may be found along the course of the inguinal canal. The gonads are comprised largely of seminiferous tubules characterized usually by the absence of spermatogenesis but frequently with a marked increase in interstitial cells.[6]

Karyotypes usually indicate a normal male (46XY) pattern. Genetic studies of families have shown an inheritance pattern with transmission through the maternal line,[5] consistent with inheritance by either a sex-linked recessive or male sex-limited autosomal dominant mechanism. Linkage studies for genes on the X-chromosome have not yet yielded conclusive results.[5,9]

The relationship of this syndrome to cancer has promulgated considerable debate in the literature. For example, Morris[4] found only one patient with cancer below the age of 20 but he did find 11 cases or 22 percent cancer frequency in patients over 30 years. Jones and Scott[10] estimate malignancies occurring in approximately 5 percent of such patients, while Hauser[11] estimates that about 8 percent of patients will develop cancer. However, the true incidence of cancer in patients with TFS is difficult to evaluate since many patients have been treated with prophylactic gonadectomy at an early age.

The most frequent form of cancer occurring in these patients is seminoma,[11] although other tumors including teratocarcinoma,[13] embryonal cell carcinoma,[12,13] as well as a gonadal sarcoma in a single patient [14] have been reported.

Genetic counseling for such patients is obviously an exceedingly delicate matter. It must be approached so that no unnecessary psychiatric or emotional burden is imposed upon the patient. Thus, in the interest of the patient, as well as her husband, the physician must guard against divulging the full implications of the XY genotype. [5,8] [14]

It is important that appropriate information be given concerning the cancer risk to the patient's gonads; details about the issue of gonadectomy should be given. In addition, the timing of prophylactic gonadectomy is important. While some authors have suggested the need for immediate gonadectomy, even in pre-pubertal patients, [15] others have been reluctant to advise prophylactic gonadectomy for any of these patients. [11]

O'Connell and associates [8] advise that bilateral gonadectomy be performed following puberty. They reported a family wherein TFS was found in three siblings, one of whom developed metastatic seminoma while a second sibling had a testicular tubular adenoma (Sertoli cell tumor). They performed prophylactic gonadectomy on two of these siblings.

In summary, we find that TFS involves a genetic defect wherein cancer of a specific type, involving the gonad, occurs in excess and wherein advice to the family in addition to genetic risk, must be tempered extremely carefully because of profound psychological and psycho-sexual implications; finally, recommendation of prophylactic gonadectomy may be of crucial importance to the patient's welfare.

Genetic Counseling and the Cancer Family Syndrome

We have studied a kindred among whom adenocarcinoma of the colon and endometrium and multiple primary malignant neoplasms have occurred with increased frequency through three generations. These findings fulfill the criteria for the cancer family syndrome [15] (see Chapter 19 for more detail on this syndrome).

This family was of interest because the proband, a 51-year-old woman, had received a diagnosis of endometrial carcinoma at the age of 40 years. She had been aware of the increased frequency of cancer in her family and when her brother received a diagnosis of carcinoma of the colon, she requested that her physician perform appropriate diagnostic studies even though she was completely asymptomatic. Findings on proctosigmoidoscopy and barium enema revealed the presence of an early adenocarcinoma of the transverse colon, and colectomy was successfully performed. Of further interest was the fact that this patient had an identical twin sister who had been completely asymptomatic at age 40 when her sister received a diagnosis of endometrial carcinoma. When she requested evaluation of her uterus because of the occurrence of endometrial carcinoma in her co-twin (and her knowledge of increased incidences of cancer in her family) a diagnosis of early endometrial carcinoma was established and a hysterectomy was successfully performed.

This family is presented because it reveals clearly the importance that certain patients, themselves, place upon the family history, and the importance of establishing good lines of communication between the patient and his physician. Obviously, genetic counseling would be of invaluable assistance for this family and many others like it. However, for reasons not completely clear to us, the family physicians caring for members of this family were apparently not directly involved in initiating cancer preventive steps which were definitely indicated. However, they did respond immediately to the request from their patients for diagnostic studies based upon correct assumptions of cancer risk. [16]

In managing patients from families who manifest an excess occurrence of cancer, the physician will not always be fortunate to have the patients bring this information to his attention. We have witnessed numerous examples in which members of cancer prone families became extremely fearful, fatalistic, and pessimistic and refused to see their physicians for cancer screening examinations. Indeed, in many circumstances, the patients manifested inordinate delay.[17]

Von Hippel-Lindau Disease

Von Hippel-Lindau's disease consists of an association of retinal angiomatoma and cerebellar hemangioblastoma. Less constant features include pancreatic and renal cysts; occasional patients develop renal cell carcinoma and pheochromocytoma. The disorder is inherited as an autosomal dominant.

Richards and associates[18] studied a family with Von Hippel-Lindau's disease in a prospective manner in order to determine the presence of renal cell carcinoma in asymptomatic members. Eleven members of the family were evaluated with excretory urograms (IVP's), renal scans, and other tests of renal function. Aortography was performed when the IVP suggested a mass lesion. Significantly, two asymptomatic patients were discovered to have findings of renal cell carcinoma. The authors concluded that genetic counseling, including diagnostic screening evaluations, are of great importance for relatives at risk for Von Hippel-Lindau disease.[18]

Medullary Thyroid Carcinoma, Pheochromocytoma, and Parathyroid Disease (Sipple's Syndrome)

The combination of medullary thyroid carcinoma, pheochromocytoma and para-thyroid disease has been referred to as Sipple's syndrome.[18a] This disorder is inherited as an autosomal dominant trait with a high degree of penetrance.[18b] In 1965 Williams[18c] identified 15 cases from the literature and added two of his own. He also showed that thyroid carcinoma occurring in this syndrome was of the medullary or solid type with amyloid stroma. Since then more than 250 cases of medullary thyroid carcinoma have been reported. There have also been several families showing the combination of thyroid carcinoma and pheochromocytoma.[18b] Parathyroid adenomas or hyperplasia have recently been shown to form an important component of this syndrome.[18d]

Medullary thyroid carcinomas have been shown to produce several functionally active compounds, including calcitonin, prostaglandins, adrenocorticotrophin (ACTH)-like substance, histaminase, and serotonin.[18b] Calcitonin has been shown to be extremely useful as a diagnostic screening study when this disorder is suspected. Measurement of serum calcitonin may be performed under basal conditions or during calcium infusion.[18e] Measurement of serum histaminase has been shown to be useful in the diagnosis of metastatic lesions as well as for postoperative follow-up.[18b] Since pheochromocytoma may also occur in this syndrome it is important that this lesion be evaluated in all patients at genetic risk for the disorder including those who have already demonstrated evidence of thyroid or parathyroid disease. When a patient and/or family is identified, diagnostic screening studies in relatives at high risk should begin at a young age. For example, Keiser and associates[18b] suggest screening of all family members beginning at five years of age or older. They advise that screening of family members for this syndrome should be conducted every year or two, and they state that a completely normal screening examination only rules out the disease at that particular moment. It in no way assures that the patient will never develop part or all of the syndrome. These authors reported a family wherein 25 cases of medullary thyroid carcinoma, 16 cases of parathyroid disease, and 11 cases of pheochromocytoma were diagnosed. Six of these patients had all three of these lesions. Eight other patients had reported but unconfirmed cases of thyroid carcinoma.

In families of the type alluded to above it is clear that genetic counseling, coupled with highly specific diagnostic evaluation could lead toward diagnosis of this disease in a potentially large number of individuals from families prone to this dominantly inherited genetic disorder. Therefore, genetic counseling is essential, and since the natural history of the disorder is one harboring a continuous risk for these specific cancers, the relatives should be counseled frequently. In our experience it is extremely important to clarify all these issues carefully with patients, so that they are fully cognizant of all manifestations of the genetic trait, and in turn, hopefully, they will cooperate fully with their physician in the total management of this and other life threatening diseases.

Discussion

The World Health Organization Expert Committee on Human Genetics has recommended increased training of medical personnel in medical genetics, with particular emphasis on genetic counseling.[19] This group emphasized their conviction that physicians should receive training in genetics at the preclinical and clinical levels and that the subject should also be dealt with in postgraduate medical education courses. The demand as well as the indications for genetic counseling are so great that existing genetic specialty clinics cannot conceivably fulfill the needs for these services at the present time. Further-more, since genetic counseling entails diagnosis, therapy, and prognosis of the patient and of his relatives at genetic risk, it is only logical that the physician providing primary family care, or the surgeon, would be expected to assume responsibility for the overall plan in order to assure continuity of this important service.[20]

A review of these several cancer genetic problems clearly indicates the important role which the physician can play in genetic counseling as a vital part of the discernment of genetic risk and subsequent management of cancer prone patients and their relatives. The physician need not have an exhaustive background in medical genetics in order to apply this important information to his interested and concerned patients. However, in many cases it will be necessary that he expand the family history portion of the clinical examination, collecting a richer account of specific histologic varieties of cancer, associated diseases, genealogic relationships, including a search for consanguinity, in order to be provided with the detailed family information which is necessary for genetic counseling. This extra effort may be amply rewarded in certain circumstances through alleviation of anxiety, guilt, apprehension, and occasional cancer phobia, when the cancer-genetic issue is clarified to the patient. Improved cancer control may also be accomplished.

We have provided a listing of genetic units in the United States and other countries of the world wherein there is interest in genetics, cancer genetics, and/or both of these activities.

It would be of value to eventually develop a national genetic register system for familial cancers which could be used in conjunction with the directory of genetic units. Through ascertainment of individuals at high familial risk for developing cancer, we would achieve a new dimension for recognition of individuals at high risk for cancer of specific anatomic organs. Thus family physicians would be armored with one extra tool for their cancer control program. A genetic register system (RAPID) is being developed at the present time by Emery and associates[21] in Edinburgh, Scotland. This is a computerized register system which is referred to by the acronym RAPID (Register for Ascertainment and Prevention of Inherited Disease). The system involves ascertainment of individuals from a high risk population determined by individuals who are at risk for having a child with a serious genetic disorder. Elaborate systems for contacting and following up individuals have been established and computer methods for recording, storage and retrieval of individuals' medical, genetic history, and other pertinent family data have been developed.

Summary

The World Health Organization Expert Committee has recommended increased training of medical personnel in medical genetics with a particular emphasis on genetic counseling. Increased patient awareness of the importance of genetics in many medical problems including cancer has served to increase the demand for genetic counseling services. We believe that genetic counseling is best handled by the physician and indeed the surgeon will find many genetic counseling implications in the management of his cancer patients. A review of the subject documents a wide variety of cancer problems which have genetic counseling implications and which could assuage the patients well being and in certain circumstances could aid in cancer control.

REFERENCES

1. Lynch, H.T.: *Dynamic Genetic Counseling for Clinicians*, Springfield, Thomas, 1969.
2. Tokuhata, G.K., and Lilienfeld, A.M.: Familial aggregation of lung cancer in humans. *J Natl Cancer Inst, 30:*289–312, 1963.
3. Lynch, H.T., and Krush, A.J.: Genetic predictability in breast cancer risk. *Arch Surg, 103:*84–88, 1971.
4. Morris, J.M., and Mahesh, V.B.: Further observations on the syndrome, "testicular feminization." *Am J Obstet Gynecol, 87:*731–748, 1963.
5. Stenchever, M.A., Ng, A.B.P., Jones, G.K., and Jarvis, J.A.: Testicular feminization syndrome: chromosomal, histologic, and genetic studies in a large kindred. *Obstet Gynecol, 33:*649–657, 1969.
6. Vaidya, P.R., and Purandare, B.N.: Testicular feminization syndrome. *J Postgrad Med, 16:*197–204, 1970.
7. Weisberg, M.D., Malkasian, G.D., Jr., and Pratt, J.H.: Testicular feminization syndrome: a review and report of 6 cases. *Am J Obstet Gynecol, 107:*1181–1187, 1970.
8. O'Connell, M.J., Ramsey, H.E., Whang-Peng, J., and Wiernik, P.H.: Testicular feminization syndrome in three sibs: emphasis on gonadal neoplasia. *Am J Med Sci, 265:*321–333, 1973.
9. Stewart, J.S.S.: Testicular feminization and color-blindness. *Lancet, 2:*592–594, 1959.
10. Jones, H.W., Jr., and Scott, W.N., (Eds.): *Hermaphroditism, Genetical Anomalies and Related Endocrine Disorders.* Baltimore, Williams and Wilkins, 1958, p. 172.
11. Hauser, G.A.: Testicular Feminization. In Overzier, K., (Ed.): *Intersexuality.* London, London Academic Press, 1963, pp. 255–276.
12. Cornet, L., Loubiere, R., and Serres, J.J., *et al.:* Gonophoric male pseudohermaphroditism with abdominal cryptorchidism and cancer of the testis: a case of seminoma associated with a testicular feminization syndrome. *Chirurgie, 97:*64–73, 1971.
13. Scully, R.E.: Gonadoblastoma: a review of 74 cases. *Cancer, 25:*1340–1356, 1970.
14. Morris, J.M.: The syndrome of testicular

feminization in male pseudohermaphrodites. *Am J Obstet Gynecol, 65:*1192–1211, 1953.

15. Gans, S.L., and Rubin, C.L.: Apparent female infants with hernias and testes. *Am J Dis Child, 104:*114–118, 1962.

16. Lynch, H.T., and Krush, A.J.: The cancer family syndrome and cancer control. *Surg Gynecol Obstet, 132:*247–250, 1971.

17. Lynch, H.T., and Krush, A.J.: Delay: a deterrent to cancer detection. *Arch Environ Health, 17:*204–209, 1968.

18. Richards, R.D., Mebust, W.K., and Schimke, R.N.: A prospective study on von Hippel-Lindau disease. *J Urol, 110:*27–30, 1973.

18a. Sipple, J.H.: The association of pheochromocytoma with carcinoma of the thyroid gland. *Am J Med, 31:*163–166, 1961.

18b. Keiser, H.R., Beaven, M.A., Doppman, J., Wells, S., Jr., and Buja, L.M.: Sipple's Syndrome: Medullary thyroid carcinoma, pheochromocytoma, and parathyroid disease: Studies in a large family. *Ann Int Med, 78:*561–579, 1973.

18c. Williams, E.D.: A review of 17 cases of carcinoma of the thyroid and phaeochromocytoma. *J Clin Pathol, 18:*288–292, 1965.

18d. Manning, P.C. Jr., Molmar, G.D., Black, B.M., *et al.*: Pheochromocytoma, hyperparathyroidism and thyroid carcinoma occurring coincidentally. *N Engl J Med, 268:*68–72, 1963.

18e. Melvin, K.E.W., Tashjian, A.H., Jr., and Miller, H.H.: Studies in familial (medullary) thyroid carcinoma, in *Recent Progress in Hormone Research,* vol. 28, Proceedings of the 1971 Laurentian Hormone Conference, edited by Astwood, E.B. New York, Academic Press, Inc., Publishers, 1972, pp. 399–470.

19. Genetic counseling: third report of the WHO expert committee on human genetics. *WHO Techn Rep Ser, 416:*5–23, 1969.

20. Lynch, H.T., Mulcahy, G.M., and Krush, A.J.: Genetic counseling and the physician. *JAMA, 211:*647–751, 1970.

21. Emery, A.E.H., Elliott, D., Moores, M., Smith, Charles: A genetic register system (RAPID). *J Med Gen, 11:*145–151, 1974.

EPILOGUE

THE EPILOGUE REPRESENTS the editor's attempt to contribute to the continuity in the stream of thought presented in the book.

Cancer genetics is an exceedingly complex and controversial subject which harbors far reaching implications for carcinogenesis. The expertise of many authorities is required for its elucidation. That fact compelled the editor to seek the assistance of colleagues in the preparation of this book, in order to probe more facets of this difficult problem. However, in any multiple author endeavor, it becomes virutally impossible for an editor to completely exclude duplication of material and to arrange for a style that is uniform throughout the text. This book is no exception and, in spite of efforts to eliminate duplication, occasional duplications have undoubtedly occurred. Some contributors with primary interests in overlapping areas have necessarily reflected them in their manuscripts. It would have been unfair and, indeed, unwise to entirely delete such specific areas of overlap, because doing so would have left gaps in the respective authors' presentations. Thus, in these situations, the editor limited discussion in order to avoid tedious duplication but nevertheless retained salient features so that the reader could profit from the full scope and breadth of the particular authors' contributions.

We should begin by acknowledging the fact that while knowledge of cancer genetic mechanisms in humans is limited to a relatively small fraction of malignant neoplasms, evidence at the infra-human level has shown clearly that genetic factors play a major role in the incidence of many cancers of specific anatomic sites. Genetic influence is often crucial regardless of whether one is concerned with spontaneously occurring cancers or whether it involves their occurrence following the administration of certain carcinogens. In humans the evidence is less clearcut for spontaneously occurring malignant neoplasms and the role of environmental factors is particularly difficult to evaluate in context with the relative importance of genetic or host factors.

Dr. Kaplan has provided a chapter on basic fundamentals in genetics. It will be well for those who have had limited recent experience with genetics to read this chapter before delving into other subject matter in this book. The reader may also find the glossary of genetic terms to be helpful.

When the full complement of cancer is considered in humans, one finds that only a relatively small proportion of tumors are transmitted in accordance with classical Mendelian inheritance patterns, i.e. familial polyposis coli, Gardner's syndrome, hereditary exostosis. On the other hand, certain cancers and precancerous disorders have been identified wherein genetic factors may be implicated, but their significance remains unclear or are in dispute. An example of this type of problem is found in systemic lupus erythematosis, although the issue of genetic and cancer association in this disease has become more clear during the past five years. In still other circumstances, differing varieties of cancer may pose an increased risk to first degree relatives of cancer probands in what is referred to as empirical risks; however, classical Mendelian inheritance patterns have not been identified for the majority of these lesions. This includes such commonly occurring malignant neoplasms as cancer of the breast, lung, stomach, colon, endometrium, prostate, and others. In many of these malignancies, environmental factors may be important. Thus, certain carcinogens may show carcinogenicity when associated with certain cancer prone genotypes. For example, recent evidence by Kellermann and Shaw have shown the importance of aryl hydrocarbon hydroxylase (AHH) in conjunction with cigarette smoking in bronchogenic carcinoma. Specifically, cigarette smokers who manifested the intermediate and high inducer phenotypes for AHH showed significant excess occurrence of bronchogenic carcinoma. These results support familial risk concepts in lung cancer espoused by Tokuhata (see Chapter 13). Specifically, Dr. Tokuhata has identified the importance of genetic factors in combination with cigarette smoking and other environmental factors in the etiology of bronchogenic carcinoma.

Tables 1-I to 1-V in the Introduction provide an overview of the several categories of hereditary and familial predisposition to cancer which are discussed throughout this book.

Many theories of carcinogenesis involve a variety of disciplines which invoke genetic influence in their etiology. Immunology is high on the list. Thus, we have incorporated viewpoints from basic (Chapter 3) and clinical immunology (Chapter 4), as well as from problems in specific histocompatibility antigens, particularly HL-A (Chapters 5 and 6). Review of this material will show immediately the complexities involved when considering genetic factors in context with the host's mode of response to a variety of environ-

mental stimuli based upon his inherent immunologic capacity.

Investigations at the biomolecular level in xeroderma pigmentosum, with particular reference to the observation that skin fibroblasts *in vitro* fail to repair DNA damage induced by ultraviolet light, is provided by Cleaver in Chapter 8. This rather complex system has implications for biomolecular repair mechanisms which may also have implications for malignant transformation of cells in other clinical disorders.

The discipline of cytogenetics has assumed a major role in the study of human malignancies, as a result, in part, of clear associations between certain precancerous disorders which have cytogenetic aberrations such as Down's syndrome, Turner's syndrome, Klinefelter's syndrome, and trisomy E and D syndromes, and others. The importance of this issue is presented in two chapters, one which emphasizes intersex problems (Chapter 10), and a second which covers the subject more broadly (Chapter 9).

Voluminous studies of viral carcinogenesis in animals has provided an impetus for human investigations. While a specific cause-effect relationship between viruses and cancer in humans has not been established, a large body of biological and epidemiologic knowledge has suggested that such relationships may in due time be established for certain forms of cancer including Hodgkins disease and Burkitt's lymphoma. It should be realized that just as in laboratory animals, theories of viral carcinogenesis in humans are also consistent with genetic etiologies. Thus, a viral-genetic hypothesis invoking an interaction between primary genetic factors, viruses, as well as other carcinogens are consistent with developing concepts in carcinogenesis. Drs. Dosik and Todaro (Chapter 7) present highlights of their extensive experience in this field with particular attention given to *in vitro* SV-40 viral transformation of skin fibroblasts from selected clinical populations such as Fanconi's anemia, Down's syndrome and others. These studies may in due time shed light on viral etiology in human cancer and may elucidate mechanisms which allow normal cells to undergo malignant transformation.

Migrant groups harbor an important potential for comprehension of cancer epidemiology. Classical are the low rates of carcinoma of the breast in inhabitants of Japan with increasing rates shown for this malignant neoplasm in the descendants of Japanese who reside in Hawaii and the continental United States. On the other hand, exceedingly high rates for gastric cancer have been demonstrated in Japan and in several other areas of the world. Kaposi's sarcoma and hepatomas occur with increased frequency amongst the Bantu of South Africa. The listing of malignant neoplasms showing marked variations in rates in differing racial and ethnic groups throughout the world are legion. Israel has provided a fertile region for the study of various migrant groups. Dr. Modan (Chapter 11) presents data on several ethnic populations residing in Israel in order to show importance for epidemiologic considerations of migrant groups in the study of cancer epidemiology.

Endocrine factors provide a major consideration for several cancers affecting man. In addition, certain Mendelian inherited cancer syndromes have been described wherein endocrinologic features are of paramount concern. Drs. Jackson and Weiss (Chapter 12) present an overview of this entire field. In addition, they emphasize their own contribution to this science stemming from their work on families with autosomal dominantly inherited medullary thyroid carcinoma and pheochromocytoma.

These investigators show the importance of calcitonin assay in cancer detection and hopefully in the control of this disorder which has such a predictable occurrence in certain families.

A series of chapters are devoted to such subjects as leukemia and lymphoma, the Wiskott-Aldrich syndrome, retinoblastoma, colon cancer, breast cancer, the cancer family syndrome, and a variety of syndromes with cutaneous manifestations. One chapter dealing with the occurrence of cancers of the central nervous system with special reference to genetic factors written by Drs. Mulcahy and Harlan (Chapter 17) was designed to serve as the prototype for an in-depth discussion of a particular system with reference to cancer and genetics. The matter has been studied intensively by the authors, who have included compilation of over 600 pertinent literature citations, and their contribution represents the most complete coverage of the subject of which the editor is aware.

A chapter has been devoted to cancer resistance in humans. This subject has received a paucity of attention in the scientific literature, possibly because it has only captured limited interest of scientists, but even more likely because of the myriad difficulties encountered in discerning a subject which at times decries comprehension. For example, with the exception of a few conditions such as diabetes mellitus, and osteogenesis imperfecta, which allegedly afford cancer resistance (but even here there is some controversy), the content of the chapter is speculative and reflects the limitations of available studies on cancer resistance in humans. However, this does not belittle its importance; we may learn much about cancer control as well as carcinogenesis through systematic study of kindreds which show a statistically significant deficit of cancer when age considerations are corrected for; and we should critically evaluate genetic and environmental factors, including major causes of morbidity and mortality in these groups.

A large variety of cancers are discussed in the chapter dealing with miscellaneous problems, cancer and genetics. This chapter was designed with the readers' interest in mind, realizing the need to receive as complete a version of the field as possible. However, while the goal of the book has been to present far reaching coverage of the subject of cancer genetics, it is obvious that explosive developments in this field will cause a book of this type to be incomplete the moment the editor rests his pen and submits it to the publisher.

The chapter on genetic counseling and cancer is deemed important since one of the major concerns of all clinicians pertains to the best way in which he can advise his patients about cancer risk, particularly when they are members of cancer prone families. This difficult subject is broached in context with myriad psychological nuances as well as cancer control implications. The authors undoubtedly permitted their own biases to creep into this presentation. A natural sequel to genetic counseling in cancer problems is found in the material pertaining to genetic counseling and cancer genetic research activities in differing units and centers throughout the world as developed and identified in the appendix. Genetic marker(s) in cancer prone subjects could prove of inestimable value for studies in etiology, carcinogenesis as well as in cancer control. Recently, Rawlings and associates (*Ann. Int. Med. 81*:771, 1974) reported two patients who had cryptogenic liver disease and alpha-1 antitrypsin deficiency of the Z phenotype. At post mortem both of these individuals were found to have hepatocellular carcinoma. These observations suggest an association between the heterozygous Z allele alpha-1 antitrypsin deficiency and this form of cancer.

Other evidence in this book has disclosed an association between heterozygous carriers of the gene for Fanconi's aplastic anemia and increased occurrences of lymphoreticular malignancies. One therefore wonders about heterozygous carriers of genes for other recessive diseases such as xeroderma pigmentosum, Wiskott-Aldrich syndrome and ataxia telangiectasia and their cancer risk. This is an area which should be the subject of future research. Detailed family studies, an issue stressed throughout this book could provide clues to these problems.

Finally, one always searches for generalities which can conveniently be used by basic scientists, clinical investigators, and practicing physicians in any particular subject. Thus, medicine is replete with triads, tetrads, major and minor criteria, and other convenient phrases used to characterize the salient aspects of a variety of medical disorders. It therefore seemed appropriate that the author attempt to develop certain criteria which could be applied to the majority of cancer genetic problems. Briefly, these are as follows:

1. All factors considered, genetic forms of cancer tend to have an earlier age of onset when compared with the usual occurrence of these same histologic varieties of cancer in the general population.

2. Bilaterality is more likely to occur in familial cancers, such as in familial breast, pheochromocystoma, nephroblastomas, acoustic neuromas, chemodectomas, and others.

3. Multiple primary malignancies occur more frequently in familial cancer problems.

4. We remain distressingly ignorant about the biological nature of familial cancer, particularly with respect to natural history and prognosis when compared to so-called sporadically occurring cancers.

APPENDIX 1

GENETIC COUNSELING AND CANCER GENETICS:
A SUMMARY OF SERVICE UNITS

IN PREVIOUS DOCUMENTATION of genetic service units throughout the world (1, 2, and 3) as published by the National Foundation—March of Dimes, there has been a dramatic increase in the total number of service units: 399 in 1968 to 892 in 1974. Of the services listed by these units, the percentage of units offering cancer genetics ("V") has remained at a constant level, but units offering genetic counseling ("J") has declined with the most recent review of units (accurate as of July 1, 1974).

The listing presented below is extracted from the updated data base established for the Fourth Edition of the International Directory of Genetic Services (4), edited by Drs. Lynch, Bergsma, and Thomas. Those units offering either J or V or both J and V were selected. Units listed with an asterisk after unit number did not respond to an updating/verification questionnaire posted September 1, 1973 which was due October 1, 1973. For your convenience, the entire list of services offered by these units are listed as well as the key to the services.

GENETIC SERVICES BY CODE

NAME OF SERVICE RENDERED	GENETIC SERVICE CODE
Behavorial Genetics	A
Biochemical Genetics	B
Birth Defects	C
Clinical Genetics	D
Computer Analysis	E
Cytogenetics	F
Dental Genetics	G
Dermatoglyphics	H
Electron Microscopy	I
Genetic Counseling	J
Hematology and Blood Groups	K
Immunogenetics	L
Molecular Genetics	M
Pharmacogenetics	N
Physical Anthropology	O
Population Genetics	P
Twin Studies	Q
Virology	R

MISCELLANEOUS SERVICES

Linkage Studies	S
Psychiatric Genetics	T
Radiation Genetics	U
Cancer Genetics	V
Social Service	W
Public Health	X
Amniocentesis	Y
No Service Specified	Z

A SUMMARY OF SERVICE UNITS

ARGENTINA

1.00   ACDFHJNPQTY
BLEIWEISS, HERMAN
GENETICA MEDICA
LAPRIDA 1204
BUENOS AIRES, ARGENTINA
  PHONE 85-4024

2.00   A-DFHKN-QS-Y
BRAGE, DIEGO
NEUROLOGY CLINIC
UNIVERSITY OF BUENOS AIRES
CARLOS PELLEGRINI 1336
BUENOS AIRES, ARGENTINA
  PHONE 41-4575

5.00   DJPTW
ORTIZ DE ZARATE, JULIO C.
DIVISION OF NEUROLOGY
FACULDADE DE MEDICINIA DEL SALVADOR
BALCACE 900 SAN MARTIN
BUENOS AIRES, ARGENTINA
  PHONE 755-2681

6.00   B-DFHJQX
PENCHASZADEH, VICTOR B.
SECCION DE GENETICA MEDICA,
  DEPARTAMENTO DE MEDICINA
HOSPITAL MUNICIPAL DE NINOS
GALLO 1330
BUENOS AIRES, ARGENTINA

7.00   DFJM
BIANCHI, NESTOR O.
DEPARTMENT OF CYTOGENETICS
COMISION DE INVESTIGACION DE LA
  PROVINCIA DE BUENOS AIRES
LA PLATA, ARGENTINA

9.00   DFHJ
ROUBICEK, MARTIN
DEPARTAMENTO DE GENETICA NESTITUTO
  DE BEOLOGIA
UNIVERSIDAD PROVINCIAL DE MAR DEL
  PLATA
ITUZAINGO 3520
MAR DEL PLATA B.A., ARGENTINA

AUSTRALIA

10.00   AHJLOQS
BENNETT, J.H.
DEPARTMENT OF GENETICS
UNIVERSITY OF ADELAIDE
ADELAIDE, AUSTRALIA
50001

12.00   DPV
DAVIS, NEVILLE
QUEENSLAND MELANOMA PROJECT
PRINCESS ALEXANDRA HOSPITAL
IPSWICH ROAD, WOOLLOONGABBA, S.2.
BRISBANE, QUEENSLAND, AUSTRALIA
  PHONE 91-0111 EXT. 474

13.00   B-DFHJ-LNPQSW-Y
KEARNEY, B.
DEPARTMENT OF PREVENTIVE SOCIAL
  MEDICINE
UNIVERSITY OF SYDNEY ROYAL
  ALEXANDRA HOSPITAL FOR CHILDREN
CAMPERDOWN, AUSTRALIA
2006   PHONE 51-0466

14.00   B-DFHJ-LNPQSW-Y
KERR, C.B.
DEPARTMENT OF PREVENTIVE SOCIAL
  MEDICINE
UNIVERSITY OF SYDNEY ROYAL
  ALEXANDRA HOSPITAL FOR CHILDREN
CAMPERDOWN, AUSTRALIA
2006   PHONE 51-0466

15.00   B-DFJ
TURNER, BRIAN
CHILDREN¤S MEDICAL RESEARCH
  FOUNDATION
ROYAL ALEXANDRA HOSPITAL FOR
  CHILDREN
CAMPERDOWN, N.S.W., AUSTRALIA
2050

16.00   B-DFHJ-LNPQSW-Y
TURNER, G.M.
DEPARTMENT OF PREVENTIVE SOCIAL
  MEDICINE
UNIVERSITY OF SYDNEY ROYAL
  ALEXANDRA HOSPITAL FOR CHILDREN
CAMPERDOWN, AUSTRALIA
2006   PHONE 51-0466

17.00   BEJKOP
KIRK, R.L.
DEPARTMENT OF HUMAN BIOLOGY
JOHN CURTIN SCHOOL OF MEDICAL
  RESEARCH
BOX 334, GPO
CANBERRA, AUSTRALIA
  PHONE 49-3086

18.00   BEFHJKOP
WALSH, R.J.
SCHOOL OF HUMAN GENETICS
UNIVERSITY OF NEW SOUTH WALES
P.O. BOX 1
KENSINGTON, N.S.W., AUSTRALIA
2033

19.00   B-DFJRY
DANKS, DAVID M.
ROYAL CHILDREN¤S HOSPITAL RESEARCH
  FOUNDATION
UNIVERSITY OF MELBOURNE
MELBOURNE, AUSTRALIA
  PHONE 357-5522

20.00   CFJY
FORTUNE, DENYS W.
DEPARTMENT OF PATHOLOGY
ROYAL WOMEN¤S HOSPITAL
MELBOURNE, AUSTRALIA

21.00   CDFHJWY
LAURIE, WILLIAM
DEPARTMENT OF PUBLIC HEALTH,
  CYTOGENETIC UNIT
STATE HEALTH LABORATORY SERVICE
BOX F 312, G.P.O.
PERTH, AUSTRALIA
6001   PHONE 86 2469 OR 86 5511

23.00   CDFJKUV
BAIKIE, A.G.
DEPARTMENT OF MEDICINE
UNIVERSITY OF TASMANIA
ROYAL HOBART HOSPITAL
TASMANIA, AUSTRALIA
  PHONE 34-2866

27.00*   CDFHJW
HAMILTON, G.J.L.
DEPARTMENT OF MENTAL HEALTH SERVICE
  OF WESTERN AUSTRALIA
IRRABEENA DIAGNOSTIC CENTER
84 THOMAS STREET
WEST PERTH, AUSTRALIA
6050   PHONE 21-9121   PERTH W.A.

28.00   C-FHVW
KIRKLAND, J.A.
DEPARTMENT OF OBSTETRICS AND
  GYNECOLOGY
QUEEN ELIZABETH HOSPITAL
WOODVILLE, AUSTRALIA
5011   PHONE 45-0222 EXT. 605

AUSTRIA

29.00   CDFJPS
ROSENKRANZ, WALTER
INSTITUTE OF MEDIZINISCHE BIOLOGIE
  UND HUMANGENETIC
UNIVERSITY GRAZ
HANS SACHS GASSE 3
GRAZ, AUSTRIA
AB010

BELGIUM

33.00   B-DFJY
LEROY, J.G.
DEPARTMENT OF GENETICS
MEDICAL GENETIC UNIT
ANTWERP STATE UNIVERSITY
ANTWERP, BELGIUM
  PHONE 03-392125 EXT. 125

34.00   B-DFHJQY
VAN BOGAERT, LUDO
DEPARTMENT OF NEUROGENETICS
FOUNDATION BORN-BUNGE
ANTWERP, BELGIUM
  PHONE 03-392125 EXT. 125

35.00   CDFHJ
DESTINE, MARIE L.
RUE ANTOINE GAUTIER, 65
BRUSSELS, BELGIUM
1040   PHONE 02-339702 EXT. 007

36.00   C-FJ-L
GOVAERTS, A.
DEPARTMENT OF IMMUNOLOGY
HOSPITAL ST. PIERRE
322 RUE HAUTE
BRUXELLES, BELGIUM
1000   PHONE 02-380000 EXT. 2580

37.00   CDFHJO-QUV
TWIESSELMANN, F.
GENETIQUE MEDICALE, FACULTE DE
  MEDECINE
UNIVERSITE LIBRE DE BRUXELLES
RUE AUX LAINES, 97
BRUXELLES, BELGIUM
1000

38.00   CFIV
VERHEST, ALAIN
DEPARTMENT OF CYTOGENETICS
INSTITUT JULES BORDET
CENTRE DES TUMEURS DE L¤UNIVERSITE
  LIBRE DE BRUXELLES
BRUXELLES, BELGIUM
1000

568

39.00   DFHJOQY
FRANCOIS, J.
DEPARTMENT OF OPHTHALMOLOGY
135 DE PINTELAAN
GENT, BELGIUM
9000   PHONE 09-226941

40.00   C-FH-JSTV-Y
VAN DEN BERGHE, HERMAN
DEPARTMENT OF HUMAN GENETICS
UNIVERSITY OF LEUVEN
MINDERBROEDERSTRAAT
LEUVEN, BELGIUM

41.00   DHJKP
DODINVAL, P.
DEPARTMENT OF HUMAN GENETICS
UNIVERSITY OF LIEGE
40 QUAI G. KURTH
LIEGE, BELGIUM
4000   PHONE 041 431905

42.00*   CFJQUY
FREDERIC, JACQUES
LABORATORY OF CYTOGENETICS
UNIVERSITY OF LIEGE
LIEGE, BELGIUM
   PHONE 32-04-420226

44.00   CFJY
KOULISCHER, LUCIEN
DEPARTEMENT DE GENETIQUE
INSTITUT DE MORPHOLOGIE
PATHOLOGIQUE
29 ALLEE DES TEMPLIERS
LOVERVAL, BELGIUM
6270   PHONE 07-364948

BRAZIL

46.00   CFJ-LPQ
AYRES, M.
LABORATORIO DE GENETICA, FALCUDADE
   DE FILOSOFIA
GENERALISSIMO DEODORO 413
CIENCIAS E LETRAS
BELEM, PARA, BRAZIL

47.00   C-FJKPQ
FREIRE-MAIA, ADEMAR
DEPARTAMENTO DE GENETICA
FACULDADE CIENCIAS MEDICAS E
   BIOLOGICAS
BOTUCATU, SAO PAULO, BRAZIL

49.00   CDFHJKOQ
BEIGUELMAN, BERNARDO
DEPARTMENT OF MEDICAL GENETICS
UNIVERSITY OF CAMPINAS
CAMPINAS, SAO PAULO, BRAZIL
   PHONE 2-5831

50.00   C-HJN-PS-V
FREIRE-MAIA, NEWTON
DEPARTAMENTE DE GENETICS
FEDERAL UNIVERSITY OF PARANA
CURITIBA, PARANA, BRAZIL

53.00   CFJ
CENTENO, JUDITH VIEGAS
LABORATORY DE GENETICA HUMANA
FACULDADE DE MEDICINA DE PELOTAS
IPESSE C.P. NO. 464
PELOTAS, RS, BRAZIL
   PHONE 2-72-28

54.00   ACDF-HJKMO-Q
SALZANO, FRANCISCO M.
DEPARTAMENTE DE GENETICS
UNIVERSIDADE FEDERAL DO RIO GRANDE
   DO SUL
CAIXA POSTAL 1953
PORTO ALEGRE, RS, BRAZIL
   PHONE 240794

55.00   CDFHJQ
LEAO, JOSE CARNEIRO
INSTITUT DE MEDICINA INFANTIL
RECIFE, BRAZIL

57.00   CDFJKV
BOTTURA, CASSIO
DEPARTMENT OF HEMATOLOGY AND

CYTOLOGY
MEDICAL SCHOOL OF RIBEIRAO PRETO
RIBEIRAO PRETO, SP, BRAZIL

58.00   CDFJ
FERRARI, IRIS
MEDICAL GENETICS II
FACULDADE MEDICINA-RIBEIRAO PRETO
CX. 301
RIBEIRAO PRETO, SP, BRAZIL

59.00   DFHJ
CABRAL DE ALMEIDA, J.C.
LABORATORY RADIOBIOLOGIA CELULAR
INSTITUTO BIOFISICA
AV. PASTEUR 458
RIO DE JANEIRO, GB, BRAZIL

60.00   B-DFHJ
CARAKUSHANSKY, GERSON
LABORATORIO GENETICA
INSTITUTO DE PUERICULTURA U.F.R.J.
AV. BRIGADEIRO TROMPOWSKY, ILHA DO
   FUNDAO
RIO DE JANEIRO, GB, BRAZIL
   PHONE 230-6355

61.00   B-DHJKO
AZEVEDO, ELIANE S.
DEPARTMENT OF PREVENTIVE MEDICINE
HOSPITAL PROF. EDGARD SANTOS
SALVADOR, BAHIA, BRAZIL
   PHONE 5-2497

62.00   B-DFJ-LPQU
PEDREIRA, CORA DE MOURA
LABORATORIO DE GENETICA HUMANA
HOSPITAL PROF. EDGARD SANTOS
60 ANDAR
SALVADOR, BAHIA, BRAZIL

63.00   CDFHJTV
PAULETE, JORGE
FACULDADE REGIONAL DE MEDICINA
CAIXA POSTAL 659
SAO JOSE DO RIO PRETO, SP, BRAZIL
15100

65.00   BFIJM
BECAK, WILLY
DEPARTMENT OF GENETICS
INSTITUTO BUTANTAN
SAO PAULO, BRAZIL
   PHONE 286-8211 R-14

66.00   CDFHJPS
FROTA-PESSOA, O.
DEPARTAMENTE BIOLOGIA, LABORATORIO
   DE GENETICA HUMANA
UNIVERSIDAD SAO PAULO
C.P. 8105
SAO PAULO, BRAZIL
   PHONE 286-0011 RAMAL 36

67.00   BDFHJT
KRYNSKI, STANISLAU
CENTRO DE HABILITACAO DA APAE DE
   SAO PAULO
RUA LOEFGREN, 2249 - VILA
   CLEMENTINO
SAO PAULO, BRAZIL
04040

68.00   ACDFHJKNPQT
SALDANHA, P.H.
FACULTY OF MEDICINE
LABORATORY OF MEDICAL GENETICS
P.O. BOX 2921
SAO PAULO, BRAZIL
   PHONE 256-4611 EXT. 70

69.00   BCFHJ
SCHMIDT, BENJAMIN J.
LABORATORIO LAVOISIER DE ANALISES
   CLINICAS
AV. ANGELICA, 2.071
SAO PAULO, BRAZIL
01227   PHONE 256-1111 OR 256-5555

BULGARIA

70.00   FV
STOYTCHKOV, JORDAN

INSTITUTE OF HAEMATOLOGY AND BLOOD
   TRANSFUSION
SOFIA 56, BULGARIA
   PHONE 72-05-55 EXT. 362

CANADA

71.00   B-DFJPSY
BOWEN, PETER
DEPARTMENT OF PEDIATRICS
4-120 CLINICAL SCIENCES BUILDING
EDMONTON 7, ALBERTA, CANADA

72.00   A-DFHJKPTY
WELCH, J. PHILIP
DEPARTMENT OF PEDIATRICS
DALHOUSIE UNIVERSITY
HALIFAX, NOVA SCOTIA, CANADA

73.00   BDJ
WHELAN, DONALD T.
MCMASTER UNIVERSITY MEDICAL CENTRE
1200 MAIN STREET WEST
HAMILTON 16, ONTARIO, CANADA
   PHONE 416 525-9140

74.00   CDFHJQUY
UCHIDA, I.A.
DEPARTMENT OF PEDIATRICS
MCMASTER UNIVERSITY
HAMILTON, ONTARIO, CANADA

75.00   BD-FHJNPQSY
SIMPSON, NANCY E.
DEPARTMENT OF PEDIATRICS
QUEENS UNIVERSITY
KINGSTON, ONTARIO, CANADA
   PHONE 613 547-6242

76.00   B-DGHJSTV-Y
SERGOVICH, F.R.
DEPARTMENT OF CYTOGENETICS
CHILDRENS PSYCHIATRIC RESEARCH
   INSTITUTE
LONDON, ONTARIO, CANADA
   PHONE 471-2540

77.00*   B-DHJNPQTX
SOLTAN, H.C.
DEPARTMENT OF PAEDIATRICS
GENETIC COUNSELING CLINIC
UNIVERSITY HOSPITAL
LONDON, ONTARIO, CANADA
N6G 2K3   PHONE 519 673-3875

78.00   CDJ
WALKER, FRANK A.
CRIPPLED CHILDRENS TREATMENT
   CENTRE
816 HEADLEY DRIVE
LONDON, ONTARIO, CANADA
   PHONE 519 471-2404

80.00   B-DFHJKY
DALLAIRE, LOUIS
MEDICAL GENETICS SECTION
SAINTE JUSTINE HOSPITAL
3175 CHEMIN ST. CATHERINE
MONTREAL 250, QUEBEC, CANADA
H3T 1C5

81.00   BDHJNP
BARBEAU, ANDRE
DEPARTMENT OF NEURO-BIOLOGY
CLINICAL RESEARCH INSTITUTE OF
   MONTREAL
110 WEST PINE AVENUE
MONTREAL, QUEBEC, CANADA
   PHONE 514 842-1481

82.00   B-FHJKPQTY
FRASER, F. CLARKE
DEPARTMENT OF MEDICAL GENETICS
MONTREAL CHILDRENS HOSPITAL
MONTREAL, QUEBEC, CANADA
   PHONE 514 937-8511 EXT. 320

83.00   B-FHJKPQT
METRAKOS, D. JULIUS
DEPARTMENT OF MEDICAL GENETICS
MONTREAL CHILDRENS HOSPITAL
MONTREAL, QUEBEC, CANADA
   PHONE 514 937-8511

84.00   B-DJ
PINSKY, LEONARD
DIVISION OF MEDICAL GENETICS
JEWISH GENERAL HOSPITAL
MONTREAL, QUEBEC, CANADA

85.00   BDJMWY
SCRIVER, C.R.
DEPARTMENT OF BIOCHEMICAL GENETICS
MONTREAL CHILDRENS HOSPITAL
MONTREAL, QUEBEC, CANADA
  PHONE 514 937-8511 EXT. 508

88.00   CDFHJWY
ROBERTS, MAUREEN H.
DEPARTMENT OF PAEDIATRICS
UNIVERSITY OF OTTAWA
OTTAWA, ONTARIO, CANADA
  PHONE 613 231-2985

90.00   BD-FHJMPX
LABERGE, CLAUDE
HUMAN GENETICS RESEARCH CENTRE
LAVAL UNIVERSITY MEDICAL CENTRE
2705 LAURIER BOULEVARD
QUEBEC 10, QUEBEC, CANADA
  PHONE 418 656-8256

91.00   B-DFHJLQW-Y
IVES, ELIZABETH J.
DEPARTMENT OF PEDIATRICS
UNIVERSITY HOSPITAL
SASKATOON, SASKATCHEWAN, CANADA
  PHONE 306 343-5940

93.00   LRV
AXELRAD, A.
DEPARTMENT OF ANATOMY
UNIVERSITY OF TORONTO, DIVISION OF
 HISTOLOGY
TORONTO, ONTARIO, CANADA
  PHONE 928-2714

94.00   CDFHJTW
BERG, J.M.
RESEARCH DEPARTMENT
MENTAL RETARDATION CENTER
TORONTO, ONTARIO, CANADA
  PHONE 416 925-5141

95.00   DFJY
GARDNER, H. ALLEN
DEPARTMENT OF PATHOLOGY
TORONTO GENERAL HOSPITAL
101 COLLEGE STREET
TORONTO, ONTARIO, CANADA

97.00   A-DF-HJQY
SIMINOVITCH, L.
DEPARTMENT OF GENETICS
HOSPITAL FOR SICK CHILDREN
TORONTO, ONTARIO, CANADA
  PHONE 416 366-7242

98.00   B-DFHJPQSXY
MILLER, JAMES R.
DEPARTMENT OF MEDICAL GENETICS,
 DEPARTMENT OF PEDIATRICS
UNIVERSITY OF BRITISH COLUMBIA
VANCOUVER, BRITISH COLUMBIA, CANADA
  PHONE 604 228-5483

99.00   CDFHJY
STYLES, SALMA
DEPARTMENTS OF MEDICAL GENETICS AND
 PATHOLOGY
ROYAL JUBILEE HOSPITAL
VICTORIA, BRITISH COLUMBIA, CANADA
  PHONE 604 386-3131

100.00*   B-DFGJL-NUV
HRUSHOVETZ, S.B.
WESTERN CYTOGENETIC LABORATORY
P.O. BOX 3687
WINNIPEG 4, MANITOBA, CANADA
  PHONE 204 589-4897

101.00   B-DFHJSY
HAMERTON, JOHN
DEPARTMENT OF MEDICAL GENETICS
HEALTH SCIENCES CHILDRENS CENTRE
WINNIPEG, MANITOBA, CANADA
R3E 0WI   PHONE 204 775-8311

CEYLON

102.00   CDFJK
WIKRAMANAYAKE, EUGENE
DEPARTMENT OF ANATOMY
FACULTY OF MEDICINE
PERADENIYA, CEYLON

CHILE

104.00   BDFHJP
ASPILLAGA, MANUEL J.
DEPARTMENT OF PEDIATRICS
HOSPITAL LUIS CALVO MACKENNA
SANTIAGO, CHILE

105.00   FHJLOP
COVARRUBIAS, EDMUNDO
DEPARTMENT OF HUMAN GENETICS
UNIVERSITY OF CHILE
SANTIAGO, CHILE

106.00   DEJOP
CRUZ-COKE, R.
DEPARTMENT OF MEDICAL GENETICS
HOSPITAL J.J. AGUIRRE
SANTIAGO, CHILE
  PHONE 373031 EXT. 11

COLOMBIA

109.00   FIRUV
OTERO-RUIZ, EFRAIM
DEPARTMENT OF RESEARCH
INSTITUTE NACIONAL DE CANCEROLOGIA
BOGOTA, COLOMBIA
  PHONE 481711

110.00   B-FH-JV
ELEJALDE, B. RAFAEL
DEPARTMENT OF PATHOLOGY
UNIVERSIDAD DE ANTIOQUIA
APARTADO AEREO 1226
MEDELLIN, COLOMBIA
  PHONE 421000

COLUMBIA

111.00   CDFHJ
AURORA, VALENCIA C.
DEPARTMENT OF PATHOLOGY
HOSPITAL UNIVERSITARIO DE CALDAS
MANIZALES, COLUMBIA
  PHONE 51400

CZECHOSLOVAKIA

113.00   CDFHJK
GETLIK, ANDREJ
PEDIATRIC CLINIC
POSTGRADUATE MEDICAL INSTITUTE
KRAMARE
BRATISLAVA, CZECHOSLOVAKIA

117.00   A-DF-HJ-LPQSXY
BRUNECKY, ZDENEK
INSTITUTE OF PEDIATRIC RESEARCH
CERNOPOLNI 9
BRNO, CZECHOSLOVAKIA
  PHONE BRNO 67-87-83

118.00   DJ
KRAJCA, KAREL
DEPARTMENT OF NEUROLOGY
DUBNICA NAD VAHOM, CZECHOSLOVAKIA

122.00   B-DF-HJLOPRVY
HOUSTEK, JOSEF
INSTITUTE OF CHILD DEVELOPMENT
 RESEARCH, FACULTY OF PEDIATRICS
CHARLES UNIVERSITY
PRAGUE 5, V UVALU 84,
 CZECHOSLOVAKIA
  PHONE 525553 OR 525558

123.00   B-DFVY
MACEK, MILAN
GENETIC DEPARTMENT
INSTITUTE OF CHILD DEVELOPMENT
 RESEARCH, FACULTY OF PEDIATRICS
CHARLES UNIVERSITY

PRAGUE 5, V UVALU 84,
 CZECHOSLOVAKIA
  PHONE 525553 OR 525558

125.00   DHJX
SALICHOVA, JOSEFINA
GENETIC DEPARTMENT
INSTITUTE OF CHILD DEVELOPMENT
 RESEARCH, FACULTY OF PEDIATRICS
CHARLES UNIVERSITY
PRAGUE 5, V UVALU 84,
 CZECHOSLOVAKIA
  PHONE 525553 OR 525558

126.00   B-DHJKPWY
SEEMANOVA, EVA
GENETIC DEPARTMENT
INSTITUTE OF CHILD DEVELOPMENT
 RESEARCH, FACULTY OF PEDIATRICS
CHARLES UNIVERSITY
PRAGUE 5, V UVALU 84,
 CZECHOSLOVAKIA
  PHONE 525553 OR 525558

DENMARK

127.00   B-DFJSY
THERKELSEN, A.J.
DEPARTMENT OF HUMAN GENETICS
UNIVERSITY OF AARHUS, INSTITUTE OF
 MEDICAL MICROBIOLOGY
AARHUS C, DENMARK
8000

128.00   DFJ
JACOBSEN, PETREA
BREJNING INSTITUTE FOR RESEARCH IN
 MENTAL RETARDATION
BREJNING, DENMARK
DK7080

131.00   BD-GJKSY
MOHR, JAN F.
INSTITUTE OF MEDICAL GENETICS
TAGENSVEJ 14
COPENHAGEN, DENMARK
2200

132.00   FJ
PHILIP, JOHN
LABORATORY OF CYTOGENETICS
UNIVERSITY OF COPENHAGEN, RIGS
 HOSPITALET
COPENHAGEN, DENMARK
  PHONE 01-393633 EXT. 4502

133.00   DGJNQ
FROLAND, ANDERS
COUNTY HOSPITAL OF COPENHAGEN
GLOSTRUP, DENMARK
  PHONE 01 964333

134.00   B-DFJSY
MIKKELSEN, MARGARETA
JOHN F. KENNEDY INSTITUTE
GI. LANDEVEJ 7-5
GOLSTRUP, DENMARK
  PHONE 01-451228 OR 452228

135.00   DGJ-LPQSTV
HAUGE, MOGENS
INSTITUTE OF CLINICAL GENETICS
UNIVERSITY OF ODENSE
SYGEHUSET
ODENSE, DENMARK
DK-5000

136.00   ACDFHJPQST
NIELSEN, JOHANNES
THE CYTOGENETIC LABORATORY
ARHUS STATE HOSPITAL
RISSKOV, DENMARK
DK-8240   PHONE 06-177777

ENGLAND

138.00   FLRV
HARNDEN, D.G.
DEPARTMENT OF CANCER STUDIES
UNIVERSITY OF BIRMINGHAM
BIRMINGHAM 15, ENGLAND
  PHONE 021-472-1301 EXT. 3342

139.00   CDFJ-LY
INSLEY, J.
INFANT DEVELOPMENT UNIT
MATERNITY HOSPITAL
BIRMINGHAM, ENGLAND
B15 2TG   PHONE 021-472-1377

140.00   BDJKM-O
LEHMANN, HERMAN
DEPARTMENT OF BIOCHEMISTRY
MEDICAL RESEARCH COUNCIL
40 UNIVERSITY
CAMBRIDGE CAMBS, ENGLAND

142.00   CFH-J
PENROSE, L.S.
KENNEDY-GALTON CENTER
HARPERBURY HOSPITAL
HARPER LANE, SHENLEY, RADLEH, HERTS
HERTFORDSHIRE, ENGLAND
WD7 9HQ

143.00   B-DFHJ-Y
CRAWFURD, M.D.A.
DEPARTMENT OF GENETICS
THE UNIVERSITY OF LEEDS
LEEDS 2, ENGLAND
  PHONE 31751 EXT. 596

144.00   BDFGJ-LNPTV
CLARKE, C.A.
DEPARTMENT OF MEDICINE
UNIVERSITY OF LIVERPOOL
LIVERPOOL, ENGLAND

145.00   FJY
WALKER, S.
NUFFIELD WING SCHOOL OF MEDICINE
P.O. BOX 147
LIVERPOOL, ENGLAND
L69 38X   PHONE 051 709-8891

146.00   DJ
JAY, BARRIE
GENETIC CLINIC
MOORFIELDS EYE HOSPITAL
CITY ROAD
LONDON E.C.1., ENGLAND
  PHONE 01-253 3411

149.00*   B-DFJQSY
HARRIS, HARRY
THE GALTON LABORATORY
UNIVERSITY COLLEGE LONDON
WOLFSON HOUSE, 4 STEPHENSON WAY
LONDON N.W.1., ENGLAND
  PHONE 01-387 7050

150.00   A-DFHJLMSY
POLANI, P.E.
PAEDIATRIC RESEARCH UNIT
GUY◻S HOSPITAL MEDICAL SCHOOL
LONDON S.E.1., ENGLAND
  PHONE LONDON 41-07 7600

153.00*   FLV
KOLLER, P.C.
CHESTER BEATTY RESEARCH INSTITUTE
INSTITUTE OF CANCER RESEARCH
ROYAL CANCER HOSPITAL
LONDON S.W.3., ENGLAND

154.00   FLV
LAWLER, SYLVIA D.
ROYAL MARSDEN HOSPITAL
FULHAM ROAD
LONDON S.W.3., ENGLAND
  PHONE 01-352 8171

155.00   EJ-LPQSVXY
RENWICK, JAMES H.
LONDON SCHOOL OF HYGEINE AND
  TROPICAL MEDICINE
KEPPEL STREET
LONDON W.C.1., ENGLAND
E   7HT   PHONE 01-637 2839

156.00   BFV
PONTECORVO, G.
IMPERIAL CANCER RESEARCH FUND
LINCOLN◻S INN FIELDS
LONDON W.C.2., ENGLAND
  PHONE 01-242 9901

157.00   DJQS
WELLS, R.S.
DEPARTMENT OF GENETICS
ST. JOHN◻S HOSPITAL
LISLE STREET, LEICESTER SQUARE
LONDON W.C.2., ENGLAND
  PHONE 01-437 8383

158.00*   BDFJ-LQR
DAVIDSON, WILLIAM M.
DEPARTMENT OF HAEMATOLOGY
KING◻S COLLEGE HOSPITAL MEDICAL
  SCHOOL
LONDON W.E.5., ENGLAND

159.00   ADFHJQ
DUBOWITZ, V.
DEPARTMENT OF CHILD HEALTH
HAMMERSMITH HOSPITAL
DU CANE ROAD
LONDON W.12, ENGLAND

160.00   A-DFHJPQWY
CLINICAL GENETICS UNIT
INSTITUTE OF CHILD HEALTH
LONDON, ENGLAND
  PHONE 01-242 9789 EXT. 4

162.00   CDFJ-LVY
HARRIS, RODNEY
DEPARTMENT OF MEDICAL GENETICS
ST. MARY◻S HOSPITAL
MANCHESTER O.J.H., ENGLAND
M13   PHONE 061-224 9633

163.00   FV
ATKIN, N.B.
DEPARTMENT OF CANCER RESEARCH
MT. VERNON HOSPITAL
NORTHWOOD
MIDDLESEX, ENGLAND
  PHONE 65-26111

164.00   BDFHJ-LO-QSY
ROBERTS, D.F.
DEPARTMENT OF HUMAN GENETICS
UNIVERSITY OF NEWCASTLE-UPON-TYNE
19 CLAREMONT PLACE
NEWCASTLE-UPON-TYNE, ENGLAND
  PHONE 28511 EXT. 3461

166.00   CHJKOPSX
STEVENSON, A.C.
POPULATION GENETICS RESEARCH UNIT
MEDICAL RESEARCH COUNCIL
OXFORD, ENGLAND
  PHONE OXFORD 62834

168.00   ADFHJP
BLANK, C.E.
CENTRE FOR HUMAN GENETICS
117 MANCHESTER ROAD
SHEFFIELD, ENGLAND
S10 5DN

169.00   CJ
LORBER, J.
DEPARTMENT OF CHILD HEALTH
CHILDREN◻S HOSPITAL
WESTERN BANK
SHEFFIELD, ENGLAND
S10 2TH

EYGPT

170.00   BDFHJKNQU
BADR, FOUAD M.
HUMAN GENETICS UNIT
NATIONAL RESEARCH CENTER
CAIRO, EYGPT
  PHONE 982433

171.00   BDFHJ-LPQSVX
HASHEM, NEMAT
DEPARTMENT OF PEDIATRICS
MEDICAL GENETICS UNIT
AIN-SHAMS MEDICAL COLLEGE
CAIRO, EYGPT
  PHONE 906267

FINLAND

172.00   BDFJKMSU
DE LA CHAPELLE, ALBERT
FOLKHALSAN INSTITUTE OF GENETICS
P.O. BOX 819
HELSINKI 10, FINLAND
SF-00101   PHONE 90-500122

173.00*   FJ
GRIPENBERG, ULLA
DEPARTMENT OF GENETICS
UNIVERSITY OF HELSINKI
POHJ. RAUTATIEKATU 13
HELSINKI 10, FINLAND
  PHONE 494-721

174.00   CDJP
NORIO, REIJO
DEPARTMENT OF MEDICAL GENETICS
VAESTOLIITTO
BULEVARDI 28
HELSINKI 12, FINLAND
SF-00120   PHONE 90-11456

176.00   B-DFJY
AULA, PERTTI
CHROMOSOME LABORATORY
CHILDREN◻S HOSPITAL
UNIVERSITY OF HELSINKI
HELSINKI 29, FINLAND
  PHONE 418411

FRANCE

179.00   BDFHJY
LARGET-PIET, LUC
DEPARTMENT OF GENETIQUE
CENTRE HOSPITALIER UNIVERSITAIRE
1 AVENUE DEL HOTEL DIEU
ANGERS 49, FRANCE
  PHONE 88-69-51 POSTE 470

180.00   J-MP
ROPARTZ, C.
CENTER AND DEPARTMENT OF
  TRANSFUSION SANGUINE
609 CHEMIN DE LA BRETEQUE
BOIS-GUILLAUME, FRANCE
76230

181.00   ACDHJQ
GILLOT, FRANCOIS A.
SERVICE DE PEDIATRIE III
C.H.U. DE NANTES 44, FRANCE

183.00   FV
TURC, CLAUDE
DEPARTEMENT D◻HISTOLOGIE,
  EMBRYOLOGIE ET CYTOGENETIQUE
CENTRE HOSPITALIER REGIONAL ET
  UNIVERSITAIRE DE DIJON
7 BOULEVARD JEANNE D◻ARC
DIJON, FRANCE
21033   PHONE 80 30-90-17

184.00   CDFH-JUV
MOURIQUAND, JALPERT P.
FACULTE DE MEDICINE
UNIVERSITY OF GRENOBLE
LA TRONCHE, FRANCE
38   PHONE 87-74-41 EXT. 338

185.00   B-DFHJ
FONTAINE, GUY
DEPARTMENT DE GENETIQUE MEDICINE
CITE HOSPITALIERE
LILLE, FRANCE
59   PHONE 57-34-02 POSTE 3429

186.00   CDFGHJS
LAURENT, COLLETE
SECTION OF CYTOGENETICS
INSTITUTE PASTEUR
LYON, FRANCE
69   PHONE 72-35-09 POSTE H5

187.00   CFIV
STAHL, ANDRE
DEPARTMENT D◻EMBRYOLOGIE ET
  CYTOGENETIQUE
FACULTE DE MEDICINE
13385 MARSEIUE CEDEX 4
MARSEILLE, FRANCE
13   PHONE 91-48-36-10

189.00* DFHJV
DE GROUCHY, JEAN
CLINIQUE DE GENETIQUE MEDICALE
HOSPITAL DES ENFANTS MALADES
PARIS XV, FRANCE
    PHONE 734-5189 EXT. 1187

190.00 BDFHJMQV
LEJEUNE, JEROME
LABORATORY DE CYTOGENETIQUE
HOSPITAL DES ENFANTS MALADES
149 RUE DE SEVRES
PARIS XV, FRANCE

193.00 FLRV
BARSKI, GEORGE
TISSUE CULTURE AND VIRUS LABORATORY
INSTITUTE GUSTAVE-ROUSSY
PARIS 94-VILLEJUIF, FRANCE

195.00 DFV
EMERIT, INGRID
LABORATORY DE CYTOGENETIQUE
FACULTE DE MEDECINE
15 RUE DE L¤ECOLE DE MEDECINE
PARIS, FRANCE
    PHONE MED 34-40 POSTE 458

196.00 CDFHJ
ROUX, CHARLES
LABORATOIRE D¤EMBRYOLOGIE
PATHOLOGIQUE ET DE CYTOGENETIQUE
C.H.U. SAINT-ANTOINE
27 RUE CHALIGNY
PARIS, FRANCE
75   PHONE 344-3333 POSTE 475

197.00 B-FHJQSWX
ROYER, PIERRE
MEDICAL GENETICS
HOSPITAL DES ENFANTS MALADES
149 RUE DE SEVRES
PARIS, FRANCE

200.00 CDFHJKWXY
SENECAL
SERVICE PEDIATRIE B
CENTRE HOSPITALIER UNIVERSITY
RENNES, FRANCE
    PHONE 16-99-591609 EXT. 211-208

GERMANY BD

206.00 FHJNPRTV
LUERS, HERBERT
INSTITUT FUR GENETIK
FREIE UNIVERSITAT
BERLIN, GERMANY BD

209.00 CDFHJOQTY
KOCH, GERHARD
INSTITUTE FUR HUMANGENETIK UND
ANTHROPOLOGY
DER UNIVERSITY ERLANGEN - NURNBERG
852 ERLANGEN BISMARCKSTRASSE
ERLANGEN, GERMANY BD
10   PHONE 09131-852318-19

210.00 BCDFHJPSUXY
DEGENHARDT, K.H.
INSTITUT FUR HUMANGENETIK
PAUL-EHRLICHSTRASSE 41-43
FRANKFURT, GERMANY BD
    PHONE 0611-63016000

211.00 BDFHJ-MPY
WOLF, ULRICH
INSTITUTE OF HUMAN GENETICS OF THE
UNIVERSITY
FREIBURG I. BR., GERMANY BD
78   PHONE 0761-203465G

212.00 CDFHJOQY
FUHRMANN, WALTER
INSTITUT FUR HUMANGENETIK
UNIVERSITAT GIESSEN
GIESSEN, GERMANY BD
D63   PHONE 0641-7021

213.00 BDFGHJKPQST
BECKER, PETER E.
INSTITUT FUR HUMANGENETIK DER
UNIVERSITAT
NIKOLAUSBERGER WEG 23
GOTTINGEN, GERMANY BD

215.00 B-DF-HJKQS-Y
PASSARGE, EBERHARD
ABTEILUNG FUR CYTOGENETIK UND
KLINISCHE GENETIK
INSTITUT FUR HUMANGENETIK,
UNIVERSITAT HAMBURG
MARTINISTRASSE 52
HAMBURG 20, GERMANY BD
2000   PHONE 040 468 436

216.00 HJW
LOEFFLER, LOTHAR
OBSTERSTRASSE 57
HANNOVER, GERMANY BD

217.00 BDFHJKPQ
VOGEL, F.
INSTITUT FUR ANTHROPOLOGIE U
HEIDELBERG, GERMANY BD
    PHONE HEIDELBERG 43750

218.00 BDFHJKPQ
LEHMANN, W.
INSTITUT FUR HUMANGENETIK
UNIVERSITAT KIEL
HOSPITALSTRASSE 42
KIEL, GERMANY BD
23   PHONE 597-3200

220.00 CDFHPV
HIENZ, HERMANN ADOLF
PATHOLOGY INSTITUT
STADT KRANKENANSTALTEN
LUTHER-PLATZ 40
KREFELD, GERMANY BD
415   PHONE 02151-8282688

221.00 CFIOSUV
GROPP, A.
INSTITUT FUR PATHOLOGIE
DER MEDIZINISCHEN HOCHSCHULE
LUBECK
KRONSFORDER ALLEE, GERMANY BD
24

223.00 CDHJK
WENDT, G.G.
DEPARTMENT OF HUMAN GENETICS
UNIVERSITAT OF MARBURG
MARBURG, GERMANY BD
    PHONE 06421-284080

224.00 FIV
LAMPERT, FRITZ H.
DEPARTMENT OF PEDIATRICS
UNIVERSITATS-KINDERKLINIK
LINDWURMSTRASSE 4
MUNCHEN 2, GERMANY BD
8   PHONE 0811-539911 EXT. 951

225.00 DJPT
ZERBIN-RUDIN, EDITH
DEPARTMENT OF GENEALOGY AND
DEMOGRAPHY
MAX-PLANCK-INSTITUT OF PSYCHIATRY
MUNCHEN 40, GERMANY BD
8   PHONE MUNCHEN 3896-435
                    KRAEPELINSKR. 2

227.00 CDFJQY
MURKEN, JAN
DEPARTMENT OF PEDIATRICS
KINDERPOLIKLINIK DER UNIVERSITAT
PETTENKOFERSTRASSE 8A
MUNCHEN, GERMANY BD
    PHONE 0811-59941

229.00 CDFJV
ZANG, KLAUS D.
DEPARTMENT OF NEUROPATHOLOGY
MAX-PLANCK-INSTITUT OF PSYCHIATRY
MUNCHEN, GERMANY BD
    PHONE 0811-3896214

230.00 CDFHJPSY
LENZ, W.
DEPARTMENT OF HUMAN GENETICS
INSTITUT OF HUMAN GENETICS
MUNSTER, GERMANY BD

231.00 CDFHJ
PFEIFFER, R.A.
DIVISION OF CLINICAL GENETICS AND
CYTOGENETICS
12-14 VESALIUS WEG
MUNSTER, GERMANY BD
44

232.00 DFJKQ
BAUKE, JOCHEN
DEPARTMENT OF INTERNAL MEDICINE,
CYTOGENETIC UNIT, DIVISION OF HEM.
UNIVERSITAT OF ULM
PARKSTRASSE 11
ULM 1, GERMANY BD
79

GERMANY DDR

234.00 FRV
WIDMAIER, R.
INSTITUT OF CANCER RESEARCH
GERMAN ACADEMY OF SCIENCE OF BERLIN
BERLIN-BUCH, GERMANY DDR
1115   PHONE 56-9851-327

236.00 C-HJN-QTV-Y
WITTWER, B.B.
MEDICAL GENETICS CENTRE
COUNSELING
KARL-MARX-STRASSE 258
MAGDEBURG, GERMANY DDR
301

237.00 CDFJ
KIRCHMAIR, H.
PEDIATRIC HOSPITAL UNIVERSITY
ROSTROCK, GERMANY DDR

238.00 CDFHJ
PELZ, L.
DEPARTMENT OF CYTOGENETICS
PEDIATRIC HOSPITAL UNIVERSITY
ROSTROCK, GERMANY DDR
25

239.00 CDFHPQTV
BETHMANN, W.
KLINIK F. GESICHTSCHIRURGIE
THALLWITZ, GERMANY DDR
7251   PHONE WURZEN 3912

GHANA

240.00 B-FI-KN-QSWX
KONOTEY-AHULU, FELIX I.D.
DEPARTMENT OF MEDICINE
KORLE BU TEACHING HOSPITAL
ACCRA, GHANA
    PHONE ACCRA 65401

GREECE

241.00 B-DFHJKNPW
DOXIADIS, SPYROS A.
INSTITUTE OF CHILD HEALTH
AGHIA SOPHIA CHILDREN¤S HOSPITAL
ATHENS, GREECE
608   PHONE 771 811

242.00 ADFHJKNPQ
MATSANIOTIS, N.
ST. SOPHIE¤S CHILDREN¤S HOSPITAL
ATHENS UNIVERSITY
ATHENS, GREECE
608

HONG KONG

243.00 B-DFHJKNRV
KNEEBONE, G.M.
PAEDIATRICS UNIT
GENETIC SERVICES
QUEEN MARY HOSPITAL
HONG KONG, HONG KONG

HUNGARY

246.00 CDFHJY
LASZLO, HORVATH

MATERNITY CARE CENTRE
LABORATORY OF GENETICS
KNEZICH-U 14,
BUDAPEST 5, HUNGARY
H-1092

249.00   DFKUV
ECKHARDT, S.
DEPARTMENT OF CHEMOTHERAPY
NATIONAL CANCER INSTITUTE
BUDAPEST, XII RATH GY U7, HUNGARY
  PHONE 354-350

250.00   B-EJM-QS
FORRAI, GEORGE
BUDAPEST, ALIG U.5., HUNGARY
1132

251.00   CDHJO-Q
GYENIS, G.Y.
UNIVERSITY INSTITUTE ANTHROPOLOGY
EMBERTANI TANSZEK
BUDAPEST, PUSKIN U.3, HUNGARY
H-1088

252.00   CDFHJKNOQ
LENART, GEORGE
JANOS KORHAZ CLINIC
BUDAPEST, XII DIOSAROK U1, HUNGARY

253.00   DFHJV
SCHULER, D.
SECOND DEPARTMENT OF PEDIATRICS
MEDICAL SCHOOL OF BUDAPEST
BUDAPEST, IX TUZOLTO U7, HUNGARY

254.00   BFJM
SZABO, G.
BIOLOGICAL INSTITUTE
MEDICAL UNIVERSITY
DABRECEN 12, HUNGARY
  PHONE 11-600-191

255.00   CDFJVY
PAPP, Z.
DEPARTMENT OF OBSIETRICS AND
GYNECOLOGY
CYTOGENETIC LABORATORY
UNIVERSITY MEDICAL SCHOOL
DEBRECEN, HUNGARY

256.00   BDFHJP
MEHES, K.
GENETIC LABORATORY, DEPARTMENT OF
  PEDIATRICS
COUNTY HOSPITAL MEGYEI KORHAZ
GYOR, HUNGARY
H-9002

257.00   B-DFHJ
VARGA, F.
DEPARTMENT OF PEDIATRICS
UNIVERSITY MEDICAL SCHOOL
PECS, JOZSEF A11, HUNGARY

258.00   CDFHJLOP
KISZELY, GYORGY
BIOLOGIAI INTEZET
SZOTE
SZEGED, HUNGARY
  PHONE 14-000

INDIA

262.00   CKPV
SANGHVI, L.D.
EPIDEMIOLOGY DIVISION
CANCER RESEARCH INSTITUTE
TATE MEMORIAL CENTER
BOMBAY 12, INDIA
  PHONE 442703

263.00   BFJKPV
UNDEVIA, J.V.
EPIDEMIOLOGY DIVISION
CANCER RESEARCH INSTITUTE
TATE MEMORIAL CENTRE
BOMBAY 12, PAREL, INDIA
  PHONE 442703

266.00   CDFJK
TALUKDER, GEETA
DEPARTMENT OF PATHOLOGY, UNIT OF
  GENETICS

INSTITUTE OF POSTGRADUATE MEDICAL
  EDUCATION AND RESEARCH
6 MULLEN STREET
CALCUTTA 6, INDIA

267.00   ABHJKO-Q
SHARMA, J.C.
DEPARTMENT OF ANTHROPOLOGY
PANJAB UNIVERSITY
CHANDIGARH, INDIA
  PHONE 29541 OR 26285

270.00   DFJ
SADASIVAN, G.
DEPARTMENT OF ANATOMY COLLEGE
HYDERAB, 1-A.P., INDIA
  PHONE 45692 EXT. 10

272.00   B-DFH-JLPV-Y
GHAI, OM.P.
DEPARTMENT OF PEDIATRICS, GENETICS
  UNIT
ALL INDIA INSTITUTE OF MEDICAL
  SCIENCES
ANSARI NAGAR
NEW DELHI 16, INDIA

273.00   FHJKPSV
GREWAL, M.S.
DEPARTMENT OF ANATOMY
UNIT OF HUMAN GENETICS AND
  DEVELOPMENT
ALL INDIA INSTITUTE OF MEDICAL
  SCIENCES
NEW DELHI 16, INDIA
  PHONE 619481 EXT. 216

276.00   CGHKOPSV
GULATI, R.K.
DEPARTMENT OF ANTHROPOLOGY
DECCAN COLLEGE
POONA, INDIA
  PHONE 22145 25973

278.00   CFJPU
PUTTANA, CHAMARA R.
INSTITUTE OF CELL BIOLOGY
NO. 2 YADAVGIRI 1 MAIN ROAD
VANIVILASPURAM, MYSORE-2, INDIA

280.00   B-DFHJKO-Q
CHAKRAVARTTI, M.R.
DEPARTMENT OF HUMAN GENETICS AND
  PHYSICAL ANTHROPOLOGY
ANDHRA UNIVERSITY
WALTAIR, A.P., INDIA

IRAN

281.00   DFJP
MAHLOUDJI, MOHSEN
NEMAZEE HOSPITAL
SHIRAZ, IRAN

IRELAND

282.00   C-FH-LP
MASTERSON, JOSEPH
DEPARTMENT OF PATHOLOGY, SECTION
  MEDICAL GENETICS
UNIVERSITY COLLEGE
EARLSFORT TERRACE
DUBLIN 2, IRELAND

ISRAEL

283.00   DFHJ
DAR, H.
GENETIC UNIT
ROTHSCHILD HOSPITAL
HAIFA, ISRAEL

284.00   B-DFHJKMOPTY
COHEN, MAIMON M.
DEPARTMENT OF HUMAN GENETICS
HADASSAH-HEBREW UNIVERSITY MEDICAL
  CENTER
P.O. BOX 499
JERUSALEM, ISRAEL
  PHONE 02-38211 EXT. 509

285.00   B-DGJKN-P
COHEN, T.
DEPARTMENT OF HUMAN GENETICS
HADASSAH-HEBREW UNIVERSITY MEDICAL
  CENTER
JERUSALEM, ISRAEL
  PHONE 02-38211 EXT. 509

286.00   A-HJ-LQY
FRIED, KALMAN
DEPARTMENT OF HUMAN GENETICS
31 HABANAI
JERUSALEM, BETH-HAKEREM, ISRAEL
  PHONE 02-526642

288.00   B-DFI-LNPQVY
HALBRECHT, ISAAC G.
FETAL DEVELOPMENT AND GENETICS UNIT
HASHARON HOSPITAL
PETAH TIQUA, ISRAEL

289.00   CDFHJ-LPRWX
CHEMKE, JUAN
CLINICAL GENETICS UNIT
KAPLAN HOSPITAL
REHOVOT, ISRAEL
  PHONE 03-953-632 OR 03-950-244

290.00   B-DFHJW-Y
LEGUM, CYRIL P.
CHILD DEVELOPMENT ASSESS. CENTER
  AND TEL AVIV UNIVERSITY
MEDICAL CENTER AT ROKACH HOSPITAL
14 BALFOUR STREET
TAL-AVIV-YAFFO, ISRAEL
  PHONE 623401

292.00   BV
BRACHA, RAMOT
DEPARTMENT OF HAEMATOLOGY
TEL-HASHOMER GOVERNMENT HOSPITAL
TEL-HASHOMER, ISRAEL
  PHONE 751323

293.00   BFJY
GOLDMAN, BOLESLAW
DEPARTMENT OF CYTOGENETICS
TEL-HASHOMER HOSPITAL
TEL-HASHOMER, ISRAEL

294.00   B-DHJP
GOODMAN, RICHARD M.
DEPARTMENT OF HUMAN GENETICS
TEL-HASHOMER HOSPITAL
TEL-HASHOMER, ISRAEL

295.00   BDJKMNP
SZEINBERG, ARIEH
DEPARTMENT OF CHEMICAL PATHOLOGY
TEL-HASHOMER HOSPITAL
TEL-AVIV UNIVERSITY MEDICAL SCHOOL
TEL-HASHOMER, ISRAEL
  PHONE 03-75 52 12

ITALY

296.00   CDFHJV
DALLAPICCOLA, BRUNO
LABORATORIO DI CITOGENETICA UMANA
CLINICA MEDICA
UNIVERSITA DI FERRARA
FERRARA, ITALY
44100   PHONE 25024

297.00   CDFJQ
BIGOZZI, UMBERTO
CENTRO GENETICA MEDICA
CLINICA MEDICA
VIALE MORGAGNI
FIRENZE, ITALY
50134   PHONE 411106

298.00   B-DFJKPUV
GIANFERRARI, LUISA
CENTRO DI STUDI DI GENETICA AMANA
  ED EUGENICA
CARSO VENEZIA 55
MILAN, ITALY
20121

302.00   B-DFJPV
FRACCARO, MARCO
EURATOM UNIT FOR HUMAN RAD. AND
  CYTOGENETICS

VIA FORLANINI 14
PAVIA, ITALY
27100   PHONE 33267

303.00   FJMOPS
POLSINELLI, MARIO
INSTITUTO DI GENETICA
VIA S. EPIFANIO 14
PAVIA, ITALY
27100   PHONE 31036 OR 31037

305.00   CDFHJKQTW
GEDDA, LUIGO
INSTITUT DI GENETICA MEDICA E
  GEMELLOLOGIA G. MENDEL
PIAZZA GALENO 5
ROME, ITALY
00161

306.00   ABD-FIJMPSTY
SERRA, ANGELO
UNIVERSITA A CATTOLICA DEL SACRO
  CUORE
INSTITUTO DE GENETICA UMANA
VIA DELLA PINETA SACHETTI 644
ROME, ITALY
00168   PHONE 3875-127

307.00   BDJKMPSWX
SILVESTRONI, EZIO
CENTRO DI STUDI D. MICROCITEMIA
CITTA UNIVERSITARIA
ROME, ITALY
  PHONE 490470

308.00   BDFJMPQ
CEPPELLINI, RUGGERO
DEPARTMENT OF MEDICAL GENETICS
UNIVERSITY OF TURIN
TORINO, ITALY

309.00   AFH-LOP
CHIARELLI, B.
DEPARTMENT OF ANTHROPOLOGY
VIA ACCADEMIA ALBERTINA 17
TORINO, ITALY
10123   PHONE 832196

JAPAN

312.00   CGJ
FUJINO, HIROSHI
DEPARTMENT OF ORAL SURGERY
KYUSHU UNIVERSITY
FUKUOKA, JAPAN

313.00   DIJLP
KUROIWA, YOSHIGORO
DEPARTMENT OF NEUROLOGY
KYUSHU UNIVERSITY
FUKUOKA, JAPAN
  PHONE 092 64-1151

314.00   DFI-LQRUV
AWANO, ISAMU
DEPARTMENT OF INTERNAL MEDICINE
FUKUSHIMA MEDICAL COLLEGE
FUKUSHIMA-SHI, JAPAN
  PHONE 21-1211

316.00   FJKPQV
TSUJI, YOSHITO
DEPARTMENT OF PUBLIC HEALTH
FUKUSHIMA MEDICAL COLLEGE
FUKUSHIMA, JAPAN

319.00   FJVY
FUJIWARA, ATSUSHI
DEPARTMENT OF OBSTETRICS AND
  GYNECOLOGY
HIROSHIMA UNIVERSITY
HIROSHIMA, JAPAN
  PHONE 0822 51-111 EXT. 297

323.00   B-FJ-MOPTY
FUJIKI, NORIV
DEPARTMENT OF GENETICS
INSTITUTE AND GENERAL HOSPITAL FOR
  DEVELOPMENTAL RESEARCH
AICHI COLONY FOR MENTAL AND
  PHYSICAL HEALTH
KASUGAI CITY, AICHI PREFECTURAL,
  JAPAN
  PHONE 0568-88-0811 EXT. 587

324.00   CDJ
MURAKAMI, UJIHIRO
INSTITUTE FOR DEVELOPMENTAL
  RESEARCH
AICHI PREFECTURAL COLONY
KAMIYA-CHO
KASUGAI, JAPAN
480-03

325.00   DPQV
MIYAO, SADANABU
DEPARTMENT OF GERIATRICS
INSTITUTE OF CONSTITUTIONAL
  MEDICINE
KUMAMOTO UNIVERSITY
KUMAMOTO CITY, JAPAN
  PHONE 0963-63-1111

328.00   BDFJKOP
MASUDA, MASASUKE
DEPARTMENT OF INTERNAL MEDICINE
DIVISION OF HEMATOLOGY AND GENETICS
KYOTO PREFECTURAL UNIVERSITY OF
  MEDICINE
KYOTO, JAPAN
  PHONE 375-231-2311 EXT. 247

332.00   FHJ
MATSUNAGA, EI
DEPARTMENT OF HUMAN GENETICS
NATIONAL INSTITUTE OF GENETICS
MISHIMA, JAPAN
  PHONE 0559-75-0771

336.00   B-DFJ-LN
YAGAMI, YOSHIAKI
DEPARTMENT OF OBSTETRICS AND
  GYNECOLOGY
KAWASUMI-CHO MIZUHO-KU
NAGOYA, JAPAN

338.00   B-FIJPR
KONDO, KIYOTARO
DEPARTMENT OF NEUROLOGY
NIIGATA UNIVERSITY HOSPITAL
NIIGATA, JAPAN
  PHONE 0252-23-6161 EXT.891

343.00   ADFHJQT
MITSUDA, HISATOSHI
DEPT. OF NEUROPSYCHIATRY
OSAKA MEDICAL COLLEGE
OSAKA, TAKATSUKI, JAPAN

344.00   CFHJVY
SASAKI, MOTOMICHI
CHROMOSOME RESEARCH UNIT
FACULTY OF SCIENCE
HOKKAIDO UNIVERSITY
SAPPORO, JAPAN
060   PHONE 711-2111 EXT. 2752

345.00   BFLSVY
YOSHIDA, MICHIHIRO C.
CHROMOSOME RESEARCH UNIT
FACULTY OF SCIENCE
HOKKAIDO UNIVERSITY
SAPPORO, JAPAN
  PHONE 011-711-2111 EXT. 2619

347.00   BDFJMPQ
MIYOSHI, KAZUNO
DEPARTMENT OF MEDICINE
TOKUSHIMA UNIVERSITY
TOKUSHIMA, JAPAN

348.00   BFHKLOQV
FURUHATA, TOTTORI
NATURAL RESEARCH INSTITUTE OF
  POLICE SCIENCE
6 SANBAN-CHO, CHIYODA-KU
TOKYO, JAPAN
  PHONE 261-9986-9

349.00   CDFJT
HIDANO, AKIRA
GENETIC COUNSELING SECTION
TOKYO METROPOLITAN POLICE HOSPITAL
FUJIMI, CHIYODAKU
TOKYO, JAPAN
102   PHONE 263-1371

350.00   ACDFHJQT
INOUYE, EIJI
DEPARTMENT OF HUMAN GENETICS AND
  CRIMINOLOGY

INSTITUTE OF BRAIN RESEARCH
UNIVERSITY OF TOKYO FACILITY OF
  MEDICINE
TOKYO, JAPAN
  PHONE 03-812-2111 EXT. 7763

355.00   DJP
NAKAJUMA, AKIRA
DEPARTMENT OF OPTHALOMOLOGY
JUNTENDO UNIVERSITY
TOKYO, JAPAN
  PHONE 03-813-3111-618

357.00   CJOP
SHINOZAKI, N.
DEPARTMENT OF POPULATION QUALITY
INSTITUTE OF POPULATION PROBLEMS
TOKYO, JAPAN

359.00   C-EGJPQSUV
TANAKA, KATUMI
DEPARTMENT OF HUMAN GENETICS
TOKYO MEDICAL AND DENTAL UNIVERSITY
TOKYO, JAPAN
113   PHONE 03-813-6111

360.00   CDFGJPSU
TONOMURA, AKIRA
DEPARTMENT OF HUMAN CYTOGENETICS
TOKYO MEDICAL AND DENTAL UNIVERSITY
TOKYO, JAPAN

362.00   B-DGHJRY
KONISHI, SHUNZO
DEPARTMENT OF PEDIATRICS
YAMAGUCHI UNIVERSITY
SCHOOL OF MEDICINE
UBE, JAPAN
  PHONE 0836-31-3121

364.00   CDFHJVY
YANAGISAWA, SATOSHI
DEPARTMENT OF PEDIATRICS
YAMAGUCHI UNIVERSITY, SCHOOL OF
  MEDICINE
UBE, JAPAN
  PHONE 0836-31-3121

365.00   BDFHJOP
HANDA, YOSHITOSHI
DEPARTMENT OF ANATOMY
WAKAYAMA MEDICAL COLLEGE
WAKAYAMA-SHI, JAPAN

366.00   DFHJ
MATSUI, ICHIRO
DEPARTMENT OF PEDIATRICS AND
  CYTOGENETIC LABORATORY
KANAGAWA CHILDRENS MEDICAL CENTER
MUTSUKAWA
YOKOHAMA, MINAMIKU, JAPAN
2-138-4   PHONE 045-711-235

LEBANON

370.00   CFJY
BARAKAT, BASSAM Y.
DEPARTMENT OF OBSTETRICS AND
  GYNECOLOGY
AMERICAN UNIVERSITY HOSPITAL
BEIRUT, LEBANON
  PHONE 340460

371.00   B-DFI-KMSWY
DER KALOUSTIAN, VAZKEN
DEPARTMENT OF PEDIATRICS
AMERICAN UNIVERSITY MEDICAL CENTER
BEIRUT, LEBANON

372.00   B-DJKP
LOISELET, JACQUES
DEPARTMENT BIOCHIMIE MEDICALE
FACULTE FRANCAISE DE MEDECINE
BEIRUT, LEBANON

373.00   CDFHJ
NAFFAH, JOSETTE
LABORATOIRE DE CYTOGENETIQUE
FACULTE FRANCAISE DE MEDECINE
B.P. 5076
BEIRUT, LEBANON

MEXICO

375.00　　　　　　　　CDFHJ-LPQ
ARMENDARES, SALVADOR S.
DEPARTMENT OF MEDICAL GENETICS
HOSPITAL DE PEDIATRIA
MEXICO CITY, MEXICO

376.00　　　　　　　　DFJK
RAMOS, MARIO GONZALEZ
UNIDAD DE GENETICA
HOSPITAL INFANTIL DE MEXICO
DR. MARQUEZ NO. 162
MEXICO CITY, D.F., MEXICO

377.00　　　　　　　　ABDFJMPU
DE GARAY, A.L.
DEPARTMENT OF GENETIC PROGRAMS
COMM. NACIONAL DE ENERGIA NUCLEAR
APDO. POSTAL NO 27-190
MEXICO 18, D.F., MEXICO
　PHONE 5-63-60-11

378.00　　　　　　　　DFHJLNPV
LISKER, RUBEN
DEPARTMENT OF GENETICS
INSTITUTO NACIONAL DE LA NUTRICION
MEXICO 22, D.F., MEXICO
　PHONE 573-12-00

379.00　　　　　　　　CDFJNW
CHAPA, RAUL GARZA
DEPARTMENT OF GENETICS
UNIVERSITY AUTONOMA DE NUEVO LEON
APARTADO POSTAL 1563
MONTERREY, NL, MEXICO
　PHONE 46-68-71 EXT. 38

NETHERLANDS

380.00　　　　　　　　CDFHJQQ
DE FROE, A.
DEPARTMENT OF HUMAN BIOLOGY AND
　GENETICS
ANTHROPOBIOLOGICAL LABORATORY
MAURITSKADE 61
AMSTERDAM, NETHERLANDS

383.00　　　　　　　　J
AULBERS, B.J.M.
DEPARTMENT OF GENETIC COUNSELING
HOF. VAN DELFTLAAN 126
DELFT, NETHERLANDS
　PHONE 01730-22040

384.00　　　　　　　　BDFHJ
ANDERS, G.J.P.A.
DEPARTMENT OF HUMAN GENETICS
ANTHROPOGENETIC INSTITUTE
GRONINGEN, NETHERLANDS

386.00　　　　　　　　DJK
DIRECTOR
HEMOPHILIA CLINIC
FLEVOLAAN 71
HUIZEN, NH, NETHERLANDS
　PHONE 02159-45182

387.00　　　　　　　　BFJKMPQS
FRASER, G.A.
DEPARTMENT OF HUMAN GENETICS
UNIVERSITY OF LEIDEN
LEIDEN, NETHERLANDS

392.00　　　　　　　　BFHJ
GEERTS, S.J.
DEPARTMENT OF HUMAN GENETICS
FACULTY OF MEDICINE
UNIVERSITY OF NYMEGEN
NYMEGEN, NETHERLANDS

393.00　　　　　　　　CDFHJQQ
JONGBLOET, P.H.
INSTITUTE FOR MENTAL RETARDATES
OTTERSUM, NETHERLANDS
　PHONE 08851-3900

397.00　　　　　　　　BDJQQ
VISSER, H.K.A.
DEPARTMENT OF PEDIATRICS, ERASMUS
　UNIVERSITY
SOPHIA CHILDRENS HOSPITAL AND
　NEONATAL UNIT
ROTTERDAM, NETHERLANDS
　PHONE 010-656566

399.00　　　　　　　　BDHJQQ
HUIZINGA, JOHN
DEPARTMENT OF HUMAN BIOLOGY
STATE UNIVERSITY OF UTRECHT
UTRECHT, NETHERLANDS

NEW ZEALAND

401.00　　　　　　　　BD-FHJPQSVY
VEALE, A.M.O.
DEPARTMENT OF COMMUNITY HEALTH
UNIVERSITY OF AUCKLAND MEDICAL
　SCHOOL
AUCKLAND, NEW ZEALAND
　PHONE 33-105

404.00　　　　　　　　BJM
CARRELL, R.W.
DEPARTMENT OF CLINICAL BIOCHEMISTRY
CHRISTCHURCH HOSPITAL
CHRISTCHURCH, NEW ZEALAND

405.00　　　　　　　　FHJUVY
FITZGERALD, PETER H.
DEPARTMENT OF CYTOGENETICS
CHRIST CHURCH HOSPITAL
CHRISTCHURCH, NEW ZEALAND
　PHONE 66591

NORTH IRELAND

408.00　　　　　　　　C-FJKPY
NEVIN, NORMAN C.
DEPARTMENT OF MEDICAL STATISTICS
HUMAN GENETICS UNIT
QUEENOS UNIVERSITY AND ROYAL
　BELFAST HOSPITAL FOR SICK CHILDREN
BELFAST, NORTH IRELAND
　PHONE BELFAST 40503 EXT. 392

NORWAY

409.00　　　　　　　　CDFJY
AARSKOG, DAGFINN
DEPARTMENT OF PEDIATRICS
UNIVERSITY OF BERGEN
BARNEKLINIKKEN
BERGEN, NORWAY
5000　PHONE 298060

413.00　　　　　　　　B-FH-MPQSVXY
BERG, KARE
INSTITUTE OF MEDICAL GENETICS
UNIVERSITY OF OSLO
BLINDERN
OSLO 3, NORWAY
　PHONE 466 800 EXT. 9139

414.00　　　　　　　　FIKPSUV
BROGGER, ANTON
GENETICS LABORATORY
NORSK HYDROOS INSTITUTE FOR CANCER
　RESEARCH
OSLO 3, MONTEBELLO, NORWAY

416.00　　　　　　　　EFUV
IVERSEN, O.H.
DEPARTMENT OF PATHOLOGY
RIKSHOSPITALET
OSLO, NORWAY
　PHONE 20-10-50 EXT. 92

PERU

421.00　　　　　　　　CDFHJY
FORTON, JULIO ANIBAL ESCALANTE
URBANIZACION SAN BORJA
JIRON MIGUEL ANGEL 310
LIMA, PERU

422.00　　　　　　　　DFHJT
NUNEZ, TERESA PEREZ
DEPARTMENT OF PATHOLOGY
UNIVERSITY PERUANA CAYETANO HEREDIA
BOX 6195
LIMA, PERU

PHILLIPPINES

423.00　　　　　　　　BFGJNPQVX
BAYANI-SIOSON, PELAGIA S.
BASIC SCIENCES AND RESEARCH
　SECTION, COLLEGE OF DENTISTRY
UNIVERSITY OF PHILLIPPINES, PADRE
　FAURA
MANILA, PHILLIPPINES
D-406　PHONE 50-16-84

POLAND

428.00　　　　　　　　DFHJS
BOCZKOWSKI, K.
SECTION OF GENETICS
MEDICAL ACADEMY
WARSAW, POLAND
PHONE 29-12-40

429.00　　　　　　　　B-DFHJUW-Y
CZERSKI, PRZEMYSLAW
DEPARTMENT OF HUMAN GENETICS
NATIONAL RESEARCH INSTITUTE OF
　MATERNAL AND CHILD HEALTH
WARSAW, KASPRZAKA 17, POLAND
01-211　PHONE 32-21-82

431.00　　　　　　　　B-DFHJPT
WALD, IGNACY
DEPARTMENT OF GENETICS
PSYCHONEUROLOGICAL INSTITUTE
SOBIESKIEGO 1/9
WARSAW, PRUSZKOW, POLAND
02957　PHONE 43-66-11

ROMANIA

432.00　　　　　　　　BFMUV
ANTOHI, STEFAN
DEPARTMENT OF GENETICS
VICTOR BABES INSTITUTE OF PATH. AND
　GENETICS
SPL. INDEPENDENTEI GG-101
BUCAREST 35, ROMANIA
　PHONE 370400

434.00　　　　　　　　CDFHJOP
MILCU, ST.M.
DEPARTMENT OF ENDOCRINOLOGY
INSTITUTE OF ENDOCRINOLOGY
BUCAREST, ROMANIA
　PHONE 33-06-02

438.00　　　　　　　　ACDF-HJ-LOT
SCRIPCARU, G.
DEPARTMENT OF FORENSIC MEDICINE
INSTITUTE OF MEDICINE
1430 TULANE AVENUE
IASSY, ROMANIA

SCOTLAND

439.00　　　　　　　　DFHJ
JOHNSTON, A.W.
ABERDEEN ROYAL INFIRMARY
ABERDEEN, SCOTLAND
AB9 2ZB　PHONE 0224-23423 EXT.
　　　　　　　　　　　　　　　2122

441.00　　　　　　　　B-EIJLPSWY
EMERY, ALAN
DEPARTMENT OF HUMAN GENETICS
UNIVERSITY
EDINBURGH, SCOTLAND
　PHONE 031-332-1311

442.00　　　　　　　　A-CEFILMPRSUV
EVANS, H.J.
MRC. CLINIC AND POPULATION
　CYTOGENETIC UNIT
WESTERN GENERAL HOSPITAL
CREWE ROAD
EDINBURGH, SCOTLAND
EH4 2XU　PHONE 031-332-1361

443.00　　　　　　　　CDFHJKSVY
FERGUSON-SMITH, MALCOLM A.
MEDICAL GENETICS DEPARTMENT
ROYAL HOSPITAL FOR SICK CHILDREN
GLASGOW, SCOTLAND
G38 SJ

SINGAPORE

445.00   B-DFJKY
BOON, WONG HOCK
DEPARTMENT OF PAEDIATRICS
UNIVERSITY OF SINGAPORE
C/O OUTRAM ROAD GENERAL HOSPITAL
SINGAPORE, SINGAPORE

SOUTH AFRICA

446.00   CDFJSY
BEIGHTON, PETER
DEPARTMENT OF HUMAN GENETICS
MEDICAL SCHOOL, OBSERVATORY
P.O. BOX 594
CAPE TOWN, CAPE PROVINCE, SOUTH
   AFRICA
   PHONE 55-4707

448.00   CDFHJQTV
HURST, LEWIS A.
DEPARTMENT OF PSYCHIATRY AND MENTAL
   HYGIENE
MEDICAL SCHOOL, JOHANNESBURG
   HOSPITAL
ESSELEN STREET
JOHANNESBURG, SOUTH AFRICA
   PHONE 724-1121 EXT. 265

449.00   CDF-HJPTY
WILTON, EUGENE
CYTOGENETIC UNIT
SOUTH AFRICAN INSTITUTE FOR MEDICAL
   RESEARCH
P.O. BOX 1038, HOSPITAL STREET
JOHANNESBURG, SOUTH AFRICA
   PHONE 724-1781

450.00   CDFJLNP
ANDERSON, INGRAM F.
DEPARTMENT OF MEDICINE
PRETORIA GENERAL HOSPITAL
PRETORIA, SOUTH AFRICA
   PHONE 29741 EXT. 4

SPAIN

451.00   CDFHJ
MARTINEZ, FRANCISCA BALLESTA
DEPARTAMENTO DE GENETICA
HOSPITAL CLINICO
C/O CASANOVA 143
BARCELONA 11, SPAIN

452.00   CDFHJ
ANTICH, JAIME
DEPARTMENT OF HUMAN GENETICS
INSTITUTE PROVINCIAL DE BIOQUIMICA
BARCELONA C-ROBERTO BASSAS 1
BARCELONA 14, SPAIN
   PHONE 211-74-02

454.00   CDFJ
PRATS, JORGE
HOSPITAL INFANTIL, SEGURIDAD
BARCELONA, SPAIN
   PHONE 250-88-59

455.00   BCFHJKPT
ABRISQUETA, JOSE A.
DEPARTAMENTO DE GENETICA HUMANA
INSTITUTO DE GENETICA
VELAZQUEZ 144
MADRID 6, SPAIN
   PHONE 2-61-18-00

456.00   B-DFHJKNPQY
CASCOS, ANDRES SANCHEZ
DEPARTAMENTO DE HUMAN GENETICS
FUNDACION JIMENEZ DIAZ
MADRID, SPAIN
   PHONE 2-44-16-00 EXT. 379

457.00   CFHJ
GONGORA, LUIS IZQUIERDO
DEPARTMENT DE GENETICA
HOSPITAL CLINICO
MADRID, SPAIN
   PHONE 2-44-15-00

458.00   CFHJ
MIRANDA, EMILIA BARREIROS

DEPARTMENT DE GENETICA HUMANA
CLINICA INFANTIL
LA PAZ
MADRID, SPAIN

460.00   DFH-KM
BOVER, GERONIMO FORTEZA
DEPARTMENT DE INVEST. CITOLOGICAS
DE LA CAJA DE AHORROS
AMADEO DE SOBOYA 4
VALENCIA 10, SPAIN
   PHONE 698500

461.00   B-DFH-KM
BAGUENA CANDELA, RAFAEL
DEPARTMENT OF MEDICAL GENETICS
FACULTY OF MEDICINE
PASEO VALENCIA AL MAR 17
VALENCIA 5, SPAIN
   PHONE 69-04-00

SWEDEN

465.00   BCFJP
LARSON, CARL A.
DEPARTMENT OF MEDICAL GENETICS
INSTITUTE OF GENETICS
LUND, SWEDEN

466.00   CDFGJNY
LINDSTEN, J.
DEPARTMENT OF CLINICAL GENETICS
KAROLINSKA HOSPITAL
STOCKHOLM 60, SWEDEN
10401

469.00   BDFJMPT
BOOK, JAN A.
UPPSALA UNIVERSITY, INSTITUTE OF
   MEDICAL GENETICS
24 V AGATAN
UPPSALA, SWEDEN
TS-752 20   PHONE 018-14-71-68

470.00   CDFJ
GUSTAVSON, K.H.
DEPARTMENT OF PEDIATRICS
AKADEMISKA SJUKHUSET
UPPSALA, SWEDEN
75014

SWITZERLAND

471.00   B-DFHJKRY
STALDER, G.R.
UNIVERSITY CHILDRENS HOSPITAL
ROMERGASSE 8
BASEL, SWITZERLAND
   PHONE 061-32-10-10

472.00   DEJ
MOSER, HANS
UNIVERSITY CHILDRENS HOSPITAL
FREIBURGSTRASSE 23, BERN,
   SWITZERLAND
CH-3008   PHONE 031-642711

473.00   CFJY
KAJII, TADASHI
LABORATORY OF EMBRYOLOGY AND
   CYTOGENETICS
UNIVERSITY CLINIC OF GYNECOLOGY AND
   OBSTETRIC 1211
RUE ALCIDE-JENTZER 20
GENEVA 4, SWITZERLAND
1200   PHONE 46-92-11 EXT. 2648

474.00   CDFJKPQSTY
KLEIN, DAVID
DEPARTMENT OF MEDICAL GENETICS
UNIVERSITY OF GENEVA
CHEMIN THURY 8
GENEVA, SWITZERLAND
   PHONE 022-468363

475.00   CDFHJVY
JUILLARD, EDOUARD
GENETIQUE MEDICALE
HOPITAL CANTONAL UNIVERSITAIRE
LAUSANNE, SWITZERLAND
1011

477.00   CDJK
TONZ, OTMAR
KINDERSPITAL
SPITALSTRASSE
LUCERNE, SWITZERLAND
   PHONE 041 25 1125

479.00   CDFJUXY
SCHMID, WERNER
DEPARTMENT OF PAEDIATRICS, DIVISION
   OF MEDICAL GENETICS
UNIVERSITY CHILDRENS HOSPITAL
STEINWIESSER 75
ZURICH, SWITZERLAND
   PHONE 051-479090

THAILAND

481.00   DJKNP
NA-NAKORN, SUPA
DEPARTMENT OF HEMATOLOGY
SIRIRAJ HOSPITAL
BANGKOK, THAILAND

TURKEY

483.00   B-DFHJ-LPQ
SAY, BURHAN
DEPARTMENT OF PEDIATRICS
HACETTEPE UNIVERSITY
ANKARA, TURKEY
   PHONE 242240 EXT. 1171

486.00   ACDFJKPTWX
SAYLI, BEKIR SITKI
MEDICAL FACULTY
UNIVERSITY OF ANKARA
SIHHIYE ANKARA, TURKEY
   PHONE 108303 EXT. 394

URUGUAY

488.00   FHJ
DRETS, MAXIMO EDUARDO
HUMAN CYTOGENETICS LABORATORY
INSTITUT DE CIENCIAS BIOLOGICAS
CASILLA DE CORREO NO 1.076 SUBCENT
MONTEVIDEO, URUGUAY

UNITED STATES

ALABAMA

489.00   B-DFJVY
FINLEY, WAYNE H.
LABORATORY OF MEDICAL GENETICS
UNIVERSITY OF ALABAMA MEDICAL
   CENTER
BIRMINGHAM, AL
35294   PHONE 205 934-4968

ALASKA

490.00   CDFHJ
AASE, JON M.
DYSMORPHOLOGY UNIT
1135 WEST 8TH AVENUE, SUITE 3
ANCHORAGE, AK
99501   PHONE 274-1842

491.00   B-DFHJX
LYONS, RICHARD B.
PUBLIC HEALTH SERVICE GENETICS
   CLINICS
UNIVERSITY OF ALASKA
BOX 95753
FAIRBANKS, AK
99701   PHONE 479-7731

ARIZONA

492.00   CDFJKW
COHEN, MELVIN L.
GENETIC COUNSELING CENTER
ST. JOSEPHS HOSPITAL AND MEDICAL
   CENTER
P.O. BOX 2071
PHOENIX, AZ
85001

493.00 CJOP
WOOLF, CHARLES M.
DEPARTMENT OF ZOOLOGY
ARIZONA STATE UNIVERSITY
TEMPE, AZ
85281

494.00 B-DFJKRWY
GILES, HARLAN R.
COLLEGE OF MEDICINE, OBSTETRICS AND
GYNECOLOGY
UNIVERSITY OF ARIZONA
TUCSON, AZ
85724

ARKANSAS

495.00 CDFHJKWY
MERRILL, ROBERT E.
BIRTH DEFECTS CENTER
UNIVERSITY OF ARKANSAS
4301 MARKHAM
LITTLE ROCK, AR
72201 PHONE MO4-5000 EXT. 274

CALIFORNIA

496.00 B-DFHJWX
DAENTL, DONNA
GENETIC COUNSELING CLINIC
KERN COUNTY HEALTH DEPARTMENT
1700 FLOWER STREET
BAKERSFIELD, CA
93305

498.00 J
STERN, CURT
DEPARTMENT OF ZOOLOGY
UNIVERSITY OF CALIFORNIA
BERKELEY, CA
94720 PHONE 415 642-2919

499.00 B-DF-NS-Y
COMINGS, DAVID E.
DEPARTMENT OF MEDICAL GENETICS
CITY OF HOPE MEDICAL CENTER
DUARTE, CA
91010 PHONE 359-8111 EXT. 220

501.00 CDFHJ
HALL, BRYAN D.
GENETIC COUNSELING CLINIC
VALLEY CHILDREN¤S HOSPITAL
3151 NORTH MILLBROOK
FRESNO, CA
93703 PHONE 209 227-2961

502.00 J
BARISH, NATALIE
DEPARTMENT OF BIOLOGY
CALIFORNIA STATE COLLEGE AT
FULLERTON
FULLERTON, CA
92631 PHONE 714 870-2546

503.00 CDFJKY
WEINSTEIN, DAVID
DEPARTMENT OF PEDIATRICS
SOUTHERN CALIFORNIA PERMANENTE
MEDICAL GROUP
1050 WEST PACIFIC COAST HIGHWAY
HARBOR CITY, CA
90710 PHONE 213 325-5111

504.00 CDFHJ-WY
DUMARS, KENNETH W.
DEPARTMENT OF PEDIATRICS, GENETICS
CLINIC
UNIVERSITY OF CALIFORNIA AT IRVINE
IRVINE, CA
92650 PHONE 714 633-9393 EXT. 150

505.00 B-FJMNVY
JONES, OLIVER W.
MEDICAL GENETICS UNIT
UNIVERSITY OF CALIFORNIA, SCHOOL OF
MEDICINE
LA JOLLA, CA
92037 PHONE 714 453-2000 EXT.
2523

506.00 B-DFH-JMNSY
NYHAN, WILLIAM L.
BIOCHEMICAL GENETICS LABORATORY
UNIVERSITY OF CALIFORNIA, SCHOOL OF
MEDICINE
LA JOLLA, CA
92037

507.00 B-DIJMWXY
O¤BRIEN, JOHN S.
NEUROSCIENCES DEPARTMENT
UNIVERSITY OF CALIFORNIA, SCHOOL OF
MEDICINE
LA JOLLA, CA
92037 PHONE 714 453-2000 EXT.
2242

508.00 J
SCHNEIDERMAN, L.J.
DEPARTMENT OF COMMUNITY MEDICINE
SAN DIEGO COUNTY PUBLIC HEALTH
CLINICS
UNIVERSITY OF CALIFORNIA AT SAN
DIEGO
LA JOLLA, CA
92037 PHONE 714 453-2000 EXT.
1792

509.00 A-DF-HJP-RTXY
CENTERWALL, WILLARD R.
DEPARTMENT OF PEDIATRICS
GENETICS, BIRTH DEFECTS, AND
CHROMOSOME SERVICE
LOMA LINDA UNIVERSITY MEDICAL
CENTER
LOMA LINDA, CA
92354

511.00 B-DF-HJN
ALFI, OMAR S.
DIVISION OF MEDICAL GENETICS
CHILDREN¤S HOSPITAL OF LOS ANGELES
4650 SUNSET BOULEVARD
LOS ANGELES, CA
90054 PHONE 213 663-3341 EXT.
2603

512.00 B-FHJKSY
CRANDALL, BARBARA F.
DEPARTMENT OF PEDIATRICS AND
PSYCHIATRY
UNIVERSITY OF CALIFORNIA, CENTER
FOR THE HEALTH SCIENCES
760 WESTWOOD PLAZA
LOS ANGELES, CA
90024 PHONE 213 825-0109

513.00 B-DFGHJN
DONNELL, GEORGE N.
DIVISION OF MEDICAL GENETICS
CHILDREN¤S HOSPITAL OF LOS ANGELES
4650 SUNSET BOULEVARD
LOS ANGELES, CA
90054 PHONE 213 663-3341 EXT.
2603

514.00 B-DFHJRTWY
EBBIN, ALLAN J.
L.A. COUNTY-USC MEDICAL CENTER
GENETICS BIRTH DEFECTS CENTER
1200 NORTH STATE STREET
LOS ANGELES, CA
90033 PHONE 213 225-3115 EXT.
73881

515.00 ADFJQT
JARVIK, L.F.
DEPARTMENT OF PSYCHIATRY
U.C.L.A.
760 WESTWOOD PLAZA
LOS ANGELES, CA
90024

516.00 B-DFJKY
KAROW, WILLIAM G.
DEPARTMENT OF MEDICAL GENETICS
SOUTHERN CALIFORNIA FERTILITY
INSTITUTE
12300 WILSHIRE BOULEVARD
LOS ANGELES, CA
90025 PHONE 213 826-8313

518.00 B-FHJ-LNPQSVY
SPARKES, ROBERT S.
DEPARTMENTS OF MEDICINE AND
PEDIATRICS
UCLA SCHOOL OF MEDICINE
760 WESTWOOD PLACE
LOS ANGELES, CA
90024 PHONE 213 825-5720

520.00 B-DFHJLNRSWY
WILSON, MIRIAM G.
DEPARTMENT OF PEDIATRICS
UNIVERSITY OF SOUTHERN CALIFORNIA
MEDICAL SCHOOL
1200 NORTH STATE STREET
LOS ANGELES, CA
90033

521.00 CDFHJK
BACHMAN, RONALD
DEPARTMENTS OF PEDIATRICS AND
GENETICS
KAISER FOUNDATION HOSPITAL
280 WEST MACARTHUR BOULEVARD
OAKLAND, CA
94611 PHONE 415 645-5816

522.00 CFJW
SHERMAN, SANFORD
DEPARTMENT OF BIRTH DEFECTS
MEDICAL CENTER
CHILDREN¤S HOSPITAL
OAKLAND, CA
94609 PHONE 415 654-5600

523.00 J
ROSENFELD, MARTIN
REGIONAL CENTER FOR MENTALLY
RETARDED
1109 WEST LA VETA AVENUE
ORANGE, CA
92666

524.00 B-DFHJKNQRW-Y
BASS, HAROLD N.
DEPARTMENT OF PEDIATRICS
KAISER-PERMANENTE MEDICAL CENTER
13652 CANTARA STREET
PANORAMA CITY, CA
91402 PHONE 213 781-2361

526.00 CDFJX
EPSTEIN, CHARLES J.
GENETIC EVALUATION AND COUNSELING
CLINIC
ROSS GENERAL HOSPITAL
1150 SIR FRANCIS DRAKE BOULEVARD
ROSS, CA
94957 PHONE 415 666-2981

527.00 CFJ
ABILDGAARD, CHARLES F.
SACRAMENTO MEDICAL CENTER
2315 STOCKTON BOULEVARD
SACRAMENTO, CA
95817

528.00* A-DFJK
ALLEN, IRVING E.
DEPARTMENT OF PEDIATRICS
ST. BERNARDINE¤S HOSPITAL
SAN BERNARDINO, CA
92404

529.00 FJK
DESANTO, DOMINI A.
MERCY HOSPITAL AND MEDICAL CENTER
CLINIC
4077 FIFTH AVENUE
SAN DIEGO, CA
92103 PHONE 714 298-4141

530.00 B-DFHJW-Y
FRYE, FREDERICK A.
BIRTH DEFECTS CENTER
CHILDRENS HEALTH CENTER
8001 FROST STREET
SAN DIEGO, CA
92123 PHONE 714 277-5808

531.00*   A-DFJ-NQRWY
GLUCK, LOUIS
SAN DIEGO COUNTY
UNIVERSITY HOSPITAL
P.O. BOX 3548
SAN DIEGO, CA
92103   PHONE 453-2000 EXT. 2587

532.00   B-DFHJUW-Y
PETERSON, RAYMOND
CHILD DEVELOPMENT CENTER
SAN DIEGO REGIONAL CENTER FOR THE
 MENTALLY RETARDED
8001 FROST STREET
SAN DIEGO, CA
92123   PHONE 277-5808 EXT. 203 OR
                                     209

533.00   B-DFGIJY
EPSTEIN, CHARLES J.
DEPARTMENT OF PEDIATRICS
UNIVERSITY OF CALIFORNIA
SAN FRANCISCO, CA
94143

534.00   B-DFJY
GRUMBACH, MELVIN M.
DEPARTMENT OF PEDIATRICS
UNIVERSITY OF CALIFORNIA
SAN FRANCISCO, CA
94143   PHONE 415 666-2101

539.00   CDFJ
EPSTEIN, CHARLES
GENETIC COUNSELING CLINIC
SANTA BARBARA COUNTY HEALTH
 DEPARTMENT
4440 CALLE REAL
SANTA BARBARA, CA
93105   PHONE 805 965-1619

540.00   CDFHJY
MANN, JOHN
PEDIATRICS CLINIC
KAISER HOSPITAL
900 KIELY BOULEVARD
SANTA CLARA, CA
95051

541.00   JKW
HOLVE, LESLIE M.
ST. JOHN°S HOSPITAL
1328 22ND STREET
SANTA MONICA, CA
90404   PHONE 829-5511 EXT. 745

542.00   B-FHJKPQSWY
CANN, HOWARD M.
DEPARTMENT OF PEDIATRICS
STANDFORD UNIVERSITY SCHOOL OF
 MEDICINE
STANFORD, CA
94605   PHONE 415 321-1200 EXT.
                                     5997

543.00   B-FHJ-LW-Y
LUZZATTI, LUIGI
DEPARTMENT OF PEDIATRICS
BIRTH DEFECTS CENTER
STANFORD UNIVERSITY MEDICAL CENTER
STANFORD, CA
94305   PHONE 415 321-1200 EXT.
                                     5358

544.00   B-DF-NQV-Y
RIMOIN, DAVID L.
DIVISION OF MEDICAL GENETICS
HARBOR GENERAL HOSPITAL
1000 WEST CARSON STREET
TORRANCE, CA
90509   PHONE 213 328-2380

546.00   CDHJX
WEBER, FELICE
VENTURA COUNTY HEALTH DEPARTMENT
GENETIC COUNSELING CENTER
VENTURA, CA
93001

  COLORADO

549.00   B-FH-MPRW-Y
O°BRIEN, DONOUGH
DEPARTMENT OF PEDIATRICS

UNIVERSITY OF COLORADO
4200 EAST 9TH AVENUE
DENVER, CO
80220   PHONE 303 394-7430

550.00   CDFJKV
REIQUAM, C.W.
DEPARTMENT OF PATHOLOGY
PRESBYTERIAN MEDICAL CENTER
DENVER, CO
80218

551.00   B-FH-NQ-SV-Y
ROBINSON, ARTHUR
DEPARTMENTS OF BIOPHYSICS AND
 GENETICS, BIRTH DEFECTS CENTER
UNIVERSITY OF COLORADO MEDICAL
 CENTER
4200 EAST 9TH AVENUE
DENVER, CO
80220   PHONE 303 394-7919

552.00   CHJKO-QSTW
SIEMENS, GEORGE J.
DEPARTMENT OF HUMAN GENETICS
UNIVERSITY OF COLORADO
1100 FOURTEENTH STREET
DENVER, CO
80202   PHONE 892-1117 EXT. 205

554.00   FJPV
WINCHESTER, A.M.
DEPARTMENT OF BIOLOGY
UNIVERSITY OF NORTHERN COLORADO
GREELEY, CO
80631

  CONNECTICUT

556.00   B-DF-RT-Y
GREENSTEIN, ROBERT M.
DEPARTMENT OF PEDIATRICS,
 CYTOGENETICS LABORATORY
UNIVERSITY OF CONNECTICUT SCHOOL OF
 MEDICINE
2 HOLCOMB STREET
HARTFORD, CT
06111   PHONE 203 243-2531 EXT. 351

557.00   A-EJPQVWX
HONEYMAN, MERTON S.
DEPARTMENT OF HEALTH
CONNECTICUT TWIN REGISTRY
79 ELM STREET
HARTFORD, CT
06115

558.00   A-FJKMPR-TWY
ROSENBERG, LEON
DEPARTMENTS OF HUMAN GENETICS
YALE MEDICAL SCHOOL
NEW HAVEN, CT
06520   PHONE 203 436-3654

560.00   FJU
MICKEY, GEORGE
DEPARTMENT OF CYTOGENETICS
NEW ENGLAND INSTITUTE FOR MEDICAL
 RESEARCH
P.O. BOX 308
RIDGEFIELD, CT
06877   PHONE 203 438-6591

  DELAWARE

562.00   CDFHJY
ROSENBLUM, HERMAN
DEPARTMENT OF PEDIATRICS
WILMINGTON MEDICAL CENTER
P.O. BOX 1668
WILMINGTON, DE
19899

  DIST. OF COLUMBIA

563.00   C-FHJLPRUW-Y
BAUMILLER, ROBERT
UNIVERSITY AFFILIATED CENTER FOR
 CHILD DEVELOPMENT

GEORGETOWN UNIVERSITY MEDICAL
 CENTER
3900 RESERVOIR ROAD, N.W.
WASHINGTON, DC

564.00   A-DFHJKNP-R
CLAYTON, ROBERT J.
DEPARTMENTS OF PEDIATRICS AND
 OBSTETRICS
GEORGETOWN UNIVERSITY HOSPITAL
3800 RESERVOIR ROAD, N.W.
WASHINGTON, DC
20007

565.00   B-DFJ
FREEMAN, MAHLON V.R.
DEPARTMENT OF OBSTETRICS-GYNECOLOGY
ARMED FORCES INSTITUTE OF PATHOLOGY
WALTER REED GENERAL HOSPITAL
WASHINGTON, DC
20306   PHONE 202 576-2934

568.00   CDFJY
JACOBSON, CECIL B.
DEPARTMENT OF OBSTETRICS,
 GYNECOLOGY AND REPRODUCTIVITY
THE GEORGE WASHINGTON UNIVERSITY
 CLINIC
2150 PENN AVENUE, N.W.
WASHINGTON, DC
20037   PHONE 202 331-6186

570.00   B-DFHJKNQX
MURRAY, JR., ROBERT F.
DEPARTMENT OF PEDIATRICS
HOWARD UNIVERSITY COLLEGE OF
 MEDICINE
DIVISION OF MEDICAL GENETICS
WASHINGTON, DC
20001   PHONE 202 797-1766

571.00   B-DFH-KW-Y
PLATT, MARK
DEPARTMENT OF NEUROLOGY
CHILDREN°S HOSPITAL
2125 13TH STREET, N.W.
WASHINGTON, DC
20009

  FLORIDA

572.00   B-DFHJKRY
FRIAS, JAIME L.
BIRTH DEFECTS CENTER
J. HILLIS MILLER HEALTH CENTER
GAINESVILLE, FL
32610   PHONE 904 392-2958

573.00   B-FH-KNRY
RENNERT, OWEN M.
DEPARTMENT OF PEDIATRICS
DIVISION OF GENETICS, ENDOCRINOLOGY
 & METABOLICS
SHANDS TEACHING HOSPITAL,
 UNIVERSITY OF FLORIDA
GAINESVILLE, FL
32601   PHONE 305 392-3331

574.00   B-DFHJ-MW-Y
WARREN, RICHARD J.
CYTOGENETICS LABORATORY
MIAMI CENTER FOR CHILD DEVELOPMENT
BOX 6 BISCAYNE ANNEX
MIAMI, FL
33152   PHONE 305 350-6870

  GEORGIA

577.00   AC-HJKO-QS-UX
FALEK, ARTHUR
DEPARTMENT OF PSYCHIATRY
GEORGIA MENTAL HEALTH INSTITUTE
EMORY UNIVERSITY
ATLANTA, GA
30306   PHONE 404 873-6661

578.00   CDJ
FREEMAN, MALCOLM
DIVISION OF PERINATAL PATHOLOGY
EMORY UNIVERSITY SCHOOL OF MEDICINE
80 BUTLER STREET, S.E.
ATLANTA, GA
30303   PHONE 404 659-1212 EXT.
                                     4051

579.00   FJK
GODWIN, JOHN T.
DEPARTMENT OF PATHOLOGY
ST. JOSEPH¤S HOSPITAL
265 IVY STREET, N.E.
ATLANTA, GA
30303

580.00   CFVX
HEATH, JR., CLARK W.
BUREAU OF EPIDEMIOLOGY
CENTER FOR DISEASE CONTROL
1600 CLIFTON ROAD
ATLANTA, GA
30333   PHONE 404 633-3311 EXT.
                                3961

581.00   CDFJQY
BYRD, J. ROGERS
DEPARTMENT OF ENDOCRINOLOGY
MEDICAL COLLEGE OF GEORGIA
AUGUSTA, GA
30902

583.00   CDFJKQY
MCDONOUGH, PAUL G.
DEPARTMENT OF OBSTETRICS AND
 GYNECOLOGY
MEDICAL COLLEGE OF GEORGIA
AUGUSTA, GA
30902

584.00   ADFHJ
KEELER, CLYDE
CENTRAL STATE HOSPITAL
MILLEDGEVILLE, GA
31601

          HAWAII

585.00   CDFHJKPWY
BINTLIFF, SHARON
DEPARTMENT OF BIRTH DEFECTS,
 DEPARTMENT OF PEDIATRICS
KAUIKEOLANI CHILDREN¤S HOSPITAL,
 UNIVERSITY OF HAWAII
HONOLULU, HI
96817   PHONE 531-3511 EXT. 164

586.00   A-HJ-MPVX
MI, M.P.
DEPARTMENT OF GENETICS
UNIVERSITY OF HAWAII SCHOOL OF
 MEDICINE
HONOLULU, HI
96822   PHONE 808 948-8552

587.00   DEJKPS
MORTON, NEWTON E.
POPULATION GENETICS LABORATORY
UNIVERSITY OF HAWAII
2411 DOLE STREET
HONOLULU, HI
96822

          IDAHO

588.00   B-DFHJW
MARKS, J.R.
IDAHO MEDICAL REGIONAL PROGRAM
BOISE, ID
83701

590.00   B-FHJW
MCKEAN, ROBERT S.
MENTAL RETARDATION PROGRAM
IDAHO STATE SCHOOL AND HOSPITAL
BOX 47
NAMPA, ID
83651

          ILLINOIS

591.00   B-DFJ-MY
ALPERN, WILLIAM
AMNIOCENTESIS SERVICE
MICHAEL REESE HOSPITAL AND MEDICAL
 CENTER
530 EAST 31ST STREET
CHICAGO, IL
60616   PHONE 312 791-2261 EXT. 40

592.00   CDFJNT-V
AMAROSE, ANTHONY P.
DEPARTMENTS OF OBSTETRICS AND
 GYNECOLOGY
UNIVERSITY OF CHICAGO
5841 SOUTH MARYLAND AVENUE
CHICAGO, IL
60637   PHONE 312 947-5310

593.00   B-DFHJY
BERMAN, JULIAN L.
DEPARTMENT OF PEDIATRICS
COOK COUNTY HOSPITAL
1825 WEST HARRISON ST.
CHICAGO, IL
60612   PHONE 312 633-7498

594.00   A-FH-Q
CARSON, PAUL E.
DEPARTMENTS OF PHARMACOLOGY AND
 GENETICS
RUSH PRESBYTERIAN-ST. LUKE¤S
 MEDICAL CENTER
CHICAGO, IL
60601

595.00   BCFIJPRWY
DORFMAN, ALBERT
DEPARTMENT OF PEDIATRICS
UNIVERSITY OF CHICAGO
950 EAST 59TH STREET
CHICAGO, IL
60637   PHONE 947-6211

596.00   ACJST
GARRON, DAVID C.
PRESBYTERIAN-ST. LUKE¤S HOSPITAL
1753 W. CONGRESS PARKWAY
CHICAGO, IL
60091   PHONE 312 942-6652

598.00   B-FH-KNRUVXY
KROMPOTIC, EVA
DEPARTMENT OF EXPERIMENTAL
 PATHOLOGY
MOUNT SINAI HOSPITAL MEDICAL CENTER
CALIFORNIA AVENUE AT 15TH STREET
CHICAGO, IL
60608   PHONE 312 542-2469

599.00   BDFIJMY
MATALON, REUBEN
DEPARTMENT OF PEDIATRICS
UNIVERSITY OF CHICAGO
CHICAGO, IL
60637   PHONE 312 947-6344

601.00   B-DFIJMY
NADLER, H.L.
DEPARTMENT OF GENETICS
CHILDREN¤S MEMORIAL HOSPITAL
CHICAGO, IL
60614   PHONE 312 D1 8-4040

602.00   B-DFHJ
SCHULZ, JEANETTE
ILLINOIS STATE PEDIATRIC INSTITUTE
1640 WEST ROOSEVELT ROAD
CHICAGO, IL
60608

603.00   CJ
SINGER, JACK D.
DEPARTMENT OF PEDIATRICS
RESURRECTION HOSPITAL
7435 WEST TALCOTT AVENUE
CHICAGO, IL
60631

604.00   B-DFH-J
SMITH, GEORGE F.
DEPARTMENT OF PEDIATRICS GENETICS
 AND HUMAN DEVELOPMENT SECTION
RUSH - PRESBYTERIAN SAINT LUKE¤S
 MEDICAL SCHOOL
1750 WEST HARRISON STREET
CHICAGO, IL
60612

605.00   B-DFH-KRW
BURNS, DONALD C.
DEPARTMENT OF RESEARCH
EVANSTON HOSPITAL
2650 RIDGE AVENUE
EVANSTON, IL
60201   PHONE 312 492-6486

606.00   A-DGHJ-LQ
COHEN, CARL
DEPARTMENT OF ZOOLOGY
UNIVERSITY OF ILLINOIS, CENTER FOR
 GENETICS
URBANA, IL
61801   PHONE 996-4970

607.00   A-DFJP
DANIEL, WILLIAM L.
GENETICS COUNSELING SERVICE
SCHOOL OF BASIC MEDICAL SCIENCES
UNIVERSITY OF ILLINOIS
URBANA, IL
61801   PHONE 217 333-8172

          INDIANA

608.00   B-HJ-NPQSY
MERRITT, A. DONALD
DEPARTMENT OF MEDICAL GENETICS
INDIANA UNIVERSITY MEDICAL SCHOOL
INDIANAPOLIS, IN
46207

          IOWA

612.00   B-DFHJ-NW-Y
ZELLWEGER, HANS
DEPARTMENT OF PEDIATRICS
UNIVERSITY HOSPITAL
IOWA CITY, IA
52240   PHONE 319 356-2674

          KANSAS

614.00   B-DFIJNVY
SCHIMKE, R.N.
DEPARTMENT OF MEDICINE
KANSAS UNIVERSITY MEDICAL CENTER
KANSAS CITY, KS
66103   PHONE 913 236-5252

615.00   B-DFJKVY
GRAY, DAVID E.
THE LATTIMORE-FINK LABORATORIES,
 INC.
MEDICAL ARTS BUILDING, WEST
WEST 10TH STREET
TOPEKA, KS
66604

616.00   BCFI-MRV
CAWLEY, LEO P.
DEPARTMENT OF CLINICAL PATHOLOGY
WESLEY MEDICAL RESEARCH FOUNDATION
WICHITA, KS
67214

          KENTUCKY

618.00   ACDJPTVX
ABRAMSON, FREDRIC
DEPARTMENT OF COMMUNITY MEDICINE
UNIVERSITY OF KENTUCKY MEDICAL
 CENTER
LEXINGTON, KY
40506

619.00   B-DFJKM
MABRY, C.C.
DEPARTMENT OF PEDIATRICS
UNIVERSITY OF KENTUCKY MEDICAL
 CENTER
LEXINGTON, KY
40506

622.00   A-DF-HJTWY
WEISSKOPF, BERNARD
CHILD EVALUATION CENTER
UNIVERSITY OF LOUISVILLE MEDICAL
 SCHOOL
540 SOUTH PRESTON STREET
LOUISVILLE, KY
40202   PHONE 584-6197

          LOUISIANA

623.00   CDFHJKMPVW
ANDERSON, ESTHER E.

DEPARTMENT OF PEDIATRICS, HERITABLE
DISEASE EVALUATION CENTER
LOUISIANA STATE UNIVERSITY, SCHOOL
OF MEDICINE
1542 TULANE AVENUE
NEW ORLEANS, LA
70112   PHONE 504 527-8233

625.00   AC-FH-KO-QSTV
KLOEPFER, H.W.
DEPARTMENT OF ANATOMY
TULANE UNIVERSITY
NEW ORLEANS, LA
70112

626.00   B-DFHJMP
THURMON, T.F.
DEPARTMENT OF PEDIATRICS, HERITABLE
DISEASE CENTER
LOUISIANA STATE UNIVERSITY, SCHOOL
OF MEDICINE
1542 TULANE AVENUE
NEW ORLEANS, LA
70112   PHONE 504 527-8233

627.00   C-FHJKO-QXY
JUBERG, RICHARD C.
DEPARTMENT OF PEDIATRICS
L.S.U. SCHOOL OF MEDICINE IN
SHREVEPORT, BIRTH DEFECTS CENTER
P.O. BOX 3932
SHREVEPORT, LA
71130   PHONE 318 635-6495

MAINE

628.00*   J
VAN PELT, JOHN C.
MAINE GENETIC COUNSELING CENTER
50 UNION STREET
ELLSWORTH, ME
04605

629.00   CDJ
STOCKS, JOSEPH F.
BIRTH DEFECTS CLINIC
MAINE MEDICAL CENTER
22 BRAMHALL STREET
PORTLAND, ME
04101

MARYLAND

631.00   BKLPQSV
BIAS, W.B.
IMMUNOGENETICS LABORATORY
JOHN HOPKINS UNIVERSITY SCHOOL OF
MEDICINE
BALTIMORE, MD
21205   PHONE 301 955-3600

632.00   B-DFJW
BURGAN, PAUL
DEPARTMENT OF PEDIATRICS
SINAI HOSPITAL
BALTIMORE, MD
21215   PHONE 301 367-7800 EXT.
                                   8630

633.00   B-LPQSVY
MCKUSICK, VICTOR A.
THE MOORE CLINIC
THE JOHNS HOPKINS HOSPITAL
BALTIMORE, MD
21205

634.00   BDFJ
THOMAS, GEORGE H.
HUMAN GENETICS LABORATORY
JOHN F. KENNEDY INSTITUTE
707 NORTH BROADWAY
BALTIMORE, MD
21205   PHONE 301 955-4173

636.00   AC-EHJ-LN-TX
MYRIANTHOPOULOS, N.C.
NATIONAL INSTITUTE OF NEUROLOGICAL
DISEASES AND STROKE
NATIONAL INSTITUTES OF HEALTH
BETHESDA, MD
20014   PHONE 301 496-5821

MASSACHUSETTS

642.00   BDJM
BADEN, HOWARD P.
DEPARTMENT OF DERMATOLOGY,
CUTANEOUS GENETICS UNIT
MASSACHUSETTS GENERAL HOSPITAL
32 FRUIT STREET
BOSTON, MA
02114   PHONE 617 726-3993

644.00   A-FHJ-OQRTW-Y
COCHRAN, WILLIAM
BOSTON HOSPITAL FOR WOMEN
221 LONGWOOD AVENUE
BOSTON, MA
02115

645.00   C-HJKY
FEINGOLD, MURRAY
CENTER FOR GENETIC COUNSELING AND
BIRTH DEFECT EVALUATION
TUFTS--NEW ENGLAND MEDICAL CENTER
171 HARRISON AVENUE
BOSTON, MA
02111

646.00   A-DFJ-LSY
GERALD, P.S.
CLINICAL GENETICS DIVISION
CHILDREN₅S HOSPITAL MEDICAL CENTER
BOSTON, MA
02115   PHONE 617 734-6000 EXT. 35

650.00   CDF-HJW
PASHAYAN, HERMINE M.
BIRTH DEFECT EVALUATION CENTER AND
CLEFT PALATE CENTER
TUFTS-NEW ENGLAND MEDICAL CENTER
HOSPITAL
NO. HARRISON AVE.
BOSTON, MA
02111   PHONE 617 482-2800

651.00   BDEJMPQ
SOELDNER, J. STUART
E.P. JOSLIN RESEARCH LABORATORY
170 PILGRIM ROAD
BOSTON, MA
02215

652.00   A-DFHJMNPTVXY
TISHLER, PETER V.
DEPARTMENT OF PEDIATRICS
HARVARD MEDICAL UNIT
BOSTON CITY HOSPITAL
BOSTON, MA
02118   PHONE 617 424-4757

656.00   B-KMRW-Y
MILUNSKY, AUBREY
GENETICS LABORATORY
EUNICE KENNEDY SHRIVER CENTER
200 TRAPELO TOAD
WALTHAM, MA
02154   PHONE 617 893-4909

MICHIGAN

658.00   B-DFJUY
BLOOM, ARTHUR D.
DEPARTMENT OF HUMAN GENETICS
UNIVERSITY OF MICHIGAN
1137 E. CATHERINE STREET
ANN ARBOR, MI
48104   PHONE 212 579-2934

661.00   B-DF-QSWY
NEEL, JAMES
DEPARTMENT OF HUMAN GENETICS
UNIVERSITY OF MICHIGAN
ANN ARBOR, MI
48108   PHONE 313 763-2532

662.00   B-DFJWY
SCHMICKEL, ROY
DEPARTMENT OF PEDIATRICS
UNIVERSITY OF MICHIGAN MEDICAL
CENTER
ANN ARBOR, MI
48104

663.00   J
FORSTHOEFEL, PAULINUS F.

DEPARTMENT OF BIOLOGY
UNIVERSITY OF DETROIT
DETROIT, MI
48221   PHONE 313 342-1000

664.00   B-DFJPY
KOEN, ANN
BIRTH DEFECTS CENTER, DEPARTMENT
GYNECOLOGY AND OBSTETRICS
WAYNE STATE UNIVERSITY SCHOOL OF
MEDICINE
275 EAST HANCOCK
DETROIT, MI
48201

665.00   B-DFHJ-LRST
WEISS, LESTER
DEPARTMENT OF PEDIATRICS
HENRY FORD HOSPITAL
2799 WEST GRAND BOULEVARD
DETROIT, MI
48202   PHONE 313 876-3121

666.00   B-DJV
BAUGHMAN, JR., FRED A.
PEDIATRIC NEURO-MUSCULAR DISEASE
CLINIC
BLODGETT MEMORIAL HOSPITAL
1810 WEALTHY S.E.
GRAND RAPIDS, MI
49506   PHONE 616 454-5951

668.00   CFJQV
REIMER, SUSAN
BUTTERWORTH HOSPITAL
GRAND RAPIDS, MI
49503

669.00   B-DFHJOPQW
HIGGINS, JAMES V.
DEPARTMENT OF ZOOLOGY
MICHIGAN STATE UNIVERSITY
LANSING, MI
48901   PHONE 517 353-4520

670.00   B-DF-HJKW
BERKER, ISAK O.
DEPARTMENT OF MENTAL HEALTH
LAPEER STATE HOME AND TRAINING
SCHOOL
LAPEER, MI
48446   PHONE 313 664-2951

671.00*   B-DFHJLO
WEIR, HOMER
DEPARTMENT OF MENTAL HEALTH
PLYMOUTH STATE HOME AND TRAINING
SCHOOL
NORTHVILLE, MI
48167   PHONE 313 453-1500 EXT. 32

672.00   DFIJUVY
SAADI, A. AL
DEPARTMENT OF ANATOMIC PATHOLOGY
WILLIAM BEAUMONT HOSPITAL
ROYAL OAK, MI
48072   PHONE 313 549-7000 EXT. 675

MINNESOTA

673.00   CDFGJVY
CERVENKA, JAROSLAV
CYTOGENETIC LABORATORY AND GENETIC
CLINIC
SCHOOL OF DENTISTRY AND HEALTH
SCIENCE CENTER
UNIVERSITY OF MINNESOTA
MINNEAPOLIS, MN
55455

674.00   B-DI-KY
DESNICK, R.J.
DEPARTMENT OF PEDIATRICS
UNIVERSITY OF MINNESOTA HOSPITAL
BOX 231, MAYO
MINNEAPOLIS, MN
55455   PHONE 612 373-4529

675.00   B-DF-HJY
GORLIN, ROBERT J.
HUMAN GENETICS CLINIC
UNIVERSITY OF MINNESOTA HOSPITAL
MINNEAPOLIS, MN
55455

676.00   ABDFJPQ
REED, SHELDON C.
DIGHT INSTITUTE FOR HUMAN GENETICS
UNIVERSITY OF MINNESOTA
MINNEAPOLIS, MN
55455

677.00   B-DFHJQXY
SCHACHT, LEE E.
HUMAN GENETICS UNIT
MINNESOTA DEPARTMENT OF HEALTH
MINNEAPOLIS, MN
55440   PHONE 612 378-1150 EXT. 26

678.00   B-DFGI-KPY
WITKOP, CARL
SCHOOL OF DENTISTRY
UNIVERSITY OF MINNESOTA
MINNEAPOLIS, MN
55415   PHONE 612 373-5006

679.00   B-DFHJMVY
YUNIS, JORGE J.
DEPARTMENT OF LABORATORY MEDICINE
 AND PATHOLOGY
MEDICAL GENETICS DIVISION
UNIVERSITY OF MINNESOTA HOSPITAL
MINNEAPOLIS, MN
55415   PHONE 373-8635

680.00   BDFHJNPQVX
GORDON, HYMIE
GENETICS CONSULTING SERVICE
MAYO CLINIC
200 1ST STREET, S.W.
ROCHESTER, MN
55901   PHONE 507 282-2511

MISSISSIPPI

682.00   B-DFHJK
EDWARDS, ROBERT H.
HUMAN GENETICS SERVICE
KEESLER USAF MEDICAL CENTER
BILOXI, MS
39534   PHONE 601 377-6546

683.00   B-FI-LPRUVXY
JACKSON, JOHN F.
DEPARTMENT OF PREVENTIVE MEDICINE
UNIVERSITY OF MISSISSIPPI MEDICAL
 CENTER
2500 NORTH STATE STREET
JACKSON, MS
39216   PHONE 601 362-4411

MISSOURI

684.00   B-DFJK
BROOKE, CLEMENT E.
DEPARTMENT OF PEDIATRICS
UNIVERSITY OF MISSOURI MEDICAL
 CENTER
COLUMBIA, MO
65201   PHONE 314 442-5111

686.00   CDFJR
FRANCISCO, C.B.
NEUROLOGY DEPARTMENT
CHILDREN¤S MERCY HOSPITAL
KANSAS CITY, MO
64108   PHONE 816 471-0626

687.00   B-DFHJY
MONTELEONE, PATRICIA L.
CARDINAL GLENNON HOSPITAL
1465 SOUTH GRAND BOULEVARD
ST. LOUIS, MO
63104   PHONE 314 865-4000

688.00   B-DFHJ-LNQSTWY
SLY, WILLIAM S.
DEPARTMENT OF PEDIATRICS AND
 MEDICINE, DIVISION OF MEDICAL GEN.
ST. LOUIS CHILDREN¤S HOSPITAL &
 WASHINGTON UNIVERSITY MEDICAL SCH.
500 SOUTH KINGSHIGHWAY BOULEVARD
ST. LOUIS, MO
63110   PHONE 314 367-6880 EXT. 35

690.00   B-DFHJY
VOLK, SISTER LEO RITA
DEPARTMENT OF CYTOGENETICS

SAINT MARY¤S HEALTH CENTER
6420 CLAYTON ROAD
ST. LOUIS, MO
63117   PHONE 314 644-3000

MONTANA

691.00   B-DF-HJOTWX
PALLISTER, PHILIP
BOULDER RIVER SCHOOL AND HOSPITAL
BOULDER, MT
59632

NEBRASKA

692.00   A-DF-JMW
AMATO, R. STEPHEN
DEPARTMENT OF PEDIATRICS
UNIVERSITY OF NEBRASKA MEDICAL
 CENTER, MOLECULAR GENETICS LAB.
OMAHA, NE
68105   PHONE 541-4612 OR 541-4633

693.00   B-DFJWY
EISEN, JAMES D.
UNIVERSITY OF NEBRASKA MEDICAL
 CENTER
42ND AND DEWEY AVENUE
OMAHA, NE
68105   PHONE 402 541-4570

694.00   B-DFHJKWX
LOMBARDO, A.J.
BIRTH DEFECTS CLINIC
CHILDREN¤S MEMORIAL HOSPITAL
OMAHA, NE
68105

695.00   AC-EJTV-X
LYNCH, H.T.
DEPARTMENT OF PREVENTIVE MEDICINE
CREIGHTON UNIVERSITY SCHOOL OF
 MEDICINE
2500 CALIFORNIA STREET
OMAHA, NE
68178   PHONE 402 536-2942

696.00   B-DFHJKMO-QSWY
MYERS, TERRY L.
CENTER FOR GENETIC EVALUATION
CHILDREN¤S MEMORIAL HOSPITAL
44TH AND DEWEY
OMAHA, NE
68105   PHONE 402 553-5400

NEW HAMPSHIRE

697.00   B-DFHJ-NQSWY
HOEFNAGEL, D.
DEPARTMENT OF MATERNAL AND CHILD
 HEALTH
DARTMOUTH-HITCHCOCK MEDICAL CENTER
HANOVER, NH
03755   PHONE 603 646-2734

NEW JERSEY

699.00   B-DFHJKV
HUDSON, PHOEBE
HACKENSACK HOSPITAL ASSOCIATION
CHILD EVALUATION CENTER
251 ATLANTIC STREET
HACKENSACK, NJ
07601   PHONE 201 487-4000 EXT. 555

703.00   B-DFHJW
KUSHNICK, THEODORE
DEPARTMENT OF PEDIATRICS
NEW JERSEY COLLEGE OF MEDICINE AT
 NEWARK
100 BERGEN STREET
NEWARK, NJ
07103   PHONE 201 877-4499

NEW YORK

706.00   A-RVXY
PORTER, IAN H.
DEPARTMENT OF PEDIATRICS, NY STATE
 DEPARTMENT OF HEALTH

BIRTH DEFECTS INSTITUTE
ALBANY MEDICAL COLLEGE, ROOM MS234
ALBANY, NY
12208

707.00   CDFJ-LQRUVY
DOSIK, HARVEY
DIVISION OF HEMATOLOGY
JEWISH HOSPITAL OF BROOKLYN
555 PROSPECT PLACE
BROOKLYN, NY
11238   PHONE 240-1211

708.00   BDFJ
FELDMAN, FELIX
PEDIATRIC SERVICE
CONEY ISLAND HOSPITAL
OCEAN PARKWAY AND AVENUE Z
BROOKLYN, NY
11235   PHONE 212 743-4100

710.00   CDFHJ
QAZI, QUTUB H.
DEPARTMENT OF PEDIATRICS
DOWNSTATE MEDICAL CENTER
450 CLARKSON AVENUE
BROOKLYN, NY
11203

711.00   B-DFIJMPW-Y
SCHNECK, LARRY
BIRTH DEFECTS
 CENTER-SPHINGOLIPIDOSES
ISAAC ALBERT RESEARCH INST.,
 KINGSBROOK JEWISH MED. CENTER
86 EAST 49TH STREET
BROOKLYN, NY
11203   PHONE 212 756-9700 EXT.
                               2628

712.00   CDFJ
SCHUTTA, EDWARD J.
DEPARTMENT OF PEDIATRICS
BROOKDALE HOSPITAL MEDICAL CENTER
LINDEN BOULEVARD AT BROOKDALE PLAZA
BROOKLYN, NY
11212   PHONE 212 240-5883

715.00   DFJ
STIEFEL, FREDERICK H.
PEDIATRICS SERVICE
CONEY ISLAND HOSPITAL
OCEAN & SHORE PARKWAYS
BROOKLYN, NY
11235   PHONE 212 743-4100

716.00   CDFJY
VALENTI, CARLO
DEPARTMENT OF OBSTETRICS AND
 GYNECOLOGY
STATE UNIVERSITY OF NEW YORK,
 DOWNSTATE MEDICAL CENTER
450 CLARKSON AVENUE
BROOKLYN, NY
11203   PHONE 212 270-2066

717.00   B-DFIJMPSW-Y
VOLK, BRUNO W.
ISAAC ALBERT RESEARCH INSTITUTE
KINGSBROOK JEWISH MEDICAL CENTER
RUTLAND ROAD AND EAST 49TH STREET
BROOKLYN, NY
11203   PHONE 212 756-9700 EXT.
                          2601-2602

718.00   B-DFJ-LY
WEXLER, IRVING B.
DEPARTMENT OF PEDIATRICS
JEWISH HOSPITAL AND MEDICAL CENTER
 OF BROOKLYN
GREENPOINT AFFILIATION
BROOKLYN, NY
11211   PHONE 212 387-3010 EXT.
                          341, 412

719.00   BDJ-LPQSX
WIENER, ALEXANDER S.
64 RUTLAND ROAD
BROOKLYN, NY
11225

720.00   BDFHJKPSW
BANNERMAN, R.M.
DEPARTMENT OF MEDICINE
BUFFALO GENERAL HOSPITAL

100 HIGH STREET
BUFFALO, NY
14203   PHONE 716 845-6467

721.00   B-FHJ-LNPRSWY
CORTNER, JEAN A.
DEPARTMENT OF PEDIATRICS
STATE UNIVERSITY OF NEW YORK
CHILDRENᵤS HOSPITAL
BUFFALO, NY
14222

722.00   B-FJ-LNPRSWY
DAVIDSON, RONALD G.
DEPARTMENT OF PEDIATRICS
STATE UNIVERSITY OF NEW YORK AT
  BUFFALO
CHILDRENᵤS HOSPITAL
BUFFALO, NY
14222

724.00   CDFH-LRWX
SHERMAN, JACK
GENETICS UNIT, DEPARTMENT OF
  PEDIATRICS
NASSAU COUNTY MEDICAL CENTER
P.O. BOX 175
EAST MEADOW, NY
11554   PHONE 542-0123 EXT. 2356

725.00   ABDFIJNTWX
WHITTIER, JOHN R.
CLINICAL SCIENCES DIVISION
CREEDMOOR INSTITUTE
STATION 60
JAMAICA, NY
11427   PHONE 212 464-7500

726.00   B-DF-HJKOWY
MIRKINSON, ARTHUR E.
GENETICS LABORATORY
NORTH SHORE HOSPITAL
MANHASSET, L.I., NY
11030   PHONE 516 562-2458

727.00   B-DFHJKY
PERGAMENT, EUGENE
DEPARTMENT OF PEDIATRICS
DIVISION OF HUMAN GENETICS
LONG ISLAND JEWISH--HILLSIDE
  MEDICAL CENTER
NEW HYDE PARK, NY
11040   PHONE 212 343-6700

729.00   A-DFHJT-VY
BARTALOS, MIHALY
14 EAST 60 STREET
NEW YORK, NY
10022

730.00   B-DFHJLY
BEARN, ALEXANDER G.
DIVISION OF HUMAN GENETICS
NEW YORK HOSPITAL - CORNELL
  UNIVERSITY MEDICAL CENTER
525 EAST 68TH STREET
NEW YORK, NY
10021

732.00   BCDFHJKW
BINGOL, NESRIN
DEPARTMENT OF PEDIATRICS
NY MEDICAL COLLEGE-FLOWER AND FIFTH
  AVENUE HOSPITAL
5TH AVENUE AT 106 STREET
NEW YORK, NY
10029

733.00   B-DFHJKRTWXY
COOPER, LOUIS Z.
DEPARTMENT OF PEDIATRICS
RUBELLA BIRTH DEFECTS EVALUATION
  PROJECT
NEW YORK UNIVERSITY MEDICAL SCHOOL
NEW YORK, NY
10006   PHONE 212 679-3200 EXT. 35

735.00   JW
FRANCIS, Y. FAY
FOUNDATION FOR REHABILITATION AND
  EDUCATION IN SICKLE CELL DISEASE
423 WEST 120TH STREET
NEW YORK, NY
10027

736.00   CDFJY
GENDEL, EDWARD
DEPARTMENT OF PATHOLOGY
NEW YORK MEDICAL COLLEGE-METRO.
  HOSPITAL
97 STREET AND FIRST AVENUE
NEW YORK, NY
10029   PHONE 360-6454 OR PL 3-3055

737.00   DFJKSV
GERMAN, J.
THE NEW YORK BLOOD CENTER
310 EAST 67TH STREET
NEW YORK, NY
10021   PHONE 212 879-7470

738.00   BCEFH-KMTY
HARRIS, RUTH C. AND COLLEAGUES
DEPARTMENT OF LIVER RESEARCH
BABIES HOSPITAL
3975 BROADWAY
NEW YORK, NY
10032

739.00   B-DFHJ-LQVY
HIRSCHHORN, KURT
DEPARTMENT OF PEDIATRICS
MT. SINAI SCHOOL OF MEDICINE
NEW YORK, NY
10029   PHONE 212 876-1000 EXT. 82

740.00   B-DFJS
KLINGER, H.P.
DEPARTMENT OF GENETICS
ALBERT EINSTEIN COLLEGE OF MEDICINE
1300 MORRIS PARK AVENUE
NEW YORK, NY
10461   PHONE 212 430-2451

741.00   CDFHJWY
LIEBER, ERNEST
MEDICAL GENETICS
BETH ISRAEL MEDICAL CENTER
10 NATHAN D. PERLMAN PLACE
NEW YORK, NY
10003   PHONE 212 673-3000

743.00   A-DFSVY
MILLER, ORLANDO J.
COLUMBIA UNIVERSITY
NEW YORK, NY
10032

746.00   B-DFHJKMSWY
NITOWSKY, HAROLD M.
GENETIC COUNSELING PROGRAM
ALBERT EINSTEIN COLLEGE OF MEDICINE
BRONX MUNICIPAL HOSPITAL CENTER
NEW YORK, NY
10461   PHONE 212 430-2501

747.00   ADFHJPQST
RAINER, JOHN D.
DEPARTMENT OF MEDICAL GENETICS
NEW YORK STATE PSYCHIATRIC
  INSTITUTE
722 WEST 168 STREET
NEW YORK, NY
10032   PHONE 212 568-4000 EXT. 267

748.00   CJ
STARK, RICHARD BOIES
CLEFT PALATE CLINIC
ST. LUKEᵤS HOSPITAL CENTER
NEW YORK, NY
10025

749.00   BCJK
WAELSCH, SALOME GLUECKSOHN
ALBERT EINSTEIN COLLEGE OF MEDICINE
EASTCHESTER ROAD AND MORRIS PARK
  AVENUE
NEW YORK, NY
10461

750.00   FHJ
WARBURTON, DOROTHY
PRESBYTERIAN HOSPITAL
NEW YORK, NY
10032   PHONE 212 579-6460

751.00   KLV
WULFF, JAMES A.
DEPARTMENT OF PEDIATRICS

BABIES HOSPITAL
3975 BROADWAY
NEW YORK, NY
10032

752.00   CDFHJV
WOLMAN, SANDRA R.
DEPARTMENT OF PATHOLGY
NEW YORK UNIVERSITY MEDICAL CENTER
550 FIRST AVENUE
NEW YORK, NY
10016   PHONE 212 OR 9-3200 EXT. 36

754.00   A-NPQSY
TOWNES, PHILIP L.
DIVISION OF GENETICS
ROCHESTER UNIVERSITY MEDICAL SCHOOL
ROCHESTER, NY
14620   PHONE 716 275-3463

755.00   CDFJ-LV
TIERSTEN, DAVID
ST. JOHNᵤS EPISCOPAL HOSPITAL
RT. 25A
SMITHTOWN, NY
11787

756.00   B-DFJP
JENKINS, EDMUND C.
NEW YORK STATE DEPARTMENT OF MENTAL
  RETARDATION
INSTITUTE FOR BASIC RESEARCH IN
  MENTAL RETARDATION
1050 FOREST HILL ROAD
STATEN ISLAND, NY
10314

757.00   B-DFJP
JERVIS, GEORGE A.
NY STATE DEPARTMENT OF MENTAL
  RETARDATION
INSTITUTE FOR BASIC RESEARCH IN
  MENTAL RETARDATION
1050 FOREST HILL ROAD
STATEN ISLAND, NY
10314

758.00   B-DFJSY
GARDNER, L.I.
DEPARTMENT OF PEDIATRICS
UPSTATE MEDICAL CENTER HOSPITAL
SYRACUSE, NY
13210

759.00   CDFHJQY
SHAPIRO, LAWRENCE R.
CYTOGENETICS LABORATORY
LETCHWORTH VILLAGE
THIELLS, NY
10984   PHONE 914 947-3487 OR
                    947-1000 EXT. 444

760.00   C-FH-KQSW-Y
FARNSWORTH, PETER B.
BIRTH DEFECTS CENTER
GRASSLANDS HOSPITAL
VALHALLA, NY
10595   PHONE 914 LY 2-8500

761.00   B-DFHJ
OIKAWA, KIYOSHI
DEPARTMENT OF PEDIATRICS AND
  GENETICS
M.R. INSTITUTE OF N.Y. MEDICAL
  COLLEGE
VALHALLA, NY
10595   PHONE 914 347-5353

NO. CAROLINA

763.00   B-LPR
HERRINGTON, ROBERT T.
DEPARTMENT OF PEDIATRICS
BIRTH DEFECTS CLINIC
CHAPEL HILL, NC
27515

765.00   CFJ
PARKE, JR., JAMES C.
DEPARTMENT OF PEDIATRICS
CHARLOTTE MEMORIAL HOSPITAL
P.O. BOX 2554
CHARLOTTE, NC
28201

766.00 CDFJ
CHRISTAKOS, A.C.
DEPARTMENT OF OBSTETRICS AND
 GYNECOLOGY
DUKE MEDICAL CENTER
BOX 3274
DURHAM, NC
27706

768.00 FHJK
HASSELL, CHARLES M.
MOSES H. CONE MEMORIAL HOSPITAL
1200 NORTH ELM STREET
GREENSBORO, NC
27405   PHONE 919 397-4073

769.00 BCFJKPW
THOMAS, JAMES J.
BIRTH DEFECTS EVALUATION CLINIC
WESTERN CAROLINA CENTER
MORGANTON, NC
28655   PHONE 437-8717 EXT. 744

771.00 BDFJY
GOODMAN, HAROLD O.
MEDICAL GENETICS SECTION,
 DEPARTMENT OF PEDIATRICS
BOWMAN GRAY SCHOOL OF MEDICINE
WAKE FOREST UNIVERSITY
WINSTON-SALEM, NC
27103

NO. DAKOTA

773.00* BDFHKLVY
WASDAHL, W.A.
DEPARTMENT OF PATHOLOGY
UNIVERSITY OF NORTH DAKOTA
GRAND FORKS, ND
58202   PHONE 777-2561

OHIO

774.00 B-DFHJKQR
WARKANY, JOSEF
DEPARTMENT OF PEDIATRICS
CHILDRENS HOSPITAL RESEARCH
 FOUNDATION
CINCINNATI, OH
45229

775.00 B-DFJ
COTTON, JAMES E.
DEPARTMENT OF MEDICAL GENETICS
CLEVELAND PSYCHIATRIC INSTITUTE
1708 AIKEN AVENUE
CLEVELAND, OH
44109   PHONE 216 661-6200 EXT. 262

779.00 B-DFHJRW-Y
SCHAFER, IRWIN A.
DEPARTMENT OF PEDIATRICS
CASE WESTERN RESERVE MEDICAL SCHOOL
CLEVELAND METROPOLITAN GENERAL
 HOSPITAL
CLEVELAND, OH
44109   PHONE 216 398-6000

780.00 B-DFGJLPSWY
STEINBERG, A.G.
DEPARTMENT OF BIOLOGY
CASE WESTERN RESERVE UNIVERSITY
CLEVELAND, OH
44106   PHONE 216 368-3700

781.00 CDFHJ
KONTRAS, STELLA B.
DEPARTMENT OF PEDIATRICS
CHILDRENS HOSPITAL
COLUMBUS, OH
43205   PHONE 614 253-8841

782.00 CDFJPY
TEGENKAMP, THOMAS R.
SEARLE DIAGNOSTIC INC.
P.O. BOX 2440
COLUMBUS, OH
43216   PHONE 614 224-5633

783.00 B-DFHJKOW
ROBINOW, MEINHARD
BIRTH DEFECTS EVALUATION CENTER

CHILDRENS MEDICAL CENTER
1735 CHAPEL STREET
DAYTON, OH
45404   PHONE 513 461-4790

784.00 CDFHJQVY
YAREMA, WILLARD A.
MEDICAL GENETICS LABORATORY
601 MIAMI BOULEVARD
DAYTON, OH
45408   PHONE 513 223-3141 EXT. 205

785.00 FJ
WALZ, DONALD V.
CYTOGENETICS LABORATORY
MOUNT VERNON STATE INSTITUTE
BOX 762
MOUNT VERNON, OH
43050   PHONE 614 397-1010

OKLAHOMA

788.00 B-HJ-MSY
SEELY, J.R.
DEPARTMENT OF PEDIATRICS
UNIVERSITY OF OKLAHOMA
CHILDRENS HOSPITAL
OKLAHOMA CITY, OK
73104   PHONE 405 236-1366 EXT. 60

OREGON

790.00 B-NPQSV-Y
PRESCOTT, GERALD H.
DEPARTMENT OF PEDIATRICS
SACRED HEART HOSPITAL
EUGENE, OR
97401   PHONE 503 344-1411

791.00 DJ
STUART, RONALD R.
CRIPPLED CHILD DIVISION, GENETICS
 CLINIC
ROGUE VALLEY MEMORIAL HOSPITAL
2825 BARNETT ROAD
MEDFORD, OR
97501   PHONE 503 773-6281 EXT. 18

792.00 B-NPQSV-Y
HECHT, FREDERICK
GENETICS CLINIC
CRIPPLED CHILD DIVISION
UNIVERSITY OF OREGON MEDICAL SCHOOL
PORTLAND, OR
97201   PHONE 503 225-8344

PENNSYLVANIA

794.00 CFH-JNQ
CHANG, PHILIP
DEPARTMENT OF BIOLOGY
CALIFORNIA STATE COLLEGE
CALIFORNIA, PA
15419   PHONE 412 938-2281 EXT. 255

795.00 BCFJ
MALCOLM, JOHN A.
DEPARTMENT OF PATHOLOGY
GEISINGER MEDICAL CENTER
DANVILLE, PA
17815   PHONE 717 784-4660 EXT. 333

796.00 JNQ
VESELL, ELLIOT S.
M.S. HERSHEY MEDICAL CENTER,
 DEPARTMENT OF PHARMACOLOGY
PENNSYLVANIA STATE UNIVERSITY,
 COLLEGE OF MEDICINE
HERSHEY, PA
17033

797.00 B-DF-HJ-LNQ
DIGEORGE, ANGELO M.
DEPARTMENT OF PEDIATRICS
ST. CHRISTOPHER HOSPITAL FOR
 CHILDREN
2600 NORTH LAWRENCE STREET
PHILADELPHIA, PA
19133

798.00 B-DFH-NRU-WY
JACKSON, LAIRD G.

DIVISION OF GENETICS
JEFFERSON MEDICAL COLLEGE
1025 WALNUT STREET
PHILADELPHIA, PA
19107   PHONE 215 829-6955

799.00 CDFJM
KAUFMANN, B.N.
DEPARTMENT OF ANATOMY
HAHNEMANN MEDICAL COLLEGE, SECTION
 OF GENETICS
PHILADELPHIA, PA
19102   PHONE 215 LO 4-5000 EXT. 4

800.00 B-DFHJY
MELLMAN, WILLIAM J.
DEPARTMENT OF HUMAN GENETICS
UNIVERSITY OF PENNSYLVANIA SCHOOL
 OF MEDICINE
PHILADELPHIA, PA
19174   PHONE 215 662-3232 OR
                              662-3227

803.00 B-DFJY
GARVER, KENNETH L.
DEPARTMENT OF OBSTETRICS-GYNECOLOGY
 AND PEDIATRICS
UNIVERSITY OF PITTSBURGH,
 MAGEE-WOMENS HOSPITAL
HALKET STREET AND FORBES AVENUE
PITTSBURGH, PA
15213

805.00 B-DFJMV
STEELE, MARK W.
CHILDRENS HOSPITAL
PITTSBURGH, PA
15213   PHONE 412 681-7700 EXT. 561

806.00 DFJPX
TURNER, J. HOWARD
DEPARTMENT OF OBSTETRICS AND
 GYNECOLOGY
MAGEE-WOMENS HOSPITAL
PITTSBURGH, PA
15213

RHODE ISLAND

808.00 A-FH-JKQRV-Y
LAMARCHE, PAUL H.
DEPARTMENT OF PEDIATRICS
RHODE ISLAND HOSPITAL
PROVIDENCE, RI
02902   PHONE 401 277-5072

SO. CAROLINA

809.00 J
LIEBERMAN, ALLAN D.
1409 ASHLEY RIVER ROAD
CHARLESTON, SC
29407

811.00 DFHJWY
SINGH, D.N.
STATE DEPT. OF MENTAL RETARDATION &
 DEPTS. OF PEDIATRICS AND PATHOLOGY
MEDICAL UNIVERSITY OF SOUTH
 CAROLINA
80 BARRE STREET
CHARLESTON, SC
29401   PHONE 803 792-4186

TENNESSEE

814.00 CDFHJUWY
LOZZIO, CARMEN B.
BIRTH DEFECTS EVALUATION CENTER
UNIVERSITY OF TENNESSEE MEMORIAL
 RESEARCH CENTER AND HOSPITAL
1924 ALCOA HIGHWAY
KNOXVILLE, TN
37916   PHONE 615 971-3184

815.00 B-FH-QSY
SUMMITT, ROBERT L.
DEPARTMENT OF PEDIATRICS
UNIVERSITY OF TENNESSEE
860 MADISON AVENUE
MEMPHIS, TN
38103   PHONE 901 527-6641 EXT. 122

817.00   B-DF-HJ-LNV-X
CRUMP, E. PERRY
DEPARTMENT OF PEDIATRICS
HUBBARD HOSPITAL
1005 18TH AVENUE NORTH
NASHVILLE, TN
37208

818.00   CDF-HJKPY
ENGEL, ERIC
DEPARTMENT OF MEDICINE
VANDERBILT HOSPITAL
NASHVILLE, TN
37203

819.00   B-DFHJKSWY
HARA, SABURO
DEPARTMENT OF PEDIATRICS
MEHARRY MEDICAL COLLEGE
NASHVILLE, TN
37208   PHONE 256-3631

    TEXAS

822.00   BCFI-MW-Y
GOLDSTEIN, JOSEPH L.
DIVISION OF MEDICAL GENETICS,
    INTERNAL MEDICINE DEPARTMENT
UNIVERSITY OF TEXAS, SOUTHWESTERN
    MEDICAL SCHOOL AT DALLAS
5323 HARRY HINES BOULEVARD
DALLAS, TX
75235

823.00   FI-KRY
HELGESON, NORMAN G.P.
DEPARTMENT OF PATHOLOGY
BAYLOR UNIVERSITY MEDICAL CENTER
3500 GASTON AVENUE
DALLAS, TX
75246   PHONE 214 820-3308

824.00   CDFJW
MANKINEN, CARL B.
DENTON STATE SCHOOL
BOX 368
DENTON, TX
76202   PHONE 817 387-3831

825.00   BDFJKM
LOCKHART, LILLIAN H.
DEPARTMENT OF PEDIATRICS AND HUMAN
    GENETICS
UNIVERSITY OF TEXAS MEDICAL BRANCH
GALVESTON, TX
77550

826.00   B-DFJ-MPRSWY
BEAUDET, ARTHUR L.
BIRTH DEFECTS CENTER
TEXAS CHILDRENS HOSPITAL, BAYLOR
    COLLEGE OF MEDICINE
HOUSTON, TX
77025   PHONE 713 521-3261

827.00   B-DFJ-MPRSWY
CASKEY, C. THOMAS
SECTION OF MEDICAL GENETICS
BAYLOR COLLEGE OF MEDICINE
HOUSTON, TX
77025   PHONE 713 529-4951 EXT. 420

828.00   B-FH-MR-V
HAAS, FELIX L.
DEPARTMENT OF BIOLOGY
M.D. ANDERSON HOSPITAL
HOUSTON, TX
77025

829.00   CFHJM
HOWELL, R. RODNEY
DEPARTMENT OF PEDIATRICS, DIVISION
    OF GENETICS
UNIVERSITY OF TEXAS MEDICAL SCHOOL
TEXAS MEDICAL CENTER
HOUSTON, TX
77025   PHONE 713 527-4555

830.00   B-DFHJLMRWY
MCNAMARA, DAN G.
DEPARTMENT OF PEDIATRICS

BAYLOR UNIVERSITY COLLEGE OF
    MEDICINE
HOUSTON, TX
77025   PHONE 713 521-3261

833.00   B-DFHJLMRWY
SCHWANECKE, REBECCA P.
NEWBORN NURSERIES
ST. JOSEPH HOSPITAL
1919 LA BRANCH
HOUSTON, TX
77002

834.00   ACDFHJ
TIPS, ROBERT
DEPARTMENT OF MEDICAL GENETICS
PASADENA GENERAL HOSPITAL
1017 MOUND STREET
NACOGDOCHES, TX
77501

835.00   BD-FJY
FARRELL, PATRICIA
GENETIC SERVICE
WILFORD HALL USAF MEDICAL CENTER
LACKLAND AFB, HOSPITAL
SAN ANTONIO, TX
78236   PHONE 512 536-3584

836.00   CDFJKPUW
LOURO, JOSE M.
DEPARTMENT OF PEDIATRICS, SECTION
    OF GENETICS AND CYTOGENETICS
UNIVERSITY OF TEXAS MEDICAL SCHOOL
    AT SAN ANTONIO
7703 FLOYD CURL DRIVE
SAN ANTONIO, TX
78229   PHONE 512 696-6251

837.00   J
MCNUTT, WALLACE
DEPARTMENT OF ANATOMY
UNIVERSITY OF TEXAS HEALTH SCIENCE
    CENTER
7703 FLOYD CURL DRIVE
SAN ANTONIO, TX
78229   PHONE 512 696-6535

838.00   BD-FJY
PRINCE, JOHN E.
GENETIC SERVICE
WILLFORD HALL USAF MEDICAL CENTER
BROOKS AFB, BOX 35313
SAN ANTONIO, TX
78235   PHONE 512 536-3584

    UTAH

839.00   CFJWX
MYERS, GARTH G.
BIRTH DEFECTS CLINIC
PRIMARY CHILDRENS HOSPITAL
320 12TH AVENUE
SALT LAKE CITY, UT
84103

840.00   CDFHJVY
SCOTT, CHARLES D.
DEPARTMNET OF INTERNAL MEDICINE
COLLEGE OF MEDICINE, UNIVERSITY OF
    UTAH
50 NORTH MEDICAL DRIVE
SALT LAKE CITY, UT
84112   PHONE 581-7761

    VERMONT

841.00   B-DFJKPY
HODGKIN, WILLIAM E.
DEPARTMENT OF PEDIATRICS
MARY FLETCHER HOSPITAL
BURLINGTON, VT
05401   PHONE 802 864-7441 EXT. 21

    VIRGINIA

843.00   ACDFHJTVWY
NACCASH, EDMUND P.
DEPARTMENT OF MEDICAL GENETICS
ARLINGTON HOSPITAL
16TH STREET AND GEORGE MASON DRIVE
    NORTH
ARLINGTON, VA
22205

844.00   B-FJKP
CARPENTER, JOHNSON T.
DEPARTMENT OF INTERNAL MEDICINE
UNIVERSITY OF VIRGINIA HOSPITAL
CHARLOTTESVILLE, VA
22901

845.00   B-DFHJKPUWY
MILLER, JAMES Q.
CHROMOSOME RESEARCH LABORATORY
UNIVERSITY OF VIRGINIA MEDICAL
    SCHOOL
CHARLOTTESVILLE, VA
22901

847.00   CDFHJ-LV
GOODWIN, A. RAY
DEPARTMENT OF PATHOLOGY
DEPAUL HOSPITAL
NORFOLK, VA
23505

849.00   BFH-JMNVXY
CHEN, ANDREW
DEPARTMENT OF GENETICS
CYTOGENETICS LABORATORY
BOX 33, MCV STATION
RICHMOND, VA
23219

851.00   CE-GJ-LP
GRUNBACHER, F.J.
DEPARTMENTS OF BIO. AND GENETICS
MEDICAL COLLEGE OF VIRGINIA
RICHMOND, VA
23219   PHONE 770-4647

852.00   B-DFHJ-LY
YOUNG, REUBEN B.
DEPARTMENT OF PEDIATRICS
MEDICAL COLLEGE OF VIRGINIA
RICHMOND, VA
23219

    WASHINGTON

854.00   CDFHJ
THULINE, HORACE
CYTOGENETICS SERVICE LABORATORY
RAINIER SCHOOL
BOX 600
BUCKLEY, WA
98321

855.00   D-FHJ-NSV
FIALKOW, PHILIP J.
DEPARTMENT OF MEDICINE
UNIVERSITY OF WASHINGTON
SEATTLE, WA
98195   PHONE 206 543-1705

856.00   A-FHJ-NPSTVWY
MOTULSKY, ARNO G.
DEPARTMENT OF MEDICINE
UNIVERSITY OF WASHINGTON
SEATTLE, WA
98105   PHONE 206 543-3573

857.00   CDFJY
SMITH, DAVID W.
DEPARTMENT OF PEDIATRICS
DYSMORPHOLOGY UNIT
UNIVERSITY OF WASHINGTON, MEDICAL
    SCHOOL
SEATTLE, WA
98105   PHONE 206 543-6676

858.00   CDFJ
EGGEN, ROBERT R.
DEPARTMENT OF PATHOLOGY AND
    CLINICAL PATHOLOGY
ST. LUKES MEMORIAL HOSPITAL
SOUTH 711 COWLEY
SPOKANE, WA
99210   PHONE 509 TE 8-4771

859.00   DFHJKWX
SCHERZ, ROBERT G.
DEPARTMENT OF PEDIATRICS
MADIGAN GENERAL HOSPITAL
TACOMA, WA
98431

WEST VIRGINIA

860.00   B-DF-HJNUVY
THOMPSON, HAVELOCK
DEPARTMENT OF PEDIATRICS
WEST VIRGINIA UNIVERSITY HOSPITAL
MORGANTOWN, WV
26506

WISCONSIN

864.00   EJOPS
DENNISTON, CARTER
DEPARTMENT OF MEDICAL GENETICS
UNIVERSITY OF WISCONSIN MEDICAL
   SCHOOL
MADISON, WI
53706

865.00   CDJ
HERRNAMM, JURGEN
DEPARTMENT OF PEDIATRICS
UNIVERSITY OF WISCONSIN MEDICAL
   SCHOOL
MADISON, WI
53706

866.00   CFVX
INHORN, STANLEY L.
STATE LABORATORY OF HYGIENE
UNIVERSITY OF WISCONSIN
MADISON, WI
53706

867.00   CJ
KAVEGGIA, ELISABETH
CENTRAL WISCONSIN COLONY AND
   TRAINING SCHOOL
317 KNUTSON DRIVE
MADISON, WI
53704

868.00   CFVX
MEISNER, LORRAINE F.
STATE LABORATORY OF HYGIENE
UNIVERSITY OF WISCONSIN
MADISON, WI
53706

869.00   CDFJ
OPITZ, JOHN
DEPARTMENT OF MEDICAL GENETICS
UNIVERSITY OF WISCONSIN MEDICAL
   SCHOOL
MADISON, WI
53706

871.00   CDFJY
SARTO, GLORIA E.
DEPARTMENT OF GYNECOLOGY-OBSTETRICS
UNIVERSITY OF WISCONSIN MEDICAL
   SCHOOL
1300 UNIVERSITY AVENUE
MADISON, WI
53706

USA, COMMONWEALTH OF

872.00   J
COMAS, ADOLFO PEREZ
PEDIATRIC ENDOCRINOLOGY AND MEDICAL
   GENETICS SECTION
MAYAGUEZ MEDICAL CENTER
P.O. BOX 1868
MAYAGUEZ, PUERTO RICO, USA,
   COMMONWEALTH OF
00708

873.00   BDFJKPS
CINTRON-RIVERA, A.A.
DEPARTMENT OF CLINICAL RESEARCH
UNIVERSITY OF PUERTO RICO
SAN JUAN, PUERTO RICO, USA,
   COMMONWEALTH OF

USSR

874.00   BDFJPQU
BOCHKOV, N.P.
INSTITUTE OF MEDICAL GENETICS
ACADEMY OF MEDICAL SCIENCES OF USSR
BALTIYSKAYA UI 8
MOSCOW, USSR
A-315   PHONE 151-1721

875.00   ACFHJNQUY
KERKIS, JUL I.
RADIATION GENETICS LABORATORY
INSTITUTE OF CYTOLOGY AND GENETICS
NOVOSIBIRSK, USSR
630090

876.00   ABFILMPRUV
MARTYNOVA, R.P.
LABORATORY OF CANCER GENETICS
INSTUTUTE OF CYTOLOGY AND GENETICS
SIBERIAN DEPT USSR ACAD SCIENCE
NOVOSIBIRSK, USSR
630090   PHONE 656-456

VENEZUELA

878.00   CDFHJPY
MURO, LUIS A.
DEPARTMENT DE MEDICINA 3
UNIVERSITY HOSPITAL LAB DE
   INVESTIGACIONES
CARACAS, VENEZUELA
PHONE 719328

WALES

880.00   B-DHJPSV-Y
HARPER, PETER S.
DEPARTMENT OF MEDICINE, SECTION OF
   MEDICAL GENETICS
UNIVERSITY HOSPITAL OF WALES
HEATH PARK
CARDIFF, WALES
CF4 4XW   PHONE 0222-755944

881.00   CDFHJPY
LAURENCE, K.M.
DEPARTMENT OF CHILD HEALTH
LLANDOUGH HOSPITAL
PENARTH, GLAMORGAN, WALES

WEST INDIES

882.00   FI-LR-TWX
THORBURN, MARIGOLD J.
DEPARTMENT OF PATHOLOGY
UNIVERSITY OF THE WEST INDIES
MONA
JAMAICA, KINGSTON 7, WEST INDIES
PHONE 967-6621 EXT. 275

YUGOSLAVIA

883.00   BDFHJKOX
AVCIN, MARIJ
DEPARTMENT OF PEDIATRICS
UNIVERSITY CHILDRENS HOSPITAL
LJUBLJANA, YUGOSLAVIA
PHONE 061-312-255

885.00   CDFJQU
ZERGOLLERN, LJILJANA
DEPARTMENT OF PEDIATRICS
UNIVERSITY OF ZAGREB-REBRO
ZAGREB, YUGOSLAVIA

REFERENCES

1. Lynch, H.T., and Bergsma, Daniel, (Eds.): *International Directory of Genetic Services.* The National Foundation—March of Dimes. New York, 1968.

2. Lynch, H.T., and Bergsma, Daniel, (Eds.): *International Directory of Genetic Services, 2nd ed,* The National Foundation—March of Dimes. New York, 1969.

3. Lynch, H.T., and Bergsma, Daniel, (Eds.): *International Directory of Genetic Services, 3rd ed,* The National Foundation—March of Dimes. New York, 1971.

4. Lynch, H.T., Bergsma, Daniel, and Thomas, Robert J., (Eds.): *International Directory of Genetic Services, 4th ed,* The National Foundation—March of Dimes. New York, 1974.

APPENDIX 2

GLOSSARY OF GENETIC TERMS

acentric

Descriptive term referring to a chromosome segment without a centromere.

acrocentric

Descriptive term referring to a chromosome in which the centromere is located very close to one end, so that one chromosome arm is relatively vary small and the other one is much larger.

additive genes

Genes which interact with each other in trait manifestations (e.g. show cumulative effects rather than dominance-recessiveness).

allele

Shortened term for alleomorph. One of two or more alternate forms of a gene occupying the same locus or point on a particular chromosome. The activities of alleles involve the same biochemical and/ or developmental process(es). A haploid cell has only a single representative for each locus. A diploid cell has two representatives for each locus, two alleles. If the two alleles at a given locus are identical, the individual is homozygous for the locus involved; if the two alleles at a given locus are different, then the individual is heterozygous for that locus.

allelomorph

See: allele.

analysis of covariance

The simultaneous analysis of the sums of squares and cross-products of two or more variates.

analysis of variance

Statistical technique that allows the partitioning of the total variation observed in an experiment among several statistically independent possible causes of the variation. A technique for the isolation of particular components of variation for assessment by comparison with error variation.

anamnesis

Collected data concerning a patient, his family, previous environment, and experiences.

aneuploid

Individual or cell characterized by having one, two, or a few whole chromosome(s) more or less than the basic diploid number of the particular species.

aneuploidy

See: aneuploid.

arithmetic mean

Mean or average. The sum of the values recorded in a series of observations divided by the number of observations.

assortment, independent

See: independent assortment.

average

See: arithmetic mean.

autosome

Any chromosome other than a sex chromosome (i.e. any chromosome other than an X chromosome or a Y chromosome).

balanced load

That which depresses the overall fitness of a *population* owing to the segregation of inferior or defective genotypes, the component genes of which are maintained in the population because they add to fitness in different combinations, e.g. as heterozygotes. See: balanced polymorphism.

balanced polymorphism

A condition in which different alleles of the same genetic locus occur in relatively high frequencies in a population, and in which the disadvantages produced by a double does of one allele (homozygosity) are balanced by the advantages produced by a single dose of the allele (heterozygosity). Genetic polymorphism can be maintained in a population of the heterozygotes for the alleles under consideration manifest a high adaptive value than either homozygote.

balanced translocation

Chromosomal structural change characterized by the change in position (location) of one or more chromosome(s) or chromosome segment(s), within the normal chromosome complement. That is, some of the chromosome material is abnormally located, but the chromosome complement involves no duplication or deletion of any chromosome material.

Barr body

Sex chromatin. The condensed single X chromosome seen in the nucleus of a somatic cell in a female mammal; named for Murray Barr, its discoverer.

Barr-negative

See: sex-chromatin-negative.

Barr-positive

See: sex-chromatin-positive.

biometry

Statistical study of biological observations and phenomena.

catamnesis

The follow-up medical history of a patient.

centromere

Region of a chromosome which is attached to a spindle fiber during mitosis and meiosis, and at which the two not-completely-divided daughter chromosomes (i.e. the pair of chromatids) are attached before producing two independent daughter chromosomes.

centromeric index

An expression of the position of the centromere of a chromosome, determined as length of the short arm divided by total length of the entire chromosome.

chiasma

An x-shaped configuration of chromosomal material, caused by the breakage and exchange and reciprocal fusion of equivalent segments of homologous chromatids during meiosis.

chimera

Individual organism consisting of two or more genetically different lines of cells within the same tissue type; a genetic mosaic, in which mosaicism occurs in a particular tissue type. The condition may result from a somatic mutation in a cell during mitosis, or from a fusion (i.e. grafting) of cells from one individual upon another individual. (See: mosaic).

chi-square

The ratio of an observed sum of squares to the corresponding variance fixed by hypotheses.

chromatids

Individual threads which are the result of lengthwise duplication of a chromosome are called chromatids as long as the threads remain joined to each other at the centromere.

chromatin

Nuclear substance which takes basic stain and becomes incorporated in the chromosomes; so called because of the readiness with which it becomes stained with certain dyes (i.e. chromaticity). Chromatin is that part of the nuclear material that makes up the genetic material and contains the genetic information (i.e. genes) of the cell. The chromatin of a cell is considered to organize and contract into the stainable chromosomes during cell division. Larger chromatin bodies are called chromocenters.

chromatin-negative
See: sex-chromatin-negative.

chromatin-positive
See: sex-chromatin-positive.

chromomeres
Areas of different optical density and/or different diameters along the length of a chromosome, expecially clearly detectible during the prophase of a cell division.

chromosomal aberration
Chromosomal abnormality; a deviation from the normal morphology or number of the chromosomes.

chromosomal deficiency
See: deletion, chromosomal.

chromosomal depletion
See: deletion, chromosomal.

chromosomal mosaicism
Mosaicism in which the genetically different cell lines contain observable morphological differences in the chromosome complements. (See: mosaicism).

chromosomal mutation
Any morphologically visible structural change in the chromosomal complement, involving the gain, loss, or relocation of chromosomal segments. Descriptively, all such structural changes include deletions or deficiencies, duplications, inversions and other translocations. (See: mutation).

chromosomal translocation
See: translocation.

chromosome
Microscopically observable nucleoprotein bodies, darkly stained with basic dyes, observable in the cell during division. The chromosomes carry the genes of the cell, arranged in a specific linear order. They are autoreduplicating structures whose number per cell, shape, and organization, are species-specific characteristics. Chemically, a chromosome is a DNA-histone thread residing in the nucleus of a cell.

chromosome complement
Group of chromosomes derived from a particular gametic (i.e. haploid), or zytotic or somatic (i.e. diploid), nucleus.

chromosome disjunction
Assortment of chromosomes during the first meiotic division.

chromosome fusion
Union of two or more chromosomes by means of chromosome structural changes to form a single chromosome. The change in the chromosome material which occurs with chromosome fusion is one form of chromosomal mutation. Among chromosomes with localized centromeres, such unions are stable if the fusion takes place in the centromere region.

chromosome map
Graphic, linear representation of a chromosome in which the genes belonging to particular linkage groups (i.e. genetic markers) are plotted according to their relative distances. There are two kinds of chromosome maps, genetic maps and cytological maps. (See: genetic maps, cytological maps).

coefficient of variation
Standard deviation expressed as a percentage of the mean, or one hundred times the dividend obtained through dividing the standard deviation by the mean.

cohort
A group of individuals, or vital statistics about them, having a statistical factor in common in a demographic study. A group of related families.

complete penetrance
Situation in which a dominant gene always produces a particular phenotypic effect or a recessive gene in the homozygous state always produces a detectable effect. (See: penetrance).

concordance
Occurrence of a particular trait in both members of a pair of individuals. Agreement between the two members of a pair

regarding presence or absence of a particular character.

congenital

Present at birth. The etiology of a congenital condition may or may not involve genetic factors, as well as other variables relevant to embryonic and fetal development and the birth process.

consanguinous union

Union between related individuals, i.e. individuals having one or more ancestors in common.

consanguinity

Involving genetic relationship (i.e. at least one common ancestor in the preceeding few generations).

constant

A quantity whose value is assumed fixed during an investigation.

constitution

The physical and psychological makeup of an individual, determined by the genetic and nongenetic (i.e. environmental) factors, and modified by interactions with environmental factors.

contingency table

A table of frequencies distinguishing two classifications simultaneously.

continuous distribution

Manifestation, by a collection of data, of a continuous spectrum of values. Graphic distribution of the data in a population is monomodal, i.e. includes only a single mode in the distribution curve. (See: discontinuous distribution.)

correlation

The interdependence of two variates. The opposite of independence.

correlation coefficient

The ratio of the covariance of two variates to the geometrical mean of their variances. Measure of the degree of association found between two characteristics in a series of observations, on the assumption that the relationship between the two

characteristics is adequately described by a straight line. A positive value indicates that an upward movement of one characteristic is accompanied by an upward movement of the other, and a negative sign indicates that an upward movement of one is accompanied by an upward movement of the other, and a negative sign indicates that an upward movement of one is accompanied by a downward movement of the other.

covariance

The mean product of the deviations of two variates from their means. Estimated as the ratio of a sum of cross-products to the corresponding number of degrees of freedom.

covariance analysis

See: analysis of covariance.

criss-cross inheritance

Mode of inheritance involving transmission of a gene which occurs on the X chromosome (i.e. a sex-linked gene.)

crossing over

Reciprocal exchange of segments at corresponding positions along pairs of homologous linkage units (i.e. chromatids, chromosomes) by symmetrical breakage and cross-wise rejoining. Crossing over results in an exchange of genes and therefore produces combinations which are different from the combinations characteristic of the parents.

cross-products, sum of

Sum of the products of corresponding deviations of two variates from their individual means.

cytogenetics

Biological discipline concerned with chromosomes and their implications in genetics i.e. the behavior of the chromosomes during mitosis and meiosis, their origin, and their relation to the transmission and recombination of genes.

cytokinesis

Cytoplasmic division and other changes exclusive of nuclear division which are a part of mitosis or meiosis. Cell division involves both nuclear division (i.e. mitosis or meiosis) and cytokinesis.

cytological map

Graphic, linear representation of a chromosome in which the genes belonging to particular linkage groups (i.e. genetic markers) are plotted according to their relative distances. The distances are determined on the basis of cytological observations obtained with the aid of chromosome mutations (i.e. deletions, inversions, and other translocations) experimentally induced by mutagenic agents. Another method of preparing cytological maps is based upon microscopic analysis of the giant chromosomes of Diptera, in which the position and extent of the chromosomal structural changes may be determined morphologically.

cytology

Study of the structure and function of the cell.

cytoplasm

Protoplasm of a cell outside the nucleus, i.e. all living parts of the cell except the nucleus.

cytoplasmic inheritance

Hereditary transmission dependent on the cytoplasm or structures in the cytoplasm rather than the nuclear genes, i.e. extranuclear inheritance.

deficiency, chromosomal

See: deletion, chromosomal.

deletion, chromosomal

Actual loss of a portion or portions of one or more chromosome(s) and the included genes.

deoxyribonucleic acid

See: DNA.

dermatoglyphics

Patterns of the ridged skin of palms, fingers, soles, and toes; the study and systematic classification of such patterns.

desoxyribonucleic acid

See: DNA.

developmental genetics

Branch of genetics primarily concerned with transmission of genetic variables which control or modulate developmental processes.

deviation, standard

See: standard deviation.

dichotomy

Sharp distinction.

diploid

Containing two homologous sets of chromosomes, one of paternal origin and the other of maternal origin, in which each type of chromosome except the sex chromosomes of the heterogametic sex (i.e. the male sex in mammals) is normally represented in duplicate.

discontinuous distribution

Manifestation, by a collection of data, into discontinuous groups of values. Graphic distribution of the data is bimodal or multimodal. (See: continuous distribution.)

discordance

Disagreement between the two members of a pair regarding the presence or absence of a particular character.

disjunction

See: chromosome disjunction.

distribution, frequency

The distribution obtained when the frequencies with which observations fall into certain classes are plotted against those classes.

dizygotic twins

Fraternal twins. Twins brought about by fertilization of two different ova by different spermatozoa.

DNA

Abbreviation for deoxyribonucleic acid (desoxyribonucleic acid), one of the key chemical compounds governing life functions. DNA is found in the cell nucleus and is an essential constituent of the genes. Structurally, DNA consists of complementary but oppositely polarized polynucleotide chains, which are hydrogen-bonded together and wound helically around a common axis in a double helix. Genetic information is apparently encoded in the sequence of the nucleotides. Replication is believed to be accomplished by separation of the complementary nucleotide chains, with each single chain retaining its integrity while serving as a template against which new complementary chains are built for the four nucleotide components (i.e. adenine and thymine, guanine and cytosine). The antiparallel strands form a right-handed helix which undergoes one complete revolution with each ten nucleotide pairs. DNA molecules are the largest biologically active molecules known, having molecular weights greater than 1×10^8. In the translation of the genetic information contained in DNA, it is commonly assumed that RNA molecules are synthesized, which then serve as templates to form specific proteins.

dominance

In *genetics*, dominance is a manifestation of a gene's ability to be expressed in the phenotype of an individual, even though that (dominant) gene is paired with a different gene. A dominant gene is manifested in the heterozygote (i.e. the individual whose genotype includes the dominant gene and another allele); a recessive gene is not manifested in the heterozygote, but only in the homozygote (i.e. the individual whose genotype includes a pair of the same recessive genes). "Dominance" and "recessiveness" are not properties of the genes per se, but result from action of the particular gene within the total reaction system of the particular genotype. (See: recessive.)

double-blind study

Research procedure in which both the investigator and the subject are unable to discriminate between the experimental factor and the control factor at the time of administering the test to obtain data for evaluating differences in effects of the two factors.

double helix

See: DNA

Drosophila

A genus of flies containing about nine hundred described species, which is the most extensively studied of all general genera from the standpoint of genetics and cytogenetics.

duplication, chromosomal

Chromosomal structural change which involves presence of a group of genes (i.e. of a chromosome or chromosomal segment) more than once in the haploid genotype or more than twice in the diploid genotype. A chromosomal duplication may result from a chromosomal structural change (i.e. mutation) resulting in the doubling of some chromosomal material in a cell and in cells derived from that cell.

dyad

Pair of chromatids connected at the centromere, derived from one chromosome in the first meiotic division.

dysgenic

Tending to be harmful to the hereditary qualities of a species.

DZ

Dizygotic

Ecology

Study of relations between individuals and their environments.

empiric risk

Prediction of the probability that a particular abnormality will occur in a particular individual. The risk that an individual, who is characterized by a particular genetic relationship to an affected individual, will manifest the trait (i.e. will be affected). Empiric risk figures are utilized in human genetics for traits which apparently involve genetic predisposition, but for which no definitive pattern of genetic transmission can be demonstrated. Empiric risk figures are based upon recurrence histories in families characterized by occurrence of affected members, and they are predictions of the probabilities that the abnormality will recur in the families in which it has already occurred.

endogenous

Arising from internal structural and/or functional causes; originating in the individual's own psychodynamics and/or neuroendocrine - metabolicmorpholigic content rather than through external causes.

environmentalist

One who emphasizes the importance of environmental factors in development and deemphasizes the importance of genetic factors.

epidemiology

Study of the incidence, distribution, prevalence, and control of a particular disorder or trait in a given population.

epigenetic

Developmental. Referring to the interaction of genetic factors during the developmental process.

epistasis

Gene interaction whereby one gene interferes with the phenotypic expression of another nonallelic gene, or of other nonallelic genes, so that the phenotype is determined effectively by the former and not by the latter when both genes occur together in the genotype. A form of interaction between genes situated at different loci, where one gene masks or prevents expression of another gene at a different locus.

euchromatin

Chromatin which shows the staining behavior characteristic of the majority of the chromosomal complement. It is uncoiled during interphase and condenses during mitosis and meiosis, reaching a maximum density at metaphase.

eugenic

Descriptive term relevant to measures or trends which improve the genetic endow-

ment of a human population, as opposed to dysgenic.

euploid

Descriptive term to specify occurrence of one complete chromosome set (i.e. monoploidy, haploidy) or whole multiples (e.g. diploidy, polyploidy) of the basic monploid (haploid) number of chromosomes characteristic of the species.

exogenous

Produced from without; originating from or resulting from external causes. Having a cause external to the body; not primarily resulting from structural or functional failure of the body.

expressivity

Degree of phenotypic expression or severity or manifestation of a penetrant gene or genotype. Expressivity refers to the degree of expression of a trait controlled by a particular penetrant gene, which may produce different degrees of expression in different individuals. Thus, expressivity of a particular penetrant gene in a particular individual may be slight or severe and may be described in qualitative and/or quantitative terms. Some genes show variable expressivities in different individuals and some genes are relatively consistent in their manifestations.

extrachromosomal

Descriptive term to describe structures that are not part of the chromosomes.

extranuclear

Descriptive term to describe structures or processes which occur outside the nucleus.

F_1

First filial generation, the first generation of descent from a given mating.

factor analysis

Statistical technique for evaluations of intercorrelations between different items in the data. Factor analysis identifies the items which are correlated with each other and those which are independent of each other. The various items of the intercorrelation matrix are examined for indications of occurrence of different clusters of items. The identification of different clusters may facilitate interpretations of data as measuring several different and unrelated variables, with each of the different variables reflected by one of the clusters.

familial

Refers to the occurrence of two or more affected individuals in a family group or pedigree.

fecundity

Reproductive potential, as measured by the quantity of gametes, particularly ova, produced.

fertility

Reproductive potential, as measured by the quantity or percentage of developing eggs or of fertile matings or offspring produced.

Feulgen procedure

A cytochemical test that utilized Schiff's reagent as a stain and is specific for DNA.

Feulgen-positive

DNA-containing.

forme fruste

An atypical or aborted form of a disease or disorder (French).

fraternal twins

Dizygotic or two-egg twins.

frequency distribution table

Table of values constructed from a series of records of individuals, showing the frequency with which individuals are present with a particular defined characteristic or group of characteristics.

gamete

Mature reproductive cell. The gametes are produced from gametocytes during the process of gametogenesis, during which a diploid cell undergoes meiosis and produces haploid gametes. The female's gametes are ova and the male's gametes are spermatozoa.

Gaussian distribution

See: normal distribution.

gene

Ultimate unit of genetic material, not further subdivisible by either genetic recombination or chromosomal structural rearrangement. A gene is composed of DNA and may be defined as a specific sequence of nucleotides. Genes are arranged in characteristic linear order on chromosomes within cells. The total complement of genes makes up the genotype. Genes in diploid organisms occur as pairs of alleles. Gene action is manifested by control of the specificity and rate of biosynthetic processes. The gene is the fundamental unit of biological heredity.

gene expression

Phenotypic manifestation of genes by the process of gene action.

gene flow

Spread of genes from one breeding population to others through the dispersal of gametes. Exchange of genetic factors between populations.

gene frequency

Proportion of one particular type of genetic allele among the total of all alleles at the particular genetic locus in a breeding population; or the probability of finding the particular gene when a gene is randomly chosen from the population.

gene interaction

Interaction between allelic or non-allelic genes of the same genotype in the production of particular phenotypic characters.

gene locus

The point or position occupied by a gene in the chromosome. Different genes which may occupy the same locus (on homoogous chromosomes) are alleles of each other.

gene, major

See: major gene.

gene mutation

Heritable change within the limits of a single gene; point mutation, as opposed to changes in chromosome structure or number. As a result of gene mutation, there are alternative states of a gene, i.e. alleles. Since the genetic information carried by a gene is encoded in a specific nucleotide sequence of DNA, and is replicated by forming complementary nucleotide chains, a gene mutation may result from any change in the normal sequence of entire nucleotides or their component bases.

gene pool

Totality of genes of a given population existing at a given time.

genetic

In biology, pertaining to genes or to traits associated with genes, transmitted from one generation to the next via the chromosomal material.

genetic drift

Change in gene frequency in a population, which may or may not be directed. Irregular and random fluctuation in gene frequency in a population from one generation to another, most likely to occur in a small breeding population; may lead to random fixation of one allele and extinction of another without regard to their adaptive values.

genetic homeostasis

Tendency of a population to equilibrate its genetic composition and to resist sudden change.

genetic isolate

Breeding population which does not exchange genes (i.e. does not interbreed with any other such group.

genetic map

Graphic, linear representation of a chromosome in which the genes belonging to particular linkage groups, i.e. genetic markers, are plotted according to their relative distances. The relative distances are based upon the frequencies of intergenic crossing-over between any two linked markers. The accuracy of genetic mapping is dependent upon the precision with which the crossing-over frequencies may be estimated from the recombination frequencies. (See: chromosome map, cytological map.)

genetic marker

Genetically controlled phenotypic difference used in genetic analysis.

genetic morphism

See: morphism.

genetic polymorphism

See: polymorphism.

genetics

Scientific study of biological heredity, transmission of genetic material from one generation to the next via the gametes. See: genetic.

genocopy

Refers to an individual who is phenotypically like another individual who is genotypically different—that is, the same phenotype is produced by a different genotype. Different combinations of different genetic and nongenetic factors may produce the same effect or character.

genotype

Sum total of the genetic material in a particular individual, i.e. the total genetic constitution.

germ line

Pertaining to the cells from which gametes are derived. The cells of the germ line, unlike somatic cells, bridge the gaps between generations.

germ plasm

Hereditary material transmitted to offspring through the germ cells or gametes.

gynandromorph

Mosaic individual whose tissues include cells of both male genotype and female genotype.

haploid

Descriptive term referring to presence of only a single set of chromosomes, such as occurs in a gamete produced by a single diploid individual.

Hardy-Weinberg Law

The principle which states that gene frequencies and genotype frequencies will both remain constant from generation to generation in an infinitely large, interbreeding population in which mating is at random and there is no selection, migration, or mutation.

hemizygous gene

Gene present in a single dose, e.g. in a haploid cell such as a gamete, or in the case of a Y-linked or X-linked gene in the heterogametic sex.

hereditarian

One who emphasizes the importance of genetic factors in development and de-emphasizes the importance of environmental factors.

heritability

Proportion of the total phenotypic variance that is genetic for a particular character in a particular population at a single generation under one particular set of conditions. Heritability is commonly expressed as a percentage and decreases with an increasing environmental component of variance for the character under observation. Mathematically, it is the genetic variance divided by the total phenotypic variance. The heritability of a particular disease or disorder may be defined as the extent to which the variation in individual risk of acquiring the disease or disorder is due to genetic differences.

hermaphroditism

Occurrence of gonads of both sexes in a single individual.

heterochromatin

Chromosome material which, unlike euchromatin, shows maximal staining in the interphase nucleus.

heterogametic

That one of the two sexes which, during meiosis, gives rise to two different types of gametes (i.e. male-determining and female determining gametes), in contrast to the homogametic sex. In humans, the male normally contains two sets of autosomes, one X chromosome, and one Y chromosome; following meiosis, the male produces haploid spermatozoa of two types, one type containing one set of autosomes and an X chromosome (i.e. female-producing), and one type containing one set of autosomes and one Y chromosome (i.e. male-producing).

heterogeneous

Mixed. Consisting of dissimilar ingredients.

heterologous

Designating an antigen and antibody that do not correspond (i.e. interact specifically) with each other. Either one, the antigen or the antibody, may be defined as being heterologous to the other.

heteromeric

Refers to genes which, in combination, control the manifestation of a particular character, when each of the interacting genes has a definite but individually different share in the production of that character.

heteromorphic chromosomes

Homologous chromosomes that differ from each other morphologically.

heteromorphosis

See: homeosis.

heteroploid

Descriptive term to specify occurrence of a chromosome number deviating from the normal number.

heterosis

Superiority of heterozygous genotypes with respect to one or more characters, (i.e. hybrid vigor) in comparison with the corresponding homozygotes; selective superiority of heterozygotes.

heterotypical

Heterotypic. Involving different kinds of arrangements or forms. Refers to the reduction division of meiosis, as contrasted with a typical mitotic division.

heterozygote
Diploid individual who has inherited two different alleles at one or more loci. An individual with different genetic factors (i.e. alleles) at the homologous (i.e. corresponding) loci of a pair of homologous (i.e. which pair during meiosis) chromosomes.

holandric
Descriptive term referring to genes occurring on the Y chromosome, completely linked to the Y chromosome.

holandric inheritance
Mode of genetic transmission involving a locus which occurs on the Y chromosome.

homeostasis
Tendency of a system to maintain a dynamic equilibrium and, in case of disturbance, to restore the equilibrium by its own regulatory mechanisms. Also, see: genetic homeostasis.

homoeosis
See: homeosis.

homogametic
Descriptive term regarding that sex which produces only one basic type of gamete, in contrast to the heterogametic sex. In humans, the female is homogametic, and normally produces only ova which are characterized by one set of autosomes and one X chromosome.

homologous
Corresponding in structure, position. Descriptive term regarding chromosomes or chromosome segments which are identical with respect to their constituent genetic loci (i.e. the same loci in the same sequence) and their structure. Homologous chromosomes are morphologically paired during the process of meiosis. The descriptive term may also be used to refer to the specificity relationship between an antigen and/ or its hapten and an antibody.

homomeric
Refers to genes which, in combination, control the manifestation of a particular character and when each of the interacting (homomeric) genes has a quantitatively similar share in the production of that character.

homotypic
See: homotypical.

homotypical
Homotypic. Involving the same kind of arrangement or form. Refers to the equational division of meiosis.

homozygote
Diploid individual who has inherited identical, rather than different, alleles in the corresponding loci of a pair of homologous chromosomes.

hybrid
A heterozygote, i.e. a diploid individual who has inherited two different alleles at one or at each of more than one locus. In common usage, an individual produced by two parents who are genetically unlike.

hyperploid
Cells or individuals which chromosome complements include, in addition to the normal complement, one or more added chromosome(s) or chromosome segment(s).

hypoploid
Cells and individuals which are deficient for one or more chromosome(s) or chromosome segment(s).

idiochromosome
Sex chromosome, i.e. X chromosome or Y chromosome.

idiogram
Diagrammatic representation of the karyotype or chromosomal complement of an individual. Idiogram construction is based upon measurements of total chromosome length, arm-length ratio, and centromere position, for each chromosome during metaphase of mitosis. The chromosomes in an idiogram are characteristically arranged in pairs in descending order of size. See: karyotype.

idiopathic

Of unknown cause.

idiotype

Sum total of hereditary determinants of an organism, consisting of its genotype (i.e. all determinants localized in the chromosomes, chromosomal genes) and plasmotype (i.e. all determinants localized extrachromosomally).

imbricate

Overlap; lie lapped over each other.

inborn error of metabolism

Genetically determined biochemical disorder resulting in an enzyme defect that produces a metabolic block which may have pathological consequences.

inbred

Result of matings between genetic relatives.

inbreeding

Crossing of genetically related individuals.

incidence

Number of cases of a particular trait or disorder in a given population over a set period of time.

independence

In statistics, the relation between two variates, each of which takes values uninfluenced by those of the other. The opposite of dependence and correlation.

independent assortment, Mendel's principle of

Members of different allele pairs assort independently of each other when germ cells are randomly formed, provided the genes in question are unlinked (i.e. not located on the same chromosome).

index case

See: proband.

induction, embryonic

Determination of the developmental fate of one cell mass by another; morphogenic effect brought about by an evocator acting upon competent tissue.

inheritance, biological

Transmission of genetic information from parents (and their ancestors) to offspring via the gametes.

interchange, chromosomal

Exchange of segments between nonhomologous chromosomes resulting in translocations.

interphase

That part of the cell cycle during which metabolism and synthesis occur without visible evidence of division, and the nucleus of the cell is not visibly engaged in mitosis or meiosis.

intersex

Individual who has sexual characteristics which are intermediate between the male and female. An intersex may arise as a result of a chromosomal aberration or a gene mutation or an aberration of gonadogenesis or from a glandular lesion or medication.

inversion, chromosomal

Chromosomal structural change characterized by reversal of a chromosome segment or chromatid segment and the gene sequence contained therein (i.e. relative to the standard arrangement of the linkage group involved). Reinsertion of a chromosomal segment into its original position but in reversed sequence.

in vitro

In isolation from the whole organism.

in vivo

Within the living organism.

irregular dominance

A condition in which a generally dominant gene is of variable expressivity and/or variable frequency of penetrance.

isoalleles

Alleles that produce such slight phenotypic differences that special techniques are required to reveal their presence.

isochromatid break

Aberration involving breaks in both sister chromatids at the same locus, followed by lateral fusion to produce a dicentric chromatid and an acentric fragment.

isochromosome

Chromosome with two identical arms,

originally the result of an anomalous division at the centromere.

isolate

Segment of a population within which assortative mating occurs.

isomorphism

Similarity in organisms of different ancestries (i.e. resulting from convergence by the two relevant lines of evolution).

karyotype

The term is used in two ways: (a) the somatic chromosomal complement of an individual or species; (b) photomicrographs of the metaphase chromosomes arranged in a standard sequence, an idiogram. See: Idiogram.

kinetochore

Centromere.

Klinefelter's syndrome

A condition in man that characteristically produces sterile males with small testes lacking spermatozoa, is sometimes associated with mental retardation, and is due to occurrence of two or more X chromosomes in addition to one or more Y chromosome(s).

late-replicating X chromosome

X chromosome which completes its replication later than the functional X chromosome and the autosomes. In the mammalian somatic cell nucleus, all X chromosomes except one apparently coil up and condense, and apparently do not function in transcription. The condensed mass of a late-replicating X chromosome in a mammalian somatic cell nucleus is believed to be the source of the sex-chromatin (i.e. Barr) body.

linkage

Occurrence of genetic loci on the same chromosome. Loci which occur on the X chromosome are termed X-linked or sex-linked; and loci which occur on the Y chromosome are termed Y-linked or holandric. Linkage refers to the association of nonallelic genes which reside on the same chromosome.

linkage group

Group of genetic loci which occur on the same chromosome.

loci

Plural of locus.

locus

See: gene locus.

Lyon hypothesis

Hypothesis advanced by Mary F. Lyon that, in mammals, one X chromosome is inactivated in some embryonic cells and their descendants, that the other is inactivated in the rest of the cells, and that mammalian females are consequently X-chromosome mosaics regarding X-chromosome manifestations. See: late-replicating X chromosome.

major gene

Gene which is individually associated with pronounced phenotypic effects. Major genes control production of discontinuous or qualitative characteris, in contrast to "minor genes" or polygenes, which manifest individually small effects. Major genes segregate clearly and are subject to Mendelian analyses. The dichotomy of genes into 'major' and 'minor' categories represents an arbitrary division in a continuous series of gene actions and interactions. See: minor gene.

male pronucleus

Generative nucleus of a male gamete.

map, genetic

See: genetic map.

maternal effect

In biology, modification of the phenotype of the progeny produced by the maternal genotype acting through the cytoplasm of the ovum. See: matrilinear inheritance.

maternal influence

The influence of the maternal environment upon which an embryo develops.

matrilinear inheritance

Transmission of cytoplasmic particles only in the female line. See: maternal effect.

matrix

A rectangular array of quantities or other symbols, convenient for representing relations between each pair of an aggregate. Strictly speaking, such an array can be treated as a generalized quantity, that is, subjected to certain rules of calculation.

maturation divisions

Series of nuclear divisions in which the chromosome complement of the nuclei is reduced from diploid to haploid number. See: meiosis.

mean

See: arithmetic mean.

mean deviation

Arithmetic average of all the differences between the observations and their mean, the differences being added without regard to their signs, i.e. ignoring whether the observation is above or below the mean.

median

The center value of a series of observations are ranged in order from the lowest value to the highest. When there is an even number of observations, the mean of the two central observations may be taken. In the frequency distribution, the median is calculated as the midpoint which divides the distribution into two halves. The median is a useful figure when the arithmetic mean is unduly affected by very large or very small outlying observations.

meiocyte

Cell in which the nucleus divides by meiosis, i.e. primary oocyte, primary spermatocyte.

meiosis

Processes involving two successive divisions of the nucleus preceding the formation of mature gametes. Homologous chromosomes pair, replicate once only, and undergo assortment so that each of the four meiotic products resulting from one complete meiosis receives one representative of each chromosome pair. Thus, the diploid chromosome number is meiotically reduced to the haploid number characteristic for the gametes or haploid phase of the life cycle.

Mendelian character

Character which, in biological inheritance or genetic transmission, follows Mendel's laws.

Mendelian genetics

The branch of genetics dealing with the study of traits and genes which behave according to the laws of Mendel.

Mendelism

Particulate inheritance of chromosomal genes according to Mendel's laws.

Mendel's laws

(a) The law of segregation: The allelic factors of a pair are segregated, i.e. the factors separate into two different gametes (and, thence, into different offspring). Segregation occurs in meiosis for the two members of each pair of alleles possessed by the diploid parental organism. (b) The law of independent assortment: The members of different pairs of allelic factors assort independently, i.e. the members of different pairs of alleles are assorted into gametes during gametogenesis independently of other pairs of alleles which reside on different chromosomes; the subsequent pairing of alleles in combinations of male and female gametes is at random.

metacentric

Refers to a chromosome in which the centromere occurs in an approximately median position, which leads to a 'V' or 'J' shape in the metaphase appearance of the chromosome. A metacentric chromosome is one in which the centromere is located at or close to the median point or midpoint of the chromosome.

metafemale
Drosophila female with three X chromosomes and a diploid set of autosomes.

mitogen
Substance which stimulates cells to undergo mitosis.

mitosis
Nuclear division whereby one nucleus duplicates itself to produce two daughter nuclei which contain identical chromosomes and which are genetically identical with each other and with the parent nucleus from which they both arose.

mitotic index
Fraction of cells undergoing mitosis in a given sample.

mode
The maximum point on the curve which most closely describes an observed frequency distribution, i.e. the measurement which occurs most frequently.

monogenic
Monomeric. Refers to character differences genetically controlled by the alleles of one particular genetic locus, i.e. as opposed to polygenic control exerted by two, three, or many nonallelic genes. The genetic transmission of a factor in monogenic inheritance involves alleles which occur at only one genetic locus, and phenotypic variation is discontinuous.

monohybrid
Refers to a cross between parents differing with respect to a single specified pair of allelic genes.

monomeric
See: monogenic.

monosomy
The abnormal condition in which one chromosome of one pair is missing, i.e. deletion of a whole chromosome from the normal chromosome number. The presence, in an otherwise normally diploid complement, of only one member of a particular chromosome pair.

monozygotic twins
Twins formed by the fission into two, at some stage in its early development, of the embryo derived from a single fertilized egg.

morbidity
Relative incidence of a disease or disorder.

morbid risk
The risk that an individual, influenced by specific variables, will develop a particular disease or disorder.

morph
One of the genetic forms or variants in a case of genetic polymorphism.

morphic gene
One of two or more different genes which occur at the same locus, i.e. one of two or more alleles.

morphism
Genetic polymorphism.

morphogenesis
Formation and differentiation of tissues and organs.

morphogenetic
Producing growth; producing form or shape.

mosaic
Organism consisting of two or more genetically different cell types, involving either the same tissue type (i.e. chimera) or different tissues. The condition may occur as a result of a somatic mutation in a cell during mitosis, or from fusion (i.e. grafting) of cells from one individual upon another, or from a double fertilization (i.e. fertilization of two different pronuclei within the same oocyte or within two attached oocytes or within an oocyte and a polar body which are attached, by two different spermatozoa). If the mosaicism involves the same tissue type, then the mosaic is a chimera. If the mosaicism does not involve the same tissue type, then the mosaic is not a chimera. (See: chimera.)

mosaicism
The occurrence of cells of two or more genotypes in the same individual.

multifactorial inheritance
See: polygenic inheritance.

multigenic inheritance

See: polygenic inheritance.

multiple allelic series

A series comprising three or more possible alleles at the same genic locus.

multiple genes

Two or more nonallelic genes (i.e. involving two or more different loci) with similar or complementary cumulative effects on a single character. See: polygenic inheritance.

multiple-factor hypothesis

Hypothesis according to which the inheritance of a particular quantitative character involves an absence of clearcut segregation into readily recognizable classes showing typical mendelian ratios. The multiple factor hypothesis assumes that quantitative characters result from the cumulative action of multiple sets of independently transmitted genes, each of which produces only a small effect. See: polygenic inheritance.

mutagen

Physical or chemical agent which significantly increases mutational events and, thus, increases mutation rates above the spontaneous background level. Mutagens include ionizing radiations, ultraviolet rays, base analogues, alkylating agents, etc.

mutagenic

Capable of inducing mutations (i.e. refers to a mutagen).

mutant

Individual resulting from mutation.

mutation

Any detectable and heritable change in the genetic material not caused by segregation or genetic recombination, which is transmitted to daughter cells and even to succeeding generations. Mutations in the germ line of sexually reproducing organisms may be transmitted by the gametes to the next generation. A mutation may be any change affecting the chemical or physical constitution, mutability, replication, phenotypic function, or recombination of one or more deoxyribonucleotides. Nucleotides may be added, deleted, inverted, or transposed to new positions with and without inversion. A chromosomal mutation involves a change in the chromosomal material which is visible with currently available cytological methods. A gene mutation or point mutation is a mutation which is not associated with any visible change in the chromosomal material.

MZ

Monozygotic

N

Number of subjects.

neo-Darwinism

The post-Darwinian concept, that species evolve by the natural selection of adaptive phenotypes caused by mutant genes.

neo-Malthusianism

The doctrine that the numbers of human beings can be controlled and the standards of living can be raised through birth control.

neomorph

Mutant gene producing a qualitatively new effect that is not produced by the normal allele.

neonatal

Relating to or affecting the newborn and especially the human infant during the first month after birth.

nondisjunction

Abnormality of nuclear division in which a pair of newly divided chromosomes fails to separate, with the result that the daughter cells contain unequal numbers of chromosomes. Nondisjunction can occur during a meiotic or mitotic division; results in one daughter cell receiving both of the unseparated mitotic division; results in one daughter cell receiving both of the unseparated chromosomes, and one daughter cell receiving none of the chromosomes involved.

nonparametric statistics

Methods of statistical analysis which are

free from assumption regarding the shape of the underlying probability distribution.

norm of reaction
Range of phenotypic reactions of a particular genotype, i.e. the variety of phenotypes which may be produced by a particular genotype interacting with different nongenetic (i.e. environmental) influences.

normal distribution
Continuous distribution of measurements, for a particular character, which is symmetrical and clusters about some central, average value. Observations become increasingly rare as one moves farther from the average. A normal distribution, for a quantitative variable in a population, is shown when the quantitative variable is measured along the abscissa and the numbers of individuals are measured along the ordinate and the distribution describes a so-called normal (i.e. bell-shaped, or Laplacian, or Gaussian) curve. A variable which shows a continuous distribution in a population would be expected to show a normal distribution.

nuclear
Refers to phenomena, processes, and constituents associated with the nucleus of the cell.

nucleic acid
Nucleotide polymer composed of subunits which are either deoxyribonucleotides (i.e. in deoxyribonucleic acid, DNA) or ribonucleotides (i.e. in ribonucleic acid, RNA).

nucleoprotein
Compound of nucleic acid and protein. Either one of two main classes of basic proteins are found combined with DNA: one of low molecular weight, protamine; and one of high molecular weight, histone. The basic amino acids of these proteins neutralize the phosphoric acid residues of the DNA.

nucleoside
Purine or pyrimidine base attached to ribose or deoxyribose. The nucleosides commonly found in DNA and RNA are: cytidine, cytosine deoxyriboside, thymidine, uridine, adenosine adenine deoxyriboside, and cytidine, uridine, adenosine, and guanosine are ribosides.)

nucleotide
Nucleoside-phosphoric acid complex. The nucleotides commonly found in DNA and RNA are cytidylic acid, deoxycytidylic acid, thymidylic acid, uridylic acid, adenylic acid, deixtadenylic acid, guanylic acid, and deoxyguanylic acid. (Thumidylic acid is a deoxynucleotide; and cytidylic, uridylic, adenylic, and guanylic acids are all ribonucleotides.)

nucleus
Spheroidal structure present in most cells which contains the chromosomes.

null hypothesis
The standard hypothesis used in testing the statistical significance of the differences between the means of samples drawn from two populations. The null hypothesis states that there is no difference between the populations from which the samples are drawn. One then determines the probability that one will find a difference equal to or greater than the one actually observed. If this probability is 0.05 or less, the null hypothesis is rejected and the difference is said to be statistically significant.

ontogenesis
Ontogeny.

ontogenetic
Pertaining to the biological development of the individual.

ontogeny
The biological development or course of development of an individual (i.e. distinguished from phylogeny).

oogamy
The union, during fertilization, of a nonmotile female gamete (i.e. egg cell) and a motile male gamete (i.e. spermatozoan).

oogenesis

Development of the female germ cell (i.e. egg cell or ovum) of an animal which takes place in the gonad; includes meiosis of the oocyte, vitellogenesis, and formation of egg membranes. An inclusive term covering both female meiosis and ovagenesis.

ooplasm

Cytoplasm of an egg cell.

ootid nucleus

One of the four haploid nuclei formed by the meiotic divisions of a primary oocyte. Three of the nuclei are normally discarded as polar nuclei, and the remaining one functions as the female pronucleus.

organizer

A living part of an embryo which exerts a morphogenetic stimulus upon another part, bringing about its determination and morphological differentiation.

organogenesis

Formation of organs.

ovulation

Release of a ripe egg from the mammalian ovarian follicle, frequently at the stimulus of a pituitary hormone.

ovum

Unfertilized egg cell.

panmictic population

Interbreeding population of individuals who mate at random, i.e. each individual is equally likely to mate with any individual of the opposite sex.

panmixis

Random mating. See: panmictic population.

parameter

A quantity whose value is necessary for the specification of a hypothetical population.

parametric statistics

Methods of statistical analysis which assume that the data follow a defined probability distribution and the results of the calculations are valid only if the data are so distributed.

partial trisomy

The presence in triplicate of a chromosome segment in an otherwise diploid complement.

pedigree

Table, chart, or diagram setting forth the ancestral or genealogical history of an individual. Diagram of a family tree, to show the occurrence of one or more traits in different members of a family.

penetrance

When a gene or an allelic pair shows an effect in the phenotype, it is said to penetrate. The penetrance of a gene is the number of individuals showing the phenotypic trait expressed as a percentage of all those possessing the gene. When a dominant gene fails to produce any effect in an individual, that is, its expressivity is nill, there is said to be a failure of penetrance. Failure of penetrance is the extreme degree of reduced expressivity of a gene. A dominant gene which fails to penetrate from time to time is an irregular dominant gene. Penetrance is the term used to indicate the frequency with which a particular gene or combination of genes is/are manifested in the phenotypes of the carriers under a set of specified environmental conditions. Expressivity of a particular gene may depend upon both the (total) genotype and the environment.

pharmacogenetics

The area of biochemical genetics dealing with genetically controlled variations in response to drugs.

phenocopy

Nonhereditary phenotypic modification, as caused by special environmental conditions, that mimics a similar phenotype caused by a specific gene or combination of genes. A modification of the phenotype, brought about by nongenetic (i.e. environmental) variables, that resembles a similar change of the phenotype caused by a particular genotype.

phenotype

The observable properties, structural and functional, of an organism, produced by the interaction of the organism's genotype (i.e. genetic potential) and the particular environment involved. The term phenotype, may be applied either to the totality of expressions of the genotype or to only particular characters or traits.

phenotypic variance

Total variance observed in a particular character.

phylogenetic

Pertaining to the evolutionary history of the species.

phylogeny

The evolutionary history of a genetically related group of organisms (i.e. as distinguished from ontogeny, the development of the individual organism).

phytohemmagglutinin

A mucoprotein derived from the string-bean Phaseolus vulgaris, which stimulates mammalian cells to undergo mitosis in culture.

plasmagene

Extranuclear hereditary determinant showing non-Mendelian inheritance or mode of biological transmission.

pleiotrophy

Production, by one particular gene, of multiple phenotypic effects.

ploidy

Refers to the number of chromosome sets per cell, i.e. haploidy, diploidy, polyploidy.

point mutation

Gene or intragenic mutation, i.e. mutation associated with genetically transmitted change in phenotype, but not observable cytologically as a gross chromosomal aberration. See: gene mutation.

Poisson distribution

A function that assigns probabilities to the sequence of outcomes of observing no events of a specified type, one event, two events, and so on, without limit. Events that followed a Poisson distribution are completely randomized, and will not be found if the events are correlated positively (i.e. in the case of clumping) or negatively (i.e. in the case of mutual repulsion). The Poisson is specific by the average number of events per observation, and its mean and variance are equal.

polar body

The minute cell produced and normally discarded during the development of an oocyte. A polar body contains one of the nuclei derived from the first or second division of meiosis, but has very little cytoplasm.

polygene

Gene which individually exerts a slight effect on the phenotype, controlling a quantitative character in conjunction with several or many other equivalent genes which involve multiple loci.

polygenic character

Quantitative variable phenotype dependent on the interaction of numerous genes located on different loci.

polygenic inheritance

Mode of genetic transmission in which the character(s) is/are affected by genes which occur on several genetic loci. Polygenic or multigenic inheritance, involving two or more different genetic loci and phenotypic continuity, may be contrasted to monogenic or simple Mendelian inheritance, involving a single genetic locus and phenotypic discontinuity. Threshold phenomena, however, may provide for a discontinuous (e.g. bimodel) distribution for a trait associated with polygenic inheritance. The different genes involved in such a trait may manifest a similar share in control of the trait, or they may manifest individually different shares (i.e. heteromeric genes).

polymorphism

Refers to the coexistence of two or more alleles in a population in frequencies which are too high to be explained merely by new mutations. See: balanced polymorphism.

polymorphism, balanced

See: balanced polymorphism

polyploid

Containing more complete sets of chromosomes than two, i.e. containing one or more complete sets of chromosomes in addition to the normal diploid complement.

polysomy

The occurrence of an abnormal number of chromosomes in which one or more pairs of chromosomes are represented by three or more homologues, instead of the usual two. If there are three homologous chromosomes, instead of the usual two, the individual is trisomic for that chromosome; if four, then tetrasomic; and so on.

population genetics

A branch of genetics dealing with the study of populations in terms of the percentages of specific genes.

position effect

In genetics, the dependence of some genic effects upon the position of the gene in the chromosome. The phenotypic effect of the gene is alerted when the position of the gene is altered. A position effect occurs when an aberration that changes the gene's position with respect to neighboring genes is accompanied by a change in the phenotypic expression of the gene.

prevalence

Number of cases of a disorder or trait that currently exists in a given population.

probability

A measure of the subjective expectancy of an event expressed as a fraction, which usually denotes the ratio of the number of ways an event can occur to the number of all possible outcomes of the situation in question.

proband

An effected individual through whom a family is first brought to the attention of the geneticist. Index case. Propositus.

proband method

A method of comparing the proportion of progeny in families, which were selected by occurrence of a proband (i.e. index case, propositus) in each family, with the proportion expected if this character were the effect of a genotype transmitted by a particular Mendelian genetic mode.

pronucleus, male

See: male pronucleus.

propositus

See: proband.

random

Arrived at by chance without the exercise of any choice.

random mating

The situation in which an individual of one sex has an equal probability of mating with another individual of the opposite sex.

random sample

A random collection from a population, selected in such a way that all items in the population are equally likely to be included in the sample.

range

Distance between the lowest and highest values observed.

range of reaction

See: norm of reaction.

recessive

Nonmanifestation of a gene which is present together with an allele which is manifested. The failure of a gene to express phenotypically its presence in the heterozygous genotype is called "recessivity," as opposed to "dominance." (See: dominance). A recessive allele is one that does not produce a phenotypic effect when heterozygous with a dominant allele.

recombination

Occurrence of progeny with combinations of genes other than those that occurred in the parents, because of independent assortment or crossing over.

regression coefficient

Amount of change that will, on the average, take place in one characteristic when the other characteristic changes by a particular unit.

regression line

A line that defines the extent of increase or decrease in one fact which may be expected from a unit increase in another factor. The line or curve showing the regression in the geometrical representation.

regulator gene

A gene whose primary function is to control the rate of synthesis of the product(s) of another or other distant gene(s).

replication

A duplication process requiring copying from a template. Repetition of an experiment or procedure.

resting cell

Cell not underoing disivion.

ribonucleic acid

See: RNA.

ribonucleoprotein

A complex macromolecule containing both RNA and protein, and symbolized by RNP.

ribonucleotide

An organic compound that consists of a purine or pyrimidine base bonded to ribose which, in turn, is esterified with a phosphate group. Such monomers are polymerized to form RNA. See: RNA.

RNA

Ribonucleic acid. Polymer of ribonucleotids which is chemically very similar to DNA. RNA is a long, unbranched molecule consisting of four types of nucleotides linked together by phosphodiester bonds. The sugar component of RNA is ribose. RNA contains no thymine, which is replaced by the closely related pyrimidine, uracil. In contrast to DNA, most RNA molecules are single-stranded, but have the potential for forming complementary helices of the DNA-type. The

RNA molecules or their descendants serve as templates against which amino acids are properly ordered to form specific proteins, the amino acids being transported to their proper site on the template by specific carrier or soluble RNA molecules. See: ribonucleotide.

RNP

See: Ribonucleoprotein.

sample

In *statistics*, a finite series of obervations of individuals taken from the hypothetical infinitely large population of possible observations or individuals.

sampling error

Variability resulting from the limited size of the samples.

satellite

In *cytogenetics*, a small segment of a chromosome connected to the main body of the chromosome by a constricted segment.

S.D.

See: standard deviation.

S.E.

See: standard error.

segregation, Mendel's principle of

Members of an allele pair separate from each other when a diploid individual forms haploid gametes, with one of the two alleles normally represented in each haploid gamete produced by meiosis of a diploid primary gametocyte.

selection

The exercise of discrimination in sampling or in arrangement, opposed to randomness.

sex cells

Gametes. Ova and spermatozoa.

sex chromatin

A condensed mass of chromatin representing an inactivated X chromosome. Each X chromosome, in excess of one X chromosome, forms a sex-chromatic body in the mammalian nucleus.

sex-chromatin-negative

Refers to a sample of cells from an individual in which the nuclei possess no sex-chromatic or Barr bodies, indicating a chromosome complement characterized by the inclusion of only one X chromosome.

sex-chromatin-positive

Refers to a sample of cells in which a significant proportion of the nuclei show sex-chromatin or Barr bodies. The characteristic presence of a sex-chromatin body within the nucleus indicates a chromosome complement characterized by the inclusion of two X chromosomes.

sex chromosomes

The homologous chromosomes that are dissimilar in the heterogametic sex (i.e. the X and Y chromosomes).

sex limited

A trait which expression is restricted to one sex or reduced in one sex.

sib

A shortened form for sibling. Full brother or sister.

sib method

In human genetics, a method of deriving the proportions of individuals with and without a particular character under observation from those members of the sibship other than the proband by whom the sibship was identified.

sibling

Term for a full brother or sister.

sibs

A single word for brothers and sisters in the same family.

sibship

Group of children resulting from the union(s) of the same two parents.

significance

The measure of reality of an apparent discrepancy between observation and expectation. A departure is said to be *statistically significant,* i.e. to be judged real, if the probability of obtaining one as large or larger is lower than some chosen level, which is then referred to as the *level of significance.*

significance test

A test designed to assess significance and so to distinguish deviation resulting from sampling error from those indicating real discrepancies between observations and hypotheses.

single-factor inheritance

See: monogenic inheritance.

skewness

Asymmetry in a frequency distribution.

soma

The body of an organism apart from the germ-line cells.

somatic

Referring to the body, or vegetative cells and tissues of an organism, as opposed to the germ-line cells which give rise to the germ cells or gametes.

somatic cells

All the body cells except the sex cells.

somatic mutation

Mutation occurring in a somatic cell, i.e. in any cell that is not destined to become a germ cell. If the mutated cell continues to divide, the individual will come to contain a patch of tissue characterized by a genotype different from the cells of the rest of the body and may manifest mosaic effects. A somatic mutation will not be transmitted to the progeny, since the germ cells are not affects.

somatotype

Body type, physique; a classification of human body-build in terms of the relative development of ectomorphic, endomorphic, and mesomorphic components.

spermatogenesis

Development of the male germ cell (i.e. spermatozoan) of an animal, which takes place in the gonad. An inclusive term covering both male meiosis and spermiogenesis.

spontaneous mutation

A naturally occurring mutation.

standard deviation

A measure of the variability in a population of items. The standard deviation of a sample is equal to the square room of the arithmetic average of the squares of the differences between the observations and their mean. The distance, measured along the abscissa, of the point of inflection, or maximum slope, from the mean in a normal curve.

standard error

Measure of the variability that a value would show in taking repeated samples from the same universe of observations, i.e. the variation which might be expected to occur merely by chance in the various characteristics of samples drawn equally randomly from one and the same population. The standard error is a measure of the variation of a population of means. It is equal to the standard deviation divided by the square root of one less than the total number of items in the population.

statistic

The estimate of a parameter arrived at from observed samples. It bears the same relation to the sample as the parameter does to the population.

statistics

The discipline concerned with the collection, analysis, and presentation of data. The analysis of data depends upon the application of probability theory. Statistical inference involves the selection of one conclusion from a number of alternatives according to the result of a calculation based on observations. See: parametric statistics, nonparametric statistics.

stochastic

Random (i.e. referring to variables, processes).

sum of cross-products

See: cross-products, sum of.

superfemale

See: metafemale.

supernumerary chromosome

A chromosome present in addition to the characteristic normal complement of chromosomes.

synapsis

The pairing of homologous chromosomes, such as occurs normally in meiosis and which permits crossing over to take place.

t The ratio of an observed deviation to its estimated standard deviation.

telecentric

Refers to chromosome or chromatid with a terminal centromere. In humans, such chromosomes may arise by centromere misdivision or breakage induced within or adjacent to the centromere region.

template

In biology, a macromolecular mold for the synthesis of another macromolecule. Through template processes, a limited number of building blocks are polymerized into macromolecular structures, whereby the actual arrangement of the building blocks is uniquely determined by a pre-existing one which is identical, complementary, or otherwise related to the newly-synthesized macromolecule.

tetratogen

Any agent that produces or increases the incidence of congenital malformations in a population.

teratogenic agent

See: teratogen.

tetrachoric correlation coefficient

The degree of association calculated between two sets of variables, with each set dichotomized into two groups, each (group) of which is assumed to show a normal distribution.

threshold character

A term used for those phenotypic characters whose segregating distributions are phenotypically discontinuous but whose inheritance is multigenic like that of continuously varying (i.e. quantitative) characters. The discontinuous segregations of such characters result from threshold effects, i.e. the characters in question have an underlying continuity with a threshold which imposes a discontinuity on their apparent expression. Threshold characters may segregate into many discontinuous phenotypic classes.

translocation

Relocation of chromosomal segment(s) within one or between nonhomologous chromosomes. A translocation which involves nonhomologous chromosomes may or may not be reciprocal (i.e. be characterized by an exchange of segments between the two different chromosomes). A translocation may or may not be balanced (i.e. characterized by a normal complement of chromosomal material despite the abnormal location of part of that complement). See: balanced translocation.

transposition

Transfer of a chromosomal segment of another position within the same chromosome, i.e. interchromosomal structural change.

triploid

Possessing three of the haploid sets of chromosomes (i.e. diploid plus haploid).

trisomy

Occurrence of a chromosome in triplicate in an otherwise diploid complement. See: partial trisomy.

trisomy, partial

See: partial trisomy.

Turner's syndrome

A condition in man resulting from monosomy for the X chromosome. An affected individual is female in phenotype, but usually sterile.

twin method

In human genetics, a method using monozygotic and dizygotic twins for evaluating the influences of heredity and environment on the phenotype.

twins

Pair of individuals who develop simultaneously within one uterus.

unilateral inheritance

See: holandric inheritance.

uracil

A pyrimidine base found only in RNA.

variable

A quantity whose value is not fixed in an investigation.

variance

Numerical calculation describing the extent of dispersion of data around a mean. When all values in a population are expressed as plus or minus deviations from the population mean, the variance is the mean of the squared deviations.

variance analysis

See: analysis of variance.

variate

A variable quantity whose measurements or frequencies from all or part of the data for analysis.

vector

A quantity which can be represented on a many-dimensional scale and is subject to mathematical analysis.

X chromosome

The sex chromosome found in double dose in the homogametic sex (i.e. in mammals, the females), and in single dose in the heterogametic sex (i.e. in mammals, the males).

Y chromosome

The sex chromosome found only in the heterogametic sex (i.e. in mammals, the males).

z The natural logarithm of the ratio of two estimated standard deviations.

zygosity

Term applied to the number of zygotes from which a pair of twins or larger set of multiple births has resulted (e.g. monozygosity, dizygosity).

zygote

The diploid cell resulting from the union of the haploid male and female gametes. The term is also used to refer to the organism that developed from a single-celled zygote.

AUTHOR INDEX

611

SUBJECT INDEX

618

F